Medical
Problems
in
Athletes

Medical Problems in Athletes

Edited by

Karl B. Fields, MD, AAFP, CAQ Sports Medicine
Professor of Medicine
Associate Chairman, Department of Family
    Medicine
University of North Carolina at Chapel Hill
Chapel Hill, North Carolina;
Director, Family Medicine Residency and
    Sports Medicine Primary Care Fellowship
Moses Cone Health System and
    Greensboro A.H.E.C.
Greensboro, North Carolina

Peter A. Fricker, OAM, MBBS, FACSP, FACSM, FASMF
(Adj.) Professor and Chair of Sports
    Medicine
University of Canberra
Canberra, Australia;
Director, Medical Services
Australian Institute of Sport
Belconnen, Australia

Associate Editors

Martha J. Delaney, MA
Research Coordinator
Moses Cone Health System and
    Greensboro A.H.E.C.
Greensboro, North Carolina;
(Adj.) Research Assistant Professor
Department of Family Medicine
University of North Carolina at Chapel Hill
Chapel Hill, North Carolina

Kieran E. Fallon, MBBS (Hons), MEx and SpSc, FRACGP, FACSP
Sports Physician
Australian Institute of Sport
Belconnen, Australia;
(Adj.) Senior Lecturer in Sports Medicine
University of Canberra
Canberra, Australia

b
Blackwell Science

JR

Blackwell Science

Editorial offices:

Commerce Place, 350 Main Street, Malden, Massachusetts
02148, USA
Osney Mead, Oxford OX2 0E1, England
25 John Street, London WC1N 2BL, England
23 Ainslie Place, Edinburgh EH3 6AJ, Scotland
54 University Street, Carlton, Victoria 3053, Australia

Other Editorial offices:

Blackwell Wissenschafts-Verlag GmbH Kurfürstendamm
57, 10707 Berlin, Germany Zehetnergasse 6, A-1140
Vienna, Austria

DISTRIBUTORS:

USA
Blackwell Science, Inc.
Commerce Place
350 Main Street
Malden, Massachusetts 02148
(Telephone orders: 800-215-1000 or 617-388-8250; fax
orders: 617-388-8270)

Canada
Copp Clark, Ltd.
2775 Matheson Blvd. East
Mississauga, Ontario
Canada, L4W 4P7
(Telephone orders: 800-263-4374 or 905-238-6074)

Australia
Blackwell Science Pty, Ltd.
54 University Street
Carlton, Victoria 3053
(Telephone orders: 03-9347-0300;
fax orders: 03-9349-3016)

Outside North America and Australia
Blackwell Science, Ltd.
c/o Marston Book Services, Ltd.
P.O. Box 269
Abingdon
Oxon OX14 4YN
England
(Telephone orders: 44-01235-465500;
fax orders: 44-01235-465555)

The Blackwell Science logo is a trade mark of Blackwell
Science Ltd., registered at the United Kingdom Trade
Marks Registry

Acquisitions: James Krosschell
Production: Irene Herlihy
Manufacturing: Lisa Flanagan

Typeset by The Composing Room of Michigan, Inc.
Printed and bound by Braun-Brumfield, Inc.
©1997 by Blackwell Science, Inc.
Printed in the United States of America

97 98 99 00 5 4 3 2 1

Library of Congress Cataloging-in-Publication Data

Medical problems in athletes / edited by Karl B. Fields,
Peter A. Fricker.
      p.   cm.
      Includes bibliographical references and index.
      ISBN 0-86542-480-2
      1. Sports medicine.   2. Athletes—Diseases.
3. Athletes—Health and hygiene. I. Fields, Karl B.
II. Fricker, Peter A., 1950–
    [DNLM: 1. Sports—physiology. 2. Physical
Examination—methods. 3. Exercise—physiology.
4. Sports Medicine. QT 261 M489 1997]
RC1210.M316 1997
617.1′027—dc21
DNLM/DLC
for Library of Congress   97-13110
                         CIP

In Memoriam

This work is dedicated to the memory of two colleagues who died suddenly, John Sutton, MBBS, MD, PhD, DSc, FACSM, FACSP in February, 1996, and David O. Hough, MD, FAAFP, FACSM, CAQ Sports Med in September, 1996. Their legacy to sports science and sports medicine is incalculable. They remain friends and an inspiration to all of us.

Table of Contents

List of Contributors

Karl Lee Barkley II, MD, CAQ Sports Medicine
University Family Physicians
Charlotte, North Carolina;
Team Physician—Davidson College
Davidson, North Carolina

Mark E. Batt, MB, BCh, Dip Sports Med (Lond.)
Consultant in Sports Medicine
Nottingham University Centre for Sports Medicine
Nottingham, United Kingdom

Kevin Boundy, BMBS, Grad Dip Ex Sp Sc, M Sports Med
Surgeon Lt. Commander
Royal Australian Navy;
Officer in Charge RAN School of Underwater
  Medicine (1990–91);
Squadron Medical Officer Australian Submarine
  Squadron (1992–93)

Peter Brukner, MBBS, DRCOG, FACSM, FACSP
Medical Director
Olympic Park Sports Medicine Centre
Melbourne, Australia;
Australian Team Physician and Medical Director
World Student Games (1983, 1985, 1987);
Team Physician—Australian Olympic Team (1996)

Louise M. Burke, BSc, Grad Dip Diet, PhD
Head of Department, Sports Nutrition
Australian Institute of Sport
Belconnen, Australia;
Visiting Lecturer in Sports Nutrition
University of Canberra
Canberra, Australia;
Team Dietitian—Australian Olympic Team (1996)

Janus D. Butcher, MD, CAQ Sports Medicine
Director of Primary Care Sports Medicine
Family Practice Residency
Eisenhower Army Medical Center
Ft. Gordon, Georgia

John F. Campbell, MD
Clinical Associate Professor of Medicine
University of North Carolina at Chapel Hill
Chapel Hill, North Carolina;
Internal Medicine Training Program Faculty
Moses Cone Health Systems

Greensboro, North Carolina;
Physician Consultant—World T.E.A.M. Sports
Charlotte, North Carolina

Chris N. Christakos, MD, CAQ Sports Medicine
Practicing Physician
Salem Family Practice
Forsyth Memorial Hospital;
Team Physician—North Forsyth High School
Winston-Salem, North Carolina;
Volunteer, Clinical Faculty
The Moses H. Cone Primary Care Sports Medicine
  Fellowship

Robert Doolittle, MD
Practicing Physician
Urgent Medical Care Center and Grimsley High
  School Adolescent Clinic;
Consulting Staff, Adolescent Medicine
Moses H. Cone Memorial Hospital
Greensboro, North Carolina

M. Anne Duncan, PhD
(Adj.) Clinical Instructor
University of North Carolina at Chapel Hill
Chapel Hill, North Carolina;
Director of Behavioral Medicine, Family Medicine
  Residency
Moses Cone Health System and Greensboro A.H.E.C.
Greensboro, North Carolina

M. Patrice Eiff, MD, CAQ Sports Medicine
Associate Professor of Family Medicine
Oregon Health Sciences University School of
  Medicine;
Team Physician—Portland State University
Portland, Oregon

Kieran E. Fallon, MBBS (Hons), MEx & SpSc, FRACGP, FACSP
Sports Physician
Australian Institute of Sport
Belconnen, Australia;
(Adj.) Senior Lecturer in Sports Medicine
University of Canberra
Canberra, Australia;
Team Physician—Australian Women's Soccer Team

Karl B. Fields, MD, CAQ Sports Medicine
Professor of Medicine
Associate Chairman, Department of Family
    Medicine
University of North Carolina at Chapel Hill
Chapel Hill, North Carolina;
Director, Family Medicine Residency and
    Sports Medicine Primary Care Fellowship
Moses Cone Health System and Greensboro A.H.E.C.;
Team Physician—Grimsley High School and
    Guilford College;
Greensboro, North Carolina

John P. Fricker, BDS, MDSc, Grad Dip Adult Ed, FRACDS
Consultant Orthodontist
Australian Institute of Sport
Belconnen, Australia;
Orthodontist and Visiting Lecturer in Dentistry
University of Canberra
Canberra, Australia

Peter A. Fricker, OAM, MBBS, FACSP, FACSM, FASMF
(Adj.) Professor and Chair of Sports Medicine
University of Canberra
Canberra, Australia;
Director, Medical Services
Australian Institute of Sport
Belconnen, Australia;
Team Physician—Australian Olympic Team (1988,
    1992, 1996)

Robert C. Gambrell, MD, CAQ Sports Medicine
Assistant Professor
Departments of Family Medicine and
    Orthopedics
Center of Sports Medicine
Medical College of Georgia
Augusta, Georgia

David F. Gerrard, OBE, MBChB (Otago), FACSP, FSMNZ
Senior Lecturer in Sports Medicine
University of Otago
Otago, New Zealand;
Team Physician—Medical Director and Chef de
    Mission
New Zealand Olympic Team (1984–1996);
Member, Medical Committee
FINA (Federation Internationale de Natation
    Amateur)

Peter N. Gilchrist, MBBS, FRANZCP, Dip Psychotherapy
Consultant Psychiatrist, Clinical Director, Weight
    Disorder Unit
Flinders Medical Centre
Adelaide, Australia;
Visiting Lecturer
Australian Institute of Sport
Belconnen, Australia

Kori A. Graves, BS
Research Assistant
Family Medicine
Moses Cone Health Systems and Greensboro
    A.H.E.C.
Greensboro, North Carolina

Wayne A. Hale, MD, MS, ABFP
Associate Professor
Department of Family Medicine
University of North Carolina
Chapel Hill, North Carolina;
Faculty Physician, Family Medicine Residency
Moses Cone Health Systems and Greensboro A.H.E.C.
Greensboro, North Carolina

John A. Hawley, PhD, BSc (Hons), Cert Ed, MA, FACSM
Senior Lecturer
University of Cape Town Medical School;
Director
High Performance Laboratory
Sports Science Institute of South Africa
Cape Town, South Africa

William A. Hensel, MD, ABFP
Clinical Associate Professor
University of North Carolina at Chapel Hill
Chapel Hill, North Carolina;
Associate and Medical Director, Family Medicine
    Residency
Moses Cone Health System and Greensboro A.H.E.C.
Greensboro, North Carolina

Greg Hickey, MBBS (Melbourne), Dip RACOG, FACSP
Sports Physician
Melbourne, Australia;
Physician Consultant—Victorian Institute of Sport
Victoria, Australia

David O. Hough, MD, CAQ Sports Medicine
(*deceased*)
Professor, Family Practice
Director, Sports Medicine
College of Human Medicine
Michigan State University
Head Team Physician—Michigan State University
Lansing, Michigan

David Hughes, B Med, Dip Sports Medicine (Lond.), FACSP
Sports Physician
Canberra, Australia;
Consultant Sports Physician
Australian Institute of Sport
Belconnen, Australia;
Team Physician—ACT Brumbies Rugby Union
    (International)

Prentiss Jones, MS
South Bend Medical Foundation
South Bend, Indiana

James S. Kramer, MD, ABFP, CAQ Sports Medicine
Family and Sports Medicine Physician
Sports Medicine Center, Murphy/Wainer
    Orthopedic Specialists
Greensboro, North Carolina;
Assistant Director, Sports Medicine Fellowship
Moses Cone Family Medicine Residency
Team Physician—Greensboro College, Dudley High
    School, Monarchs (AHL) Hockey, Bats (Yankees
    Farm Team) Baseball
Greensboro, North Carolina

Daniel Larson, MD
Medical Director
Upper Hudson Primary Care Consortium
Albany, New York;
Staff Physician
Division of Family Practice
Glens Falls Hospital
Glens Falls, New York

Wade A. Lillegard, MD, CAQ Sports Medicine
Assistant Clinical Professor
University of Minnesota Center for Sports Medicine
Duluth Clinic
Duluth, Minnesota

John M. MacKnight, MD
Assistant Clinical Professor of Internal Medicine
University of Virgina
Charlottesville, Virginia

Warren McDonald, BSc, MBBS, FACSP
Visiting Senior Lecturer in Sports Medicine
University of Canberra
Canberra, Australia;
Sports Physician
Australian Institute of Sport
Belconnen, Australia;
Team Physician—Australian Olympic Team (1996)

Christopher A. McGrew, MD
Associate Professor
Department of Orthopedics/Sports Medicine
Division and Department of Family and Community
    Medicine
University of New Mexico Health Sciences Center
Albuquerque, New Mexico

Henry S. Miller, Jr., MD
Professor of Internal Medicine and Cardiology
Bowman Gray School of Medicine of Wake Forest
    University
North Carolina Baptist Hospitals
Winston-Salem, North Carolina

James Moriarity, MD, CAQ Sports Medicine
Physician, University Health Services and Team
    Physician
University of Notre Dame
Notre Dame, Indiana

David B. Pyne, B AppSc, M AppSc, PhD
Exercise Physiologist
Australian Institute of Sport

Belconnen, Australia;
Visiting Lecturer in Exercise Physiology
University of Canberra
Canberra, Australia;
Exercise Physiologist
Australian Swimming Team

Curtis D. Reimer, MD
Practicing Physician
Physicians Building Family Practice;
Team Physician—Hastings College and Hastings
    Senior High School
Hastings, Nebraska

Brent S. E. Rich, MD, ATC
Practicing Physician
Arizona Orthopaedic and Sports Medicine
    Specialists
Phoenix, Arizona;
Team Physician—Arizona State University
Tempe, Arizona

Edward N. Robinson, Jr., MD
Clinical Professor
Department of Medicine
University of North Carolina
Chapel Hill, North Carolina;
Infectious Diseases
Internal Medicine Training Program
Moses Cone Health System and Greensboro A.H.E.C.
Greensboro, North Carolina

Thomas R. Sachtleben, MD
Sports Medicine Fellow, Family Medicine
Moses Cone Hospital
Greensboro, North Carolina;
Team Physician—Elon College
Elon College, North Carolina;
Ben L. Smith High School
Greensboro, North Carolina

Edward Shahady, MD, ABFP, CAQ Sports Medicine
Professor of Family Medicine
University of Florida
Gainsville, Florida;
Director
North Broward Family Practice Residency Program
Fort Lauderdale, Florida

Bryan W. Smith, MD, PhD, CAQ Sports Medicine
Clinical Assistant Professor of Pediatrics and
    Orthopaedics
University of North Carolina School of Medicine;
Head Team Physician
University of North Carolina at Chapel Hill
Chapel Hill, North Carolina

Henry W. B. Smith III, MD
Clinical Associate Professor of Medicine
University of North Carolina at Chapel Hill
Chapel Hill, North Carolina;
Moses Cone Health System and Greensboro
    A.H.E.C.
Greensboro, North Carolina

Struan Sutherland, MBBS, MD, DSc, FRACP, FRCPA
Associate Professor
University of Melbourne
Melbourne, Australia;
Foundation Director
Australian Venom Research Unit;
Consultant to World Health Organisation
   (Envenomation)

David Andrew Tate, MD
Associate Professor of Medicine (Cardiology)
Associate Director of Cardiac Catheterization Lab
University of North Carolina at Chapel Hill
Chapel Hill, North Carolina

John A. Williamson, O St J, Bsc, MBBS, DA FRANZCA, Dip DHM, FACTM
Associate Professor in Anaesthesia
University of Adelaide;

Director of Hyperbaric Medicine
Royal Adelaide Hospital
Adelaide, Australia;
Consultant to World Lifesaving on Marine
   Envenomation

Michael J. Woods, DO
Practicing Physician—Arlington Group Sports
   Medicine
Harrisburg, Pennsylvania;
Team Physician—Harrisburg Heat (Professional)
   Soccer;
Team Physician, Dickerson College
Carlisle, Pennsylvania;
Sports Medicine Fellow, 1995–1996
Department of Physical Medicine and
   Rehabilitation
Michigan State University
East Lansing, Michigan

Introduction: Medical Assessment Prior to Sports

Karl B. Fields

Sports require intense effort and place the body under extreme physical stress. The growing number of accounts of sport-associated tragedies led to concerns about the safety of athletes. In the United States, the "Athletes' Bill of Rights" arose as a response to several deaths of young athletes and called for every athlete to have a comprehensive evaluation before sports participation (1). The irony that the healthiest appearing individuals in society die while participating in a contest glorifying the physical accomplishments of man has been appreciated since ancient times. Even in the second century A.D. Galen placed limitations on certain individuals when he observed, "For some I have forbidden to exercise at all, even the most suitable exercises, wishing them to be satisfied with only the activities essential to life" (2).

Fortunately, death during sports participation rarely occurs in athletes under 30 years of age, with estimates of 1 death in every 200,000 participants (3). Most fatalities in younger athletes are caused by congenital cardiac anomalies, whereas coronary artery disease accounts for the majority of deaths in athletes over 30 years of age. Occlusions of coronary vessels may be a gradual process that, while developing for years, causes clinical symptoms only when luminal diameter of the vessels is reduced to a critical point. Unfortunately, deaths occur before athletes recognize symptoms. Other chronic medical conditions such as diabetes mellitus and hypertension cause complications that arise over time. Sports participation in the early phase of the disease may not be problematic. However, after the individual has had the disease 10 years or more, end-organ damage, which may change the advisability of certain sports, is likely.

Special factors influence the screening process for athletes prior to their sports participation. Age is a major consideration in whether a disease is likely to occur in the athlete. Because of the known causes of sudden cardiac death, the cardiac history for athletes under 30 years of age focuses on questions that screen for congenital heart disease and worrisome symptoms. For athletes 30 to 50 years of age, the history assesses known cardiac risk factors that would indicate a higher likelihood of coronary artery disease. However, in athletes over age 50, who have a higher prevalence of coronary artery disease, even a negative history may not be sufficient reassurance of the absence of disease. For these individuals careful pre-exercise screening for vigorous sport necessitates an objective measure of cardiac status, such as an exercise tolerance test.

Some diseases trouble athletes more frequently than the general population. Exercise-induced asthma is perhaps the best example of this. While less than 10% of the general population experiences asthma, bronchospasm associated with physical activity in various sports occurs in 10% of elite athletes, up to 20% of high school athletes, and perhaps 50% of figure skaters. Sports that require a high minute ventilation may provoke bronchospasm. Some sports place susceptible individuals in environmental conditions in which precipitating factors are more common. For example, the intense cold and dry air of winter sports is the key trigger of bronchospasm in figure skaters, cross-country skiers, and other winter athletes (4). Runners bothered by pollens or air pollutants may inhale as much of these substances in one hour of vigorous distance running as other individuals would in one day. Swimmers with a sensitivity to chlorine inhale toxic concentrations over the duration of prolonged workouts even when pool conditions are safe for the recreational swimmer (5).

Sports may also place demands on the body that worsen an existing chronic disease. An example of this is hypertension, as isometric or resistance exercises may cause marked elevations of blood pressure. However, a balanced program that integrates aerobic activity with strength conditioning has a beneficial effect on blood pressure.

Sports can increase the athlete's risk of complications from a chronic illness. For example, any disease that leads to splenomegaly increases the risk of traumatic splenic injury in contact or collision sports. Infectious mononucleosis, which has precipitated splenic rupture in a number of participants, is the disease in which this concern has been most worrisome. However, hemoglobinopathies, malaria, hemolytic anemias, lymphoma, and a variety of metabolic, infectious, collagen vascular, and neoplastic diseases also cause splenomegaly and would also place an athlete at greater risk. Another example of sport placing an athlete at greater risk of a disease complication is the increased risk of retinal hemorrhage in an athlete with diabetic retinopathy who attempts power lifting.

Thus, medical screening prior to participation focuses on three priorities: 1) identifying athletes at particular risk of having a medical problem; 2) understanding whether the athlete with a medical illness faces an unacceptable risk in sport participation; and 3) determining whether participation in a given sport will worsen control of a particular illness. This information generally may be obtained from a careful medical history. In fact, in most studies of preparticipation evaluations, approximately 70% of problems are identified in the history portion of the examination (6). In addition, a good history directs the physician to include specific components in the physical examination that make detection of a problem more likely.

SPECIFIC CONCERNS BEFORE AN ATHLETE BEGINS PARTICIPATION

Infectious Disease
The athlete with a history of infectious disease generally falls into one of two categories—recovering from an acute process or troubled with a chronic infection. For the athlete who has experienced an acute infection, the physician attempts to make several judgments. Has the individual recovered completely from the effects of the illness? This determines the extent to which the athlete can return to training. Were there any sequelae or complications that may affect return to sport? An individual who has recently had a viral syndrome should not have any residual cardiac dysfunction suggesting a myocarditis. Similarly, someone recuperating from a pulmonary infection should have regained nearly normal lung function. Has the risk of the athlete infecting others ended? Obviously, someone with a contagious process places other team members at risk.

Chronic infections typically restrict the athlete to a greater degree than do acute. However, a number of athletes with HIV infection now compete. While their risk to others remains low, the effect of participation on their long-term prognosis remains unclear. Chronic active hepatitis raises the specter of hepatic injury. Chronic pyelonephritis poses a risk to kidney function, particularly if the athlete might worsen the condition through extreme dehydration or trauma.

Cardiovascular Disease
Hypertension is the most common cardiovascular disease, and a family history or personal history of past problems raises the index of concern. Hypertension typically causes few if any symptoms. Thus this condition is the exception to the rule that most problems may be detected in the history. Careful assessment of blood pressure at rest, and perhaps during exercise, remains the best method of identifying hypertensive athletes.

In the younger athlete any history that suggests a risk for congenital heart disease stimulates a more in depth evaluation. A family history of sudden death under age 50 may relate to hypertrophic cardiomyopathy, premature coronary artery disease, or a number of cardiac conditions. Symptoms of dizziness, syncope, palpitations, excessive fatigue, or chest pain may be other indications of disease (and may require explanation). A history of a heart murmur also merits concern, although a benign flow murmur may be detected on examination of many athletes (7).

Athletes over 30 years of age need to be questioned regarding any symptoms of coronary artery disease. Exertional chest pain, shortness of breath, diaphoresis, nausea, and pain radiating to the jaw, arm, or shoulder all heighten the concern for angina. Atypical chest pain in the individual with multiple risk factors still indicates a high risk for disease. In addition, any of the myriad of cardiac symptoms can occur with ischemia so that a positive history of cardiovascular symptoms should lead to further evaluation and, usually, an exercise tolerance test. However, for the older asymptomatic athlete, the key historical features concern the type of physical exertion planned and the overall risk of disease. Thus, women under age 50 with risk factors but no symptoms and women over age 50 doing only moderate intensity activity still have a relatively low risk of coronary artery disease and for them exercise tolerance testing is optional. However, men aged 30 to 40 years with two or more major cardiac risk factors, and all men over age 40 who wish to pursue vigorous exercise, should be considered candidates for exercise tolerance testing (8).

Pulmonary Disease

Pulmonary problems occur with relative frequency in athletes primarily because of the high number of individuals who have exercise-induced asthma. Any past history of asthma, allergic rhinitis, or atopic disease makes the athlete a likely candidate for bronchospasm during exercise. Symptoms may be subtle, such as a decline in performance, but particularly worrisome is a history of frequent coughing after exertion. Chest tightness and pain are often manifestations of asthma. Frank wheezing is a less common presentation. Symptoms suggesting bronchospasm prompt an objective evaluation of pulmonary function with and without an exercise challenge. While pulmonary problems limit performance, only rarely do they prevent participation.

Chronic pulmonary diseases present a different side of the spectrum of lung problems and sports participation. Whether the athlete has chronic obstructive disease, chronic bronchitis, severe asthma, restrictive disease, sarcoidosis, or an immune condition, the current status of the disease determines the extent to which the individual may participate in sports. In many patients with advanced lung disease, the purpose of sport may be to maintain independent function and strength at the best possible level with little emphasis on performance or competition. For these individuals the evaluation requires objective measurement of their capability, for example, determining whether the patient has oxygen desaturation with certain activities. In addition, the physician optimizes the treatment regimen to allow ongoing physical activity.

Neurology

Safety remains a primary goal of most preparticipation evaluations. In this regard certain patients with a history of epilepsy should not participate in sports that place them at undue risk. Sports that have greater intrinsic danger and that carry the risk of a fatal consequence if the participant experiences a seizure during participation should be discouraged. For example, weightlifting, swimming, scuba diving, rock-climbing, vehicular sports, skiing, and certain gymnastic events pose high risks. Any sport that would place others at risk, including archery, shooting, shot put, discus, and javelin, may also be inadvisable. Patients with well-controlled seizure disorders can pursue most other athletic endeavors. After a prolonged seizure-free interval, certain physicians may return athletes to some of the higher risk sports under close observation. The history regarding seizure disorders should document specifics about the type of seizure, the frequency of occurrence, medications used for control, precipitating factors, past experience with exercise, and its effect on seizures.

Other neurologic concerns include a history of headaches. A change in onset or pattern of headaches adds to the concern that they may be outward manifestations of intracranial pathology. Because up to 10% of individuals have recurrent headaches, only those with enough symptoms or an abnormal finding on examination should be screened with imaging. Postconcussion headaches fall into a special category, since the literature raises the specter of potentially fatal second impact syndrome. Other symptoms compatible with neuropathies, specific muscle weaknesses, or unusual disorders may merit assessment before sports activity.

Chronic Medical Illnesses

Chronic medical illnesses require a careful history to assess their stability and impact on physical activity. Many symptoms occur with sports participation; for example, runners may experience abdominal pain and cramping during marathons. However, when the history of gastrointestinal symptoms seems extreme, further evaluation for a significant illness may be warranted. Some sports may worsen reflux symptoms and the use of nonsteroidal anti-inflammatory drugs by athletes may trigger gastritis or peptic ulcer disease. Nephrologic conditions can be worsened by activity, so appropriate care must be taken to ensure safe participation.

Both diabetes mellitus and thyroid disease are not uncommon amongst athletes. Well-controlled diabetics have participated and succeeded at the highest level of sport. However, those in poor control can worsen their disease. Similarly, thyroid conditions can greatly impair sports performance until appropriate treatment restores normal thyroid function.

Otolaryngologic and ophthalmologic conditions may pose greatest difficulties when they interfere with vision or equilibrium. Thus, the history needs to explore symptoms and determine whether additional testing is necessary. Dermatologic conditions, when contagious, preclude participation when there is a risk of spread to other athletes. Many chronic skin conditions may worsen with the stresses, equipment used, or environmental exposures common to sport. Anemias may limit oxygen-carrying capacity to the extent that vigorous sport cannot be endured until normal hemoglobin levels are restored.

Arthritis poses a unique challenge to sports play. Since the joints are integral to the function of the entire musculoskeletal system, their degree of inflammation and chronic degeneration determines what an individual can reasonably do. Certainly some judgment is needed to decide when a given physical stress may worsen the condition.

Finally, special situations such as high altitude sports, scuba diving, work in extreme environments, pregnancy, cancer, or psychological conditions require individualization as to what activity can be safely pursued. Each condition must be considered unique and assessment should include physical capabilities of the individual who plans to participate. In almost every situation some physical activity is possible and, generally, beneficial. One of the worst aspects of any chronic medical condition is for the individual to lose control over what he or she wishes to do in life. Athletes can derive major psychological benefits from mastering a chronic illness and still achieving sports excellence.

SUMMARY

Each individual has the potential to participate in some athletic endeavor. Few absolutes exist, so that sports participation remains possible even for some patients with advanced illness. No simple set of rules can guide the physician for any medical problem; thus, clinicians must turn to an emerging literature base in sports medicine and the field's growing experience in treating athletes with specific conditions. Each chapter of this book reviews a medical condition and how it affects athletes. The text is intended to serve as a guide for physicians to assist athletes in participating safely and in achieving their full potential.

REFERENCES

1 O'Donoghue DH. Treatment of injuries to athletes. Philadelphia: WB Saunders, 1970:iv.
2 Green R, trans. Galen's hygiene. Springfield, IL: Charles Thomas, 1951:187
3 Epstein SE, Maron BJ. Sudden death and the competitive athlete: perspectives on preparticipation screening studies. J Am Coll Cardiol 1986;7:220–230.
4 Fields KB. Three common medical problems in sports. In: Richmond JC, Shahady EJ, eds. Sports medicine for primary care. Boston: Blackwell Science, 1995:541–554.
5 Drobnic F, Freixa A, Casan P, et al. Assessment of chlorine exposure in swimmers during training. Med Sci Sports Exerc 1996;28:271–274.
6 AAFP, AAP, AMSSM, AOSSM, AOASM. Preparticipation physical evaluation. Monograph, 1992.
7 Rich BS. Sudden death screening. Med Clin North Am 1994;78:267–288.
8 American College of Sports Medicine. Guidelines for exercise testing and prescription. 4th ed. Philadelphia: Lea & Febiger, 1991:8.

PART I
INFECTIOUS PROBLEMS IN ATHLETES

Chapter 1
Infectious Problems in Athletes: An Overview

Peter A. Fricker

Infectious conditions constitute a significant proportion of those problems that hinder an athlete—recreational or elite—who enjoys training, exercising, competing, or performing. In athlete care, medical problems are as important as injuries, and the practitioner must thoroughly understand the range of these ailments to promote recovery, minimize complications, and prevent contagion. As illustrated by the discussions in this book on team care and travel, the good sports medicine practitioner must first be a good primary care physician with skills in general medicine and, especially, in the treatment of infections.

INFECTION AND ATHLETES

To demonstrate the size of the problem that infectious conditions pose to athletes, the Sports Medicine Department of the Australian Institute of Sport (AIS) reviewed 588 serial consultations of medical practitioners by athletes-in-residence and athletes attending training camps at the AIS (1). This largely adolescent population of elite athletes consists of approximately 350 who reside on a 12-month (renewable) basis, and approximately 50 athletes who are in residence on short-stay (training camp) programs. Of the total number of consultations, 41.8% ($n = 246$) were for medical conditions, not injuries. Males and females were approximately evenly represented (males for 136 consultations, females for 110). For males, 43.3% of consultations were for medical conditions; for females, 40.2% of consultations were medical; infectious conditions were the top diagnosis for both genders. Table 1-1 lists the most common diagnoses and frequencies for these athletes.

The Impact of Infectious Disease on Exercise Capacity

Few good studies describe the impact of infectious illness on an athlete's capacity to exercise. One study, however, has examined aerobic capacity after the athlete has contracted infectious mononucleosis (2). Sixteen cadets from the United States Military Academy (West Point) who were recovering from infectious mononucleosis had their aerobic capacity determined immediately after becoming afebrile. Nine of these cadets undertook a low intensity exercise program over 2 weeks while the others remained inactive; all 16 then were permitted to exercise at their own discretion for a further 2 weeks. Aerobic capacity was measured again at this time. The authors found no differences between the groups on $\dot{V}o_2max$, METS, or run time to exhaustion, and concluded that athletes recovering from infectious mononucleosis can begin an exercise program as soon as they become afebrile. Notably, this study did not focus on aerobic capacity after such illness, but rather on "simply seeing if one, once afebrile, could begin exercising without a detrimental side effect." A possible confounder of these results was that the athletes studied carried strong aerobic fitness ($\dot{V}o_2max$ approx. 60 mL/kg/min for males, and 50 mL/kg/min for females) prior to their illness, and that any decline in aerobic fitness over 2 weeks of inactivity may have been minimal. One individual had had aerobic capacity assessed prior to his illness, and showed no change before or after his illness.

A prospective study on virus infections and sports performance was reported on 68 athletes in the United Kingdom in 1988 (3). Track and field athletes training for the Commonwealth Games were screened for viral infection during winter

Table 1-1   Medical Conditions at the Australian Institute of Sport

Diagnosis	Frequency	
	Male ($n = 136$)	Female ($n = 110$)
Upper respiratory infection	47	36
Chest infection	38	18
Generalized viral infection	17	21
Gastroenteritis	12	15
Asthma/allergy	12	10
Skin rash/fungal infection	7	4
Lassitude, lethargy	4	4
Otitis externa	5	1

training; their form was assessed by questionnaire and an analogue scale. Static elevated titers of neutralizing antibody to coxsackie B1 to B5 were present in 54% of the athletes; 79% had serologic evidence of past viral infection (including coxsackie B, Ebstein-Barr virus, cytomegalovirus, adenovirus) and/or *Mycoplasma pneumoniae*. The raised titers did not, however, relate to poor performance, and the authors concluded that there was no evidence that loss of form was related to subclinical infection. This emphasizes that clinicians should interpret elevated antibody levels to viruses with great caution when assessing athletes complaining of a drop in performance.

These studies, however, should not lead the reader to believe that infection can be disregarded or taken lightly. Active infection and, in particular, febrile illness produce well-documented effects on athletes, both short term and long term (complications included), and these are discussed more fully in this chapter and in the chapters that follow.

Does Exercise Predispose to Infections?

In an overview of exercise and immunity, Pedersen and Bruunsgaard (4) addressed the question of whether exercise predisposes an athlete to infection. Chapter 32 in this book, on immunology and exercise, also provides a useful guide to understanding the implications of exercise intensity on predisposition to infection.

Pedersen and Bruunsgaard state that after prolonged intense exercise, the number of lymphocytes in the blood is reduced, as is the function of natural killer cells. The latter are mainly responsible for viricidal and antitumor activity. Secretory (mucosal) immunity is also impaired, and these changes all create a window of opportunity over a period of an hour or two for pathogenic microorganisms to do their damage. On the other hand, for those who undertake regular moderate exercise, the immune system is enhanced and this may in fact protect individuals from infection.

A recent review by Brenner et al. (5) agrees with this summary and makes the point that skin lacerations, heavy sweating, and associated softening and maceration of the dermis impair the defense usually provided by the skin, and contribute to the development of skin infections in athletes.

"Overtraining" is a rather nebulous term, and strict definitions are still being developed. However, the term covers the concept of training beyond the individual's capacity to recover, and it is thus associated with the predisposition to infection described above. In a paper on overtraining, Fitzgerald (6) alludes to several studies that demonstrate that exercising during the incubation phase of an infection can increase the severity of the illness, and thus advises athletes who feel they may be getting ill to reduce training "for a day or two."

Exercise and Disease States

The chapters that follow discuss the impact of exercise on progress of disease—ranging from infectious conditions, to disorders such as those that affect the musculoskeletal system, to considerations of cancer. In brief, mild to moderate exercise is generally considered beneficial, provided appropriate care is taken of the primary condition.

Certainly, specific conditions such as acute febrile illness require care in the management of exercise programs. Primos (7) has provided a very useful guide for clinicians in this context. In a discussion of viral infections and complications such as myocarditis, he recommends a "neck check" of symptoms:

- If the patient has symptoms *above* the neck—such as nasal congestion, runny nose, and sore throat—he or she can probably continue to exercise at a reduced level of intensity.
- If the patient has symptoms *below* the neck—such as chest congestion, hacking cough, fever, or chills—then abstinence from exercise (particularly intense exercise) is recommended.

Infections of the upper and lower respiratory tract have also been implicated in the development and manifestations of asthma. A Norwegian study by Heir et al. (8) examined the influence of respiratory tract infection and bronchial responsiveness in elite cross-country skiers compared with inactive controls. All subjects were nonsmokers and none suffered asthma or other chronic lung disease. The researchers found that on methacholine challenge, there was a transient increase in bronchial responsiveness in athletes who undertook physical exercise during the symptomatic period of their (upper and/or lower) respiratory tract infections, but not in the inactive controls. The authors concluded that exercise during the symptomatic period of respiratory illness may intensify or generate mechanisms leading to enhanced bronchial responsiveness, or asthma. This serves to warn medical practitioners that athletes are at special risk—especially in colder climates—when they exercise during infection.

CONCLUSION

Athletes present with a range of medical conditions to their treating practitioners, and infectious diseases head the list. Almost half of the problems evaluated at a national sports institute during a survey were for medical conditions, not injury. Similar experiences have been reported by doctors working at major sporting events such as the Olympic Games.

Management of infectious conditions requires an understanding of the effects of the disease, its complications, its potential for spread, and its effects on the capacity to exercise. Athletes present special problems because they exercise, and wish to continue to do so even when sick; they therefore necessitate special counseling and careful observation by their medical practitioners.

REFERENCES

1 Fricker PA, Orchard J. Injuries and illnesses at the Australian Institute of Sport—a survey, 1993. Unpublished.
2 Welch MJ, Wheeler L. Aerobic capacity after contracting infectious mononucleosis. J Orthop Sports Phys Ther 1986;8:199–202.
3 Roberts JA, Wilson JA, Clements GB. Virus infections and sports performance—a prospective study. Br J Sports Med 1988;22:161–162.
4 Pedersen BK, Bruunsgaard H. How physical exercise influences the establishment of infections. Sports Med 1995;19:393–400.
5 Brenner I, Shek PN, Shephard RJ. Infection in athletes. Sports Med 1994;17:86–107.
6 Fitzgerald L. Overtraining increases the susceptibility to infection. Int J Sports Med 1991;12:55–58.
7 Primos WA. Sports and exercise during acute illness. Recommending the right course for patients. Physician Sports Med 1996;24:44–46,51–53.
8 Heir T, Aanestad G, Carlsen KH, Larsen S. Respiratory tract infection and bronchial responsiveness in elite athletes and sedentary control subjects. Scand J Med Sci Sports 1995;5:94–99.

Chapter 2
Upper Respiratory Tract Infections

Warren McDonald

The upper respiratory tract is the most common site of infection in humans, accounting for more than half of all acute illnesses. In Western societies, upper respiratory tract infections (URTIs) account for 30% to 50% of time lost from work by adults and 60% to 80% of time lost from school by children. Typically, the highest rates occur in children under 1 year of age, who average 6 to 8 episodes per year; the rates remain high through early childhood. A progressive decrease occurs after age 6, and adults average 3 to 4 episodes per year (1).

The literature regarding upper respiratory tract infection lacks clarity, mainly because nomenclature problems tend to distort epidemiological data. Part of the difficulty is that upper respiratory infections cover several anatomically distinct regions (although all are obviously part of the respiratory tract) such as the nose, mouth, sinuses, and throat. Infections that involve all or some of these structures are grouped together by a variety of terms, such as "common cold," "flu," influenza, or URTIs.

Conversely, anatomically specific infections such as sinusitis and pharyngitis are also part of the URTI spectrum, although, as in this text, they are often discussed separately. Therefore, this chapter focuses on the viral URTIs, which account for 66% to 90% of all URTIs, and are generally referred to as the common cold.

OVERVIEW OF VIRAL URTIs

Over 200 viruses from eight different genera cause URTIs. The most common agents are rhinoviruses (of which there are over 100 serotypes) followed by coronaviruses, respiratory syncytial virus, para-influenza virus, and adenoviruses. Table 2-1 summarizes these viruses, their incidence, peak season, incubation period, and usual length of infection. Differentiation between viral groups is usually difficult on clinical grounds alone. Similarly, viral URTIs are difficult to distinguish clinically from bacterial respiratory infections.

Viral URTIs occur throughout the year, although seasonal peaks are noted in autumn and spring in temperate climates. The reason for these peaks is not well understood, although closer human contact in inadequately ventilated spaces (as the autumn weather becomes colder) and exposure to cold, wet weather are possible factors. The incubation period for viral URTIs is only a few days, with the length of illness lasting from a few days up to 2 weeks. Transmission of the infectious agent occurs by aerosol and droplet inhalation, direct saliva spread, indirect saliva spread by intermediate eating or drinking implements, or infected hands. No one particular mode of transmission appears to be responsible for all colds (2).

Viruses infect epithelial cells of the nasopharynx via attachment to specific cellular receptors. The virus causes spotty destruction of the nasal mucosa, with edema, hyperemia, and mucoid discharge. There is mild infiltration with inflammatory cells and hyperactivity of mucus-secreting glands in the submucosa. Epithelial cells may slough, and subsequently the entire epithelium may disintegrate. Destruction of epithelial cells impairs nasociliary clearance. Therefore a purulent nasal discharge may result, and does not necessarily indicate infection by a pathogenic bacterium. Engorgement of the nasal turbinates may obstruct openings of sinuses, and subsequent changes within sinuses have been demonstrated

Table 2-1   Common Viruses Causing Upper Respiratory Tract Infections

Virus	Percentage of Common Cold–Like Illnesses	Predominant Season	Incubation Period (days)	Length of Illness (mean)
Rhinovirus	15–40	Early autumn, early spring	1–2	4–9 days
Coronavirus	10–20	Late autumn, winter, early spring	3	6–7 days
Respiratory syncytial virus	Infants/children: 20–25	Late autumn, winter, spring	4–6	Up to 2 weeks
Parainfluenza	Adults: 5 Children: 4.3–22	Spring	3–6	3–4 days
Adenoviruses	Adults: <2 Children: 3–5	Autumn, winter, spring	A few days	1–2 weeks

SOURCE: Adapted from Dolin R. Common viral respiratory infections. In: Isselbacher KJ, Braunwald E, Wilson JD, et al., eds. Harrison's principles of internal medicine. Vol 1. 13th ed. New York: McGraw-Hill, 1994:803–807.

with both MRI and CT scanning. These changes are variable and may last beyond the time taken for clinical symptoms to resolve (1,3).

Viral URTIs produce local symptoms and signs (related directly to the upper respiratory tract) such as enlarged cervical lymph nodes, nasal congestion, and mild sore throat. In addition, systemic symptoms and signs such as malaise, headache, fever, raised resting pulse rate, myalgia, and arthralgia develop with some URTIs. Their presence often signifies a more serious infection, either in terms of severity or of organ involvement.

As noted previously, most viral URTIs have a short incubation period of a few days, and the duration of illness spans 4 to 14 days. Prolonged infections, especially in the young, trigger concern for involvement of the lower respiratory tract, obstruction of sinus openings or eustachian tubes, and subsequently more severe illness from bacterial secondary infection (e.g., acute sinusitis, otitis media).

Diagnosis of viral URTI is clinical, with little useful information obtained from diagnostic tests. Viruses can be isolated in tissue culture from nasal washes or nasal secretions, but in practice this is done only for epidemiological purposes as it does not aid treatment regimens. If a bacterial URTI is suspected, one may see a rise in the patient's white cell count, C-reactive protein, and erythrocyte sedimentation rate (ESR). In addition, nasal or throat swabs, or sputum culture may provide diagnosis of the pathogen and antibiotic sensitivities, allowing for specific antibiotic treatment.

A typical clinical picture does not always emerge, and it is possible for mild infections (with only one or two signs or symptoms) or subclinical infections to occur. Definitive laboratory proof of this is difficult because of the large number of viral serotypes with a similar clinical picture. Theoretically, these mild or subclinical infections may still negatively affect performance during the incubation period and after clinical symptoms have disappeared. Such changes in performance have been demonstrated in typical viral URTIs (2,4).

SPECIAL CONSIDERATIONS IN ATHLETES

Coaches, athletes, and treating physicians have long suspected a link between exercise, the immune system, and infection. Regular moderate exercise has been accompanied by anecdotal reports of improvements in one's generalized sense of well-being, with less infectious episodes. Conversely, coaches and high-level athletes have reported an increased susceptibility to infection (especially viral URTIs) at times of high intensity or volume training, during precompetition phases of training, during major competitions, and in the immediate postcompetition phase. Furthermore, one of the most common features of the overtraining or burnout syndrome is recurrent URTI.

In recent years, well-controlled scientific experiments tend to support this anecdotal evidence. Changes in parameters of the immune system occur with both short-term exercise and long-term training (see Chapter 32). Cross-sectional data looking at major mass-participation sporting events have shown a significant increase in the risk of URTI with greater training volumes and intensity of effort (5). Prospective data comparing high-level exercising groups with nonexercising groups have shown increased numbers of infection episodes and prolonged duration of infection episodes in the exercising groups. Additionally, fewer subjects in the exercising groups had *no* episodes of infection and their distribution of infection throughout the year was more even (i.e., no seasonal variation). Other prospective work on runners has shown an increased risk of URTI with increasing distances run. On the other hand, some small studies have confirmed the belief that moderate aerobic exercise enhances immune function, with a fewer number of URTIs in previously sedentary subjects who commenced a moderate aerobic ex-

ercise program compared with those who remained sedentary. These results have been modeled in what is known as the J curve (Fig 2-1).

The effects of exercise during an infection are variable. Animal studies have shown that, in some cases, exercise at the time of or just after inoculation increased the severity and effects of infection. In particular, viral infections showed increased viremia, and in some cases (e.g., coxsackievirus infection) increased titers in heart muscle. However, such results have not been the case in all situations (6). In humans, anecdotal evidence and individual case studies have documented the risk of exercising while seriously infected, with numerous cases of acute myocarditis (viral cardiomyopathy) resulting in sudden death. On the other hand, exercising during mild infections apparently presents no significant risks of increasing the severity or spread of infection. As discussed in Chapter 1, the determining factor appears to be the development of systemic symptoms, in particular fever and raised resting pulse rate, but also malaise, myalgia, arthralgia, and generalized lymphadenopathy. As previously mentioned, such symptoms represent a significant increase in the severity of infection, and exercise may worsen this and prolong recovery. Rest is generally advised until such symptoms are

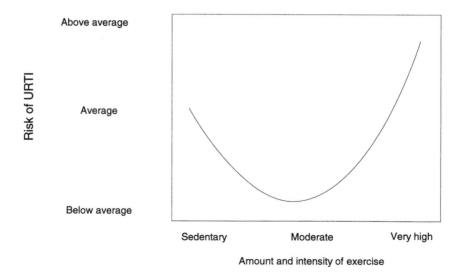

Figure 2-1.   The J curve.

settled. If, however, a viral URTI is limited to local symptoms only, moderate exercise appears to be safe, and perhaps even beneficial.

As noted earlier, both clinical and subclinical infections may present as poor performance. In athletes, this is translated to poor training or competitive efforts. Therefore, investigation of a sudden decline in performance by an athlete should include investigation for a viral URTI. If viral URTI is indeed the cause of deteriorating performance, appropriate management (including exercise) needs to be prescribed.

Treatment Strategies in Athletes
Treatment regimens for viral URTIs are numerous and varied. Various medications are available, mostly as over-the-counter preparations. Consumers utilize these preparations freely, supporting a multimillion dollar industry. However, the effectiveness of these preparations has rarely been verified. The following is a summary of the most commonly used medications (2,7).

Antihistamines Antihistamines are thought to be effective in relieving symptoms of URTIs and are used either alone or as part of many "cold" preparations. Their effects are thought to be due to the atropinelike drying action on the mucus membranes, rather than by antagonism of histamine. The major clinical benefits appear to include reductions in nasal congestion, sneezing, postnasal drainage, and nasal discharge. The major side effect is drowsiness, although the newer antihistamines (e.g., loratadine, terfenadine) do not cross the blood–brain barrier and are therefore nonsedating. Antihistamines are not proscribed by the International Olympic Committee (IOC).

Decongestants Decongestants are primarily sympathomimetic agents, which cause vasoconstriction of the nasal mucosa and thus a reduction of rhinorrhea. They can be administered either orally or by nasal spray. Their administration causes a noticeable reduction in nasal symptoms including congestion, sneezing, and discharge. Side effects include elevated pulse rate and diastolic blood pressure, palpitations, fatigue, and dizziness. As stimulants, these medications, including pseudoephedrine, ephedrine, phenylephrine,

phenylpropanolamine, and oxymetazoline, are banned by the IOC for sports competition in their oral form, although some nasal sprays are permitted.

Expectorants and Antitussives Expectorants aim to reduce the viscosity of sputum, allowing more effective removal of secretions from the respiratory tract. Their effect in reducing frequency of coughing has not been proven. They are legitimate for sporting use. Antitussives act centrally to suppress the cough center; although their effect has not been proven, they are often found in combination therapy. Examples include codeine, dextromethorphan, and diphenhydramine, which are all allowed for use in competitive sport.

Anticholinergics Anticholinergics antagonize the parasympathetic nervous system and therefore reduce rhinorrhea and other nasal symptoms. Ipratropium nasal spray reduces nasal discharge and sneezing and is permitted for sport.

Analgesic and Antipyretic Medications This group includes aspirin (salicylates), paracetamol (acetaminophen), and nonsteroidal anti-inflammatory drugs. Analgesic/antipyretic medications aim to reduce headache, muscle aches, and generalized discomfort, as well as any fever. Interestingly, recent studies have suggested that, although aspirin and paracetamol (acetaminophen) are effective in suppressing the serum antibody response, they increase nasal symptoms and signs and increase the duration of virus shedding, when compared with ibuprofen (2). None of these medications is proscribed by the IOC.

Combination Treatments Combination medications present multiple active medications, which theoretically have the advantage of treating various symptoms simultaneously. The most effective combination treatments use a decongestant and an antihistamine to reduce nasal symptoms, together with an analgesic to reduce headache and general discomfort. From a drugs-in-sport perspective, such medications are banned for competition because of the stimulant effects of the decongestants. However, their use is permitted for training situations.

Vitamin and Mineral Supplements Vitamin and mineral supplements are often used as adjunct therapy, both as preventive measures and as treatment. In particular, vitamin C and zinc supplements have been regularly used because of their supposed protective effects against oxidative damage caused by infection. Neither vitamin C nor zinc appears to prevent infection, but large doses of both (especially vitamin C) may reduce the duration and severity of viral URTIs (8,9).

All the above medications provide symptomatic relief and systemic support to the immune system. However, if there are signs and symptoms of bacterial infection, then specific antibiotic therapy is necessary. Unfortunately, specific antiviral treatments (e.g., topical interferon) have been disappointing in their effects thus far (2). Some mild reduction in symptoms have been reported in some studies, but such benefits have been negated by side effects. Symptomatic treatments, such as inhalation of warm humidified air, provide some symptomatic relief, but do not conclusively alter the course of the disease. Many people believe that milk and milk products aggravate colds by stimulating mucus production, but this has not been proven scientifically.

Drug Treatment and Exercise

Using the above drug information and knowledge of the effects of exercise on infection, the following approach to viral URTIs in athletes may be recommended. If symptoms are localized then symptomatic treatment with combination decongestants—antihistamines (if out of competition) or antihistamines (if in competition) plus an analgesic agent is recommended. The appropriate medication depends on the predominant symptoms. Exercise is permitted in most cases, altho. gh moderate aerobic training is recommended while symptoms are severe.

However, if systemic symptoms, particularly fever and raised resting pulse rate, are present, then rest from exercise is paramount. Regular analgesic/antipyretics are used to reduce fever while combination medications or antihistamines reduce nasal symptoms. A return to exercise is guided by cessation of fever, resting pulse rate approaching normal, and diminution of other symptoms. This may take up to 14 days to occur.

In the initial stages of resumption of exercise, moderate aerobic exercise is recommended to stimulate the immune response. As the patient tolerates this exercise, the duration and intensity may be increased, until full return to normal training occurs.

SUMMARY

Treatment of viral URTIs is aimed at symptomatic relief. The choice of medications depends on the prominent symptoms and the timing of competition. If symptoms are localized to the upper respiratory tract, then exercise is permitted; however, systemic symptoms, particularly fever and raised resting pulse rate, require the patient to rest. Return to full training depends on diminution of symptoms and return of temperature and resting pulse rate to normal.

REFERENCES

1 Dolin R. Common viral respiratory infections. In: Isselbacher KJ, Braunwald E, Wilson JD, et al., eds. Harrison's principles of internal medicine. 13th ed., vol 1. New York: McGraw-Hill, 1994:803–807.
2 Hilding DA. Literature review: The common cold. ENT J 1994;73:639–647.
3 Gwaltney JM Jr, Phillips CD, Miller RD, Riker DK. Computed tomographic study of the common cold. N Engl J Med 1994;330:25–30.
4 Smith AP. Respiratory virus infection and performance. Phil Trans R Soc Lond B 1990;327:519–528.
5 Nieman DC. Immunology and sports. In: Johnson RJ, Lombardo J, eds. Current review of sports medicine. Philadelphia: Current Medicine, 1994:304–314.
6 Mackinnon LT, Thomasi TB. Immunology of exercise. In: Appenzeller O, ed. Sports medicine: fitness, training, injuries. 3rd ed. Baltimore: Urban and Schwarzenberg, 1988:273–289.
7 Smith MBH, Feldman W. Over-the-counter cold medications: a critical review of clinical trials between 1950 and 1991. JAMA 1993;269:2258–2263.
8 Hemild H. Does vitamin C alleviate the symptoms of the common cold? A review of current evidence. Scand J Infect Dis 1994:26:1–6.
9 Pyne DB, Gray AB, McDonald WA. Exercise and immunity. In: Bloomfield JA, Fricker PA, Fitch K, eds. Science and medicine in sport. 2nd ed. Sydney: Blackwell Scientific, 1995:601–615.

Chapter 3
Pharyngitis and Mononucleosis

Robert Doolittle

Consider a 16-year-old volleyball player complaining of a sore throat with nasal congestion, a low-grade fever, and a mild cough for the past 2 days. Your examination finds a red pharynx with scanty exudate, tender and moderately enlarged anterior cervical lymph nodes, and a temperature of 38.3 °C (101 °F). The rapid strep antigen test is negative. At this point many clinicians would perform a culture for streptococcus and would then be faced with the unresolved questions of whether to start an antibiotic, which antibiotic to choose, and how long to treat this patient. These questions take on added importance when caring for individuals who are athletes in a team setting or who live in dormitories or other close quarters.

Pathogens identified as playing a role in pharyngitis syndromes are named in Table 3-1. Most cases of acute pharyngitis are of viral origin (1). Clinical emphasis since the 1950s has been on finding those few cases that are due to group A β-hemolytic streptococcus so that appropriate treatment could prevent the significant morbidity and mortality from the suppurative and nonsuppurative complications. Recent serologic evidence has suggested additional bacterial etiologies, particularly *Mycoplasma pneumoniae*, *Chlamydia pneumoniae*, and *C. trachomatis* (2,4). Whether these bacteria are primary or secondary in their roles as pathogens, and whether antibiotic therapy is helpful or curative, is not clear. Most nonstreptococcal causes of acute pharyngitis are either self-limited or rare.

The most common complaints of patients with pharyngitis are listed in Table 3-2, and the most common physical findings in Table 3-3. Although most physicians base their decisions regarding etiology on their subjective interpretation of signs and symptoms (5,6), such decision making is notoriously inaccurate (7,8) and generally results in inappropriate treatment with antibiotics. Attempts at developing clinical scoring systems for identifying streptococcal infections have been unsuccessful (9,10).

CAUSES OF PHARYNGITIS

Streptococcal Tonsillopharyngitis

The incidence of streptococcal pharyngitis is highest in the 5- to 15-year-old age group and most commonly occurs during the winter and spring months. Spread occurs by large aerosolized droplets from an infected person's respiratory tract and by direct transfer of oropharyngeal secretions. Occasional epidemics occur via contamination of food items. After 24 hours of an effective antibiotic, individuals with this illness are no longer contagious (11). The few who become streptococcal carriers harbor fewer and less virulent organisms and are probably not an important source of disease (12). Because treatment of streptococcal pharyngitis prevents the sequelae of acute rheumatic fever (13) and the suppurative complications of peritonsillar and retropharyngeal abscess (14), the physician must identify these infections and emphasize compliance with therapy.

Streptococcal pharyngitis in those who live, play, and attend class together is often manifested by the abrupt onset of severe throat pain with fever and tender cervical nodes. Cough, rhinorrhea, and hoarseness are not typically associated, whereas headache and abdominal pain are frequently present, especially in younger children. Swollen tonsils are progressively covered with exudate. The

Table 3-1   Pathogens Identified in Patients Presenting with Pharyngitis

VIRAL	
Pharyngitis as a Prominent Symptom	**Pharyngitis as a Secondary Symptom**
Adenovirus	Rhinovirus
Enterovirus: Coxsackie A, B	Coronavirus
Echo	Influenza viruses
Epstein-Barr virus (EBV)	Parainfluenza viruses
Herpes simplex virus: I & II (HSV)	Respiratory syncytial virus
Human immunodeficiency virus (HIV)	Measles virus
	Rubella virus
BACTERIAL	
Streptococcus: groups A, C, G	
Mycoplasma	
Chlamydia pneumoniae and *trachomatis*	
Neisseria gonorrhoeae	
Arcanobacterium (Corynebacterium)	
haemolyticum	
Corynebacterium diphtheriae	
Yersinia enterocolitica	

soft palate may exhibit petechiae or small raised red follicular lesions with yellow centers (doughnut lesions). At first, the tongue has strawberry-red papillae protruding through a white surface, but it becomes beefy red by the fourth day of illness. If the causative organism is a lysogenic strain producing erythrogenic toxin and the host has no neutralizing antibody, the rash of scarlet fever appears 2 days after the sore throat begins. Occurring first on the face and neck, the rash becomes gener-

Table 3-2   Common Presenting Complaints of Patients with Pharyngitis

Sore throat
Fever
Swollen, tender neck glands
Skin rash
Symptoms often associated with streptococcus
   abrupt onset of illness
   headache
   malaise
   abdominal pain
   nausea, vomiting
Symptoms rarely associated with streptococcus
   rhinorrhea
   cough
   conjunctivitis
   stridor
   hoarseness
   diarrhea

Table 3-3   Common Physical Findings in Patients with Pharyngitis

Red pharynx
Fever
Findings often associated with streptococcus
   pharyngeal edema and exudate
   cervical lymphadenopathy
   strawberry tongue
   palateal petechiae or doughnut lesions
   scarlet fever rash
Findings not associated with streptococcus
   rhinitis
   conjunctivitis
   generalized adenopathy
   oropharyngeal ulcers
   bullous myringitis
   splenomegaly
   hepatomegaly

alized in the next 24 hours, spreading over the trunk and extremities while sparing the palms and soles. This rash lasts 4 or 5 days and is followed, days or even weeks later, by a desquamation of affected skin. Composed of very small erythematous papules, the rash blanches and may become confluent and petechial in the axillary and inguinal areas (Pastia's lines). Illnesses to consider when faced with scarlet fever include measles, Kawasaki's disease, and staphylococcal toxic shock syndrome (15). The newly reported invasive toxin producing streptococcus that causes necrotizing fasciitis is associated with a primary cutaneous rather than pharyngeal focus of infection (16).

A milder illness is seen in endemic infections away from group settings (17). Only one-half of such children with positive cultures have pharyngeal exudate, and only one-third have fever or leukocytosis. The disease is also milder following tonsillectomy (14). Patients under 2 years of age with streptococcus usually have rhinorrhea, excoriated nares, moderate to low-grade fever, and a more protracted course. Acute rheumatic fever is rare as a sequel in those under age 3 and in adults. Streptococcal pharyngeal infection may be associated with otitis media, sinusitis, and pneumonia.

Rapid diagnostic tests of group A streptococcus are in widespread use and are highly specific; however, reports of their sensitivity vary from 60% to 95%. The accuracy of the rapid test is influenced by specimen collection technique, length of illness at presentation, and laboratory handling; in clinical practice, the test produces far too many false negatives to base a decision not to treat on these results alone (18–22). If a rapid streptococcal test is negative but definitive exclusion of group A streptococcus is important, a swab of the posterior pharynx and both tonsils should be cultured in the traditional fashion.

Antibiotic therapy for streptococcal pharyngitis reduces contagion, shortens the disease course, prevents suppurative sequelae, and reduces the incidence of acute rheumatic fever (23–28). Suggestions that early treatment may blunt the immune response and increase the recurrence rate have proven false (29). Treatment does not appear to prevent poststreptococcal glomerulonephritis. In 1996, penicillin is still the drug of choice with ei-

ther a full 10-day oral course or a single intramuscular injection of benzathine penicillin. However, clinical relapses and failure to eradicate streptococcus from the pharynx with penicillin raise questions about this approach (30–33). Evidence for beta-lactamase producing copathogens including *Staphylococcus aureus, Haemophilus influenzae, Moraxella catarrhalis,* and anaerobes in treatment failures (34–36) has not been correlated with improved outcome after more specific therapy for these bacteria (37). Within the United States there is no documented resistance or tolerance to penicillin among group A streptococci (38–40).

Positive throat cultures after treatment in asymptomatic patients imply a chronic carrier state rather than a treatment failure. There is no reason to exclude these carriers from school or sports activities (12). When a patient has multiple episodes of culture positive pharyngitis that are mild or atypical, chronic carriage should be suspected and identified as benign to alleviate patient (and parent) anxiety (15).

Although resistance of group A streptococcus to erythromycin has been found in Japan, France, Spain, and Finland (41), this has not been identified as a problem in the United States (38), and this drug is still the main alternative for penicillin-allergic patients. The new long-acting macrolide azithromycin requires once-a-day dosing for only 5 days and should be strongly considered for use when compliance is an issue (42). Streptococci are generally sensitive to cephalosporins, and there are a number of advocates for their use (32,34), although published studies are not large or rigorous enough to prove any advantage over penicillin (33). Clindamycin is also effective against streptococcus, whereas sulfonamide, tetracycline, and chloramphenicol have no role in treatment.

Other Bacterial Causes

Of particular interest is emerging consideration of nonstreptococcal bacterial causes of pharyngitis. One-half to three-fourths of patients with *Mycoplasma pneumoniae* infection initially complain of sore throat and have an erythematous pharynx, usually without an exudate. By the end of the first week of illness, the cough has become the most prominent symptom, and headache, malaise, and fever are continuing rather than resolving. A cold agglutinin titer rises to 1:64 in 70% of patients by the second week. Reactive airway disease symptoms, most notably exercise-induced bronchospasm, are often present with this infection and may persist for several weeks. Mycoplasma does not respond to cephalosporin or penicillin and requires erythromycin or tetracycline for proper treatment (43). Several studies suggest that this bacteria is at least as common as streptococcus in older teens and adults with pharyngitis (2,44).

Both *Chlamydia trachomatis* and *Chlamydia pneumoniae* have been implicated as potential causes in studies using antibody titers to document infection (2,4,44,45), but clinical identification is difficult and current knowledge is insufficient to outline a clinical approach.

Neisseria gonorrhoeae may be cultured from the throat, although it is unclear whether it causes disease or is a colonizing reservoir for oro-genital transmission (46). Suspicion for this organism is heightened by a history of oral intercourse or of same-sex male partners in patients whose sore throat does not follow a typical course. Current guidelines suggest that single-dose therapies with ceftriaxone, quinolones, or cefixime are adequate (47).

Three other bacterial infections are uncommon but should be remembered especially when treating international athletes. Diphtheria, extremely rare in those countries with high rates of childhood immunizations, might be a consideration when patients are from areas where immunizations are not required or not available (48). *Arcanobacterium* (formerly *Corynebacterium*) *haemolyticum* is a Gram-positive rod that causes acute pharyngitis with a scarlet fever–like rash, most often found in teenagers and young adults (49). *Yersinia enterocolitica* is an infrequent cause of a toxic febrile pharyngitis with or without gastrointestinal symptoms, which progressively worsens until the need for hospitalization is obvious (50,51).

There are also well-documented epidemics of food-borne group C and group G streptococcal pharyngitis, although these infections appear to be self-limiting and do not require treatment (52–54).

Viral Infections

Although often difficult to distinguish from streptococcal infections by clinical examination, viruses are the most prevalent cause of pharyngitis in all age groups. Symptoms of cough, rhinitis, hoarseness, conjunctivitis, stridor, and diarrhea are common with viral infection but rare in streptococcal disease. Respiratory syncytial virus (RSV), parainfluenza, rhinovirus, coronaviruses, measles, and rubella may all cause an erythematous pharynx, but other symptoms and signs usually overshadow the throat complaints. The association of high fever, conjunctivitis, cervical adenitis, and exudative pharyngitis in patients under 3 years of age is the classic description of adenovirus infection, but this clinical picture is rarely seen after childhood (1).

The presence of oropharyngeal ulcers with fever and pharyngitis is common to a number of infections, particularly enteroviruses and herpes simplex. Enteroviruses are active in summertime and are spread by both fecal–oral and respiratory transmission. After a 3- to 6-day incubation, abrupt onset of fever with variable exanthematous and enanthematous changes develop (55,56). Herpangina refers to small (1 to 4 mm) papulovesicular or ulcerated lesions on the tonsillar pillars, palate, uvula, and posterior pharyngeal wall with only occasional lesions on the posterior tongue or buccal mucosa. Accompanied by fever, pharyngitis, malaise, and anorexia, this syndrome is caused by coxsackie A and B and echovirus, and usually resolves in less than a week without any complications (57). Slightly larger ulcers (4 to 8 mm), appearing primarily on the buccal mucosa and posterior tongue with similar lesions on the palms and soles, is pathognomonic for hand-foot-and-mouth disease caused by coxsackie A16 (and rarely 5, 7, 9, and 10), which is self-limited to a 4- to 6-day period (58).

In contrast with the enteroviruses, herpes simplex virus is primarily an anterior oral cavity disease of less abrupt onset and more prolonged course with recurrent episodes. Following direct contact with the source and a short incubation period (1 to 3 days), vesicular lesions appear on the lips, buccal mucosa, gingiva, and tongue and evolve rapidly to form shallow erythematous, painful ulcers. The nares, cheeks, lips, and chin may be involved, as well as tender regional adenopathy. New lesions may appear over the next 5 days, with complete resolution over 1 to 2 weeks without scarring. It is very important to note that primary herpes simplex virus (HSV) infection may involve the entire oral cavity and pharynx and may cause exudative pharyngitis without obvious ulcers (59). Two recent studies document HSV as the pathogen in up to 11% of cases of acute pharyngitis in university students (60,61). The role of acyclovir in the prevention and treatment of oropharyngeal HSV is not established but appears to reduce symptoms (62).

Epstein-Barr Virus (EBV)   If the 16-year-old patient described above returned after 7 days of illness with continued fever, pharyngitis, and adenopathy plus malaise and anorexia, this would represent a classic presentation of infectious mononucleosis (IM or glandular fever). Finding a lymphocytosis of greater than 50% with at least 10% atypical lymphocytes and a positive mono spot test establishes the diagnosis. The patient can expect a mostly benign course and resolution over the ensuing 2 or 3 weeks. However, EBV titers indicate that this classic presentation occurs in less than one-third of those who seroconvert.

In industrialized countries, around 50% of EBV infections occur prior to adolescence and are generally mild without prompting a healthcare visit (63). In lower socioeconomic groups and developing countries, EBV seropositive rates approach 90% by the age of 10 years (64). The peak incidence of classic IM in the United States is 15 to 19 years of age and is associated with onset of intimate oral contact between those shedding the virus and those still susceptible to it (63). In all populations the prevalence of EBV antibodies exceeds 90% by the end of the third decade of life (65).

EBV, a member of the herpesvirus family, shares with other herpesviruses the characteristic of persistent latent infection for life. Transmission through contact with infected oropharyngeal cells or B lymphocytes is followed by spread to regional lymph nodes, viremia, B cell proliferation, and spread to distant lymphoid sites. The disease represents the immune response to the infected B

cells with the reactive lymphocytosis consisting of cytotoxic T cells. The mechanism of spread must be relatively inefficient, as susceptible roommates of students with IM do not experience seroconversion at a greater frequency than the general college population (66).

Table 3-4 is a compilation of clinical features from several studies. Most typically, after an incubation period of 30 to 50 days, a prodrome of malaise, headache, and anorexia for 3 to 5 days is followed by the onset of fever, sore throat, and tender cervical lymphadenopathy in a majority of the adolescents who seek medical attention. The pharyngitis may be only mild erythema of the tonsillar pillars, but most often is a cryptic hyperplasia with palatal edema and a yellow-gray tonsillar exudate. Fever up to 39 to 40 °C with evening peaks may persist for up to 10 to 14 days. Splenomegaly is present at least 50% of the time and peaks during the second or third week of the illness. Ultrasound imaging documents enlargement in far more cases than are apparent with clinical exam, suggesting that the spleen is a very difficult organ to palpate

Table 3-4   Clinical Findings in Infectious Mononucleosis

Symptoms	Percentage of Patients
Sore throat	70–80
Malaise	43–76
Headache	37–62
Nausea, vomiting, anorexia	7–43
Myalgia	12–21

Signs	
Fever	65–98
Lymphadenopathy	90–100
Pharyngitis	83–91
Exudative pharyngitis	22–69
Splenomegaly	50–63
Palpebral edema	5–36
Palatal petechiae	13–47
Rash	3–25
Jaundice	0–10

SOURCE: Adapted from Cheeseman SH. Infectious mononucleosis. Semin Hematol 1988;25:262.

(67). Hepatic tenderness is a frequent finding, but not hepatic enlargement. Most patients have elevated liver enzymes, although jaundice is unusual. Transient maculopapular eruptions occasionally arise on the trunk, but if these patients receive amoxicillin or ampicillin almost 100% develop this rash within 24 to 72 hours. Studies have reported a 30% incidence of group A β-hemolytic streptococcus (GABHS) with IM but more recent data indicate that this rate is closer to 5% and is no more common than in a population without IM (68).

The acute phase of this illness resolves over a 3-week period, with the patient gradually increasing activity during this time. Generalized malaise, weakness, and an inability to sustain a hard training program may persist for several weeks. It appears that well-conditioned young adults have fewer symptoms and return to activity more quickly than the general college population. To reach a pre-illness level of fitness and competitiveness, however, athletes may require 2 to 3 months (69).

Table 3-5 summarizes reported complications of IM. Although EBV affects most organ systems, complications occur in fewer than 5% of cases. Splenic rupture (in 0.1% to 0.5% of cases) during the period of splenomegaly—the 4th to 21st day of illness—may occur spontaneously or after mild trauma, and is the most frequent reason cited for delaying a return to athletics (69). Most cases of splenic rupture occur during normal daily activities such as lifting, bending, and straining at defecation. Patients should be warned to seek immediate attention for the sudden onset of left upper-quadrant pain that radiates to the left shoulder or worsens with inspiration. Ultrasound or CT scan should establish the diagnosis of splenic rupture, and the treatment of choice in most cases remains splenectomy (70,71). No cases of splenic rupture have occurred after 4 weeks from the onset of illness; however, if any doubt about splenomegaly exists, then diagnostic imaging should be used to confirm resolution before allowing return to play (67).

Airway obstruction from massive tonsillar and adenoid enlargement is a life-threatening complication and may require emergency intubation or tonsillectomy. With early recognition, these conditions usually respond within several hours to oral

Table 3-5 Reported Complications of Infectious Mononucleosis

Splenic	Rupture, wandering spleen
Hematologic	Aplastic anemia, hemolytic anemia, thrombocytopenia, thromboasthenia, agranulocytosis
Neurologic/ Psychiatric	Encephalitis, aseptic meningitis, seizures, Guillain-Barré syndrome, cranial neuropathy, peripheral neuropathy, depression, psychosis, subacute sclerosing panencephalitis
Respiratory	Upper airway obstruction, pneumonia, pleural effusion, mediastinal lymphadenopathy
Cardiac	Conduction disturbances, myocarditis, pericarditis
Gastrointestinal	Hepatitis, Reye's syndrome, pancreatitis, mesenteric lymphadenopathy, malabsorption
Renal	Glomerulonephritis, renal hypertrophy, hemolytic uremic syndrome
Ophthalmologic	Conjunctivitis, uveitis, visual impairment
Other organs	Orchitis, arthritis
Dermatologic	Maculopapular exanthems, petechiae, jaundice, urticaria
Infectious	Streptococcal pharyngitis, systemic bacterial infection

SOURCE: Fleisher GR. Epstein-Barr virus. In: Belshe RB, ed. Textbook of human virology. Littleton, MA: PSG Publishing Co., 1984, with permission.

or parenteral corticosteroids. In adults over 40 years, hepatitis and neurologic problems such as Bell's palsy and Guillain-Barré syndrome may result from EBV infection without pharyngitis or cervical adenopathy (72). Seroepidemiologic studies demonstrate that chronic fatigue syndrome is not caused by EBV (73,74).

In cases with a classic presentation in an adolescent or young adult, rapid mono spot tests are believed to be 90% sensitive by the third week of illness. Infected children and older adults are less likely to have a positive spot test. In cases where the presentation is confusing and EBV infection is an important part of the differential diagnosis, se-

Table 3-6   Interpretation of EBV Serum Antibody Patterns

	IgG VCA	IgM VCA	EBV–NA
Susceptible	−	−	−
Acute infection	+	+	−
Convalescent phase	+	±	+
Chronic or reactivated	+	−	+
Old infection	+	−	+

Plus sign, antibody present; minus sign, antibody absent; NA, nuclear antigen.
IgG VCA peaks during acute illness and is sustained for several weeks. Acute/convalescent comparisons are therefore of minimal value during the weeks after onset unless seroconversion is detected. The antibody level declines slightly over several months and usually persists for life. High levels can be present in reactivation; however, the stable levels found in quiescent infections can vary greatly among individuals. A single high anti–IgG VCA result cannot be interpreted as evidence of acute infection or reactivation but only as evidence of infection at an undetermined time.
IgM VCA rises quickly in primary infection and lasts approximately 1 month in children under 4 years of age and 1–3 months in older children and adults. It is generally not detected in reactivation and is a valuable serologic marker for acute EBV infection when used with clinical correlation.
EBV–NA appears 6–8 weeks after onset of symptoms and is detectable indefinitely.

rologic studies should be relied upon. Table 3-6 summarizes EBV serum antibody responses. In most clinical situations the measurement of immunoglobulin M and G (IgM and IgG) to viral capsid antigen (VCA) will provide the most information. Both antibodies develop early in the disease (85% in the first week and 100% by the third week), and while IgM VCA is usually not detectable by the third to fourth month following the acute infection, IgG VCA persists for life (64).

Infectious organisms other than EBV that have been reported to cause mono-like illnesses include cytomegalovirus, toxoplasmosis, hepatitis B, rubella, herpes simplex virus, human immunodeficiency virus (HIV), mumps, and adenovirus (75). Seronegative cases of mononucleosis are most often caused by cytomegalovirus (CMV) and have a more insidious and prolonged course (63). Acute HIV infection most commonly presents as an IM-like syndrome from 6 days to 6 weeks following the date of exposure. Seroconversion to HIV antibody positive occurs from 8 days to 10 weeks after this acute illness (76).

Treatment of IM is mainly supportive and addresses the variable symptoms of each patient. Clinicians are frequently asked for specific relief from the throat discomfort, the misery of the malaise, and the inability to breathe normally. Acetaminophen, NSAIDs, nasal decongestant sprays, and similar over-the-counter medications may provide some relief, and occasionally viscous xylocaine or codeine may be needed for throat pain. Although there is no evidence that bed rest hastens recovery, continued activity seems to worsen the febrile response and fatigue. Isolation from teammates, roommates, or family members is not necessary because spread of infection requires intimate oral contact or shared eating utensils (66). Restriction from heavy lifting and contact sports for 4 weeks or until splenomegaly resolves is reasonable (65, 69,77).

Oral prednisone (subject to International Olympic Committee restrictions and banned at time of competition) in tapered doses starting at 60–80 mg effectively reverses airway obstruction from lymphoid swelling throughout Waldeyer's throat ring, but is not thought to reduce splenic size (78). Corticosteroids also help with complications such as hemolytic anemia, thrombocytopenia, myocarditis, severe hepatitis, and neurologic disorders, although the response is less predictable. The clinical course, including fever and lymphadenopathy, may be shortened by a tapered course of corticosteroid (65,79), but most authorities do not advocate their routine use because of the uncertainty of long-term effects (1).

Acyclovir has not proven clinically useful at this point, but early success with fulminant IM treated by acyclovir plus prednisolone has prompted a double-blind placebo-controlled study (80,81). Antibiotics are indicated only for secondary bacterial complications or concurrent infections.

RETURN TO PLAY

Most illnesses, including IM, negatively affect maximum athletic performance during both the acute phase and recovery. Scientific evidence is being gathered on the deleterious effects of fever and viral infection on cardiac, respiratory, and muscle function (69). Training during and after an illness should be approached with caution to prevent both injuries and prolongation of the condition. Exercise when fever is present should be prohibited, and infectious athletes should be kept out of the team setting. A resting tachycardia (or relative tachycardia in the conditioned athlete) or signs of dehydration should also argue against athletic participation. Resumption of training with reduced intensity and duration after the fever and systemic symptoms have resolved should be safe if athletes are allowed to set their own submaximal pace for 10 to 14 days (and potentially longer after mononucleosis) before returning to a maximal training effort. In general, IM patients should not return to contact and collision sports in less than 1 month, although moderate training may begin in the third week after illness. Clinicians may well need to act as advocates for recovering athletes in discussions with trainers and coaches to prevent a "too much, too soon" approach.

REFERENCES

1 Denison MR. Viral pharyngitis. Semin Pediatr Infect Dis 1995;6:62–68.
2 Komaroff AL, Aronson MD, Pass TM, et al. Serologic evidence of chlamydial and mycoplasmal pharyngitis in adults. Science 1983;222:927–929.
3 Van Cauwenberge PB, Vander Mijnsbrugge A. Pharyngitis: a survey of the microbiologic etiology. Pediatr Infect Dis J 1991;10(suppl):S39—S42.
4 Huovinen P, Lahtonen R, Ziegler T, et al. Pharyngitis in adults: the presence and coexistence of viruses and bacterial organisms. Ann Intern Med 1989;110:612–616.
5 Schwartz B, Fries S, Fitzgibbon AM, Lipman H. Pediatricians' diagnostic approach to pharyngitis and impact of CLIA 1988 on office diagnostic tests. JAMA 1994;271:234–238.
6 Tanz RR, Hofer C. A survey of U.S. pediatricians' strategies for managing group A streptococcal (GABS) pharyngitis. Abstracts of the XII Lancefield International Symposium on Streptococci and Streptococcal Diseases, St. Petersburg, Russia, 1993 (abstract L3).
7 Poses RM, Cebul RD, Collins M, Fager SS. The accuracy of experienced physicians' probability estimates for patients with sore throats. Implications for decision making. JAMA 1985;254:925–929.
8 Breese BB, Disney FA. Accuracy of diagnosis of beta streptococcal infections on clinical grounds. J Pediatr 1954;44:670–673.
9 Komaroff AL, Pass TM, Aronson MD, et al. The prediction of streptococcal pharyngitis in adults. J Gen Intern Med 1986;1:1–7.
10 Seppala H, Lahtonen R, Ziegler T, et al. Clinical scoring system in the evaluation of adult pharyngitis. Arch Otolaryngol Head Neck Surg 1993;119:288–291.
11 Randolph MF, Gerber MA, DeMeo KK, Wright L. Effect of antibiotic therapy on the clinical course of streptococcal pharyngitis. J Pediatr 1985;106:870–875.
12 Kaplan EL. The group A streptococcal upper respiratory tract carrier state: an enigma. J Pediatr 1980;97:337–345.
13 Dajani A, Taubert K, Ferrieri P, et al. Treatment of acute streptococcal pharyngitis and prevention of rheumatic fever: a statement for health professionals. Pediatrics 1995;96:758–764.
14 Chamovitz R, Rammelkamp CH Jr, Wannamaker LW, Denny FW Jr. The effect of tonsillectomy on the incidence of streptococcal respiratory disease and its complications. Pediatrics 1960;26:355–367.
15 Tanz RR, Shulman ST. Diagnosis and treatment of group A streptococcal pharyngitis. Semin Pediatr Infect Dis 1995;6:69–78.
16 Stevens DL, Tanner MH, Winship J, et al. Severe group A streptococcal infections associated with a toxic shock-like syndrome and scarlet fever toxin A. N Engl J Med 1989;321:1–7.
17 Bisno AL. Streptococcal infections. In: Harrison TR, Wilson JD, eds. Harrison's principles of internal medicine. 12th ed. New York: McGraw-Hill, 1991:563–569.
18 Gerber MA, Spadaccini LJ, Wright LL, Deutsch L. Latex agglutination tests for rapid identification of group A streptococci directly from throat swabs. J Pediatr 1984;105:702–705.
19 Berkowitz CD, Anthony BF, Kaplan EL, et al. Co-

operative study of latex agglutination to identify group A streptococcal antigen on throat swabs in patients with acute pharyngitis. J Pediatr 1985;107:89–92.

20 Lieu TA, Fleisher GR, Schwartz JS. Clinical performance and effect on treatment rates of latex agglutination testing for streptococcal pharyngitis in an emergency department. Pediatr Infect Dis 1986;5:655–659.

21 Gerber MA, Randolph MF, Chanatry J, et al. Antigen detection test for streptococcal pharyngitis: evaluation of sensitivity with respect to true infections. J Pediatr 1986;108:654–658.

22 Dobkin D, Shulman ST. Evaluation of an ELISA for group A streptococcal antigen for diagnosis of pharyngitis. J Pediatr 1987;110:566–569.

23 Randolph MF, Gerber MA, DeMeo KK, Wright L. Effect of antibiotic therapy on the clinical course of streptococcal pharyngitis. J Pediatr 1985;106: 870–875.

24 Krober MS, Bass JW, Michels GN. Streptococcal pharyngitis. Placebo-controlled double-blind evaluation of clinical response to penicillin therapy. JAMA 1985;253:1271–1274.

25 Hall CB, Breese BB. Does penicillin make Johnny's strep throat better? Pediatr Infect Dis 1984;3:7–9.

26 Denny FW. Current problems in managing streptococcal pharyngitis [review]. J Pediatr 1987;111: 797–806.

27 Denny FW, Wannamaker LW, Brink WR, et al. Prevention of rheumatic fever: treatment of the preceding streptococcic infection. JAMA 1950;143: 151–153.

28 Wannamaker LW, Rammelkamp CH Jr, Denny FW, et al. Prophylaxis of acute rheumatic fever by treatment of the preceding streptococcal infection with various amounts of depot penicillin. Am J Med 1951;10:673–695.

29 Gerber MA, Randolph MF, DeMeo KK, Kaplan EL. Lack of impact of early antibiotic therapy for streptococcal pharyngitis on recurrence rates. J Pediatr 1990;117:853–858.

30 Feldman S, Bisno AL, Lott L, et al. Efficacy of benzathine penicillin G in group A streptococcal pharyngitis: Reevaluation. J Pediatr 1987;110: 783–787.

31 Gastanaduy AS, Kaplan EL, Huwe BB, et al. Failure of penicillin to eradicate group A streptococci during an outbreak of pharyngitis. Lancet 1980;2:498–502.

32 Pichichero ME. Cephalosporins are superior to penicillin for treatment of streptococcal tonsillopharyngitis: Is the difference worth it? Pediatr Infect Dis J 1993;12:268–274.

33 Shulman ST, Gerber MA, Tanz RR, Markowitz M. Streptococcal pharyngitis: the case for penicillin therapy. Pediatr Infect Dis J 1994;13:1–7.

34 Pichichero ME, Margolis PA. A comparison of cephalosporins and penicillins in the treatment of group A beta-hemolytic streptococcal pharyngitis: a meta-analysis supporting the concept of microbial copathogenicity. Pediatr Infect Dis J 1991:10:275–281.

35 Simon HJ, Sakai W. Staphylococcal antagonism to penicillin-G therapy of hemolytic streptococcal pharyngeal infection. Effect of oxacillin. Pediatrics 1963;31:463–469.

36 Brook I. Role of beta-lactamase-producing bacteria in the failure of penicillin to eradicate group A streptococci. Pediatr Infect Dis 1985;4:491–495.

37 Tanz RR, Shulman ST, Sroka PA, et al. Lack of influence of beta-lactamase-producing flora on recovery of group A streptococci after treatment of acute pharyngitis. J Pediatr 1990;117:859–863.

38 Coonan KM, Kaplan EL. In vitro susceptibility of recent North American group A streptococcal isolates to eleven oral antibiotics. Pediatr Infect Dis J 1994;13:630–635.

39 Smith TD, Huskins WC, Kim KS, Kaplan EL. Efficacy of beta-lactamase-resistant penicillin and influence of penicillin tolerance in eradicating streptococci from the pharynx after failure of penicillin therapy for group A streptococcal pharyngitis. J Pediatr 1987;110:778–782.

40 Stjernquist-Desatnik A, Orrling A, Schalen C, Kamme C. Penicillin tolerance in group A streptococci and treatment failure in streptococcal tonsillitis. Acta Otolaryngol Suppl (Stockh) 1992;492:68–71.

41 Seppala H, Nissinen A, Jarvinen H, et al. Resistance to erythromycin in group A streptococci. N Engl J Med 1992;326:292–297.

42 Still JG. Management of pediatric patients with group A beta-hemolytic streptococcus pharyngitis: treatment options. Pediatr Infect Dis J 1995;14:557–561.

43 Clyde WA Jr. Clinical overview of typical mycoplasma pneumoniae infections. Clin Infect Dis 1993;17(suppl):S32–S36.

44 Komaroff AL, Branch WT Jr, Aronson MD, Schachter J. Chlamydial pharyngitis [letter]. Ann Intern Med 1989;111:537–538.

45 Hashiguchi K, Ogawa H, Kazuyama Y. Seroprevalence of *Chlamydia pneumoniae* infections in otolaryngeal diseases. J Laryngol Otol 1992;106:208–210.

46 Hutt DM, Judson FN. Epidemiology and treatment of oropharyngeal gonorrhea. Ann Intern Med 1986;104:655–658.

47 Drugs for sexually transmitted diseases. Med Lett Drugs Ther 1995;37:117–122.

48 Expanded programme on immunization. Outbreak of diphtheria, update. Wkly Epidemiol Rec 1993;68:134–140.

49 Waagner DC. *Arcanobacterium haemolyticum*: biol-

ogy of the organism and diseases in man. Pediatr Infect Dis J 1991;10:933–939.

50 Tacket CO, Davis BR, Carter GP, et al. *Yersinia enterocolitica* pharyngitis. Ann Intern Med 1983;99: 40–42.

51 Rose FB, Camp CJ, Antes EJ. Family outbreak of fatal *Yersinia enterocolitica* pharyngitis. Am J Med 1987;82:636–637.

52 Hill HR, Caldwell GG, Wilson E, Hager G, Zimmerman RA. Epidemic of pharyngitis due to streptococci of Lancefield group G. Lancet 1969;2:371–374.

53 Group C streptococcal infections associated with eating homemade cheese—New Mexico. MMWR Morb Mortal Wkly Rep 1983 Oct 7;32:510,515–516.

54 Gerber MA, Randolph MF, Martin NJ, et al. Community-wide outbreak of group G streptococcal pharyngitis. Pediatrics 1991;87:598–603.

55 Cherry JD. Enteroviruses: polioviruses (poliomyelitis), coxsackieviruses, echoviruses and enteroviruses. In: Feigin RD, Cherry JD, eds. Textbook of pediatric infectious diseases. Philadelphia: WB Saunders, 1990:1705–1753.

56 Forman ML, Cherry JD. Enanthems associated with uncommon viral syndromes. Pediatrics 1968;41:873–882.

57 Cherry JD. Herpangina. In: Feigin RD, Cherry JD, eds. Textbook of pediatric infectious diseases. Philadelphia: WB Saunders, 1990:230–232.

58 Froeschle JE, Nahmias AJ, Feorino PM, et al. Hand, foot and mouth disease (Coxsackievirus A16) in Atlanta. Am J Dis Child 1967;114:278–283.

59 Kohl S. Postnatal herpes simplex virus infection. In: Feigin RD, Cherry JD, eds. Textbook of pediatric infectious diseases. Philadelphia: WB Saunders, 1990:1558–1583.

60 Glezen WP, Fernald GW, Lohr JA. Acute respiratory disease of university students with special reference to the etiologic role of *Herpesvirus hominis*. Am J Epidemiol 1975;101:111–121.

61 McMillan JA, Weiner LB, Higgins AM, Lamparella VJ. Pharyngitis associated with herpes simplex virus in college students. Pediatr Infect Dis J 1993;12:280–284.

62 Brunell PA. Indications for oral acyclovir in children. Pediatr Infect Dis J 1993;12:970.

63 Schooley RT. Epstein-Barr virus infections, including infectious mononucleosis. In: Harrison TR, Wilson JD, eds. Harrison's principles of internal medicine. 12th ed. New York: McGraw-Hill, 1991:689–692.

64 Radetsky M, Overturf GD. Epstein-Barr infections in adolescents and young adults. In: Adolescent medicine: state of the art reviews, vol. 6. Philadelphia: Hanley and Belfus, 1995:91–99.

65 O'Brien RF. Infectious mononucleosis. In: Adolescent medicine: state of the art reviews, vol. 2. Philadelphia: Hanley and Belfus, 1991:459–471.

66 Schooley RT, Dolin R. Epstein-Barr virus (infectious mononucleosis). In: Mandell GL, Douglas RG Jr, Benett JE, eds. Principles and practice of infectious diseases. 3rd ed. New York: Churchill Livingstone, 1990:1172–1185.

67 Dommerby H, Stangerup SE, Stangerup M, Hancke S. Hepatosplenomegaly in infectious mononucleosis, assessed by ultrasonic scanning. J Laryngol Otol 1986;100:573–579.

68 Collins M, Fleisher GR, Fager SS. Incidence of beta hemolytic streptococcal pharyngitis in adolescents with infectious mononucleosis. J Adolesc Health Care 1984;5:96–100.

69 Sevier TL. Infectious disease in athletes. Med Clin North Am 1994;78:389–412.

70 Safran D, Bloom GP. Spontaneous splenic rupture following infectious mononucleosis. Am Surg 1990;56:601–605.

71 Konvolinka CW, Wyatt DB. Splenic rupture and infectious mononucleosis. J Emerg Med 1989;7: 471–475.

72 Bailey RE. Diagnosis and treatment of infectious mononucleosis. Am Fam Physician 1994;49:879–888.

73 Buchwald D, Sullivan JL, Komaroff AL. Frequency of "chronic active Epstein-Barr virus infection" in a general medical practice. JAMA 1987;257:2303–2307.

74 Hellinger WC, Smith TF, Van Scoy RE, et al. Chronic fatigue syndrome and the diagnostic utility of antibody to Epstein-Barr virus early antigen. JAMA 1988;260:971–973.

75 Jones JF. Epstein-Barr virus infections. In: McAnarney ER, et al., eds. Textbook of adolescent medicine. Philadelphia: WB Saunders, 1992: 873–879.

76 Crowe SM, McGrath MS. Acute HIV infection. In: Cohen PT, Sande MA, Volberding PA, eds. The AIDS knowledge base. 2nd ed. Boston: Little, Brown, 1994:4.2-1–4.2-7.

77 Haines JD Jr. When to resume sports after infectious mononucleosis. How soon is safe? Postgrad Med 1987;81:331–333.

78 Cheeseman SH. Infectious mononucleosis. Semin Hematol 1988;25:261–268.

79 Brandfonbrener A, Epstein A, Wu S, Phair J. Corticosteroid therapy in Epstein-Barr virus infection. Effect on lymphocyte class, subset, and response to early antigen. Arch Intern Med 1986;146:337–339.

80 Andersson J, Britton S, Ernberg I, et al. Effect of acyclovir on infectious mononucleosis: a double-blind, placebo-controlled study. J Infect Dis 1986;153:283–290.

81 Andersson J, Ernberg I. Management of Epstein-Barr virus infections. Am J Med 1988;85:107–115.

Chapter 4
Sinusitis, Otitis Media, Otitis Externa, and Conjunctivitis

Janus D. Butcher
Wade A. Lillegard

Infections of the upper respiratory tract and special sense organs occur commonly in the athlete. These illnesses are similar in presentation to those seen in the general population, but they are of particular concern in the competitive athlete. The increased incidence in certain sports (particularly water sports), the risk of spread to other athletes, and the potential impact on performance demand prompt recognition by the team physician. In addition, because many medications commonly used in treating these conditions are banned by the International Olympic Committee (IOC) and national governing bodies such as the National Collegiate Athletic Association (NCAA), healthcare providers must have up-to-date information regarding treatment options.

SINUSITIS

Sinusitis is a very common infection, accounting for approximately 4.6% of physician visits by young adults (1). Athletes involved in water sports such as swimming, diving, surfing, and water polo appear to have a particularly high risk of developing this infection (2,3). The primary pathology in sinusitis is obstruction of the ostial openings from allergies, upper respiratory tract infections (URTIs), or anatomic anomalies (polyps, septal deviation, foreign bodies, or tumors). This leads to decreased oxygen tension in the sinuses, decreased clearance of foreign material, secondary infection, mucosal edema, further ostial obstruction, and accumulation of fluid or pus (4). The most common organisms involved in acute sinusitis are the aerobic bacteria *Streptococcus pneumoniae*, *Haemophilus influenzae*, and *Branhamella catarrhalis*. Approximately 10%

are due to anaerobic organisms (5). Aspirated sinus fluid in sinusitis is sterile in up to 30% of cases, indicating either a viral or allergic etiology (4).

Presentation
Patients with acute sinusitis present with a purulent nasal discharge and/or a productive cough, which is worse at night or when supine. Associated symptoms include headache, facial pain, upper dental pain, or fever. Physical examination reveals red and swollen nasal mucosa with a purulent discharge from the meatus. Malodorous breath may also be present. Percussion often reveals maxillary or frontal sinus tenderness and further evaluation may show abnormal transillumination. Radiographs are generally not necessary unless the patient appears toxic or is febrile, or there is concern of acute frontal sinusitis.

Treatment
The goals of treatment are threefold: to open the sinus ostia, restore mucociliary clearance, and treat the underlying disorder (allergy and/or bacterial infection). Ostial obstruction from mucosal swelling is best treated with a topical decongestant such as oxymetazoline (allowed by the IOC and NCAA [6]), twice a day for up to 3 days, or oral pseudoephedrine (banned by the IOC, allowed by the NCAA [6]), 30–60 mg four times daily. Mucolytics such as guaifenesin (allowed by the IOC and NCAA [6]), 600–1200 mg twice a day, can facilitate drainage in some patients. Antihistamines are only useful if there is a strong allergic component to the disease. They should otherwise be avoided, as they tend to thicken secretions and hinder drainage. Sedative antihistamines are not allowed by the IOC for shooters (6). Antibiotic treatment with ampi-

cillin, amoxicillin, or trimethoprim–sulfameth-oxazole is the most cost effective first-line therapy (4). Standard treatment courses are 7 to 10 days, although some authors advocate regimens as short as 3 to 5 days and others suggest courses of 2 to 3 weeks or until symptoms have ceased for a certain period of time (7). If there is incomplete resolution or early relapse, the diagnosis should be confirmed with sinus radiographs. The patient is then treated for one more week with either an extension of the same medication or a penicillinase-resistant drug (e.g., amoxicillin—clavulanate or a second or third generation cephalosporin).

Chronic sinusitis may require extending the therapy until all signs and symptoms have been absent for a duration of 5 days. This can result in a total of 3 to 4 weeks of therapy. Patients with persistent symptoms should be evaluated with a computerized tomogram of the sinuses (to assess for ethmoid/sphenoid disease or obstructive lesions) and referred to an otolaryngologist for further evaluation.

Athletic performance can be adversely affected by both the fever associated with sinusitis and the medications used for its treatment. Isometric and dynamic strength as well as endurance have all been shown to decrease in febrile subjects (8). Further, the severity of myalgia has been correlated with reduced muscle function. Fever itself increases oxygen consumption by 13% for every degree increase over 37 °C (9). Antihistamines may cause adverse central nervous system symptoms (drowsiness and decreased reaction time), but these have not been shown to either enhance or inhibit the athlete's physical performance (10).

There are no firm guidelines on when an athlete with sinusitis can safely return to full activity. Roberts (11) has put forth reasonable recommendations for athletes with febrile URTIs: exercise may be resumed a few days after symptoms clear if there are no systemic symptoms, but a full month of recovery should be allowed with symptoms of extreme fatigue or myalgia. Diving should not be allowed until the sinusitis is resolved, as the atmospheric–sinus pressure disequilibrium from an obstructed ostia can cause sinus wall mucosal damage and bleeding (barosinusitis) (12).

OTITIS MEDIA

Otitis media refers to an infection of the middle ear and the mucosally lined air spaces of the temporal bone. Eustachian tube dysfunction, following a viral upper respiratory infection or in response to environmental allergens, results in the collection of fluid in the middle ear canal. This fluid then acts as a growth medium for bacteria, and the characteristic symptoms result from a bacterial superinfection. The most common pathogens involved in adults are *Streptococcus pneumoniae*, *Haemophilus influenzae*, *Streptococcus pyogenes*, *Mycoplasma pneumoniae*, and *Moraxella catarrhalis*.

Presentation

Typical presenting complaints include otalgia with occasional vertigo and hearing impairment. Fever and other symptoms of an upper respiratory infection may or may not be present. Physical examination reveals an erythematous tympanic membrane (TM) (Plate 1) with decreased mobility on pneumo-otoscopy or tympanogram. Fluid pressure may cause the TM to spontaneously rupture, resulting in resolution of pain followed by otorrhea. Tenderness in the mastoid area is common with acute otitis media, and does not usually represent mastoiditis (13).

Treatment

Acute otitis media is generally treated with antibiotics with the presumption of a bacterial etiology. Amoxicillin (250–500 mg), three times a day for 10 days, or erythromycin (250 mg), four times a day for 10 days, are effective first-line agents. Resistant cases will usually respond to amoxicillin–clavulanate (250–500 mg) three times a day for 7 to 10 days, or cefixime (400 mg) daily for 7 days. Treatment with decongestants and/or antihistamines (if there are associated allergies) may improve eustachian tube function and help to drain the collected middle ear fluid.

Many over-the-counter preparations include pseudoephedrine or ephedrine, both of which are banned by the IOC but allowed by the NCAA (6). Sedating antihistamines are banned by the IOC for shooting sports. Tympanocentesis using a 20-

gauge needle is effective in relieving symptoms but should only be done by those experienced with the procedure. Diving should be avoided until there is normal TM mobility by Valsalva or tympanogram because of the risk of TM rupture at depths greater than 4.3 ft when there is eustachian tube dysfunction (13).

Grommets Tympanostomy tubes (grommets) are commonly used in the treatment of chronic otitis media. The patient frequently asks his or her primary care physician questions regarding continued participation in water sports. Most studies done on active swimmers with grommets have shown no increase in the development of otorrhea and in fact have shown lower rates of infection in swimmers compared with nonswimmers (14). Wearing ear plugs does not prevent infection in swimmers with grommets; however, the use of polymyxin B-neosporin-hydrocortisone (two drops at night after swimming) does decrease the incidence of otorrhea (15). It is important to warn these patients to restrict their activities to surface swimming and avoid any diving activities, as the increased pressure may result in a higher rate of infection (14).

OTITIS EXTERNA (SWIMMER'S EAR)

Otitis externa or "swimmer's ear" is an infection of the external ear canal frequently affecting individuals involved in sports with repetitive water exposure or mechanical trauma to the external ear. This may be a greater threat to outdoor athletes such as swimmers, sail-boarders, kayakers, and surfers participating in polluted bodies of water (16). Barotitis externa is a separate, noninfectious process exclusive to divers. The most commonly isolated organisms are Gram-negative rods, particularly *Pseudomonas aeruginosa* and *proteus* sp. (17) and fungi *(Aspergillus)*.

Presentation
Typical presenting complaints for otitis externa are otalgia, pruritus, and a purulent discharge from the ear. Otoscopic examination reveals a tender, erythematous and edematous external

meatus, frequently with purulent material obstructing the canal. The tympanic membrane may be erythematous, but generally exhibits normal motion on pneumo-otoscopy (17).

Treatment
Treatment of this condition involves careful removal of the purulent debris by irrigation, followed by protection from exposure to water and mechanical trauma (e.g., avoiding ear plugs). Corticosporin drops (polymyxin B, neosporin, and hydrocortisone), a combination of an anti-inflammatory agent and antibiotic that is allowed by both the IOC and NCAA (6), should be applied liberally over a cotton wick to retain the medication. Resistant cases are frequently due to pseudomonas and respond to ciprofloxacin ear drops (2 mg/mL) applied over a wick twice a day for 7 days (18). Swimming can be resumed when symptoms resolve and there is no clinical evidence of infection, usually in 5 to 7 days. Individuals with frequent recurrences should use an acidic and/or drying agent such as acetic acid, or aluminum sulfate and calcium acctate, before and after swimming (19). Swimmers should also be advised to tilt the head and shake the water from the ear canals after swimming and dry the area with a hair dryer.

CONJUNCTIVITIS

Presentation
Conjunctival inflammation may be due to allergies, toxic insult, or infection, with conjunctival hyperemia the common finding in all cases (Fig 4-1). Characteristics of the discharge and associated symptoms help to differentiate the specific etiology of conjunctivitis. Allergic conjunctivitis typically presents with pruritus, redness, and a scant watery discharge. In this type, a slit-lamp examination may show a cobblestone appearance of the conjunctiva.

Viral and bacterial conjunctivitis both cause ocular irritation with a discharge, pain, and photophobia. The discharge in viral conjunctivitis is generally clear to yellow and watery and is usually associated with a viral prodrome. Bacterial conjunctivitis, on the other hand, manifests as a pro-

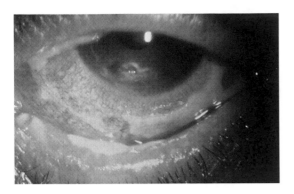

Figure 4-1. Conjunctivitis with hyperemia and discharge. (Courtesy of Brad Pearman, MD.)

fuse yellow to green exudate. The most commonly involved bacterial organisms are *Staphylococcus aureus, Staphylococcus epidermidis,* and *Streptococcus* and *Haemophilus* species (20). One of the most severe forms of conjunctivitis is caused by *Neisseria gonorrhoeae* infection. This must be considered in any sexually active adolescent or young adult presenting with a prominent purulent discharge. Culture and Gram's stain should be used to confirm the diagnosis, as parenteral antibiotic treatment with close observation is required in this form of conjunctivitis.

The herpes simplex virus also poses special risks to the athlete because of the ease of transmission and potential for severe complications, including dendritic keratitis and corneal scarring (21). This infection is most common in wrestling and rugby, but can be spread in any contact sport. The transmission results through direct contact with an active herpes lesion, which can remain infectious up to 5 days following crust formation. This infection typically presents with a clear watery discharge, vesicular lesions on the lids, and preauricular nodes (22). Frequently the patient has other active herpes skin lesions.

Treatment

Allergic conjunctivitis is best treated by avoidance of the allergen and applying topical vasoconstrictor and antihistamine solutions. Naphazoline HCL with antazoline, two drops every 4 hours, is often effective and allowed by both the IOC and NCAA (6). Ketorolac tromethamine (0.5%) drops effectively relieve symptoms of allergic conjunctivitis and are an allowed drug for athletes. Ophthalmic corticosteroids are also unrestricted and very effective, but should only be prescribed by an ophthalmologist due to the risks of glaucoma and cataracts.

Culture-guided therapy for infectious conjunctivitis is generally not warranted unless there is a suspicion of gonococcal infection. Broad spectrum antibiotic solutions or ointments such as trimethoprim sulfate and polymyxin B sulfate cover both Gram-negative and Gram-positive organisms (20). Gentamicin sulfate, tobramycin, and sulfacetamide sodium are also effective, but the latter frequently causes a stinging sensation. Drops or ointment should be applied every 1 to 2 hours while the patient is awake until clinical evidence of the infection resolves. Herpes keratoconjunctivitis is treated topically with trifluridine (Viroptic), one drop (1% solution) every 2 hours for up to 21 days. The associated skin lesions should be treated with acyclovir (Zovirax), 200 mg five times a day for 10 days.

Another important consideration in the treatment of conjunctivitis is avoiding the infection of other athletes. Prevention of transmission is best accomplished through careful screening of athletes before competition in high-contact sports such as wrestling; infectious athletes should be excluded from competition until they have been adequately treated and their symptoms are completely cleared. Swimmers with conjunctivitis should be held from participation because of the potential spread of viral agents (adenovirus 3) in chlorinated swimming pools (22).

REFERENCES

1 Noffby R. Clinical aspects on bacterial infections in the upper respiratory tract. Scand J Infect Dis 1983;39(suppl):14–18.
2 Slavin RG. Sinusitis. J Allergy Clin Immunol 1984;5:712–716.
3 Bailey BJ, Strunk CL, Smith CW. Otolaryngology. In: Rakel RE, ed. Textbook of family practice. 4th ed. Philadelphia: WB Saunders, 1995:441–480.

4 Willett L, Carson J, Williams J. Current diagnosis and management of sinusitis. J Gen Internal Med 1994;9:38–45.

5 Josephson J, Rosenberg S. Sinusitis. CIBA Clin Symp 1994;46:1–32.

6 Fuentes R, Rosenberg J, Davis A. Athletic drug reference '95. Research Triangle Park, NC: Clean Data, 1995.

7 Williams JW, Hollerman DR, Samsa GP, Simel DL. Randomized controlled trial of 3 vs 10 days of trimethoprim/sulamethoxazole for acute maxillary sinusitis. JAMA 1995;273:1015–1021.

8 Friman G, Wright J, Ilback N, et al. Does fever or myalgia indicate reduced physical performance capacity in viral infections? Acta Med Scand 1985;217:353–361.

9 Dinarello C, Wolf S. Pathogenesis of fever. In: Bennett JC, Plum F, eds. Cecil's textbook of medicine. 19th ed. Orlando, FL: WB Saunders, 1992:462–464.

10 Mongomery L, Deuster P. Effects of antihistamine medications on exercise performance: implications for sportspeople. Sports Med 1993;15:179–195.

11 Roberts J. Viral illnesses and sports performance. Sports Med 1986;3:296–303.

12 Kizer K. Scuba diving and dysbarism. In: Auerbach P, ed. Wilderness medicine: management of wilderness and environmental emergencies. 3rd ed. St Louis: Mosby, 1995:1176–1208.

13 Jackler RK, Kaplan MJ. Ear, nose, and throat. In: Tierne LM, McPhee SJ, Papadakis MA, eds. Current medical diagnosis and treatment. 34th ed. Norwalk, CT: Appleton & Lange, 1995:169–202.

14 Pringle MB. Grommets, swimming, and otorhea—a review. J Laryngol Otol 1993;107:190–194.

15 Cohen HA, Kauschansky A, Ashkenasi A, et al. Swimming and grommets. J Fam Pract 1994;38:30–32.

16 Dewailly E, Poirier C, Meyer FM. Health hazards associated with windsurfing on polluted water. Am J Public Health 1986;76:690–691.

17 Schuller DE, Bruce RA. Ear, nose, throat, and eye. In: Strauss RH, ed. Sports medicine. 2nd ed. Philadelphia: WB Saunders, 1991:189–203.

18 Arnes FL, Dibb W. Otitis externa: clinical comparison of local ciprofloxacin versus local oxytetracycline, polymyxin B, hydrocortisone combination treatment. Curr Med Res Opin 1993;13:182–186.

19 Rosenfeld J. Otitis media and externa. In: Taylor RB, ed. Family medicine, principles and practice. 4th ed. New York: Springer-Verlag, 1994:555–567.

20 Snyder R, Glasser D. Antibiotic therapy for ocular infection. West J Med 1994;161:579–594.

21 Holland EJ, Mahanti RL, Belongia EA, et al. Ocular involvement in an outbreak of herpes gladiatorum. Am J Ophthalmol 1992;114:680–684.

22 Weinberg SK. Medical aspects of synchronized swimming. Clin Sports Med 1986;5:159–167.

Chapter 5
Infectious Bronchitis and Pneumonia in Athletes

Karl B. Fields

Bronchitis and pneumonia often follow viral upper respiratory tract infections. As upper respiratory infections account for more lost time from sport than all other medical illnesses combined, bronchitis and pneumonia are relatively frequent problems for athletes (1). Viral infections cause most cases of bronchitis and pneumonia, along with a lesser number of bacterial illnesses. Little difference exists between the types of bronchitis experienced by nonathletes versus athletes. However, most pneumonias in athletes fall into two less serious categories: community-acquired and atypical. The more serious pneumonias that relate to nosocomial spread or to immunocompromised hosts rarely develop in athletic individuals.

ACUTE BRONCHITIS

Overview of the Disease

Acute bronchitis is defined as a respiratory infection characterized by inflammatory change of the bronchial tree leading to recurrent cough. To label an infection as bronchitis, physicians must exclude pneumonia or an upper respiratory source such as sinusitis. In spite of multiple etiologies—including viral, bacterial, asthmatic, chemical, or irritant—bronchitis results in the same complex of symptoms. The hallmark is a cough that is persistent and sometimes productive of clear mucus or purulent sputum. Typically, the coughing interrupts daily activities and disturbs sleep.

Physical findings in bronchitis are often unimpressive. Fever is usually absent, but when present remains low grade. The lung findings consist of rhonchi, or coarse breath sounds, or in many cases a normal auscultation. The presence of rales or other signs of pulmonary infiltrate suggest a localized process such as pneumonia and are inconsistent with the diagnosis of bronchitis. In addition, neither sinus tenderness nor purulent nasal discharge occurs. This is an important distinction as drainage from sinusitis ranks among the most common causes of persistent cough in primary care medicine.

Laboratory testing reveals minimal if any elevation of the total white blood cell count. Typically, since most of the infections are viral, the counts are low with the differential showing a lymphocytosis. Acute phase reactants such as ESR or CRP remain in the low category. Sputum Gram's stain in acute bronchitis typically shows a mixture of the normal oral flora. Likewise, sputum cultures grow a variety of oral flora, so neither of these tests helps direct the clinician toward a specific diagnosis or treatment. Chest radiographs may demonstrate some hyperinflation, but should not show infiltrates.

The primary etiologic agents in bronchitis are the common respiratory viruses. Epidemic outbreaks occur secondary to rhinovirus, respiratory syncytial virus (RSV), influenza A, coronavirus, and others. Bacteria are felt to be a less common cause of acute bronchitis. Once an inflammatory process disrupts the mucoprotective barrier of the respiratory tree and impairs function of the ciliated respiratory cells, bacteria can invade the mucosa. The same bacteria that account for most pneumonias and sinusitis cause acute bronchitis as well. The five key pathogens detected are *Streptococcus pneumoniae*, *Haemophilus influenzae* (particularly nontypeable strains), *Moraxella catarrhalis*, *Mycoplasma pneumoniae*, and *Chlamydia pneumoniae*. Anaerobes do not cause acute bronchitis since the respiratory bronchioles are a high oxygen tension environment (2).

A key differential diagnostic concern centers around excluding irritants or bronchospasm as the cause of symptoms as opposed to an infectious etiology. The distinction between acute bronchitis and asthma is often blurred. This is particularly true for certain infectious agents such as RSV that typically cause extensive wheezing. Inhaling caustic substances such as hydrochloric acid or smoke can precipitate an irritant bronchitis resembling a burn, which causes extensive coughing with or without associated wheezing.

Controversies in Acute Bronchitis

More questions than answers exist regarding acute bronchitis. Controversy continues with the following issues: What determines the appropriate diagnosis of bronchitis? Do antibiotics make a difference in the treatment of bronchitis? Is bronchitis a variant of asthma and not a primarily infectious problem? What outcome measure determines the response to bronchitis? Do existing studies have enough validity that clinicians can rely on them to direct therapy for these patients? Considering the many uncertainties in the general literature, it is not surprising that little information has arisen to help direct the treatment of athletes with acute bronchitis.

Studies of Etiology   Historical features continue to form the basis for the diagnosis. Prior symptoms of an upper respiratory infection point more strongly toward an infectious etiology than does a sudden onset of productive cough without a precipitating illness. If the patient has known allergic problems, a history of asthma, or symptoms that primarily occur with exercise, acute bronchitis becomes less likely than does an asthmatic condition. Similarly, high fever, shaking chills, and a more debilitating infection strongly suggest a pneumonia, even when physical examination and chest radiograph fail to demonstrate the diagnosis. Diagnostic uncertainty increases when the patient seems too ill for a typical acute bronchitis or when the cough continues to persist much longer than the 7 to 10 days expected. Particularly when the cough changes from productive to a dry, irritative quality, the physician must question

whether the original infection is still the primary reason for continuing symptoms.

Recently, researchers have labeled a group of patients who develop persistent cough and sometimes wheezing following an acute episode of bronchitis as having "acute asthmatic bronchitis" (3). This adult diagnosis parallels the coining of "wheezing associated respiratory infection" (WARI) for a similar pediatric process that typically follows RSV epidemics. Cough and signs of bronchospasm may persist for as long as 3 months after the original infection. These are patients who have no prior history of asthma and, after resolving their acute process, may not have subsequent asthmatic episodes. This type of ongoing problem may develop in 15% to 30% of acute bronchitis patients, and even a greater number of individuals may show some residual changes on pulmonary function tests that continue to be present for several months. These types of findings raise the question of whether we should focus on acute bronchitis as an infectious process or as an inflammatory process triggering acute bronchospasm.

Chlamydia infections potentially are the trigger for adult asthmatic syndromes. One study demonstrated increased chlamydia titers in adults who had developed a wheezing illness after an acute respiratory illness (4). Data from Finland implicate *Chlamydia pneumoniae* in 43% of hospitalized pneumonia patients during epidemics (5). During nonepidemic times, chlamydia is thought to account for about 10% of lower respiratory tract infections. A treatment trial using azithromycin or doxycycline for patients with adult asthmatic bronchitis resulted in significant improvement in 50% of the individuals (6).

Studies of Treatment   Debate has sharpened because studies that have focused on trying to establish a bacterial etiology for bronchitis have been uniformly unsuccessful. Similarly, no convincing evidence has emerged that antibiotics are clearly indicated for acute bronchitis. Some of this uncertainty stems from the fact that attempts to study acute bronchitis are fraught with confounding variables: because the etiology of acute bronchitis cannot quickly be determined, who should be included in a study? And, lacking a clear etiology, how does one determine a clinical cure? Thus, clinical outcome studies typically focus on duration of cough or sputum production as the criterion for improvement—neither being a very objective measure for disease modification. In addition, most studies cannot completely exclude sinusitis, pneumonia, allergic diseases, or other potential diagnoses as causes for the symptom complex we define as acute bronchitis.

The studies of acute bronchitis rarely have had large sample sizes, and they offer only limited insight about treatment. For example, studies that examined the effect of antibiotics on duration of cough showed little difference with or without treatment. A large number of studies have examined the effect of treatment on productive sputum, but only a minority of these have been double-blinded with control groups.

The general results of prospective studies show, at best, some symptomatic response to antibiotics, such as earlier resolution of productive cough and improvement of general symptoms. Doxycycline, which receives endorsement as a rational empiric therapy for acute bronchitis, has shown benefits in only one placebo controlled study. A critical analysis of the value of various studies led separate authors to conclude that no study offered clear support for the use of antibiotics in acute bronchitis (7,8).

Many antibiotics are used to treat acute bronchitis, including amoxicillin, extended spectrum macrolides, cephalosporins, amoxicillin/clavulanate, and quinolones (9–11). Although multiple studies of these agents have been published, they compare efficacy to amoxicillin or cefaclor as the "gold standards." Most show clinical resolution rates of 90% with a standard course of therapy (usually 10 days). But unfortunately, even the gold standards have not been evaluated against placebos in well-designed trials. Increasing resistance of *Streptococcus pneumoniae,* nontypeable *H. influenzae,* and *M. catarrhalis* has been demonstrated and may relate to overuse of antibiotics. The lack of convincing trials has led some infectious disease specialists to conclude that acute bronchitis does not warrant antibiotic treatment (8). Because of the small evidence of any benefit, the clinician should limit use of antibiotics to those patients who have a more severe clinical course.

As cough is often the key clinical symptom of both acute bronchitis and asthma, speculation suggests that acute bronchitis may represent an inflammatory, rather than an infectious, disease. Cough may be the marker for an immune reaction triggered by inflammation, foreign bodies, bacteria, viruses, or chemical irritants. Limited evidence for this theory comes from several small studies that have compared erythromycin versus albuterol in the treatment of acute bronchitis (12,13). In these trials, patients responded more favorably to albuterol than to the antibiotic.

Special Considerations in Athletes with Acute Bronchitis

Athletes depend on excellent pulmonary function to perform at maximal levels. For this reason even mild impairments of flow dynamics brought on by acute bronchitis potentially have greater consequences in athletes than in nonathletes. The demands of sport may lead clinicians to use the peak flow as an objective measure of how a respiratory infection influences the pulmonary capacity of a given athlete. This testing can help decide how quickly an athlete can return to intense training and competition. The athlete with documented impairment needs to return to training with a less intense workout schedule while recovering. Excess stress could promote relapse or a secondary complication of an otherwise minor infectious process.

In addition, physical activity requires very high minute ventilation. Rapid air flow is key to some of the known triggers for exercise-induced asthma such as airway drying, cooling, and exposure to irritants or antigens. If acute bronchitis triggers airway hyper-reactivity, these same effects of increased minute ventilation more likely will trigger bronchospasm in the athlete recovering from acute bronchitis.

Intense exercise depresses immune function for brief periods (14), and evidence points toward impairment of mucociliary clearance after extreme exertion (15). For these reasons athletes who attempt to train vigorously through bouts of acute bronchitis place themselves at risk for lowering their resistance to secondary bacterial infections. Olympic rowers who needed antibiotics for respiratory infections had prolonged illnesses causing an average of 10.6 days missed from training (16). This raises the question of whether athletes allow themselves enough rest to recover adequately from acute infections, but specific advice is difficult to offer as the effect of exercise on the duration of pulmonary function changes following acute bronchitis has not been determined.

Approaches to Treatment of Acute Bronchitis in the Athlete

With symptomatic care, athletes will typically recover from acute bronchitis. As a group, athletes are healthier, have less chronic illnesses, and are less likely to smoke than nonathletes. Antibiotic treatment is appropriate for more severe infections or ones in which symptoms do not abate after 7 to 10 days. When antibiotics are prescribed, amoxicillin, erythromycin, tetracycline, doxycycline, or trimethoprim/sulfamethoxazole are all considered first-line agents. If atypical organisms are suspected, erythromycin or tetracycline class antibiotics work best. Extended spectrum macrolides, such as azithromycin or clarithromycin, are more expensive but provide an alternative that covers all common bacteria, resistant bacteria, and the atypical organisms that cause acute bronchitis. Extended spectrum macrolides also cause less gastrointestinal irritation than do erythromycin preparations (17).

Empiric antibiotic therapy is also appropriate during the height of a competitive season or the final weeks of preparation for a major competition. Under these circumstances, observation to see if the clinical course worsens may cause too much lost time from training. Thus, the small risk of antibiotic therapy is outweighed by the potential competitive benefit to the athlete. Typically, athletes will show significant improvement within 3 days of beginning treatment with antibiotics. If not, a chest radiograph and reexamination seem appropriate. At that point, antibiotic selection should be reviewed, and bronchodilator or anti-inflammatory therapy should be considered as well.

Return to training cannot be rushed and certainly should not occur if the athlete continues to have a low-grade fever or myalgia. Generally, two easy training days should be allowed for every one day missed with acute illness, although this must be individualized. As albuterol or similar beta agonists may help resolve cough and some of the airway obstruction experienced during and after acute bronchitis, screening peak flow rates may identify the athletes who need beta agonists and also the frequency which they should use a bronchodilator (see also Chapter 22).

Failure to demonstrate a diminished peak flow does not exclude the possibility of an asthmatic-type process. In fact, an empiric use of beta agonists may be required even when screening tests show little response to inhalation of a bronchodilator. Use of inhaled nedocromil, cromolyn sodium, or corticosteroids has not been studied in acute bronchitis. Since these anti-inflammatory agents are becoming the mainstay of asthma treatment, logic dictates that empiric therapy with them is reasonable in the "acute asthmatic bronchitis" patients. Similarly, in any athletes with a prior history of allergy, allergic rhinitis, or asthma, inhaled anti-inflammatory agents or even a short course of oral corticosteroids may be warranted (subject to IOC regulation).

PNEUMONIA IN THE ATHLETE

Pneumonia is a lower respiratory infection characterized on the chest radiograph by interstitial or alveolar infiltrates. Classic symptoms include fever, tachypnea, and cough as well as rales, rhonchi, or signs of consolidation on lung examination. Chest radiographs demonstrate a new infiltrate in one or more areas of the lungs. While these symptoms and findings usually indicate pneumonia, the differential diagnosis remains extensive and includes diverse conditions such as pulmonary embolus, malignancy, collagen vascular disease, immune lung disease, atelectasis, and asthma. For this reason, a more extensive workup may be required in patients who do not respond promptly to treatment.

An adult who enters the physician's office for treatment of respiratory symptoms has approximately a 3% chance of having pneumonia (18). Tests that suggest a higher likelihood of a bacterial pneumonia include elevated white blood cell counts, particularly with an increase in the polymorphonuclear leukocyte cells and bands, and elevation of erythrocyte sedimentation rates (ESR) and C-reactive proteins (CRP). Sputum Gram's stains and cultures are most helpful when they identify one predominant bacterium; however, they usually show contamination with normal mouth flora. Chest radiographs that have very specific findings such as air bronchograms or classic lobar infiltrates strongly suggest pneumonia in the otherwise healthy individual who has no prior history of a lung abnormality.

Certain clinical parameters predict pneumonia just as well as laboratory or radiologic testing. These parameters include a patient with a productive cough who has an elevated respiratory rate, temperature greater than 37.7 °C (100 °F), localized rales, and decreased breath sounds, while having no viral prodrome or history of asthma (18).

Pneumonia consistently ranks among the top ten causes of mortality in Western nations, but athletes rarely experience the more serious pneumonias. High-risk pneumonias affect hospitalized or institutionalized patients, individuals with HIV disease, the elderly, or the immunosuppressed, or may occur following influenza A or varicella infections. Athletes commonly develop typical community-acquired pneumonias or pneumonias from atypical organisms. In studies of healthy young adults who develop pneumonia, five pathogens cause over 90% of the cases. The most common bacteria are *Streptococcus pneumoniae* and *Haemophilus influenzae,* which cause between 25% and 40% of cases. The two most frequent atypical organisms—*Mycoplasma pneumoniae* and *Chlamydia pneumoniae* (TWAR strain)—typically cause 20% to 30% of cases and a higher percentage during epidemics. Common respiratory viruses cause 30% to 50% of pneumonias with some variation based on time of year.

Some differences in the clinical picture occur based on the etiologic agent causing a given pneumonia. For example, a sudden onset of symptoms including elevated temperature and a single episode of a shaking chill suggests *Streptococcus pneumoniae* as the etiologic agent. A dry cough, insidious onset over 2 to 3 weeks, and diarrhea suggest a *Mycoplasma pneumoniae.* Pharyngitis and otitis media can also occur in association with a mycoplasma pneumonia. Chlamydia pneumonias of-

ten mimic mycoplasma and occur sporadically or as outbreaks in groups of young adults in school or military settings. Chlamydia, however, may fail to respond to erythromycin. Another clue may be the association of sinusitis or laryngitis, either of which is much more common with chlamydia (18,19).

Diagnosis of a given pneumonia may hinge on confirmatory testing. Bacterial processes may have an associated bacteremia, and, as such, blood cultures can lead to a definitive diagnosis. Mycoplasma causes elevated cold agglutinin titers in about two-thirds of patients, but these are nonspecific. However, cold agglutinin titers significantly higher than 1:64 more commonly point to mycoplasma than to viral pneumonia. Enzyme-linked immunosorbent assay (ELISA) testing for mycoplasma typically relies on IgG antibodies, and thus does not distinguish past from present infection. However, elevated IgM titers indicate acute disease, and new tests under development may help speed diagnosis by testing for IgM. The chest radiograph usually shows interstitial infiltrates and no consolidation; but, even with extensive cough, the chest radiograph may show minimal changes. Conversely, relatively well-appearing patients may have markedly abnormal chest radiographs. Inconsistencies between the clinical appearance and the radiographic picture are one of the atypical features of mycoplasma pneumonias. Microimmunofluorescence techniques for acute antibody rises are the most accurate tests in chlamydia pneumonia but are not definitive. Rapid tests relying on new technologies, such as DNA probes and polymerase chain amplification of respiratory secretions, hold promise for more specific immediate diagnosis for both chlamydia and mycoplasma (19; Fig 5-1).

Clinical Course and Return to Activity After Pneumonia

Pneumonia causes a much greater insult to pulmonary function than does bronchitis. Rapid return to training and competition should not be the primary goal of any therapeutic program, rather the physician should focus on complete resolution of the infection. Without taking appropriate recovery time, the athlete may face a greater risk of complications such as persistent infection, abscess, or

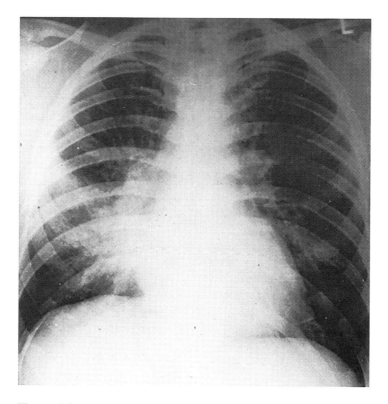

Figure 5-1. Perihilar infiltrates secondary to mycoplasma pneumonia. (Reprinted by permission of Wolfe Medical Publications, Ltd. from Emonde RTD, Rowland HAK. The Miles color atlas of infectious disease. Vol. 4, 2e. 1987:371.)

empyema, which typically occur only in more debilitated patients.

In a healthy host, such as most athletes, appropriate antibiotic treatment leads to dramatic improvement in clinical symptoms within 72 hours. When this is not the case, additional diagnostic evaluation and an empiric change in antibiotics seem warranted. Radiographs rarely return to normal as rapidly as clinical symptoms, and even in uncomplicated cases may take 6 weeks to completely clear (20). The spectrum of symptomatology also varies with the severity of the original infection and the pathogenic organism.

Mycoplasma pneumonia may occur in epidemics in college-age students including those who are athletes. Fortunately, this is the shortest duration of any common pneumonia and often all pulmonary changes resolve completely in 2 to 4 weeks.

Relatively little pulmonary scarring occurs, and thus training recovery may proceed relatively rapidly so that after the acute phase resolves, the athlete will need 1 to 2 reduced-training days for each day of acute infection. Pulmonary changes in pneumococcal pneumonia, on the other hand, resolve more gradually and typically require 4 to 6 weeks for a complete resolution. However, a proportion of patients, even when previously healthy, may take a full 3 months to return to normal pulmonary status. Few data exist on *Haemophilus influenzae, Chlamydia pneumoniae,* and different respiratory viruses that would allow the clinician to predict the recovery phase for the athlete (21).

Since the chest radiograph clears so slowly, many athletes may be able to resume light training before films are completely normal, although an objective measure of near-normal pulmonary function is desirable. In addition, monitoring heart rate response to exercise and subjective measures such as perceived exertion may help to guide the intensity of workouts.

Treatment of Pneumonia in the Athlete

In all but a few cases, athletes are healthy enough that they can do well with outpatient treatment for their pneumonia. Athletes who come for care appearing sicker than expected usually have a complicating factor. This may include asthma or a delay in diagnosis, as when when the athlete has tried to deny that he or she was sick enough to require formal medical treatment. When individual athletes become sick enough to merit hospitalization, they should be managed using the same criteria for treatment of any patient with community-acquired pneumonia. This means oxygen supplementation if they show desaturation; full workup including chest radiographs, blood cultures, and other confirmatory diagnostic tests; and parenteral antibiotics with supplemental intravenous fluids.

For athletes stable enough for oral treatment, several options exist. Common oral antibiotics such as amoxicillin, trimethoprim/sulfamethoxasole, erythromycin, cefaclor, or cephalexin have been used for years in respiratory infections, but generally do not cover all the possible pathogens. Ideally, the clinician wants an agent that covers each of the common bacteria and atypical organisms that cause most pneumonias. Doxycycline at a dosage of 200 mg every 12 hours for 10 days offers coverage against *Streptococcus pneumoniae*, *Haemophilus influenzae*, *Mycoplasma pneumoniae*, and *Chlamydia pneumoniae*. This becomes an attractive first-line antibiotic choice with advantages of low cost and coverage of the four most common treatable organisms. Increased sun sensitivity may pose a problem for athletes in certain outdoor sports, and gastrointestinal side effects are a problem for a minority of patients.

Azithromycin, while more costly, covers the same organisms equally well. One advantage with this preparation is that after a loading dose of 500 mg, the athlete only takes one 250-mg tablet daily for 4 days, which may help promote compliance. Another benefit is that the 5-day treatment provides bactericidal antibiotic levels for 10 days because of this antibiotic's long half-life and pharmacokinetics. Azithromycin has fewer gastrointestinal side effects than standard erythromycin products and does not sensitize the athlete to sunburn (6,17,22,23).

A third alternative oral preparation is ofloxacin, which at a dosage of 400 mg every 12 hours for 10 days, effectively eliminates most community-acquired pneumonias (23). Tolerance to quinolones is very good, with few reported side effects. Quinolones are contraindicated in young athletes with open epiphyses, because animal studies show that they may damage growing cartilage. Some infectious disease specialists hesitate to use quinolones in community-acquired pneumonias because of the concern that they may not effectively treat pneumococcal infections. Case reports show that ciprofloxacin failed to eliminate serious pneumococcal, anaerobic, and mycoplasma infections; this suggests it is not a good choice for most common respiratory infections (24). Ofloxacin, however, appears to have good activity against the pneumococcus infection; is virtually completely absorbed on oral administration; and is a reasonably priced product for treatment.

SUMMARY

Acute bronchitis and pneumonia occur in individuals of all ages, including athletes. The potential impairment of respiratory function poses the greatest problem for athletes with regard to their return to sport. Controversy exists as to whether acute bronchitis arises from inflammatory changes associated with bronchospasm and cough or from a prolonged infectious process. Antibiotic efficacy in the treatment of acute bronchitis has not been clearly established, but neither has the efficacy of treatment with inhaled bronchodilators or anti-inflammatory agents. Thus, in most cases the physician must make a clinical judgment regarding the use of medication and may choose to use objective respiratory function data to help the athlete return to training.

Pneumonia virtually always takes an athlete out of physical activity for a minimum of 2 weeks, usually for even longer periods. Bronchodilators and anti-inflammatory agents have a limited role in most pneumonias and do not often affect the time elapsed until the athlete can return to training. Three agents provide broad coverage for the outpatient oral treatment of pneumonia: doxycycline, azithromycin, and ofloxacin. Fortunately, these antibiotics are well tolerated and allow most athletes to be treated as outpatients.

REFERENCES

1 Weidner TG. Literature review: upper respiratory illness and sport and exercise. Int J Sports Med 1994;15:1–9.

2 Davis AL, Hahn DL, Niederman MS, O'Connell EJ. Acute bronchitis in adults and children. Patient Care 1996;30:102–124.

3 Hahn DL. Acute asthmatic bronchitis: a new twist on an old problem. J Fam Pract 1994;39:431–435.

4 Hahn DL, Dodge RW, Golubjatnikov R. Association of *Chlamydia pneumoniae* (Strain TWAR) infection with wheezing, asthmatic bronchitis, and adult-onset asthma. JAMA 1991;266:225–230.

5 Kauppinen MT, Herva E, Kujala P, et al. The etiology of community-acquired pneumonia among hospitalized patients during a *Chlamydia pneumoniae* epidemic in Finland. J Infect Dis 1995;172:1330–1335.

6 Hahn DL. Treatment of *Chlamydia pneumoniae* infection in adult asthma: a before-after trial. J Fam Pract 1995;41:345–351.

7 Orr PH, Scherer K, Macdonald A, Moffatt MEK. Randomized placebo-controlled trials of antibiotics for acute bronchitis: a critical review of the literature. J Fam Pract 1993;36:507–512.

8 Gonzales R, Sande M. What will it take to stop physicians from prescribing antibiotics in acute bronchitis? Lancet 1995;345:665–666.

9 Dere WH, Farlow D, Therasse DG. Loracarbef versus cefaclor in the treatment of acute bacterial bronchitis. Clin Ther 1992;14:41–53.

10 Dark D. Multicenter evaluation of azithromycin and cefaclor in acute lower respiratory tract infections. Am J Med 1991;91 (suppl 3A):31–35.

11 Safran C. Cefpodoxime proxetil: dosage, efficacy and tolerance in adults suffering from respiratory tract infections. J Antimicrob Chemother 1990;26 (suppl):E93–E101.

12 Hueston WJ. Albuterol delivered by metered-dose inhaler to treat acute bronchitis. J Fam Pract 1994;39:437–440.

13 Hueston WJ. A comparison of albuterol and erythromycin for the treatment of acute bronchitis. J Fam Pract 1991;33:476–480.

14 Nieman D. Exercise, upper respiratory infection, and the immune system. Med Sci Sport Exerc 1994;26:128–139.

15 Muns G, Singer P, Wolf F, Rubinstein I. Impaired nasal mucociliary clearance in long-distance runners. Int J Sports Med 1995;16:209–213.

16 Budgett RGM, Fuller GN. Illness and injury in international oarsmen. Clin Sports Med 1989;1:57–61.

17 Piscitelli SC, Danziger LH, Rodvold KA. Clarithromyin and azithromycin: new macrolide antibiotics. Clin Pharmacy 1992;11:137–152.

18 File TM, Tan JS, Plouffe JF. Community-acquired pneumonia: What's needed for an accurate diagnosis. Postgrad Med 1996;99(1):95-102,105–107.

19 Cunha BA, Ortega AM. Atypical pneumonia: extrapulmonary clues guide the way to diagnosis. Postgrad Med 1996;99:123–128,131–132.

20 Jay SJ, Johanson WG Jr, Pierce AK. The radiographic resolution of *Streptococcus pneumoniae* pneumonia. N Engl J Med 1975;293:798–801.

21 Cassiere H, Rodrigues JC, Fein AM. Delayed resolution of pneumonia: when is healing too slow? Postgrad Med 1996;99:151–154,157–158.

22 Marrie TJ. Community-acquired pneumonia. Clin Infect Dis 1994;18:501–515.

23 Cunha BA. Community-acquired pneumonia: cost-effective antimicrobial therapy. Postgrad Med 1996;99:109–110,113–114,117–119.

24 Frieden TR, Mangi RJ. Inappropriate use of oral ciprofloxacin. JAMA 1990;264:1438–1440.

Chapter 6
Hepatitis in Athletes

Brent S. E. Rich

In 1994, the American Medical Society for Sports Medicine (AMSSM) and the American Academy of Sports Medicine (AASM) wrote a joint position statement, "Human Immunodeficiency Virus and Other Blood-Borne Pathogens in Sports" (1). This document establishes guidelines for practitioners to counsel patients and athletes with these disorders and to offer recommendations for sports participation. The hepatitis virus, human immunodeficiency virus (HIV), and other blood-borne pathogens continue to evolve as risks in athletic competition. This chapter reviews the clinical courses and profiles of the types of viral hepatitis that pose the greatest risk to athletes.

DEFINITIONS

Hepatitis is an inflammation of the liver, and the leading causes include alcohol, drugs, bacteria, biliary tract obstruction, exposure to toxins, as well as numerous viruses. Viral hepatitis may be transmitted by infected food or water, poor personal hygiene, sexual contact, inoculation of infected blood or blood products, or perinatal transmission from mother to child. In the United States, approximately 60,000 cases of viral hepatitis are reported to the Centers for Disease Control (CDC) each year, though this may represent only 10% to 20% of the actual cases (2).

Because the liver performs numerous functions such as storage, production, metabolism, filtration, and disposal of different substances, initial disease symptoms are very generalized (i.e., nausea, vomiting, malaise, anorexia, headaches, myalgias, fever, chills, weight loss, and aversion to smoking). Individual symptoms within the same disease syndrome may also be variable, thus making diagnosis, prognosis, and morbidity difficult to predict. With significant liver function impairment, jaundice occurs as a result of yellow pigment accumulating in the skin or eyes secondary to the inability of the liver to remove bilirubin from the blood. Laboratory studies usually reveal abnormal elevation of liver enzymes, particularly alanine aminotransferase (ALT) and aspartate aminotransferase (AST). Other serologic markers may aid in screening, diagnosis, and in determining active hepatitis from a chronic carrier state.

Hepatitis A Virus (HAV)

Transmission Hepatitis A is transmitted though the gastrointestinal system by fecal contamination and oral ingestion. Sporadic and epidemic causes arise from contaminated food or water. Person-to-person contact makes HAV common in institutional care of patients, and also poses risks in the athletic setting. Proper personal hygiene is essential to prevent spread. Rates of HAV vary by country, with lower rates in nations that have clean drinking water and efficient waste disposal methods. U.S. data estimate that 130,000 to 150,000 cases of HAV occurred in 1990 out of a population of 240 million (3).

Presentation The incubation period is 4 weeks (range: 15 to 50 days). Fever, nausea, vomiting, abdominal pain, and anorexia occur abruptly and last approximately 7 days. Jaundice is common in adults, but not in children. HAV never results in chronic hepatitis, is not life-threatening, and has no carrier state. Diagnosis is made by identifying antibody to HAV (IgM anti-HAV) in the blood serum when symptoms develop. It lasts for 3 to 6 months and confirms active or recent infection.

Total anti-HAV antibody or IgG can be identified after several months, and indicates immunity against further exposure.

Treatment   Treatment is based on the nature of symptoms and is primarily supportive (i.e., rest, fluids, and good nutrition). Although the condition rarely requires hospitalization, intravenous fluids are occasionally required for dehydration. ALT levels should be monitored twice weekly initially and with decreasing regularity as the condition dictates. Prophylaxis is accomplished by intramuscular injection of inactivated hepatitis A vaccine (Havrix) to those ≥2 years of age.

Hepatitis B Virus (HBV)

Transmission   Hepatitis B (HBV) is a viral infection of the liver transmitted by infected blood or body fluids through perinatal contact, sexual contact, and/or contaminated needles. HBV is found to be significantly more concentrated in blood than HIV; that is, there are 100 million infectious particles per milliliter of blood in HBV (4), compared with a few hundred to a few thousand particles per milliliter of blood in HIV (5). This is significant in that only one case of HBV has been documented to occur in sport: a high school Sumo wrestler in Japan contracted HBV from an opponent in 1982 (6). In addition, there was no evidence of any increased risk of HBV transmission in a study of Australian Rules football participants, a sport in which there is significant contact, collision, and risk of blood exposure (7). Not surprisingly, no cases of HIV transmission in sport have been well documented, although one possible case was reported among soccer players in Italy in 1990 (8). Without validated reports of HBV or HIV in sport, the disqualification of athletes with these conditions may not be indicated. Nevertheless, further research, education, proper wound care, and universal precautions with any exposure to body fluids should be routine in the athletic setting.

Presentation   In 1990, the United States had an estimated 300,000 annual cases of HBV (9) and an additional 750,000 to 1,000,000 HBV carriers (10). A *carrier* is defined as a person who is positive for the hepatitis surface antigen (HBsAg) on two occasions, 6 months apart, or positive for HBsAg

and negative for immunoglobulin M antibody to the core antigen on a single specimen. These individuals may transmit the virus even though they do not manifest HBV symptoms. The incubation period ranges from 25 to 160 days (average 120 days), depending on the concentration of the inoculate. Clinical symptoms are similar to HAV infection, occur insidiously, and last several weeks. Chronic HBV infection occurs in 6% to 10% of adults, 25% to 50% of children (ages 1 to 5 years), and 70% to 90% of infants. Cirrhosis, chronic liver disease, and hepatocellular carcinoma may affect these individuals later in life. The mortality rate is 1.4%.

Treatment   Serologic testing confirms the diagnosis. HBsAg is detectable 30 to 60 days after exposure, correlates with elevated liver enzymes, and indicates infectivity. When HBsAg persists longer than 6 months, a chronic carrier state is confirmed. Additionally,

> IgM anti-HBc indicates recent HBV infection.
> HBeAg marks high infectivity.
> Anti-HBe indicates recovery and decreasing infectivity.
> Anti-HBs is a protective antibody that indicates recovery and offers immunity against further infection.

Treatment   Prophylactic treatment consists of avoiding unnecessary exposure to any blood product and by intramuscular injection of hepatitis B vaccine (Engerix B) at a 0-, 1-, and 6-month schedule. HBV vaccine is recommended in infants, children, and healthcare workers. Hepatitis B immune globulin (H-BIG) provides passive protection from HBV exposure and is recommended to infants born to infected HBV mothers, healthcare workers sustaining accidental needle sticks, blood exposure, or sexual contacts of a HBsAg-positive person.

Hepatitis C Virus (HCV)

Transmission   HCV is responsible for the majority of "non-A, non-B hepatitis" (NANB) cases and 20% to 50% of sporadic viral hepatitis in the United States (11). HCV has an insidious onset of generalized symptoms and occurs with an incubation period of 2 weeks to 1 year (average 8 weeks).

Exposure occurs parenterally, sexually, and perinatally.

Presentation   Most HCV patients initially remain asymptomatic, although more than 75% develop a chronic state, which results in chronic liver disease and the possibility for liver cancer. The fatality rate is 1% to 2%.

Treatment   Anti-HCV is used to identify individuals with acute or chronic HCV. If positive for anti-HCV the individual should be considered infectious and followed with serial ALT levels for at least 12 months to determine the possibility of chronic liver disease. Treatment for HCV is with the antiviral agent interferon. No vaccine is available.

Hepatitis D Virus (HDV)

Transmission   Hepatitis D (delta virus) is an RNA virus particle that depends on HBV for replication by using the surface antigen (HBsAg) as a surface protein. This protein coating allows the virus to survive. HDV may occur concurrently with HBV infection or in an HBsAg carrier. Routes of transmission and symptoms are the same as for HBV.

Presentation   If sudden deterioration occurs in an HBV patient, HDV should be suspected. HDV infection in an asymptomatic or mildly symptomatic chronic HBsAg carrier may cause cirrhosis, chronic active hepatitis, and often fulminant hepatitis B. The incubation period is 3 to 13 weeks. Serologic testing is possible by identifying HDAg in early infection and total anti-HDV later or after the acute effects. Ten to fifteen percent of cases become chronic, and mortality ranges near 30%.

Hepatitis E Virus (HEV)

Transmission   HEV is an NANB hepatitis transmitted by the fecal-oral route and by contaminated water. HEV is prevalent in developing countries, but not in more modern nations.

Presentation   Onset is acute after an incubation period of 3 to 6 weeks. No chronic state or serologic tests are available, and a mortality rate of 20% has been seen in pregnant women.

Treatment   Prevention occurs by practicing proper hygiene and by avoiding contaminated food and water. Treatment is symptomatic.

SUMMARY

The hepatitis viruses are a family of separate and distinct diseases that cause inflammation and potential damage to the liver. Athletes are not immune from exposure or contracting these diseases. Their significance in relation to athletic participation is changing as more knowledge is gained in this area. A summary regarding details of these infections is found in Table 6-1.

Diagnosis

1 Suspicion of hepatitis should be based on exposure to pathogens and generalized clinical symptoms. Jaundice is a useful clue, but is not always present. Serum ALT is a useful screening tool and correlates with liver dysfunction.
2 Only HAV and HEV occur by the fecal-oral route or from contaminated water or food. HBV, HCV, and HDV are blood-borne pathogens.
3 Laboratory testing provides a method of differential diagnosis for the following hepatitis viruses.
   - Acute hepatitis panel (IgM anti-HAV, HBsAg, IgM anti-HBc and anti-HCV):
        Rule out HAV or HBV
        Recent HAV infection—IgM anti-HAV
        Recent HBV infection—IgM anti-HBc
        Acute HBV infection—HBsAg with IgM anti-HBc
        Chronic HBV infection—HBsAg without IgM anti-HBc
        Determine HCV infection—anti-HCV
   - Hepatitis B monitoring panel (HBsAg, HBeAg, anti-HBe):
        Chronic HBV—persisting HBsAg
        Determine infectivity—HBeAg
        Monitor resolution—conversion from HBeAg to anti-HBe
   - Chronic carrier panel (HBsAg, HBeAg, total anti-HBc):
        Chronic carrier—all three markers elevated
   - HBV immunity monitored by anti-HBs
4 Recommended guidelines for return to exercise and training have not been established, thus clinicians must use practical judgment based on the severity of the illness and any residual symp-

Table 6-1   Summary of Clinical Features of Viral Hepatitis

	HAV	HBV	HCV	HDV	HEV
Incubation	2–6 weeks	8–24 weeks	2–52 weeks	3–13 weeks	3–6 weeks
Onset	Abrupt	Insidious	Insidious	Abrupt	Abrupt
Symptoms					
Asymptomatic Patients	Most children	Most children Adults: 50%	About 75%	Rare	Rare
Jaundice	Children: 10% Adults: 70–80%	25%	25%	Varies	Unknown
Routes of transmission					
Fecal/Oral	Yes	No	No	No	Yes
Parenteral	Rare	Yes	Yes	Yes	No
Sexual	No	Yes	Possible	Yes	No
Perinatal	No	Ycs	Possible	Possible	No
Water/Food	Yes	Yes	No	No	Yes
Chronic state	No	Adults: 6–10% Children: 25–50% Infants: 70–90%	75%	10–15%	No
Case fatality rate	0.6%	1.4%	1–2%	30%	1–2% Pregnant women: 20%
Serologic testing					
Acute disease	IgM anti-HAV	IgM anti-HBc, HBsAg	Anti-HCV	HDAg	None
Chronic discase	None	HBsAg	Anti-HCV	Total anti-HD	None
Infectivity	None	HBeAg, HBsAg, HBV-DNA	Anti-HCV	Total anti-HD	None
Recovery	None	Anti-HBe, anti-HBs	None	None	None
Carrier state	None	HBsAg	None	HDAg, anti-HD	None
Screening for immunity	Total anti-HAV	Anti-HBs, total anti-HBc	None	None	None

toms. In general, athletes require 1 to 2 days of convalescence with reduced training for each day of recent illness.

REFERENCES

1 Joint Position Statement. Human immunodeficiency virus and other blood-borne pathogens in sports. Clin J Sports Med 1995;5:199–204.

2 Hepatitis learning guide. 2nd ed. Abbott Park, IL: Abbott Laboratories, 1994:3.

3 Hepatitis learning guide. 2nd ed. Abbott Park, IL: Abbott Laboratories, 1994:9.

4 Centers for Disease Control. Guidelines for pre-vention of transmission of human immunodeficiency virus and hepatitis B virus to health-care and public-safety workers. MMWR Morb Mortal Wkly Rep 1989 June 23;38(suppl 6):1–37.

5 Ho DD, Moudgil T, Alam M. Quantitation of human immunodeficiency virus type 1 in the blood of infected persons. N Engl J Med 1989;321:1621–1625.

6 Kashiwagi S, Hayashi J, Ikematsu H, et al. An outbreak of hepatitis B in members of a high school sumo wrestling club. JAMA 1982;248:213–214.

7 Siebert DJ, Lindschau PB, Burrell CJ. Lack of evidence for significant hepatitis B transmission in Australian Rules footballers. Med J Aust 1995;162:312–313.

8 Brown LS, Drotman P. What is the risk of HIV in-

fection in athletic competition? Presented at the 9th International Conference on AIDS, Berlin, June 6–11, 1993. Abstract.

9 Hepatitis learning guide. 2nd ed. Abbott Park, IL: Abbott Laboratories, 1994:14.

10 Protection against viral hepatitis. Recommenda-tions of the Immunization Practices Advisory Committee (ACIP). MMWR Morb Mortal Wkly Rep 1990 Feb 9;39 (RR-2):1–26.

11 Dolan PJ, Skibba RM, Hagan RC, Kilgore WR III. Hepatitis C: prevention and treatment. Am Fam Physician 1991;43:1347–1350,1355–1360.

Chapter 7
Urinary Tract Infections in Athletes

Wayne A. Hale
Curtis D. Reimer

Although no studies in athletes have documented the prevalence of urinary tract infections (UTIs), athletes would not be expected to differ from other healthy people of the same age and sex. Therefore, UTIs, particularly those involving the lower tract, should occur frequently in female and older athletes.

PREDISPOSING FACTORS

Factors that decrease natural barriers, or increase exposures to colonization of the periurethral area with pathogenic organisms, make ascending infection more likely. Thin, amenorrheic, or post-menopausal female athletes have less estrogenic effect and thinner periurethral tissues, which provide less resistance to contamination of their bladder. Similarly, elderly men have less genitourinary antibody secretions than they had in their youth. Athletes with an active sex life may have greater exposure to sexually transmitted diseases such as urethritis and postcoital UTIs.

Urinary retention promotes UTI by allowing bacteria time to multiply and invade lining tissues before being flushed out. Voluntary urinary retention and dehydration associated with prolonged activity during sports lead to urinary stasis. Dehydration also predisposes an individual to obstruction from renal lithiasis, causing greater risk of infection. Mechanical obstruction of the urethra from diaphragms, prostatic hypertrophy, or other causes may occasionally be a factor in UTIs of athletes. In addition, trauma to the urethra or bladder can encourage reflux, tissue damage, and invasion by organisms.

TYPES OF INFECTION

Cystitis

Cystitis in young women is the most common UTI treated by sports medicine physicians. Findings suggestive of this diagnosis are the abrupt onset of frequency, urgency, and internal dysuria. The urine specimen usually shows pyuria and often hematuria, proteinuria, and a positive nitrate test. The onset may be postcoital, and there is frequently a history of recurrent bladder infections. On a urine culture, 100 to 100,000 colonies of a single pathogenic species of bacteria can grow. However, a culture is unnecessary in the presence of classic symptoms when there are no complicating factors (e.g., diabetes, pregnancy, recurrent infection, or gynecologic symptoms).

Other conditions that mimic cystitis include vaginitis when associated with external dysuria, vaginal discharge, odor, pruritus, and dyspareunia. Urethritis also causes milder dysuria of gradual onset, sometimes associated with vaginal discharge and a history of a new sexual partner. In both conditions, examination of the perineum, introitus, vagina, and cervix may suggest the causative agent. Microscopic examination of a wet-prep of vaginal secretions may show yeast, trichomonads, or clue cells indicating bacterial vaginosis. Cultures of the cervix, urethra, or mucosal lesions may be positive for gonorrhea, chlamydia, or herpes simplex, whereas the urine culture generally grows fewer than 100 colonies of mixed species or nonpathogenic bacteria (1).

Epididymitis

Epididymitis causes an acutely painful, swollen scrotum, and can have associated dysuria or urethral discharge. In athletes less than 35 years old, epididymitis has a strong association with sexually acquired urethritis secondary to chlamydia or gonorrhea (2). Older men more often develop this condition secondary to prostatitis, with *Escherichia coli* the most common agent. Physical examination reveals a tender, indurated epididymis, while a urinalysis typically shows a positive leukocyte esterase and frank pyuria.

Urethritis

Urethritis most commonly relates to a sexually transmitted disease; however, traumatic urethritis has been reported in bicyclists. One author reported personal experience of dysuria, mild hematuria, and chills after a 150-km bicycle trip. His urinalysis showed leukocytes, erythrocytes, and bacteriuria; cystoscopy revealed urethritis with inflammation of the membranous urethra. Symptoms eventually resolved after discontinuation of long-distance rides (3).

Prostatitis

Prostatitis, also reported in bicyclists, occurs from saddle pressure. Patients complain of outlet obstruction symptoms such as frequency, dribbling, nocturia, and incomplete emptying, although dysuria is generally not present (4,5). Three male patients aged 25 to 50 years reported the onset of the above symptoms in relation to the purchase or use of a 10-speed or stationary bicycle. Voiding habits rapidly returned to normal after discontinuation of cycling or modification of the seat to reduce pressure on the perineum (4). Physical examination should include a rectal to identify any prostate findings suggestive of bacterial prostatitis, prostatic hypertrophy, or prostate cancer (5). A significantly tender prostate gland should not be vigorously palpated because of the risk of sepsis if there is bacterial prostatitis. Urine obtained after the examination should be cultured if a bacterial etiology is suspected.

Pyelonephritis

Although no specific reports have been related to exercise, acute pyelonephritis affects approximately 4% of the greater than 6 million patients consulting physicians in the United States for UTIs

(6). Classic clinical symptoms include those found in lower UTIs, along with fever, chills, flank pain, nausea, and vomiting. Costovertebral tenderness ranges from exquisite to absent (6). *E. coli* represents 80% of the causative organisms. Pregnant athletes have a 3% to 7% incidence of uncomplicated pyelonephritis, which can be prevented by closely monitoring urine samples and treating asymptomatic bacteriuria (6). For nonpregnant athletes without urinary tract obstruction or impending instrumentation, treatment of asymptomatic bacteriuria is not recommended (1).

SPORT-SPECIFIC RISK FOR UTI

Bicyclists

Bicycle-related genitourinary problems such as traumatic urethritis and prostatitis may predispose an athlete to infection or obstruction (7). Female cyclists develop cystitis following long-distance rides, presumably from pressure on the urethra, leading to urethritis, incomplete bladder emptying, and subsequent infection (5). Antibiotics almost immediately relieve the symptoms of bacterial UTIs (3). However, yeast and fungal infections, triggered by increased moisture in the perineal area, cause symptoms similar to UTIs and may worsen with standard antibiotic treatment (8).

Athletes with Spinal Cord Injures

Persons with spinal cord injuries (SCI) have an increased risk of developing UTIs from ureteral reflux of bacteria colonizing the bladder and urethra. The method of bladder drainage greatly influences colonization, with indwelling catheters causing the highest prevalence (9). Diagnosis is complicated by the poor sensitivity and specificity of symptoms and signs. For this reason, objective evidence of UTI or the presence of fever or other signs of sepsis guides antibiotic treatment. Symptomatic UTIs warrant therapy; treatment of asymptomatic bacteriuria leads to antibiotic-resistant organisms (9). Likewise, antimicrobial prophylaxis has not proven beneficial (10).

Other Sports

Although no specific documentation of UTIs is recorded in other sports, certain sports logically would carry a higher risk. Prolonged events such as ultramarathons or triathlons are commonly associated with dehydration and urinary retention. In addition, horseback riding, motorcross, and gymnastics have the potential for perineal trauma.

TREATMENT

Management of UTIs in athletes is similar to that for the general population. Proper hydration, especially during prolonged events, and mechanical adjustments of equipment such as bicycle seats can aid in prevention.

Cystitis, pyelonephritis, epididymitis in males older than 35 years, and bacterial prostatitis all respond well to trimethoprim-sulfamethoxazole (TMP-SMX) or fluoroquinolones, although other agents can be efficacious.

Cystitis

Uncomplicated cystitis requires a 3-day course of appropriate antibiotics to eradicate *E. coli* from vaginal and perineal flora, thus decreasing recurrent infections. This will not eradicate asymptomatic upper tract infections, and early recurrences should be cultured and treated for a 7- to 10-day course. Recurrent cystitis proven by culture should be treated continuously with prophylaxis, postcoital prophylaxis, or patient-initiated therapy, whichever is most appropriate to the circumstances. Estrogen replacement therapy will benefit those patients found to be deficient in the hormone (1).

Pyelonephritis

Empiric therapy for pyelonephritis should last 10 to 14 days and be guided by initial Gram's stain findings, with Gram-negative organisms treated with TMP-SMX or quinolones and Gram-positive organisms treated with amoxicillin (6). Culture and sensitivity should be obtained to screen for unusual or resistant organisms. Complicated pyelonephritis requires hospitalization for parenteral antibiotics, as determined by cultures and sensitivities and imaging studies. Pregnant patients also should be hospitalized for treatment.

Epididymitis

Epididymitis requires a 10-day course of TMP-SMX or a fluoroquinolone in individuals older than 35 years, while those athletes under age 35 should be empirically treated with doxycycline or tetracycline for 10 to 14 days. Nonpharmacologic treatment consists of scrotal elevation, ice, bed rest, and sitz baths. Risk factors such as indwelling catheters, urethral instrumentation, and urethral stricture also need to be addressed (2). Pain relief may necessitate NSAID treatment or possibly even narcotic medicines.

Prostatitis

Bacterial prostatitis requires a prolonged treatment course for 6 to 12 weeks with double-strength TMP-SMX, fluoroquinolones, or doxycycline (11). Severe, acute cases can require hospitalization for parenteral antibiotics. If an enlarged prostate is palpable on rectal examination, further evaluation may lead to surgical intervention. Prostatitis and traumatic urethritis related to bicycling is treated with relative rest and mechanical adjustments. Prevention strategies include changing the angle of the seat, switching to a wider seat with more padding, and wearing padded cycling shorts (5,7).

RETURN TO PARTICIPATION

General rules appropriate for minor illnesses should be followed when discussing the athlete's return to sports following a urinary tract infection. Athletes should be afebrile for 24 to 48 hours prior to returning. Increased hydration is recommended, and long-duration, high-intensity events should be entered with caution and close follow-up.

CONCLUSION

Urinary tract infections are common, and therefore are likely to occur in athletes being cared for by sports medicine physicians. Occasionally, the infection or a mimicking inflammation is caused directly by a specific sports activity. Determining the cause will allow the physician to recommend alterations that can prevent recurrence. Often knowledge of diagnosis and treatment of common UTIs will enable the physician to institute therapy that permits the athlete to return to competition quickly.

REFERENCES

1 Stamm WE, Hooton TM. Management of urinary tract infections in adults. N Engl J Med 1993;329:1328–1334.

2 York JB. The male genitourinary system. In: Strauss RH, ed. Sports medicine. 2nd ed. Philadelphia: WB Saunders, 1991:515–528.

3 Hershfield NB. Pedaller's penis. Can Med Assoc J 1983;128:366–367.

4 O'Brien KP. Sports urology: the vicious cycle. N Engl J Med 1981;304:1367–1368.

5 Weiss BD. Clinical syndromes associated with bicycle seats. Clin Sports Med 1994;13:175–186.

6 Bergeron MG. Treatment of pyelonephritis in adults. Med Clin North Am 1995;79:619–649.

7 Mellion MB. Common cycling injuries; management and prevention. Sports Med 1991;11:52–70.

8 Dickson TB Jr. Preventing overuse cycling injuries. Physician Sports Med 1985;13:116–123.

9 Cardenas DD, Hooton TM. Urinary tract infection in persons with spinal cord injury. Arch Phys Med Rehabil 1995;76:272–280.

10 The prevention and management of urinary tract infections among people with spinal cord injuries: National Institute on Disability and Rehabilitation Research Consensus Statement: January 27–29, 1992. J Am Paraplegia Soc 1992;15:194–204.

11 Forland M. Urinary tract infection; how has its management changed? Postgrad Med 1993;93:71–85.

Chapter 8
Sexually Transmitted Diseases

Michael J. Woods
David O. Hough

Sexually transmitted diseases (STDs) are prevalent throughout the world. In the United States, more than 12 million cases are diagnosed yearly (1). Up to two-thirds of the cases of gonorrhea reported annually occur in men and women 25 years of age or younger (2), and drug-resistant strains have spread to most nations. U.S. data show 3 million teenagers infected with STDs every year, and the incidence of syphilis in women in this age group doubled from 1985 to 1991 (3). Coinfection with human immunodeficiency virus (HIV) must also be considered in STDs.

A recent study looking at sexual behavior in the United States (1) found that most American males have sexual intercourse by 16 to 17 years of age; most females do so by 17 to 18 years of age. The majority of young adults aged 18 to 24 years have multiple serial sexual partners. With regards to prevention of STDs, the estimated frequency of appropriate condom use with every sexual encounter among adolescents is approximately 10% to 20%. In addition, collegiate athletes have been shown to have significantly higher "risky" lifestyle behavior patterns when compared to nonathletes (4). These behaviors include less consistent use of contraception, more sexual partners, and increased frequency of STDs.

Many adolescents and young adults participate in athletics and seek their primary care through the sports medicine physician or team trainer. Athletes often feel more comfortable approaching the team physician with questions regarding STDs because of easy access in the training room or on the field. In addition, many athletes develop a rapport with the team physician from frequent interaction, and are more likely to confide in him or her (2). For these reasons, sports medicine physicians need to maintain skills in the diagnosis, treatment, and counseling related to STDs.

Both common and unusual presentations of STDs have been reported in sports activities. Meier published a case of acute periostitis caused by syphilis in a 37-year-old male jogger originally thought to have shin splints (5). Transmission of pubic lice and molluscum contagiosum have occurred between wrestlers (6). Crossover has been reported between herpes simplex virus types 1 and 2 (HSV-1 and HSV-2) in an athletic setting, in which HSV-1 occasionally causes herpes genitalis and HSV-2 occasionally causes herpes labialis (7). Herpes gladiatorum, a common problem of wrestlers, is caused by HSV-1; no outbreaks caused by HSV-2 have been reported (7). Athletes involved in contact sports with any of these conditions must be held from competition until they no longer pose a risk for transmission to other athletes.

STDs CHARACTERIZED BY GENITAL ULCERS

A common presenting complaint in an athlete infected with an STD is a painful or painless genital ulcer. The diseases included in this category are primarily genital herpes, syphilis, and chancroid. In developed nations, genital herpes is the most common of these (8). STDs with genital ulcers are a marker for increased risk of HIV because the ulcers allow for easier transmission of the virus. Genital ulcers with poor healing or an inadequate response to treatment increase the suspicion for HIV (9).

Genital Herpes Simplex Virus (HSV)
Genital herpes occurs in all populations and is typically caused by HSV-2 (10). A dramatic increase in

Table 8-1 Treatment of STDs Characterized by Genital Ulcers

Genital Herpes Simplex Virus

First clinical episode	Acyclovir, 200 mg PO 5× daily for 7 to 10 days or until clinical resolution
Recurrent episodes	Acyclovir, 200 mg PO 5× daily for 5 days *or* Acyclovir, 400 mg PO TID for 5 days *or* Acyclovir, 800 mg PO BID for 5 days
Daily suppressive therapy	Acyclovir, 400 mg PO BID
Alternative	Acyclovir, 200 mg PO 3–5× daily

Syphilis

• Primary and secondary	
Adults	Benzathine penicillin G, 2.4 million units IM in a single dose
Children	Benzathine penicillin G, 50,000 units/kg IM, up to 2.4 million units in a single dose
Nonpregnant, penicillin-allergic	Doxycycline, 100 mg PO BID for 2 weeks *or* Tetracycline, 500 mg PO QID for 2 weeks
• Early latent	
Adults, children	Same as for primary and secondary syphilis
Nonpregnant, penicillin allergic	Doxycycline, 100 mg PO BID for 2 weeks *or* Tetracycline, 500 mg PO QID for 2 weeks
• Late latent (or unknown duration)	
Adults	Benzathine penicillin G, 7.2 million units total, as 3 doses of 2.4 million units IM each, at 1 week intervals
Children	Benzathine penicillin G, 50,000 units/kg IM, up to 2.4 million units, for 3 total doses
Nonpregnant, penicillin allergic	Same as for early latent syphilis
• Late (tertiary) syphilis (no neurosyphilis)	Benzathine penicillin G, 7.2 million units total, as 3 doses of 2.4 million units IM at 1 week intervals
• Neurosyphilis	Aqueous crystalline penicillin G, 12–24 million units IV every 4 hours, for 10–14 days

Chancroid

General regimens	Azithromycin, 1 g PO in a single dose *or* Ceftriaxone, 250 mg IM in a single dose *or* Erythromycin base, 500 mg PO QID for 7 days
Alternative regimens	Amoxicillin, 500 mg plus clavulanic acid 125 mg PO TID for 7 days *or* Ciprofloxacin, 500 mg PO BID for 3 days

SOURCE: 1993 Sexually transmitted diseases treatment guidelines. Centers for Disease Control and Prevention. MMWR Morb Mortal Wkly Rep 1993 Sept 24;42(RR-14):1–102.

cases since the 1960s has led to an annual incidence of 200,000 to 500,000 cases per year in the United States. Serologic studies suggest that approximately 30 million persons in the United States have genital HSV infection (8,9; Plate 2).

The initial episode of genital herpes causes systemic symptoms including malaise, fever, headache, and myalgia in 40% of men and 70% of women (10). Painful lesions are reported in 95% of men and 99% of women. Associated symptoms include pain, itching, dysuria, vaginal or urethral discharge, and tender inguinal adenopathy. Internal dysuria and external dysuria (caused by urine passing over irritated tissues) occur more often in women than men. Urethral discharge and dysuria affect one-third of men with primary HSV-2 (10).

Diagnosis hinges on clinical presentation. The most commonly used confirmatory laboratory test is the Tzanck smear. In the presence of HSV, this slide test shows multinucleated giant cells and intranuclear inclusions. Viral isolation is the most sensitive and specific method for confirming the diagnosis (10).

The initial episode of genital herpes is treated with acyclovir, 200 mg orally five times a day for 7 to 10 days or until clinical resolution (Table 8-1). Acyclovir does not eradicate latent virus or affect the risk, severity, or frequency of recurrences. Recurrent episodes are treated with acyclovir, 200 mg orally five times a day for 5 days, or with alternative regimens listed in Table 8-1. Daily suppressive therapy may be considered for frequent recurrences (8). Sexual partners of patients with genital herpes should be counseled, evaluated, and treated if symptomatic. Topical acyclovir is available, but minimally effective.

Finally, relevant to the care of athletes is the fact that latent herpes virus in the dorsal root ganglia can be reactivated from the psychological and environmental stresses of competition (11). High altitude skiers, for example, have experienced recurrences in herpes infections that are presumed to be a result of ultraviolet radiation exposure (12,13). Prophylactic use of oral acyclovir, 400 mg orally twice daily (11), should be considered prior to competition or when the first warning signs of infection appear in an athlete at risk for recurrence.

Syphilis

Syphilis is a systemic disease caused by the spirochete *Treponema pallidum*. From 1985 to 1991, a syphilis epidemic occurred in the United States (14). Syphilis infection can be primary, secondary, tertiary, or latent. As with all diseases causing genital ulcers, syphilis denotes an increased risk of HIV, and serologic testing for HIV should be included in the workup.

The incubation period for syphilis infection is 9 to 90 days, with a mean of 21 days (15). The initial skin manifestation is a small macule at the site of entry, which breaks down to form an ulcer. The ulcer, called the primary chancre, is normally solitary and painless with a well-defined margin and an indurated base. In men, the chancre is typically found on the glans, shaft, or coronal sulcus of the penis. Chancres occur on the vulva, vaginal walls, or cervix in women. The anus and rectum are other common sites. Left untreated, the chancre resolves spontaneously in 3 to 6 weeks (15). Inflammation from the ulcer and the primary syphilis infection usually leads to enlarged bilateral nontender inguinal lymph nodes.

Secondary infection is marked by rash, mucocutaneous lesions, and adenopathy. Tertiary infection is manifested by cardiac, neurologic, ophthalmic, or gummatous lesions. Latent syphilis is defined by positive serologic testing in an asymptomatic person. Patients with latent syphilis known to have been infected within the preceding year have early latent syphilis, while others have late latent syphilis, or syphilis of unknown duration. Theoretically, tertiary syphilis and late latent syphilis require a longer course of treatment because the organisms divide more slowly (see Table 8-1; Plate 3).

Direct microscopic examination provides the definitive diagnosis for early syphilis. Dark field microscopy should be done first, using exudate from the suspected lesion. Additional microscopic examination can be done by direct fluorescent antibody testing for *T. pallidum* (DFA-TP).

Serologic testing is initially done with nontreponemal antibody tests, such as RPR (rapid plasma reagin) or VDRL (Venereal Disease Research Laboratory). These tests are 78% to 85% sensitive for identifying primary syphilis. A reactive RPR or VDRL test should be confirmed with a treponemal serologic test, either the fluorescent-Treponemal antibody absorption test (FTA-ABS) or the microhemagglutination assay for antibodies to *T. pallidum* (MHA-TP) (15).

Treponemal tests usually remain reactive for a lifetime, regardless of treatment; in nontreponemal tests, antibody titers usually correlate with disease activity. A fourfold change in titer in one direction represents successful treatment, while change in the other direction indicates reinfection or recurrence. Examination of the CSF and VDRL-CSF should be done on patients with suspected neurosyphilis.

Parenteral penicillin G remains the drug of choice for treatment of all stages of syphilis (see Table 8-1). Benzathine penicillin G, 2.4 million units IM in a single dose, effectively treats either primary or secondary syphilis. A lumbar puncture is not recommended for routine evaluation in those patients who do not have clinical symptoms and signs of neurosyphilis. Nonpregnant patients with a penicillin allergy should be treated with doxycycline, 100 mg orally twice daily for 2 weeks, or with tetracycline, 500 mg orally four times daily for 2 weeks. Pregnant women or patients with neurosyphilis who are allergic to penicillin should still be treated with penicillin, after desensitization if necessary (8). Sexual partners of infected persons should be evaluated and the Centers for Disease Control (CDC) treatment guidelines followed (8).

Chancroid

Chancroid, an ulcerative STD, most often involves the genitals and frequently causes development of an inguinal bubo. This infection, caused by the *Haemophilus ducreyi* bacterium, typically occurs in lower socioeconomic settings, among groups who frequent prostitutes. Men have a much higher incidence of infection than women, and uncircumcised men are even more susceptible (10). The disease occurs in endemic areas; for example, in the United States, 90% of the reported cases occur in 5 of the 50 states (15). Throughout the world, scattered outbreaks have occurred in large cities. Up to 10% of patients with chancroid may have coexisting HSV or *T. pallidum* infection, as well as a high rate of HIV disease (8).

The incubation period for chancroid ranges from 4 to 7 days. Clinically, multiple small inflammatory papules appear and transform into pustules within 24 to 48 hours. These pustules rupture to form sharply circumscribed painful ulcers. Men develop lesions on the foreskin, penile shaft, or coronal sulcus. The most common infection sites in women are the perineum and labia (15). Tender inguinal adenitis is present in over half of the cases, and is usually unilateral with overlying erythema (bubo). These buboes can become fluctuant and rupture spontaneously, forming inguinal ulcers (10).

Definitive diagnosis necessitates identification of *H. ducreyi* and exclusion of other causes of genital ulcers. Unfortunately, cultures for *H. ducreyi* have a sensitivity of only 60% to 80% (9,15). This makes confirmation of the diagnosis difficult.

Successful treatment resolves symptoms, cures the infection, and blocks transmission, but may not prevent scarring in severe cases. The recommended treatment is a single dose of either azithromycin, 1 g orally, or ceftriaxone, 250 mg IM, or erythromycin base, 500 mg orally four times daily for 7 days (see Table 8-1). Drug resistance has not occurred with these antimicrobials. Sexual partners of infected persons should be examined and treated if they have had recent sexual contact (within 10 days), even if asymptomatic (8).

STDs CHARACTERIZED BY URETHRITIS AND CERVICITIS

Athletes infected with STDs often have urethritis or cervicitis. Symptoms and signs include penile or vaginal discharge, dysuria, proctitis, or epididymitis. These infections, even when asymptomatic, cause numerous complications in women, including pelvic inflammatory disease (PID), salpingitis, infertility, ectopic pregnancy, and chronic pelvic pain. Transmission, other than from sexual contact, may occur, such as ophthalmia neonatorum in infants from delivery in a chlamydia-infected birth canal (16).

Nongonococcal Urethritis (NGU)

Nongonococcal urethritis represents inflammation of the urethra without evidence of gonococcal infection. Distinguishing characteristics of NGU are mucoid or purulent discharge from the urethra with five or more polymorphonuclear leukocytes (PMNs) per oil immersion field on an intraurethral swab smear (8). *Chlamydia trachomatis* causes 23% to 55% of cases, with 20% to 40% being caused by *Ureaplasma* and 2% to 5% by *Trichomonas vaginalis*. HSV and unknown agents cause the remainder of cases (8).

Recommended treatment is with doxycycline, 100 mg orally twice a day for 7 days (Table 8-2 provides erythromycin regimens). Sexual partners should be evaluated and treated if indicated (8). A screening urinalysis with a dipstick leukocyte esterase test has been advocated as part of the preparticipation physical exam. If positive, this should be followed by urethral swab to identify asymptomatic male athletes infected with chlamydia (17).

Mucopurulent Cervicitis (MPC)

Mucopurulent cervicitis, a cervical infection, typically presents with a yellow endocervical exudate, but may cause abnormal vaginal bleeding (e.g., after intercourse or a vaginal exam) or be totally asymptomatic. As with NGU, an MPC diagnosis can be made by finding an increased number of PMNs via Gram's stain. The most common infectious agents are *C. trachomatis* and *Neisseria gonorrhoeae*, but in the majority of cases no organism is identified (8). In high risk populations, where results may be delayed or the patient is unlikely to return, empiric treatment should be initiated for *C. trachomatis* and *N. gonorrhoeae*. This lessens the risk for PID or continued spread of the organisms to others (9). In lower risk patients and sexual partners of infected women, treatment should be based on test results.

Chlamydial Infections

In the United States, approximately 4 million infections occur annually from *C. trachomatis*, making it the most prevalent bacterial STD (9). These infections, which are common in sexually active adolescents and young adults, often cause mild or no symptoms. Therefore, unrecognized infection is highly prevalent (16), and routine screening should be done on high risk populations. As noted previously, untreated chlamydia may cause PID, infertility, and ectopic pregnancy (9).

When symptoms do occur in women, they include vaginal discharge and dysuria. Ascending infection can cause lower abdominal pain and abnormal menstruation. Symptoms in men include urethral discharge or dysuria, which are usually milder than gonorrhea. *C. trachomatis* is responsible for most cases of NGU and can cause epididymitis and Reiter's syndrome in men (16). Left untreated, women or men may transmit the infection to others.

Cultures should be obtained from the endocervix in women and the urethra in men using swabs with plastic or wire shafts, not wooden. An endocervical brush may be used in women. Nonculture chlamydia tests are also available as Chlamydiazyme EIA test (Abbott) and MicroTak DFA test (Syva). The sensitivity of nonculture tests is 97% to 99% in women and greater than 70% in men (16).

The CDC's recommended treatment regimens for chlamydial infections are doxycycline, 100 mg orally twice a day for 7 days, or azithromycin, 1 g orally in a single dose. Neither of these is recommended during pregnancy, when erythromycin should be substituted ([8] see Table 8-2). Although azithromycin is more expensive than doxycycline, compliance will obviously be much better with the single-dose regimen. Only an estimated 60% of patients complete the full week of therapy (9). Infected patients must have their sexual partners evaluated and treated.

Gonococcal Infections

Gonococcal infections are caused by *Neisseria gonorrhoeae*, a Gram-negative diplococcus. Demographic risk factors for infection in the United States include low socioeconomic class, urban residence, early onset of sexual activity, unmarried status, and a history of past gonorrhea infection (10). In the United States the overall prevalence of gonorrhea has declined steadily since the mid-1980s, even though an estimated 1 million new infections occur annually. An increasing number of strains of *N. gonorrhoeae* are penicillinase-producing and tetracycline-resistant. Coinfection with *C. trichomatis* is very common. For this reason, effective therapy varies from region to region, but persons being treated for gonorrhea should also be treated with a regimen that is effective against chlamydia (see Table 8-2). Other STDs, including HIV and syphilis, should be excluded by serologic testing.

Table 8-2   Treatment of STDs Characterized by Urethritis and Cervicitis

Nongonococcal Urethritis

Treatment	Doxycycline, 100 mg PO BID for 7 days
Alternatives	Erythromycin base, 500 mg PO QID for 7 days
	or
	Erythromycin base, 250 mg PO QID for 14 days
	or
	Erythromycin ethylsuccinate, 400 mg PO QID for 14 days

Chlamydial Infections

Treatments	Doxycycline, 100 mg PO BID for 7 days*
	or
	Azithromycin, 1 g PO in a single dose*
	Do not use during pregnancy.
Alternatives	Ofloxacin, 300 mg PO BID for 7 days
	or
	Erythromycin base, 500 mg PO QID for 7 days
	or
	Erythromycin ethylsuccinate, 800 mg PO QID for 7 days
	or
	Sulfisoxazole, 500 mg PO QID for 10 days
	(inferior efficacy)

Gonococcal Infections

Treatments	Ceftriaxone, 125 mg IM in a single dose
	or
	Cefixime, 400 mg PO in a single dose
	or
	Ciprofloxacin, 500 mg PO in a single dose
	or
	Ofloxacin, 400 mg PO in a single dose
	PLUS
	A regimen effective against *C. trachomatis* (see above)
Alternative	Spectinomycin, 2 g IM in a single dose

SOURCE: 1993 Sexually transmitted diseases treatment guidelines. Centers for Disease Control and Prevention. MMWR Morb Mortal Wkly Rep 1993 Sept 24;42(RR-14):1–102.

Uncomplicated gonococcal infections are common in women, but they can present with vaginal discharge, urethral syndrome, Fitz-Hugh and Curtis syndrome, or with disseminated disease such as arthritis-dermatitis syndrome. Men usually present as urethritis with purulent urethral exudate and dysuria. An untreated infection can progress to urethral stricture and epididymitis (9). Women may not be symptomatic until complications like PID occur. Whether PID is symptomatic or not, infertility or ectopic pregnancy can follow as a result of tubal scarring.

Diagnosis of *N. gonorrhoeae* infection in men with urethritis is by Gram's stain. In women and asymptomatic men, it is not as useful (10). Cultures are more sensitive and specific and should be done if there is any concern about an antibiotic-resistant gonococcal strain.

The CDC recommends ceftriaxone, 125 mg IM in a single dose, for treatment of uncomplicated gonococcal infections. Other recommended regimens are listed in Table 8-2. Again, a regimen should be added that is effective against *C. trachomatis*. Ceftriaxone may also abort incubating syphilis (8). Patients should be instructed to refer their sexual partner for evaluation and treatment. Standard guidelines, such as those published for 1993 by the CDC, contain further recommendations on treatment of complicated or disseminated infections (8).

DISEASES CHARACTERIZED BY VAGINAL DISCHARGE

Female athletes often develop vaginitis, and 90% of the infections are caused by trichomoniasis, bacterial vaginosis, or candidiasis (18). Symptoms include vaginal discharge, itching, irritation, or odor. Of these, only trichomoniasis is truly sexually transmitted. Bacterial vaginosis, however, occurs more commonly in women with multiple sexual partners; treatment of male sexual partners has not helped prevent recurrence (8). Vulvovaginal candidiasis is not usually sexually transmitted, but may coexist with other STDs.

Algorithms that rely on history, physical examination, and simple laboratory tests direct the workup and diagnosis of these conditions (18,19). Typically, trichomoniasis and bacterial vaginosis produce the largest amount of vaginal discharge and cause vaginal odor (19). Itching and external dysuria suggest trichomoniasis and candidiasis. Typical physical findings include vulvar erythema in trichomoniasis and candidiasis. The vaginal discharge in each differs: bacterial vaginosis causes a thin, homogeneous, and grayish-white drainage; candidiasis produces a curdy white or "cottage cheese–like" discharge; and trichomoniasis has a thin, yellow-green, and frothy appearing discharge.

Laboratory testing reveals a vaginal pH that is elevated (>4.5) for trichomoniasis and bacterial vaginosis and normal (4.5 or less) for candidiasis. Two slides, one with two drops of normal saline and the other with 10% KOH are prepared. In the presence of bacterial vaginosis, but less so in trichomoniasis, a pungent, fishy odor will be detected on the KOH slide (the "whiff" test). The KOH slide microscopically shows the pseudohyphae of Candida. Examination of the saline slide reveals the motile *T. vaginalis* organisms in trichomoniasis, or the bacteria-coated epithelial cells (clue cells) characteristic of bacterial vaginosis. Gram's stain may also be helpful because bacterial vaginosis is caused by overgrowth of *Gardnerella vaginalis* (small Gram-variable rods) and *Mobiluncus* species (small curved Gram-negative rods) crowding out the normal prevalent *Lactobacillus* species (large Gram-positive rods) (18).

Treatment   Symptomatic female athletes, but not sexual partners, with bacterial vaginosis should be treated with regimens effective against *G. vaginalis, Mycoplasma hominis,* and the anaerobic bacteria *Bacteroides* and *Mobiluncus* species. Treatment regimens include metronidazole, 500 mg orally twice a day for 7 days, or alternatively metronidazole, 2 g orally in a single dose. Side effects include gastrointenstinal distress and a metallic taste. Patients should avoid alcohol during treatment and for 24 hours after treatment, as they risk a disulfiram-like reaction. Pregnant women should not use metronidazole in the first trimester. Topical regimens include vinegar douches or clotrimazole, 100 mg daily for 7 days (18) (Table 8-3).

Identification of the protozoan *T. vaginalis* merits treatment in women and men even though the infection typically causes symptoms only in women. Treatment of male sexual partners and avoidance of sex until treatment is completed decreases recurrences. Recommended treatment is metronidazole, 2 g orally in a single dose or 500 mg twice a day for 7 days (8).

Candida albicans, and occasionally, other *Candida* species such as *Torulopsis* species, cause yeast infections. Topical preparations are most effective in treatment ([8] see Table 8-3). Self-medication with over-the-counter (OTC) preparations should be advised only if the patient has a recurrence of the same symptoms that a physician has previously diagnosed as candidiasis (8). Patients with persistent symptoms, treatment failures, or frequent recurrences should be reevaluated by their physician rather than continue OTC medications.

Table 8-3   Treatment of Diseases Characterized by Vaginal Discharge

Bacterial Vaginosis

Treatment	Metronidazole, 500 mg PO BID for 7 days[a,b]
Alternatives	Metronidazole, 2 g PO in a single dose[b]
	or
	Clindamycin cream, 2%, 1 applicator (5 g) intravaginally at bedtime for 7 days
	or
	Metronidazole gel, 0.75%, 1 applicator (5 g) intravaginally BID for 5 days[b]
	or
	Clindamycin, 300 mg PO BID for 7 days

Trichomoniasis

Treatment	Metronidazole, 2 g PO in a single dose[b]
Alternative	Metronidazole, 500 mg BID for 7 days[b]

Vulvovaginal Candidiasis[c]

Treatment	Butoconazole, 2% cream, 5 g intravaginally for 3 days
	or
	Clotrimazole, 1% cream, 5 g intravaginally for 7–14 days[d]
	or
	Clotrimazole, 100 mg vaginal tablet for 7 days[d]
	or
	Miconazole, 100 mg vaginal suppository, one daily for 7 days[d]
	or
	Terconazole, 80 mg suppository, one daily for 3 days

[a]Patients should avoid alcohol during treatment and for 24 hours afterward.
[b]Metronidazole should not be used in the first trimester of a pregnancy.
[c]See the 1993 CDC STD treatment guidelines for more alternatives.
[d]Over-the-counter (OTC) preparations.
SOURCE: 1993 Sexually transmitted diseases treatment guidelines. Centers for Disease Control and Prevention. MMWR Morb Mortal Wkly Rep 1993 Sept 24;42(RR-14):1–102.

OTHER AREAS OF CONCERN

Pelvic Inflammatory Disease (PID)

Pelvic inflammatory disease encompasses the spectrum of endometriosis, salpingitis, tubo-ovarian abscess, and/or pelvic peritonitis. Causative agents include gonococcus, chlamydia, anaerobic flora, and *G. vaginalis*. Difficultly in diagnosis because of variable signs and symptoms (8) should lead practitioners to have a low threshold for treating PID, because tubal scarring and subsequent infer-

tility may follow these infections. In the absence of another established cause for lower abdominal tenderness, adnexal tenderness, and cervical motion tenderness, empiric treatment for PID should be started.

Studies have demonstrated clinical efficacy, but not the effects of treatment on long-term complications (8). Recommended treatment for inpatient management of PID is cefoxitin, 2 g IV every 6 hours, *or* cefotetan, 2 g IV every 12 hours plus doxycycline, 100 mg IV or orally every 12 hours

Table 8-4 Treatment of Pelvic Inflammatory Disease (PID)

Inpatient Treatment

Regimen A	**=**	Cefoxitin, 2 g every 6 hours
	Or	Cefotetan, 2 g every 12 hours
	Plus	Doxycycline, 100 mg IV or PO every 12 hours
Regimen B	**=**	Clindamycin, 900 mg IV every 8 hours
	Plus	Gentamicin, loading dose IV or IM (2 mg/kg of body weight), followed by maintenance dose 1.5 mg/kg) every 8 hours

Outpatient Treatment

Regimen A	**=**	Cefoxitin, 2 g IM plus probenecid 1 g PO in a single dose concurrently
	Or	Ceftriaxone, 250 mg IM
	Or	Another third-generation cephalosporin, such as cefotaxime (Clatoran) or ceftizoxime (Cefizox)
	Plus	Doxycycline, 100 mg PO BID for 14 days
Regimen B	**=**	Ofloxacin, 400 mg PO BID for 14 days
	Plus	(either) Clindamycin, 450 mg PO 4× a day
	Or	Metronidazole, 500 mg PO 500 mg PO BID for 14 days

SOURCE: 1993 Sexually transmitted diseases treatment guidelines. Centers for Disease Control and Prevention. MMWR Morb Mortal Wkly Rep 1993 Sept 24;42(RR-14):1–102.

and continued at least 48 hours after the patient has shown significant improvement. After parenteral treatment, oral doxycycline, 100 mg twice a day, is continued for a total of 2 weeks (Table 8-4). Outpatient treatment is appropriate for less severe cases (8). Sexual partners should be evaluated and treated empirically.

Sexually Transmitted Epididymitis

Sexually transmitted epididymitis is usually associated with symptomatic or asymptomatic urethritis. In men less than 35 years of age, *N. gonorrhoeae* and *C. trachomatis* are the usual etiologic agents. Sexually transmitted *E. coli* infection can occur in homosexual males. Men older than 35 years of age, or those with a history of recent surgery, can get nonsexually transmitted epididymitis associated with Gram-negative urinary tract infections (8).

Presenting symptoms include unilateral testicular pain with palpable swelling of the epididymis. Testicular torsion must be considered in those with a sudden onset of severe pain, as it is a surgical emergency (8).

Workup includes Gram's stain of urethral discharge, culture for *N. gonorrhoeae,* testing for *C. trachomatis,* and a Gram's stain smear of uncentrifuged urine to look for Gram-negative bacteria. Recommended treatment is with ceftriaxone, 250 mg IM in a single dose, plus doxycycline, 100 mg orally twice a day for 10 days (contraindicated for patients less than 18 years of age). Alternatively, ofloxacin, 300 mg orally twice a day for 10 days, can be used (8). Bed rest and scrotal elevation are helpful. Recent sexual partners should be evaluated and treated. Patients and partners should avoid sex until treatment is completed and they are symptom-free.

Human Papilloma Virus (HPV)

Human papilloma virus infection is associated with exophytic warts of the genital and anal tissues. Some HPV types have been strongly associated with genital dysplasia and carcinoma (8). The use of condoms may help reduce the transmission of HPV.

The goals of treatment are removing the warts

and making symptoms more tolerable. No therapy has been shown to eradicate HPV (8). Recurrence rates are high with all forms of treatment (about 25% in 3 months). Treatment should be guided by the patient's preference after he or she is given the available treatment options. These options include cryotherapy with liquid nitrogen or cryoprobe; podofilox, 0.5% solution (genital warts only) applied twice daily for 3 days, followed by 4 days of no therapy—this cycle may be repeated four times (contraindicated in pregnancy); podophyllin, 10% to 25% in compound tincture of benzoin; trichloroacetic acid, 80% to 90%; and electrodesiccation or electrocautery. The CDC guidelines contain further details on treatment methods (8).

For information about hepatitis B virus, pediculosis pubis, and scabies, all of which may be sexually transmitted, see the relevant chapters.

CONCLUSION

Counseling

Treatment of sexually transmitted diseases is part of the total care of the athlete. A recent study of 350 senior medical students (20) showed that over half felt inadequately trained to take an accurate sexual history, and one-fourth were too embarrassed. Perhaps due to the lack of these skills, only 11% to 37% of primary care physicians routinely take a sexual history from their new patients (12), even though taking a sexual history is very important, as is counseling for reducing risky behaviors.

In light of what we know about high-risk sexual behaviors in adolescents and young adults, including our athletes, sports medicine physicians have an important counseling role in prevention of STDs and the spread of HIV disease. Since risk of HIV transmission through sports is negligible, a physician's educational efforts should focus on reducing risks from sexual activity (21). To be effective, open-ended questions regarding sexual orientation and behavior are best (1,9). For example, rather than asking a male or female athlete if they are homosexual, it may be more helpful and appropriate to ask, "Are you sexually active with women, men, or both?" Answers to such questions

will help in diagnosing and treating all STDs effectively.

The athlete's confidentiality must be respected, including not disclosing their infected status to other participants or athletic staff (22). Appropriate public heath reporting of STDs should be done discreetly and be followed to conclusion by sports medicine physicians.

REFERENCES

1 Seidman SN, Rieder RO. A review of sexual behavior in the United States. Am J Psychiatry 1994;151:330–341.
2 Nelson WE, McCue FC, Friz RL, et al. Management of sexually transmitted diseases in athletes. Athletic Training 1993;Summer:126–129.
3 Kay LE. Adolescent sexual intercourse. Strategies for promoting abstinence in teens. Postgrad Med 1995;97:121–127,132–134.
4 Nattiv A, Puffer JC. Lifestyles and health risks of collegiate athletes. J Fam Pract 1991;33:585–590.
5 Meier JL, Mollet E. Acute periostitis in early acquired syphilis simulating shin splints in a jogger. Am J Sports Med 1986;14:327–328.
6 Harvy J, Magsamen B, Strauss RH. Medical problems of wrestlers. Physician Sports Med 1987;15:136–138,140–142,146,148.
7 Nelson MA. Stopping the spread of herpes simplex: a focus on wrestlers. Physician Sports Med 1992;20:116–118,123–124,127.
8 1993 sexually transmitted diseases treatment guidelines. Centers for Disease Control and Prevention. MMWR Morb Mortal Wkly Rep 1993 Sep 24;42(RR-14):1–102.
9 Hook EW III, Sondheimer S, Zenilman J. Today's treatment for STDs. Patient Care 1995;29:40–56.
10 Holmes KK, Mårdh P-A, Sparling PF, Wiesner PJ, eds. Sexually transmitted diseases. 2nd ed. New York: McGraw-Hill, 1990:149–155,263–266,392–394,403.
11 Scheinberg RS. Stopping skin assailants: fungi, yeasts, and viruses. Physician Sports Med 1994;22:33–36,38–39.
12 Spruance SL, Hamill ML, Hoge WS, et al. Acyclovir prevents reactivation of herpes simplex labialis in skiers. JAMA 1988;260:1597–1599.
13 Mills J, Hauer L, Gottlieb A, et al. Recurrent herpes labialis in skiers. Clinical observations and effect of sunscreen. Am J Sports Med 1987;15:76–78.
14 Special focus: surveillance for sexually transmit-

ted disease. Centers for Disease Control and Prevention. MMWR CDC Surveill Summ 1993 Aug 13;42(SS-3):1–39.

15 Hoffman IF, Schmitz JL. Genital ulcer disease: management in the HIV era. Postgrad Med 1995;98:67–70,73–74,76,79–80,82.

16 Recommendations for the prevention and management of *Chlamydia trachomatis* infections, 1993. Centers for Disease Control and Prevention. MMWR Morb Mortal Wkly Rep 1993 Aug 6;42(RR-12):1–39.

17 Khosla RK. Detecting sexually transmitted disease: a new role for urinalysis in the preparticipation physical exam? Physician Sports Med 1995;23:77–78,80.

18 Deutchman ME, Leaman DJ, Thomason JL. Vag-

initis: diagnosis is the key. Patient Care 1994;28:39–44,48–50,52–54,57,61.

19 Fox KK, Behets FM-T. Vaginal discharge: how to pinpoint the cause. Postgrad Med 1995;98:87–88,90,93–94,96,101,104.

20 Merrill JM, Laux LF, Thornby JI. Why doctors have difficulty with sex histories. South Med J 1990;83:613–617.

21 Goodman RA, Thacker SB, Solomon SL, et al. Infectious diseases in competitive sports. JAMA 1994;271:862–867.

22 American Academy of Pediatrics Committee on Sports Medicine and Fitness: Human immunodeficiency virus [acquired immunodeficiency syndrome (AIDS) virus] in the athletic setting. Pediatrics 1991;88:640–641.

Chapter 9
Rocky Mountain Spotted Fever and Lyme Disease

John F. Campbell

Rocky Mountain spotted fever and Lyme disease are two important tick-borne infections that have been seen with increasing frequency in recent decades. Potential reasons for this increase include increased human contact with infected ticks and better surveillance for these diseases. Athletes, particularly those who live, train, or compete in tick-infested areas, may have an increased risk for these infections.

ROCKY MOUNTAIN SPOTTED FEVER (RMSF) AND OTHER SPOTTED FEVERS

Epidemiology

The spotted fevers comprise a large group of vector-borne rickettsial infections with a worldwide distribution. Rocky Mountain spotted fever (RMSF), caused by the *Rickettsia rickettsii* organism, is confined to the western hemisphere; however, spotted fevers caused by other rickettsial species are recognized on all inhabited continents (Table 9-1). Except for rickettsialpox, these spotted fevers are transmitted to humans by ticks. Transmission usually occurs during the spring and summer months when tick activity is greatest.

RMSF is diagnosed more frequently in children and in adults whose housing or occupations lead to frequent tick exposure (1,2). Wide geographic variations and changes in RMSF rates over time have been noted. When RMSF was first described over a century ago, its range was confined to the western United States. The disease is now most common in the southeastern United States. The mean annual incidence of RMSF was 14.59/100,000 persons in a study in North Carolina (1). The epidemiology of other spotted fevers is less well understood. Recent reports of newly recognized rickettsial species causing overlapping spotted fever syndromes have contributed to our understanding of this global problem (3–5).

Presentation

The pathogenesis of the spotted fevers is systemic vasculitis induced by direct endothelial damage to small arteries, capillaries, and veins (6). RMSF is characterized by the classic triad of fever, headache, and petechial rash that begins on the extremities and spreads centrally (Plate 4). The rash usually appears 3 to 5 days after onset of fever. Therefore, during spring and summer months in endemic areas, physicians should consider RMSF in patients with high fever and headache. Other spotted fevers can manifest with eschars at the site of the tick bite, with or without a generalized rash (see Table 9-1). When rash does occur it can be petechial, like that seen in RMSF, but maculopapular and vesicular rashes have been described (2).

Clinical and epidemiologic clues remain the best diagnostic tools for RMSF and other spotted fevers. Serologic tests lack sensitivity early in illness when therapeutic decisions must be made. The specificity of these tests has also been questioned (2). False-positive serologic tests may result from remote exposure to rickettsial antigens unrelated to the acute illness or from cross reactivity with other, undefined antigens. Reliance on serologic testing can lead to overdiagnosis of RMSF. Direct staining of skin biopsy specimens can provide a rapid and accurate diagnosis of RMSF and some other spotted fevers, but this method of detection is not practiced widely. Culture and polymerase chain reaction testing for rickettsiae are largely confined to research laboratories.

Table 9-1 Synopsis of Epidemiologic and Clinical Features of Spotted Fever Group Rickettsioses

Disease	Organism	Geographic Area	Vector	Rash Distribution	Eschar
RMSF	*R. rickettsii*	Western Hemisphere	Tick	Extremities to trunk	No
Boutonneuse	*R. coronii*	Africa, Mediterranean, India	Tick	Trunk, extremities, face	Yes
Queensland Tick Typhus	*R. australis*	Australia	Tick	Trunk, extremities, face	Yes
North Asian Tick Typhus	*R. sibirica*	Siberia, Mongolia	Tick	Trunk, extremities, face	Yes
Rickettsialpox	*R. akari*	USA, USSR, Korea, Africa	Mite	Trunk, extremities, face	Yes

SOURCE: Adapted with permission from Mandell GL, Bennett JE, Dolin R. Principles and practice of infectious diseases. London: Churchill Livingstone, 1995.

Treatment

Early, empiric antibiotic therapy for the spotted fevers should be started on the basis of clinical suspicion. Doxycyline, 100 mg twice daily, or another tetracycline given for 5 to 7 days, is the preferred regimen. Chloramphenicol, 500 mg four times a day, is also effective and is used in young children and pregnant women to avoid the adverse effects of tetracyclines on bones and teeth. Ciprofloxacin has proved effective for treating Mediterranean spotted fever (7).

Prevention

Widespread efforts to eradicate tick vectors are impractical, and there are no vaccines currently available for RMSF or other spotted fevers. Thus, efforts to prevent spotted fevers and other tick-borne diseases should include patient education on ways to avoid tick exposure. Tick bites in high-risk areas can be reduced by wearing protective clothing, using DEET-containing insecticides (N,N-diethylmetatolumide), and checking frequently for ticks.

Individuals who discover an attached tick should be instructed in the proper method of tick removal. The tick's mouth parts should be grasped with tweezers at the skin surface. Gentle but steady traction should be applied to remove the intact tick, with care taken not to crush the tick. The bite site should be thoroughly cleansed.

Special Considerations in the Athlete

There is no recognized association between participation in athletics and the acquisition of any spot-

ted fever group rickettsioses. RMSF is more common in persons whose environment or occupation bring them into frequent contact with ticks (1,2). Extrapolating from these observations, RMSF and other spotted fevers pose a greater potential risk for athletes such as hikers and backpackers during spring and summer months.

Treatment Strategies Treatment of the athlete with spotted fever should be no different than with the routine patient. An early diagnosis based on clinical suspicion remains the key to successful therapy. Patients presenting with fever and rash are likely to be too ill to participate in athletics, but early treatment with appropriate antibiotics will be sufficient to cure the overwhelming majority. Convalescence is quite variable, but many athletes should be able to return to training within 2 to 3 weeks.

LYME DISEASE

Epidemiology

Since the original report in 1977 of a cluster of children with acute arthritis, Lyme disease has been recognized worldwide (8,9). Humans acquire the disease through the bite of ixodid ticks infected with spirochetes in the *Borrelia burgdorferi* complex. Disease transmission is most common in the spring and summer months when these ticks are most active. Transmission occurs most often with nymphal stage ticks. These ticks are generally no larger than the period at the end of this sentence, making recognition by the human host more difficult (10).

Lyme disease is now the most commonly reported vector-borne disease in the United States (11). Within the United States, the disease is endemic in the Northeast, upper Midwest, and parts of California and Oregon. Surveillance data suggest the disease is spreading. Focal epidemics have been reported with attack rates up to 35% in longitudinal studies of affected communities (12). Lyme borreliosis has also been reported from Europe (9,13), Asia (14,15), the former Soviet Union (16), and Australia (17).

Lyme disease is a multisystem illness caused by widespread dissemination of *B. burgdorferi* after the bite of an infected tick. Spirochetes may invade and remain latent in multiple organ sites, particularly skin, joints, and the central nervous system. Data on pathogenesis are still emerging, but it appears that tissue infiltration with lymphocytes and plasma cells and perivascular inflammation cause the clinical manifestations of Lyme disease (18).

Presentation

Lyme disease, like other spirochetal infections, occurs in stages. While the overall clinical course of untreated Lyme disease is one of relapsing, multisystem illness, great variability is seen in individual patients. Infection can be asymptomatic or limited to transient involvement of only one organ system. Symptomatic early infection (stage 1) consists of the characteristic rash, erythema chronicum migrans (ECM). The rash begins as a small macule or papule at the site of the tick bite. The lesion expands with an erythematous border and partial central clearing. Occasionally, several distinct red rings emerge, and annular satellite lesions are common (Plate 5). The erythematous border may be warm to the touch, but lesions are generally flat and painless. Malaise, fever, headache, and myalgias can also occur during stage 1.

Disseminated infection (stage 2) occurs days to weeks into illness. Patients may have migratory myalgias and arthralgias, occasionally associated with joint swelling and inflammation. Neurologic manifestations ranging from severe headache to meningoencephalitis, cranial, and peripheral neuropathies can occur during stage 2. A small percentage of untreated patients have transient cardiac conduction abnormalities.

Late manifestations of Lyme disease (stage 3) can occur after months or years of latency. Relapsing arthritis, particularly of the knees and other large joints, occurs in up to 60% of untreated individuals, but the frequency of attacks decreases with time (19). Chronic persistent arthritis develops in only a small percentage of patients. Data are emerging that suggest individuals with chronic Lyme arthritis may have a genetic predisposition to treatment-resistant disease (20).

Late neurologic complications of Lyme disease include subacute encephalopathy and sensory neuropathy. Other chronic disorders, such as chronic fatigue syndrome and fibromyalgia, have been associated with Lyme disease. Steere (21) has emphasized the differences of Lyme disease from these other disorders and points out that Lyme disease is now an overdiagnosed illness (21).

Testing

The best diagnostic test for Lyme disease remains observation of typical clinical characteristics in a person who has lived in, or traveled to, an endemic area. Serologic testing for Lyme disease is now widely available but has many pitfalls. Serologic tests are relatively insensitive for stage 1 disease, so early diagnosis depends on the recognition of the characteristic ECM rash. Serologic testing holds more potential for the diagnosis of stages 2 and 3 of the disease, but currently available tests are poorly standardized and numerous examples of false-positive and false-negative test results have been published (22,23). As a result, these tests may provide more confusion than clarity.

Serial testing with enzyme-linked imunoassays and Western blotting techniques can result in more accurate serologic results (19). Histologic observation of spirochetes in tissue, culture, and polymerase chain reaction looking for *B. burgdorferi* DNA have a role in diagnosis, but are not yet feasible for routine use.

Treatment

Successful treatment of Lyme disease can generally be accomplished with oral doxycycline, 100 mg two times a day (19). Amoxicillin is an alternative, particularly for pregnant women and children, and cefuroxime can be used in patients with penicillin allergy. Stage 1 disease can usually be treated with 10 days of therapy, but 3 to 4 weeks of treatment is generally given for later stages. Parenteral ceftriaxone is preferred for neurologic syndromes and some cases of heart block. Although some patients, particularly those with chronic arthritis, will relapse after therapy, most recommended regimens are curative. Persistence or relapse of illness after appropriate treatment should always raise suspicion for misdiagnosis.

Prophylactic antibiotic therapy for asymptomatic individuals with tick bites has raised much anxiety and controversy. A recent decision analysis concluded that antibiotic therapy would be cost effective if the risk of infection after tick bite was 3.6% or greater (24). However, another study conducted in the highly endemic community of Lyme, Connecticut showed the risk of Lyme disease after tick bite was only 1.2% in untreated individuals (25). Prophylactic therapy may be considered in individuals residing in endemic areas who remove an engorged tick or those with questionable follow-up (19).

Natural infection with *B. burgdorferi* appears to result in life-long immunity to reinfection in most people. Animal studies of vaccine-induced immunity have been successful. The current state of human vaccine trials has recently been reviewed (26).

Special Considerations in the Athlete

As with the spotted fevers, there are no clear data showing athletes to have a lesser or greater risk for developing Lyme disease. The major risk factor is exposure to the appropriate tick vector: one serosurvey in Sweden showed orienteers to have a high prevalence of Lyme antibodies (27). Athletes with extensive outdoor exposure during spring and summer in endemic areas should be aware of the risk of Lyme disease. Athletes with exposure to the grassy or wooded areas favorable to tick exposure should be educated about the preventive strategies noted earlier.

The diagnosis of Lyme disease should not pose special diagnostic dilemmas in most athletes. However, confusion may arise when athletes develop chronic Lyme arthritis, which mimics a sports-related injury. Careful questioning about tick exposure in endemic areas, signs and symptoms of

stage 1 or 2 disease, and possibly serologic testing should help with these difficult cases.

Treatment Strategies   There are no treatment requirements unique to athletes with Lyme disease. Early, appropriate antibiotic therapy is effective in eradicating infection and preventing late complications. As noted earlier, patients with persistent illness after therapy should be reevaluated to determine if the diagnosis was correct. The convalescent period varies widely, and return to training and participation in athletics should be individualized with each patient, depending on the extent of infirmity.

REFERENCES

1   Wilfert CM, MacCormack JN, Kleeman K, et al. Epidemiology of Rocky Mountain spotted fever as determined by active surveillance. J Infect Dis 1984;150:469–479.
2   Walker DH, Didier R. *Rickettsia rickettsii* and other spotted fever group rickettsioses (Rocky Mountain spotted fever and other spotted fevers). In: Mandell GL, Bennett JE, Dolin R, eds. Principles and practice of infectious diseases. 4th ed. London: Churchill Livingstone, 1995:1721–1727.
3   Fan MY, Walker DH, Yu SR, Liu QH. Epidemiology and ecology of rickettsial diseases in the People's Republic of China. Rev Infect Dis 1987;9:823–840.
4   Sexton DJ, Dwyer B, Kemp R, Graves S. Spotted fever group rickettsial infections in Australia. Rev Infect Dis 1990;13:876–886.
5   Kelly P, Matthewman L, Beati L, et al. African tick-bite fever: a new spotted fever group rickettsiosis under an old name [letter]. Lancet 1992;340: 982–983.
6   Saah AJ. Introduction to section E rickettsioses. In: Mandell GL, Bennett JE, Dolin R, eds. Principles and practice of infectious diseases. 4th ed. London: Churchill Livingstone, 1995:1719–1720.
7   Raoult D, Gallais H, De Micco C, et al. Ciprofloxacin therapy in Mediterranean spotted fever. Antimicrob Agents Chemother 1986;30:606–607.
8   Steere AC, Malawista SE, Snydman DR, et al. Lyme arthritis: an epidemic of oligoarticular arthritis in children and adults in three Connecticut communities. Arthritis Rheum 1977;20:7–17.
9   Schmid GP. The global distribution of Lyme disease. Rev Infect Dis 1985;7:41–50.
10   Roueche B. The foulest and nastiest creatures that be. New Yorker 1988 Sept 12:83–89.

11 Lyme Disease—United States, 1991–1992. MMWR Morbid Mortal Wkly Rep 1993 May 14;42:345–348.

12 Lastavica CC, Wilson ML, Berardi VP, et al. Rapid emergence of a focal epidemic of Lyme disease in coastal Massachusetts. N Engl J Med 1989;320: 133–137.

13 Gustafson R, Svenungsson B, Forsgren M, et al. Two-year survey of the incidence of Lyme borreliosis and tick-borne encephalitis in a high-risk population in Sweden. Eur J Clin Microbiol Infect Dis 1992;11:894–900.

14 Kawabata M, Baba S, Iguchi K, Yamaguti N, Russell H. Lyme disease in Japan and its possible incriminated tick vector, *Ixodes persulcatus* [letter]. J Infect Dis 1987;156:854.

15 Ai CX, Hu RJ, Hyland KE, et al. Epidemiological and aetiological evidence for transmission of Lyme disease by adult *Ixodes persulcatus* in an endemic area in China. Int J Epidemiol 1990;19: 1061–1065.

16 Dekonenko EJ, Steere AC, Berardi VP, Kravchuk LN. Lyme borreliosis in the Soviet Union: a cooperative US—USSR report. J Infect Dis 1988;158: 748–753.

17 Stewart A, Glass J, Patel A, et al. Lyme arthritis in the Hunter Valley. Med J Aust 1982;1:139.

18 Duray PH, Steere AC. Clinical pathologic correlations of Lyme disease by stage. Ann NY Acad Sci 1988;539:65–79.

19 Steere AC. *Borrelia burgdorferi* (Lyme disease, Lyme borreliosis). In: Mandell GL, Bennett JE, Dolin R, eds. Principles and practice of infectious diseases. 4th ed. London: Churchill Livingstone, 1995:2143–2155.

20 Kalish RA, Leong JM, Steere AC. Association of treatment-resistant chronic Lyme arthritis with HLA-DR4 and antibody reactivity to OspA and OspB of *Borrelia burgdorferi*. Infect Immun 1993;61:2774–2779.

21 Steere AC. Current understanding of Lyme disease. Hosp Pract (Off Ed) 1993;28:37–44.

22 Schwartz BS, Goldstein MD, Ribeiro JM, et al. Antibody testing in Lyme disease. A comparison of results in four laboratories. JAMA 1989;262:3431–3434.

23 Corpuz M, Hilton E, Lardis MP, et al. Problems in the use of serologic tests for the diagnosis of Lyme disease. Arch Intern Med 1991;151:1837–1840.

24 Magid D, Schwartz B, Craft J, Schwartz JS. Prevention of Lyme disease after tick bites. A cost-effectiveness analysis. N Engl J Med 1992;327:534–541.

25 Shapiro ED, Gerber MA, Holabird NB, et al. A controlled trial of antimicrobial prophylaxis for Lyme disease after deer-tick bites. N Engl J Med 1992;327:1769–1773.

26 Wormser GP. A vaccine against Lyme disease? Ann Intern Med 1995;123:627–629.

27 Fahrer H, van der Linden SM, Sauvain M-J, et al. The prevalance and incidence of clinical and asymptomatic Lyme borreliosis in a population at risk. J Infect Dis 1991;163:305–310.

Chapter 10
Pericarditis and Myocarditis

James S. Kramer

Chest pain is common in athletes of all ages. In the United States this symptom alone accounts for approximately 650,000 physician visits annually for patients between 10 and 21 years of age (1). The etiologies are myriad. Cardiovascular causes of chest pain are uncommon in the pediatric population but are potentially dangerous. Most often seen in this category are dysrhythmia and pericarditis (2,3). In the adult population, myopericarditis, although uncommon, is responsible for sudden death in exercising individuals (4,5) or may lead to chronic, dilated cardiomyopathy. Not infrequently, myocarditis and pericarditis occur together; hence the term myopericarditis. For the purposes of this chapter, each topic is discussed separately.

PERICARDITIS

The spectrum of pericardial disease can be divided into three pathologic conditions: pericarditis, or inflammation of the pericardial surface; pericardial effusion, an accumulation of fluid between the pericardial membranes; and tamponade, a life-threatening rampant accumulation of fluid in the pericardial space. In the United States, the most common cause of infectious pericarditis is viral (e.g., coxsackie B5, B6), although mycoplasma, bacteria, mycobacteria, and fungal organisms are sometimes implicated (6). Other generalized conditions such as connective tissue disorders, renal failure, and hypothyroidism are etiologies of pericarditis.

The symptoms of pericarditis depend on the cause. Viral pericarditis typically presents with anterior chest pain, malaise, fever, and myalgia. The pain is often worse with breathing or belching and may radiate to the shoulder. Usually pain is positional so that the patient feels worse when lying down and relieved by sitting up and leaning forward.

The most important, and often the only sign of pericarditis, is a pericardial friction rub. While this rub is pathognomonic, it may be intermittent, variable, or even absent. When no physical findings are apparent, ECG signs may be the only evidence of pericardial involvement. A common finding is ST elevation. Initially ECG changes consist of ST-T segment elevation in leads I, II, aVL, aVF, and V_2 through V_6 with preservation of the upper concavity, in contrast to the acute injury of myocardial infarction (MI) in which the ST segment has upward convexity. Additionally, reciprocal ST depression as seen in MI is absent in pericarditis. Return of the ST segment to baseline in a few days is followed by symmetric T wave inversion, which may persist indefinitely (7). Thus, ECG changes and clinical features are critical, as acute viral pericarditis must be distinguished from acute myocardial infarction (Fig 10-1).

The physical signs of pericardial effusion depend on the amount of fluid buildup. Without tamponade, vital signs are often normal, but the patient often appears anxious and dyspneic. Heart sounds are distant. ECG evidence may reveal electrical alternans and overall low voltage. Classically, a globular heart on x-rays is diagnostic of pericardial effusion. Echocardiography is confirmatory in the diagnosis.

Cardiac tamponade is the most important complication of pericardial effusion and can occur with surprising speed. This life-threatening development warrants emergent treatment since

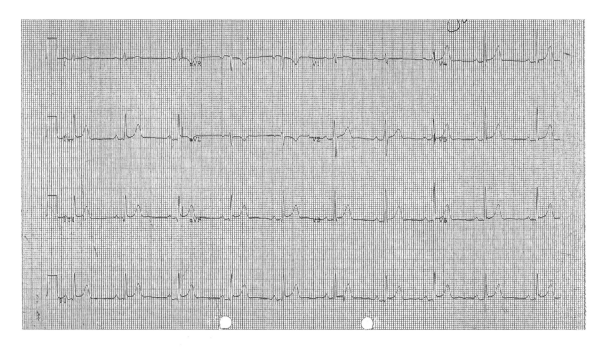

Figure 10-1. A 33-year-old female cyclist complained of shortness of breath and chest pain while riding. Evaluation revealed lupus erythematosus. ECG revealed pericarditis with diffuse elevation of ST segments.

cardiac compression leads to hypotension and shock.

Recommendations

Athletes with pericarditis, regardless of etiology, should not participate in competitive sports. Full activity may be resumed when there is no evidence of active disease by history, physical examination, appropriate diagnostic studies, exercise testing, and ambulatory and 12-lead ECG. Athletes with chronic pericardial disease that results in constriction should not participate in competitive sports (8).

MYOCARDITIS

Myocarditis, an inflammatory process involving the myocardial wall, can be precipitated by a variety of agents. Infectious etiologies include bacterial, viral, rickettsial, mycotic, or parasitic organisms. Most acute myocarditis is viral, with coxsackievirus B the most common culprit of both pericarditis and myocarditis (9). In the United

States, viral myocarditis is the most common form of inflammatory heart disease. Numerous other viruses have been implicated worldwide, including coxsackievirus A, echovirus, influenza, and human immunodeficiency virus (HIV). Less common viral agents identified are adenovirus, arbovirus, Epstein-Barr virus, herpes simplex virus 1, human cytomegalovirus, measles, rubella, respiratory syncytial virus, and varicella-zoster (10).

The pathophysiology remains obscure, but the timing of the onset of clinical changes strongly suggests activation of an autoimmune mechanism (11). Coxsackievirus infections usually occur in epidemics, particularly in the summer and early fall. Systemic signs and symptoms at the time of infection are typically mild and nonspecific, but can include fever, headache, myalgia, respiratory and gastrointestinal distress, exanthem, lymphadenopathy, splenomegaly, meningitis, and hepatitis.

No clear historical or physical findings confirm the early diagnosis of myocardial involvement. Recent myalgia is an important historical clue (12). Signs and symptoms, if any, relate to the severity of

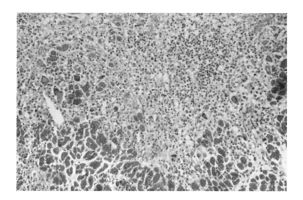

Figure 10-2. Infiltration of the myocardium with lymphocytes in viral myocarditis. (Courtesy of Gower Medical Publishing Ltd.)

myocardial necrosis and inflammation (Fig 10-2). The typical clinical picture consists of chest pain, fatigue, dyspnea, and palpitations (11). Congestive heart failure may develop in the presence of left ventricular dilatation and left ventricular dysfunction. Serious arrhythmias and heart block can also occur.

A key clinical feature of myocarditis is that the more outward clinical manifestations of myocarditis rarely occur at the height of the infectious illness, but rather become evident during convalescence as the systemic infectious symptoms subside. Acute viral myocarditis should be suspected in anyone with a recent viral syndrome who develops signs and symptoms of left ventricular dysfunction (13). However, athletes may not offer a classic history, as not all patients with viral myocarditis recall having a viral illness.

Certain diagnostic studies help confirm viral myocarditis, including leukocytosis and an elevated erythrocyte sedimentation rate or C-reactive protein (CRP). Elevation of serum cardiac enzymes varies with the extent of myocardial necrosis. Measurement of acute and convalescent antibody titers may identify a particular etiologic agent. The ECG, in contrast to that of pericarditis, is nonspecific and may show ST-T wave changes or an injury pattern. An echocardiogram is extremely useful in demonstrating diminished cardiac function.

Endomyocardial biopsy remains controversial (14,15), but does help delineate prognosis. Biopsy-proven viral myocarditis spontaneously improves, whereas this rarely happens with idiopathic dilated cardiomyopathy. The procedure, in experienced hands, has a complication rate of between 1% and 3% (16,17). Difficulties arise in the evaluation of biopsy material, such that even experienced pathologists using strict histologic criteria have found labeling viral myocarditis vexing. To help eliminate some of the confusion, cardiac pathologists have developed a standardized classification system now known as the "Dallas Criteria." These criteria judge the initial biopsy by the degree of myocarditis present, and correlate subsequent biopsies with the continuation or resolution of these pathologic changes (10). Even with established criteria, another problem with endomyocardial biopsy is that approximately 90% of patients with clinically suspected myocarditis have no histologic evidence of any myocarditis on biopsy (18).

As noted in the Dallas Criteria, the inflammation of myocarditis evolves through active, healing, and healed phases. Unfortunately, no studies relate the pathologic stage with the risk of sudden death. All stages may constitute a pathologic substrate for cardiac arrhythmias (19). For this reason, cardiac biopsy alone cannot guide the return to activity of the athlete.

Recommendations

The 26th Bethesda Conference (8) offers the following recommendations for the athlete with myocarditis in regard to return to activity:

1   The athlete should be withdrawn from all competitive sports and undergo a prudent convalescent period of about 6 months after the onset of clinical manifestations. Before the athlete may return to competitive athletic training, an evaluation of cardiac status should be undertaken, including assessment of ventricular function at rest and with exercise.

2   An athlete should be allowed to return to competition when ventricular function and also cardiac dimensions have returned to normal, and clinically relevant arrhythmias are absent on ambulatory monitoring.

3   Sufficient clinical data are not available to justify a strong recommendation to perform endo-

myocardial biopsy as a precondition for return to athletic competition after the proposed 6-month period of deconditioning. The role of invasive electrophysiologic testing in accessing the eligibility of athletes with myocarditis remains to be defined (8).

DISCUSSION

Since a viral etiology is most commonly associated with infectious myopericarditis, how does the physician advise an ill athlete with a systemic viral infection? When is rest mandatory? Is it unsafe to exercise with concerns of viral mediated cardiotoxicity?

Animal data suggest that exercise during experimentally induced septicemic viral infections may increase the risk of acute myocarditis and late cardiomyopathy. A study using mice infected with coxsackievirus B3 showed that treadmill running increased the severity of myocarditis, although not mortality (20). Similarly, another study demonstrated that swimming produced myocarditis in adult mice infected with less virulent coxsackievirus A9 (21). In a comparable study, weanling mice vigorously swam in warm water while they were acutely infected with coxsackievirus B3, and they developed a myocardial inflammation, dilatation, and necrosis. Viral titers were 500 times higher in the exercise group compared with sedentary controls. Lastly, the swimming mice were shown to have an increased risk of dilated cardiomyopathy (22).

No such studies have been performed in humans, and the degree to which animal data can be transferred to the human model is unclear. Further investigation into the relationship between exercise, systemic viral infections, and immune system response continues. However, until research offers clear guidelines about exercise during viral infections, advice relies on common sense. Research documents that acute, febrile viral infections decrease muscle strength and endurance performance (23), and thus any workout during such a time is suboptimal. Rest seems prudent during the acute phases of systemic viral infection, particularly in the presence of myalgia and fever. Upper respiratory symptoms without systemic features need not preclude exercise as tolerated. After acute systemic symptoms resolve, training can resume in a stepwise fashion. A reasonable guideline for the recovering athlete is to allow 1 to 2 days of reduced-intensity exercise for each complete rest day during the preceding illness.

SUMMARY

Pericarditis and myocarditis are uncommon infections in athletes, and primarily occur following viral infections. More specific symptoms, physical findings, and ECG changes allow the physician to identify pericarditis more confidently than myocarditis. Complete resolution of pericarditis typically allows the athlete to return to full activity.

Myocarditis, unfortunately, occurs as a more subtle disease, whose identification, evaluation, and prognosis remain obscure. Particularly worrisome is the athlete with simple viral symptoms who has myalgia, tachycardia, and low-grade fever. Clinical judgments rely on the physician's experience and intuition. Once myocarditis is confirmed, however, athletes need a minimum of 6 weeks' convalescence, and a return to activity should follow comprehensive evaluation utilizing specific guidelines.

REFERENCES

1 Coleman WL. Recurrent chest pain in children. Pediatr Clin North Am 1984;31:1007–1026.
2 Zavaras-Angelidou KA, Weinhouse E, Nelson DB. Review of 180 episodes of chest pain in 134 children. Pediatr Emerg Care 1992;8:189–193.
3 Brenner JI, Ringel RE, Berman MA. Cardiologic perspectives of chest pain in childhood: a referral problem? to whom? Pediatr Clin North Am 1984;31:1241–1258.
4 Kramer MR, Drori Y, Lev B. Sudden death in young soldiers: high incidence of syncope prior to death. Chest 1988;93:345–347.
5 Virmani R, Roberts WC. Sudden cardiac death. Hum Pathol 1987;18:485–492.
6 Agner RC, Gallis HA. Pericarditis: differential diagnostic considerations. Arch Intern Med 1979;139:407–412.
7 Goldschlager N, Goldman MJ. Principles of clinical electrocardiography. 13th ed. Norwalk, CT: Appleton and Lange, 1989.

8 Maron BJ, Isner JM, McKenna WJ. Hypertrophic cardiomyopathy, myocarditis, and other myo-pericardial diseases and mitral valve prolapse. Med Sci Sports Exerc 1994;26(suppl):S261–S267.

9 Hirschman SZ, Hammer GS. Coxsackie virus myo-pericarditis: a microbiological and clinical review. Am J Cardiol 1974;34:224–231.

10 Francis GS. Viral myocarditis: detection and management. Physician Sports Med 1995;23:63–68,83.

11 Woodruff JF. Viral myocarditis: a review. Am J Pathol 1980;101:427–484.

12 Lewes D. Viral myocarditis. Practitioner 1976;216:281–287.

13 Ramamurthy S, Talwar KK, Goswami KC, et al. Clinical profile of biopsy proven idiopathic myocarditis. Int J Cardiol 1993;41:225–232.

14 Fenoglio JJ Jr, Ursell PC, Kellogg CF, et al. Diagnosis and classification of myocarditis by endomyocardial biopsy. N Engl J Med 1983;308:12–18.

15 Parrillo JE, Aretz HT, Palacios I, et al. The results of transvenous endomyocardial biopsy can frequently be used to diagnose myocardial diseases in patients with idiopathic heart failure. Circulation 1984;69:93–101.

16 Deckers JW, Hare JM, Baughman KL. Complications of transvenous right ventricular endo-myocardial biopsy in adult patients with cardio-myopathy: a seven-year survey of 546 consecutive diagnostic procedures in a tertiary referral center. J Am Coll Cardiol 1992;19:43–47.

17 Starling RC, Van Fossen DB, Hammer DF, et al. Morbidity of endomyocardial biopsy in cardio-myopathy. Am J Cardiol 1991;68:133–136.

18 Vasiljevic JD, Kanjuh V, Seferovic P, et al. The incidence of myocarditis in endomyocardial biopsy samples from patients with congestive heart failure. Am Heart J 1990;120:1370–1377.

19 Aretz HT, Billingham ME, Edwards WD, et al. Myocarditis: a histopathologic definition and classification. Am J Cardiovasc Pathol 1986;1:3–14.

20 Illback NG, Fohlman J, Friman G. Exercise in coxsackie B_3 myocarditis: effects on heart lymphocyte subpopulations and the inflammatory reaction. Am Heart J 1989;117:1298–1302.

21 Tillcs JG, Elson SH, Shaka JA, et al. Effects of exercise on coxsackie A9 myocarditis in adult mice. Proc Soc Exp Biol Med 1964;117:777–782.

22 Gatmaitan BG, Chason JL, Lerner AM. Augmentation of the virulence of murine coxsackie virus B-3 myocardiopathy by exercise. J Exp Med 1970;131:1121–1136.

23 Daniels WL, Sharp DS, Wright JE. Effects of virus infection on physical performance in man. Mil Med 1985;150:8–14.

Chapter 11
Blood-Borne Pathogens and Sports

Christopher A. McGrew

Blood-borne pathogens are defined as disease-causing microorganisms that can be transmitted from one person to another through blood contact. Many have been identified, but in the field of sports medicine human immunodeficiency virus (HIV) and hepatitis B virus are of primary concern. This chapter highlights the current practical sports medicine issues involving these two diseases. Additionally, a brief discussion of hepatitis C is presented, although its relevance to sports is not as clear at this time.

EPIDEMIOLOGY IN THE UNITED STATES

There are 40,000 to 50,000 new HIV infections diagnosed each year in the United States, and nearly 100 percent of these patients become chronically infected. HIV infects millions of individuals worldwide, with highest numbers in Africa, the United States, and Asia. Approximately 40,000 HIV-related deaths occur each year in the United States (1).

There are approximately 300,000 new cases of hepatitis B virus (HBV) infection diagnosed each year in the United States, and 5% to 10% of these patients become chronically infected. Currently, there are approximately 1.5 million chronic HBV carriers in the United States (1). U.S. mortality estimates attribute 5,000 to 10,000 deaths each year to HBV (1).

There are approximately 150,000 new cases of hepatitis C virus (HCV) infection diagnosed each year in the United States, and 50% to 75% of these patients become chronically infected (2). Data from 1995 suggest that there are approximately 3.5 million chronic HCV carriers in the United States (3).

Transmission

Both HIV and HBV are transmitted through sexual contact; or parenteral exposure to blood and blood components; or contamination of infected blood on open wounds or mucous membranes; or perinatal transmission from infected mother to fetus or infant. HCV spreads from exposure to blood and blood components, but whether transmission occurs through other routes remains unclear. Blood transfusion and needle sharing among IV drug users efficiently transmits the virus, but transmission rarely arises from occupational exposure in the healthcare setting (4). Since similarities exist with HBV, HCV probably is transmitted by sexual contact as well. The risks of breast feeding and perinatal transmission for HCV-infected mothers are not established (5).

Hepatitis delta virus (HDV) is an unusual RNA virus that requires the presence of HBV for expression of the disease. The HDV virus results in a more virulent course of the disease than HBV alone, and may be present during initial infection with HBV or may infect persons with preexisting HBV infection. Risk factors for the two diseases are similar (6).

Both in the general population and in the healthcare setting, HBV is transmitted far more readily than HIV (1). Several factors play a role. A milliliter of blood contains hundreds to thousands of infectious particles of HIV, as opposed to the hundreds of millions of particles of HBV (7). Additionally, HIV is less "sturdy" than HBV in its capacity to resist inactivation by drying/exposure to air. Both viruses can be inactivated by a variety of cleaning agents. In the case of HBV, the chronic carrier who is e-antigen positive represents the greatest concern for transmission.

There is no evidence of transmission of these blood-borne pathogens via other routes, such as aerosol or casual household contact. Tears, sweat, saliva, sputum, and respiratory droplets have not been implicated in infection transmission. Spinal fluid, semen, and vaginal secretions, along with blood, do potentially spread infection.

The overwhelming majority of new infections for both HIV and HBV come from the well-recognized routes of sexual intercourse and sharing of intravenous needles (8). Information on transmission remains incomplete for HCV. Infection rates continue to rise at a fast rate in the adolescent population, most notably because of unsafe sexual contact. No significant information suggests that the prevalence of these infections is greater in the athletic population than in the general population. Survey evidence from the U.S. National Collegiate Athletics Association (NCAA) reveals that HIV-infected athletes participate in sports at several institutions (9).

In terms of risk for infection, limited evidence derived from a study of one small population of intercollegiate athletes noted less use of safe sex practices than in the general student population (10). Although athletes do not use intravenous drugs at any greater rate than the general population, the sharing of needles associated with the use of anabolic/ergogenic substances has been implicated in a few cases of suspected HIV transmission (11).

Potential for Transmission During Sports

Transmission of HIV during sporting activity has not been validly documented. One alleged case of HIV transmission occurred in 1990 between soccer players in Italy (12). However, this case lacked sufficient documentation: after thorough review, it was not considered to be a transmission through athletic activity (13). In 1982, one well-documented case of transmission of HBV through sports was reported in a group of high school sumo wrestlers in Japan (14). No reports concerning HCV have emerged.

HIV   The risk of transmission in the sports arena has only been investigated in a few circumstances, with American football receiving the most attention. Initially, the risk of transmission on the football field in both the National Football League (NFL) and NCAA had been conservatively estimated at a rate of less than one transmission per million games (15,16). These risk estimates were based on the prevalence of HIV in players, the number of significant bleeding incidents per game, and the transmission rate in healthcare settings for needle sticks with typical hollow-bore needles. However, typical blood exposures in football, or for that matter in other athletic events, involve superficial blood spattering on intact or nonintact skin or mucous membranes. Blood spattering is not comparable to deep needle sticks, and thus one would expect that these estimates, although representing a minute chance of transmission, actually overestimate the risk. Using data that suggest lower transmission risk, Brown et al. (15) reported a new calculation format that estimated the risk of HIV transmission at less than one per 85 million game contacts.

HBV   No estimates of the potential of HBV transmission on the athletic field have been published. Based on the risk of transmission by parenteral exposure of HBV in the healthcare setting (approximately 2% to 10% e-antigen–negative, and 30% to 40% e-antigen–positive) compared to estimates of HIV transmission risk (approximately 0.3% by parenteral exposure), extrapolation yields a rate that is 20 to 100 times greater for HBV. Thus, the chance is of one HBV infection transmitted every 10,000 to 50,000 games. Using a lower risk formula (17), extrapolation of HBV data gives an estimate of one transmission in 850,000 to 4.25 million game contacts. However, as noted with HIV risk estimates, using parenteral route transmission rates overestimates infections; a more realistic (albeit theoretical) rate could be calculated using data for transmission via mucocutaneous exposure (18).

EXERCISE CONSIDERATIONS

In general, patients with HIV infection and/or hepatitis B infection have years of good health, during which they may need guidance on many issues, including exercise and sports participation. In addition, exercise on a regular basis may be part of a comprehensive treatment plan for individuals infected with blood-borne pathogens. Regular moderate exercise appears to be beneficial to the general health of the HIV-infected persons. Exercise in some form can be continued throughout the course of the disease and seems to play an important role in improving quality of life (19). The effects of high-intensity training and competition at the elite level have not yet been studied in the HIV-infected individual.

Mixed results come from studies looking at the effects of exercise on the immune system in the general population. Some studies suggest that overtraining may increase the susceptibility of certain groups of athletes to upper respiratory tract infections (20). Conversely, other studies have shown that regular exercise may be protective against certain upper respiratory tract infections and improve certain immune system parameters (21). To date, no evidence suggests that the HIV-infected population increases their susceptibility to the characteristic opportunistic infection as a result of exercise or overtraining. Much of the research on exercise and HIV disease has focused on CD4 (lymphocyte) levels, which appear to increase with exercise (22). "Viral load" (quantitative measurement of HIV RNA) gives an indication of the amount of current viral activity and has been shown to correlate with disease progression. Research is needed to determine the usefulness of this lab test in evaluating the effect of exercise on the HIV-infected athlete.

Several variables influence the level of continued athletic participation and competition in the HIV-infected athlete. These include the athlete's current state of health, the status of the HIV infection, the nature and intensity of the HIV infection, and potential stresses from athletic competition (19). Calabrese and LaPierre (19) have suggested the following empirical guidelines to participation and competition:

- Before initiating a new exercise program (or significantly increasing the level of current program), a complete physical exam is advisable.
- Otherwise healthy, asymptomatic athletes with HIV may continue in competition and exercise

without restriction, but should avoid overtraining.

- Athletes with AIDS-related complex may continue to train, but not exhaustively and not for competition.
- Athletes with AIDS may remain physically active and continue training on a symptom-related basis, but should avoid strenuous exercise and reduce or stop training during acute illness.

Exercise Considerations for Hepatitis-Infected Athletes

In general, acute hepatitis (B or C) infection may be viewed like any other viral infection. Clinical signs and symptoms such as fatigue, fever, or organomegaly will help determine what level of exercise is possible. In the case of the asymptomatic hepatitis-infected patients, there is no evidence to suggest that intense training is deleterious to their health. This applies to both the acute or the chronic state. If there are clinical manifestations of organ impairment, all activity should be modified to reduce exercise intensity, duration, and frequency.

PRECAUTIONS FOR ATHLETICS

Testing Athletes

The consensus of published guidelines suggests that athletes do not require routine tests for blood-borne pathogens (23–27). Two main points underline the rationale for this consensus of recommendations. First, from a public health standpoint, testing would have to be justified on its likelihood to prevent transmission on the athletic field. As previously discussed, the likelihood of transmission is infinitesimally small in the athletic arena. Therefore, it is impossible to show how testing would prevent disease. Second, the frequency of testing would be indefinite. For example, an athlete with a negative test prior to the season would not be guaranteed of having a negative test 6 weeks later, given the lag time for a positive test for blood-borne pathogens.

Voluntary testing of athletes should always be explained and offered both for athletes and non-athletes. Those who have risk factors—for example, a history of multiple sexual partners, sexual contact with high-risk individuals, sexually transmitted diseases, IV drug abuse, or blood transfusions before 1985—deserve testing and education primarily to deal with personal health issues and not because of their risk to other competitors.

Educating Athletes

Blood-borne pathogen education for the athlete should first emphasize safe behavior off the field, as this is where the risk is greatest. The sports medicine provider has ample opportunity to interact with the adolescent population, one of the fastest growing groups of blood-borne pathogen–infected individuals. Preparticipation physicals, event coverage, and office evaluations of injuries all provide contact with adolescents who might not otherwise seek healthcare.

A secondary emphasis is to point out to many athletes that documented fear of the potential for transmission of blood-borne pathogens through sports is unwarranted (28). Survey data have shown that a significant number of athletes still feel that testing could prevent transmission, and thus sports medicine providers have an obligation to dispel such misconceptions. Athletes should be educated about more realistic dangers, such as sharing needles when using illicit ergogenic substances (18).

Responsibilities of the Athletic Health Care Team

Hygiene and Infection Control In athletic healthcare, as elsewhere, good hygiene practices make good sense from a public health standpoint. The following guidelines arise from modifications of universal precaution and "body substance isolation" protocols (25). Major components stress adherence to basic principles of good hygiene and infection control.

- Pre-event preparation includes proper care for existing wounds, abrasions, cuts, or weeping wounds that may serve as a source of bleeding or as a port of entry for blood-borne pathogens. These wounds should be covered with an occlusive dressing that withstands the demands of competition. Likewise, care providers with any healing wound or dermatitis should have these areas adequately covered to prevent transmission to or from a participant. Athletes may be advised to wear more protective equipment to protect high-risk areas such as elbows and hands.

- The necessary equipment and/or supplies important for compliance with these guidelines should be available to caregivers. These supplies include appropriate gloves, disinfectant bleach, antiseptics, designated receptacles for soiled equipment and uniforms, bandages and/or dressings, and a container for appropriate disposal of needles, syringes, or scalpels.

- During an event, early recognition of uncontrolled bleeding is the responsibility of officials, athletes, coaches, and medical personnel (athletic trainers, physicians, other attendant healthcare workers). In particular, athletes should be aware of their responsibility to report a bleeding wound to the proper medical personnel.

- Personnel managing an acute blood exposure should employ universal precautions, which include proper hygiene such as handwashing and proper disposal procedures, such as sharps disposal.

- In a sport where a wound poses significant potential for transmission of disease, the participant with active bleeding should be removed from the playing field or court as soon as possible. Uniforms saturated with blood, regardless of the source, must be evaluated by appropriate medical personnel for the potential likelihood of infection risk; uniforms should be changed, if necessary, before the athlete's return to the field.

- A surface contaminated with spilled blood should be cleaned according to appropriate protocol before play is resumed.

- After practices or games, all equipment or uniforms soiled with blood should be handled and laundered in accordance with hygienic methods that would be normally used for treatment of any soiled equipment or clothing before subsequent use.

- All medical and nonmedical persons involved with sports should be trained in basic first aid and infection control. This training should include coaches, equipment managers, and officials.
- Infection control guidelines of government or sporting associations may cover some members of the athletic healthcare team, and may need to be individualized. The sports medicine team should also assess the need for HBV immunization for all personnel involved with the healthcare of the athlete.

Administrative and Legal Concerns

Sports medicine practitioners need to know the various state and national regulations concerning confidentiality, not only as concerns the issue of blood-borne pathogen infection but for all aspects of care. In general, confidentiality dictates that medical information is the property of the patient, but certain exceptions include medical conditions that are reportable by law.

In the United States and Australia, AIDS and hepatitis B are reportable illnesses. HIV infection is reportable to public health agencies in most locales, but standards vary dramatically within countries. Any physician who needs more information should contact his or her city, county, state, or national health officials (27). The sports practitioner should remain current on regulations concerning body fluids, contamination, and the prevention of blood-borne pathogen transmission in the workplace. Team physicians often assist their team's institution with the development and implementation of plans to comply with such regulations. Unfortunately, data currently suggest that adherence to universal precautions in the athletic healthcare setting is less than optimal (9).

REFERENCES

1 Centers for Disease Control and Prevention. Guidelines for prevention of transmission of human immunodeficiency virus and hepatitis B virus to health care and public safety workers. MMWR Morbid Mortal Wkly Rep 1989;38 (suppl):1–37.
2 Dolan PJ, Skibba RM, Hagan RC, Kilgore WR III. Hepatitis C: prevention and treatment. Am Fam Physician 1991;43(4):1347–1360.
3 Gumber SC, Chopra S. Hepatitis C: a multifaceted disease. Review of extrahepatic manifestations. Ann Intern Med 1995;123:615–620.
4 Wormser G, Forseter G, Joline C, et al. Hepatitis C infection in the health care setting. 1. Low risk from parenteral exposure to blood of human immunodeficiency virus affectations. Am J Infect Control 1991;19:237–242.
5 Noskin G, et al. Prevention, diagnosis and management of viral hepatitis—a guide for primary care physicians. Chicago: American Medical Association, 1995.
6 Rezieeto M. The delta agent. Hepatology 1983;3: 729–737.
7 Ho D, Moudgill T, Alam M. Quantitation of human immunodeficiency virus type I in the blood of infected persons. N Engl J Med 1989;321:1621–1625.
8 National Collegiate Athletic Association 1994–95. Blood-borne pathogens and intercollegiate athletes. In: Sports medicine handbook. Overland Park, KS: 1993:24–28.
9 McGrew C, Dick R, Gikas P, et al. Survey of NCAA institutions concerning HIV/AIDS policies and universal precautions. Med Sci Sports Exerc 1993;4:917–921.
10 Nattiv A, Puffer J. Lifestyles and health risks of collegiate athletes. J Fam Pract 1991;33:585–590.
11 Nemechek P. Letter. N Engl J Med 1991;325:357.
12 Torre D. Transmission of HIV-1 via sports injury. Lancet 1990;335:1105.
13 Goldsmith M. When sports and HIV share the bill, smart money goes on common sense. JAMA 1992;267:1311–1314.
14 Kashiwagi S. Outbreak of hepatitis B in members of a high school sumo wrestling club. JAMA 1982;248:213–214.
15 Brown L, Drotman P. What is the risk of HIV infection in athletic competition? Ninth International Conference on AIDS; June 6–11, 1993. Abstract.
16 Dick R, Worthman A. Frequency of bleeding and risk of HIV transmission in intercollegiate athletics. Med Sci Sports Exerc 1995;5(suppl):S13.
17 Brown L, Drotman P, Chu A, et al. Bleeding injuries in professional football: estimates of the risk for HIV transmission. Ann Int Med 1995;122:271–275.
18 McGrew C. HIV and HBV in sports and medicine. Part II of II. Sports Med Prim Care 1995;1:35–37.
19 Calabrese L, LaPierre D. HIV infections: Exercise in athletes. Sports Med 1993;1:1–7.
20 Nieman DC. Exercise, upper respiratory tract infection and the immune system. Med Sci Sports Exerc 1994;26:128–139.
21 Eichner R. Infection, immunity, and exercise: what to tell patients? Physician Sports Med 1993;1:125–135.

22 LaPerriere A, O'Hearn P, Ironson G, et al. Exercise and immune function in healthy HIV antibody positive gay males. In: Proceedings of the 9th Annual Scientific Sessions of the Society of Behavioral Medicine. Boston, 1988:28.

23 World Health Organization International Federation of Sports Medicine. Consensus statement on AIDS in sport. Geneva, Switzerland: World Health Organization, 1989.

24 Canadian Academy of Sports Medicine Task Force on Infectious Disease in Sports. HIV as it relates to sport. Clin J Sports Med 1993;3:63–65.

25 Guideline 2H: blood-borne pathogens and intercollegiate athletics. In: NCAA sports medicine handbook 1994–95, ed. Overland Park, KS: NCAA, 1993:24–28.

26 Brown L, et al. HIV/AIDS policies in sports: the national football league. Med Sci Sports Exerc 1994;26:403–407.

27 American Medical Society for Sports Medicine and American Orthopaedic Society for Sports Medicine. Position statement on HIV and other blood-borne pathogens in sports. Clin J Sports Med 1995;5:199–204.

28 Anderson W, McKeag D, Albrecht R, et al. Second replication of a rational study of the substance use and abuse habits of college student athletes. Presented to the NCAA, July 30, 1993.

Chapter 12
The Traveling Athlete

Kieran E. Fallon
Edward N. Robinson, Jr.

Traveling athletes face significant challenges, ranging from the inconveniences of lost luggage to the fatigue associated with jet lag and the risk of life-threatening infections. Managing these risks becomes a routine part of the team physician's role in caring for athletes who participate in international competition. This chapter reviews common problems related to travel.

JET LAG

Circadian Rhythms and Performance

Many physiologic variables demonstrate circadian rhythmic oscillations. Disturbance of these rhythms by rapid airline travel across meridians can result in fatigue, malaise, sleep disturbance, gastrointestinal symptoms, and, in some individuals, decrements in sporting performance (1–3). Eastward flight is more likely to cause impairments in performance than westward flight. Realignment of individual rhythms requires a variable period of time for adjustment to new time cues, and, as a general rule, one day of adaptation should be allowed for each hour of time shift that occurs in excess of 3 hours (4). Resolution of jet lag occurs 30% to 50% faster following westward flights (2).

Diminished anaerobic capacity and dynamic strength from jet lag lasts only 3 to 4 days (3). A relative paucity of data exists relating to the duration of negative effects on other variables. Some authorities note that much of the available data relate to untrained individuals and may not be applicable to highly trained athletes (5).

Recommendations

For athletes, the recommendations for minimizing jet lag include:

1 Take a westward flight if travel involves crossing of 10 or more time zones (2).

2 Arrive 5 to 7 days before any major international level competition (1).
3 Once on board, set watches to the time of the destination and avoid comparisons with the times at home.
4 Adjust activity levels gradually to those appropriate to the current time at the destination.
5 Upon arrival at the destination, adjust sleeping and eating to local time.
6 At the destination, assist the avoidance of stiffness with a light training session, which can also prevent athletes from sleeping inappropriately.
7 Despite the fact that sleep disturbance may occur for several nights following arrival, avoid daytime sleep.
8 The ability to sleep on planes is extremely variable, but if arrival is scheduled for early morning, sleep during the later part of the flight (6).

Recently, use of melatonin has been shown to decrease the severity of a number of manifestations of jet lag in aircrew (7,8). Various dose regimens have been investigated, and it appears that 5–8 mg taken on the day of the flight and for 3 to 5 days following arrival is effective. No current studies relate melatonin use to athletes and performance. Other approaches to improving sleep after travel, such as adjustments to sleep patterns prior to departure and specific nutritional regimens, have not been extensively studied.

Advice for Plane Travel

Mental preparation for a potentially frustrating airline experience is important. The athlete's expectations and attitudes affect how he or she feels at the end of the flight. A passive, accepting mental outlook is preferred (6). Anticipation of and a plan of action for contingencies such as delays, luggage transfers, boredom, inactivity, and annoying passengers are advisable.

Seating   Long journeys by plane are often stressful, but a number of strategies can be used to assist the athlete to arrive in good condition. Seating assignments should be selected early, with large athletes or those with injuries seated adjacent to aisles or bulkheads that may allow more leg room. Athletes should always occupy nonsmoking seats. Special needs of disabled athletes should be assessed well in advance of travel.

Diet   Meals are important, and a wide variety of diets are available on most airlines. Unexpected variation from an athlete's normal diet may not be avoidable. Overeating is ill advised, and hydration needs to be maintained by liberal use of water, fruit juice, and mineral water. Coffee, tea, and cola drinks promote dehydration and insomnia. These, along with alcohol (a diuretic), are to be avoided during flight and for 48 hours before the flight (9). The risk of dehydration is increased by the low relative humidity inside the cabin, so athletes should take their own water bottles onto flights and use them frequently. Intake of 300 mL of fluid per hour is recommended (10).

Physical Comfort   Clothing should be loose and comfortable. Athletes should be encouraged to move about the cabin periodically to stretch, talk, and avoid boredom. Athletes can perform an inflight seated exercise routine discreetly. Inflight entertainment may alleviate boredom, but each athlete should take reading material and perhaps a portable CD or cassette player onboard to keep occupied (1). Sleep is often difficult but avoidance of stimulants and the use of ear plugs and eye shades may be useful. Short-acting benzodiazepines such as temazepam are appropriate for those with a history of insomnia in aircraft, but their use should be supervised by a physician. Routine use of any hypnotic medication during a flight is unwise. Alcohol is not an appropriate sedative, as it has negative effects on REM sleep (11) and causes increased disturbance in circadian rhythms.

IMMUNIZATIONS

All travelers should ensure that basic immunizations including tetanus, diphtheria, polio, mea-

sles, mumps, and rubella are up to date. Hepatitis A vaccine is the most commonly required extra immunization and is effective for 5 to 10 years. If time constraints do not allow for vaccination, passive protection against hepatitis A using Human Normal Immunoglobulin Gammaglobulin is effective, but only lasts 6 months. Hepatitis B vaccination is indicated for long-term travelers to endemic regions and for those in high-risk groups. Typhoid vaccine is indicated where unsafe water and food may be present. The oral vaccine, which lasts for 1 to 3 years, is now available and is approximately 70% effective. Cholera vaccine is no longer recommended by the World Health Organization due to its low efficacy and short duration of protection.

Some vaccines are required for entry by various countries and, in some cases, for return home. Parts of equatorial Africa, and Central and South America, are endemic areas for yellow fever. As vaccination requirements are variable, specific current information should be obtained. The live yellow fever vaccine is safe, and protection lasts up to 10 years. Japanese encephalitis, which is caused by a flavivirus and carries significant mortality and neurologic morbidity, is an example of a specific disease that requires vaccination but occurs in limited geographical areas. High-risk areas are China, Korea, Nepal, northern India, and parts of Southeast Asia.

Rabies vaccination is indicated for those likely to be exposed to infected animals while traveling in endemic areas for periods greater than 1 month. The areas of greatest risk for rabies are Africa, Central and South America, India, Sri Lanka, and Thailand.

TRAVELER'S DIARRHEA

Etiology

As many as 20% to 50% of travelers to tropical and subtropical areas can develop diarrhea, making this the most common medical problem encountered by travelers. Greater than 80% of cases have a bacterial etiology. The most common organisms, in decreasing order of importance, are enterotoxigenic *Escherichia coli* (40% to 75% of cases), *Shigella, Campylobacter jejuni, Aeromonas* species, *Pleisomonas shigelloides,* various *Salmonella* species, and noncholera *Vibrio* bacteria (12). Other causes of diarrhea include viruses such as rotavirus and protozoal infections like giardiasis. Noninfective etiologies should not be forgotten, and include dietary changes, stress, and toxins that may arise from staphylococcus or bacillus organisms.

Presentation

Traveler's diarrhea typically involves the passage of three or more unformed stools in a 24-hour period and usually lasts for 3 to 5 days. Abdominal pain and cramps are common, and associated symptoms include vomiting and nausea. Fewer than 20% of cases report fever or the passage of bloody stools (dysentery).

Prevention

The axiom "boil it, cook it, peel it, or forget it" remains a useful preventive strategy for avoiding traveler's diarrhea. Handwashing with soap and water prior to eating, drinking carbonated bottled beverages or purified water, and using effective methods of water purification are also important.

Water   The simplest method of water purification is boiling, which eliminates most enteropathogens. Iodine may be used as an alternative agent and requires 4 drops (0.2 mL of 2% tincture of iodine) per 1 liter of water. The treated water should be left for 30 minutes prior to ingestion. This method is less effective in turbid water. The taste of iodine may be particularly unpalatable to some. Similar problems can occur if chlorine (2 drops or 0.1 mL of 5% chlorine bleach per 1 liter of water) is used. Similarly, chlorine-treated water must stand for 30 minutes, and long-term use is not recommended because of the potential for production of carcinogenic trichloromethanes in the solution. Commercial water purifiers are popular and act by inactivation of organisms by iodine present in complex resins. The resultant water is palatable, little iodine is present in the final product (which is available in 5 minutes), and treatment of turbid water is not a problem (13).

Food   Food should be eaten while hot, and only boiled or well-cooked vegetables or fruit that have been peeled by the consumer should be eaten. Uncooked and reheated foods are not recommended. Tap water, milk and other dairy products, and ice should be avoided. Untreated tap water should not be used even for brushing teeth. One common mistake is to assume that water in hotel refrigerators is safe.

Antibiotics   Antibiotic prophylaxis of traveler's diarrhea is controversial. Decisions for prophylaxis must consider underlying medical illnesses, the importance of the journey, the expected compliance of the traveler with food precautions, and the wishes of the traveler. In general, prophylaxis for sport teams traveling to high-risk areas for competition is recommended. Currently, the most predictably effective drugs are the fluoroquinolones, such as norfloxacin (400 mg/day) or ciprofloxacin (500 mg/day). These should be commenced upon arrival in the foreign country and ceased 2 days after returning home. The recommended duration of prophylactic treatment is less than 3 weeks (13). A test dose prior to departure to determine allergy or intolerance may be appropriate. Trimethoprim-sulfamethoxazole and doxycycline were previously popular but resistance to these medications is common. Bismuth subsalicylate (2 tablets, four times a day) is commonly recommended but is less effective than antibiotics.

Treatment

Treatment of diarrhea includes appropriate replacement of fluids and electrolytes. Loperamide is recommended for symptomatic relief. If diarrhea is severe, dysenteric, or persists for 48 hours without improvement, antibiotics should be used. Two appropriate regimens are

1 Norfloxacin, 800 mg initially, followed by 400 mg 12 hourly for 3 days.
2 Ciprofloxacin, 1000 mg initially, then 500 mg 12 hourly for 3 days.

Should diarrhea last for more than 5 to 7 days, giardiasis should be considered: a single empiric dose of tinidazole (2 g) is reasonable (not available in the United States). More persistent diarrhea requires investigation (14).

MALARIA

Etiology and Presentation

Malaria is caused by parasites of the genus *Plasmodium*. *P. falciparum, P. vivax, P. malariae,* and *P.*

ovale are four species carried by the *Anopheles* mosquito (15). Malaria with *P. falciparum* has an incubation period that varies from 7 to 14 days, and has a mortality of 20% if left untreated (16). For *P. malariae,* the incubation period may be up to 40 days, allowing initial symptoms to develop after the traveler is home. Initial clinical features include a classical sudden feeling of cold with rigors, followed by hot flushes, headache, and marked sweating. Other common features of malaria are vomiting, diarrhea, myalgias, anemia, jaundice, and splenomegaly (16). Febrile convulsions may occur in children, especially those suffering from cerebral malaria.

Prevention

A series of simple measures can decrease the risk of malaria. Using insect repellents, wearing long-sleeved shirts and trousers, and minimizing exposure outside between dusk and dawn when mosquitos are most active are common-sense recommendations. Insect sprays and mosquito coils should be used, and travelers should sleep in screened rooms, in beds under mosquito nets impregnated with permethrin.

Malaria chemoprophylaxis is appropriate for all travelers to areas of significant risk. The currency of specific advice relating to prophylactic drugs should always be checked through access to databases.

Chloroquine has been the most commonly used drug but can now only be recommended for travel to areas where resistant strains of *P. falciparum* do not occur. The standard dose is 300 mg base, once a week for 2 weeks before, during, and for 4 weeks after returning from an endemic region.

Mefloquine is now the most widely used drug for chloroquine-resistant malaria (17). It is not recommended in pregnancy, epileptic patients, or for children weighing less than 15 kg. The standard dose is 250 mg, once a week beginning 1 week before departure, during residence, and for 4 weeks after leaving the malarious area (18).

Doxycycline is effective against chloroquine-resistant malaria. It is most commonly used for individuals unable to take mefloquine and for travelers to areas of mefloquine resistance (e.g., east-

ern Thailand and its border regions, Myanmar, and Cambodia). Doxycycline (100 mg) should be taken daily commencing several days prior to exposure and for 4 weeks following the return home. Doxycycline is not suitable for children or pregnant women. Some authorities recommend limiting its use to 8 weeks (17).

Maloprim (dapsone and pyrimethamine) and Fansidar (sulphadoxine and pyrimethamine) are not widely recommended because of resistance and potentially significant side effects (Stevens-Johnson syndrome).

THE RETURNED ATHLETE WHO IS UNWELL

In some situations it is prudent for the returned asymptomatic traveler to undergo medical screening. Reasons include the occurrence of a significant illness whilst overseas, prolonged travel to or residence in a high-risk area, a potential rabies exposure, exposure to HIV infection or other sexually transmitted diseases, or behaviors that would be considered high risk for acquiring these infections.

When the athlete returns unwell from overseas, a number of historical factors are important. These include detailed information relating to regions (and not merely the countries) visited, timing of exposures to potential pathogens, types of exposures, vaccinations and medications, health of traveling companions, and the exsistence of concurrent illnesses.

Fever

Fever is the presenting symptom that causes most concern. Once simple infections have been excluded, the common causes of fever include malaria, dengue, and enteric pathogens such as typhoid and hepatitis A. Fever in a traveler returning from a malarial area should be regarded as malaria until proven otherwise. As the risk of severe illness and death is directly related to the length of time between the onset of symptoms and initiation of therapy, early diagnosis is paramount. Examination of thick and thin blood films for the presence of malarial parasites is the appropriate diagnostic tool. A full blood count; liver function tests; electrolytes, and cultures of blood, urine, and feces;

stool examination; and relevant serology are useful in the diagnosis of other causes.

Dengue fever occurs in tropical and subtropical environments with highest risk in Southeast Asia, the Caribbean, and the Pacific Islands. It is caused by a flavivirus and is transmitted by the *Aedes* mosquito. Mild cases present with fever, myalgia, headache, and anorexia. Nonimmune subjects often experience a more severe syndrome, which includes severe headache, backache, lower limb and joint pains, lymphadenopathy, and a rash.

Enteric infections may present with undifferentiated fever but are usually heralded by diarrhea, which may or may not be bloody. Typhoid is the most important of the enteric fevers.

Amebic abscess may present with fever as the only symptom. If no cause is found following initial investigations for fever, a chest x-ray, abdominal ultrasound, and/or abdominal CT may help identify an hepatic amebic abscess.

Viral causes of hemorrhagic fevers include Lassa fever, Marburg and Ebola viruses. Their onset is usually nonspecific; the illness begins gradually in Lassa fever, and abruptly in the others (19). Early symptoms are nondiagnostic and include pharyngitis, conjunctival injection, fever, myalgia, arthralgia, and headache. These are followed by hemorrhagic manifestations, jaundice, and, in cases involving the Marburg and Ebola viruses, disseminated intravascular coagulation and pancreatitis. While these infections are fortunately rare, they are considered highly contagious and have associated high morbidity and mortality. HIV infection also causes nonspecific fevers, is a risk to all sexually active travelers, and must be suspected if symptoms similar to those of glandular fever (infectious mononucleosis) present following high-risk behavior.

Diarrhea

Chronic diarrhea may follow travel to third world countries. Nonmicrobial causes of diarrhea should be remembered, but a postinfective irritable bowel syndrome is the most common cause of persistent bowel symptoms following travel (20). *Salmonella, Shigella,* and *Campylobacter* are important bacterial pathogens. Protozoal infections such as giardiasis, amebiasis, cryptosporidiosis, and cyclosporiasis also occur. Helminthic causes include hookworm, schistosoma, and strongyloides (20). Appropriate investigations include a full blood count, electrolytes, liver function tests, relevant serology, and serial stool microscopy and culture. Treatment of chronic diarrhea depends on the specific diagnosis, but when a cause cannot be determined, an empiric course of tinidazole (or other appropriate antibiotic) seems warranted because of the significant possibility of giardiasis.

Eosinophilia may be found during routine testing of the returned traveler. This finding should trigger a search for helminthic infections, with strongyloidiasis and schistosomiasis as important suspects. Otherwise known as Katayama fever, acute schistosomiasis commences with intense itching of the skin soon after contact. Several weeks later fever, malaise, headache, abdominal pain, diarrhea, and an allergic skin eruption occur; in view of this delay, the initial presentation may occur well after return from travel. Certain drugs may also lead to eosinophilia, and a history of medications should be reviewed.

Strongyloides stercoralis is an intestinal nematode endemic to the tropics and subtropics. Infection is usually asymptomatic, but cutaneous manifestations occur. These include recurrent urticaria, particularly of the wrists and buttocks, and the classical "larva currens" in which a serpiginous, pruritic, raised, red migrating lesion occurs along the course of larval migration (21). Abdominal symptoms result from parasites residing in the lumen and mucosa of the duodenum and jejunum. Nausea, diarrhea, weight loss, and abdominal pain are common manifestations.

Jaundice

Jaundice may develop upon return to the traveler's native country. Although hepatitis is common, malaria, leptospirosis, and ascending cholangitis should be considered. A useful axiom is that "fever plus jaundice indicates ascending cholangitis until proven otherwise" (20). Presentation of this combination mandates blood cultures and early abdominal ultrasound. These symptoms should not be ascribed to viral hepatitis until other serious causes are excluded, based on standard diagnostic principles.

SUMMARY

More than 300 million people travel internationally each year, a significant proportion of whom are athletes. While some concerns about traveling relate primarily to performance (e.g., jet lag), infections can pose significant risks, including long-term morbidity or even death. Immunizations, prophylaxis, and preventive strategies lessen the risks of these occurrences.

Nevertheless, the true risks for the traveler continually change so that in each situation, before any therapy is chosen, careful assessment of the probability of acquiring an infection should be made. This can only occur if the physician has information that describes the current risk of exposure, the effectiveness of therapy, and the detailed travel plans of the individual. In many situations a change in travel plans may be more advisable than a specific medical regimen. Thus, to appropriately advise traveling athletes, the physician should access the most current medical information, relying on text sources only as a general guide for principles of treatment.

Information Resources

A chief challenge to the provider of health advice is access to accurate information on country-specific problems. As each country's endemic and epidemic health risk varies with year, season, and region, textbooks and journal articles provide insufficient detail and timeliness to be useful beyond providing broad brushstrokes (22,23). Current information, which is readily available from subscription and from electronic resources such as the Internet, should be utilized to update specific concerns about each travel locale.

The Travel Medicine Advisor
American Health Consultants Inc.
P.O. Box 740056
3525 Piedmont Road, Building 6, Suite 400
Atlanta, GA 30374 USA
Telephone: (404) 262-7436
Toll free (U.S) 1-800-688-2421
URL http://www.ahcpub.com

Bimonthly updates provide reasonably current recommendations about specific topics (e.g., malaria) and countries (e.g., Belize). The *Travel Medicine Advisor* also provides updates to the International Association for Medical Assistance to Travelers (IAMAT) directory of English-speaking medical personnel. The current yearly subscription price is $329 (US).

Centers for Disease Control
Atlanta, GA USA
URL http://www.cdc.gov

Accessible via any local or commercially available web server, the CDC web site provides detailed, travel-specific advice that is updated continually.

Summary of Health Information for International Travel
This biweekly newsletter, commonly known as the "Blue Sheet," provides updates to the CDC Yellow Book for countries reporting cholera, yellow fever, and plague. Blue sheet updates are also accessible on the CDC's Internet web site.

Health Information for International Travel, 1995
Superintendent of Documents
U.S. Government Printing Office
Washington, DC 20402 USA
Phone: 202-512-1800
URL http://www.access.gpo.gov

This CDC publication, also known as the "Yellow Book," contains advice on required immunizations and malaria prophylaxis suggestions by country. The price is $14 (US).

REFERENCES

1 Hahn AG, Martin DT, Smith DA, et al. International travel by elite athletes. Position Statement No. 2, Dept of Physiology. Australian Institute of Sport, 1996.
2 Winget CM, DeRoshia CW, Holley DC. Circadian rhythms and athletic performance. Med Sci Sports Exerc 1985;17:498–516.
3 Hill DW, Hill CM, Fields KL, Smith JC. Effects of jet lag on factors related to sport performance. Can J Appl Phys 1993;18:91–103.
4 Shepard RJ. Circadian rhythms and the athlete. Can J Sport Sci 1991;16:5.
5 O'Conner PJ, Morgan WP. Athletic performance following rapid traversal of multiple time zones: a review. Sports Med 1990;10:20–30.

6 Bond J. Minimizing jet lag and jet stress. Unpublished paper. Dept of Psychology, Australian Institute of Sport, 1995.

7 Claustrat B, Brun J, David M, et al. Melatonin and jet lag: confirmatory result using a simplified protocol. Biol Psychiatry 1992;32:705–711.

8 Petrie K, Dawson AG, Thompson L, Brook R. A double blind trial of melatonin as a treatment for jet lag in international cabin crew. Biol Psychiatry 1993;33:526–530.

9 Harcourt P. Sports travel. Sports Coach 1993; 16:3–5.

10 Warr C. The traveling athlete. Unpublished paper. Dept of Physiology, Australian Institute of Sport, 1996.

11 Loat CER, Rhodes EC. Jet-lag and human performance. Sports Med 1989;8:226–238.

12 Dupont HL, Ericsson CD. Prevention and treatment of traveler's diarrhea. N Engl J Med 1993;328:1821–1826.

13 Hudson B. Developing-country travel and endemic diseases. Aust Fam Physician 1994;23: 1666–1677.

14 Ruff T. Illness in returned travelers. Aust Fam Physician 1994;23:1711–1721.

15 Russell RC. Vector-borne diseases and their control. Med J Aust 1993;158:681–690.

16 Currie B. The diagnosis and treatment of malaria in Australia. Aust Fam Physician 1993;22:1773–1779.

17 Rogerson SJ, Biggs BA, Brown GV. Chemoprophylaxis and treatment of malaria. Aust Fam Physician 1994;23:1696–1709.

18 Wyler DJ. Malaria chemoprophylaxis for the traveler. N Engl J Med 1993;329:31–37.

19 Speed BR, Gerrard MP, Kennett ML, et al. Viral haemorrhagic fevers: current status, future threats. Med J Aust 1996;164:79–83.

20 Ruff T. Returned travelers: what to do when they present with illness. Mod Med 1996;38:44–54.

21 Liu LX, Weller PF. Intestinal nematodes. In: Isselbacher KJ, Braunwald E, Wilson JD, et al., eds. Harrison's principles of internal medicine. 13th ed. New York: McGraw-Hill, 1994:916–920.

22 Oldfield EC III, Wallace MR, Hyams KC, et al. Endemic infectious diseases of the Middle East. Rev Infect Diseases 1991;13(suppl 3):S199–S217.

23 Oldfield EC III, Rodier GR, Gray GC. The endemic infectious diseases of Somalia. Clin Infect Dis 1993;16(suppl 3):S132–S157.

PART II
CARDIOLOGIC AND OTHER REGIONAL MEDICAL CONDITIONS AND CHRONIC ILLNESSES

Chapter 13
Cardiovascular Response to Exercise

Edward Shahady

Cardiovascular fitness or conditioning is measured by the maximum amount of oxygen uptake with exercise, or $\dot{V}o_2$max. $\dot{V}o_2$max is a measure of the body's ability to extract oxygen from the air and transport that oxygen to muscle. Oxygen transport requires complex physiologic interactions among the pulmonary, cardiovascular, and musculoskeletal systems, and exercise has a profound effect on the entire system.

PHYSIOLOGIC ADAPTATION

Dynamic exercise, which involves contraction of the body's large muscle groups, stimulates the cardiorespiratory system. Cardiovascular adaptations occur throughout the whole body, primarily in the heart centrally, and the muscle peripherally. These changes occur in all populations, whether young, old, sick, or healthy. The degree of change depends on the health of the organs involved, the age of the patient, and the characteristics of the training.

Cardiac Muscle Adaptation
Untrained subjects increase cardiac output in response to exercise primarily by an increase in heart rate. This differs from the trained endurance athlete who does so mainly by increasing stroke volume. Increases in both cardiac volume and mass, compared with sedentary individuals, are characteristic physiologic adaptations of endurance-trained athletes. (This contrasts with the skeletal muscle and myocardial hypertrophy that occurs in response to speed or strength training.) As would be predicted by Starling's curve, dilation and hypertrophy of all four cardiac chambers in the en-

durance-trained athlete increase the pumping capability of the heart. A more efficient heart generates greater stroke volume and thus increases oxygen delivery to tissues during exercise (1).

Bradycardia of trained athletes increases the diastolic filling time and further augments both stroke volume and coronary blood flow. Both resting heart rate and heart rate at any level of submaximal exercise decrease progressively with endurance training, primarily reflecting augmented vagal tone. The total hemoglobin and blood volume of the endurance-trained athlete is also increased, which further enhances oxygen transport. Due to the increase in ventricular volume and the associated bradycardia, myocardial oxygen consumption decreases for the same absolute workload. Further demonstrating that these changes are caused by exercise, cardiac enlargement and bradycardia both characteristically regress when training is discontinued (2).

Hemodynamics
As has been noted, exercise produces significant changes in the heart, which correlate with altered hemodynamics. Greater left ventricular chamber size corresponds with large end-diastolic volumes at rest and during exercise. In addition, increases in left ventricular mass parallel large stroke volumes at rest and during exercise, as well as an increase in the maximal cardiac output. The nonconditioned heart has an end-diastolic volume significantly less than that of the well-conditioned heart (Fig 13-1). A typical nonconditioned heart with an end-diastolic volume of 120 mL and an end systolic volume of 50 mL has a stroke volume of 70 mL per beat and an ejection fraction of 58%. In contrast, the conditioned heart, with an end-dia-

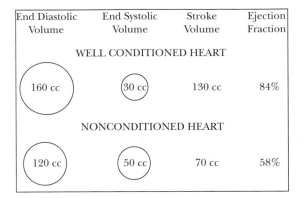

End Diastolic Volume	End Systolic Volume	Stroke Volume	Ejection Fraction
WELL CONDITIONED HEART			
160 cc	30 cc	130 cc	84%
NONCONDITIONED HEART			
120 cc	50 cc	70 cc	58%

Figure 13-1. Comparison of the well-conditioned vs. nonconditioned heart.

stolic volume of 160 mL and an end-systolic volume of 30 mL, has a stroke volume of 130 mL and an ejection fraction of 84%. The conditioned heart is 33% larger at the end of diastole, and 40% smaller at the end of systole. Thus, the exercise-induced changes in the cardiovascular system are not only manifest by cardiac dimensions but also by efficiency of the cardiorespiratory system.

In addition to increased cardiac output, there is a redistribution of the blood flow during exercise. For example, in an individual with a cardiac output at rest of 5900 mL whose cardiac output with exercise increases to 24,000 mL, the following changes occur:

- Coronary blood flow increases from 240 mL at rest to 1000 mL during exercise.
- Cerebral flow stays the same at 750 mL, both at rest and during exercise.
- Flow to the kidneys, gastrointestinal tract, and liver decreases from 3100 mL at rest to 600 mL at maximum exercise.
- Marked shunting of blood away from these organs to muscle flow shows an increase from 1300 mL at rest to over 20,000 mL at maximum exercise.

Especially during hot environmental conditions, the increased cardiovascular output must also account for the shunting of blood to the skin capillary system to allow for necessary cooling to counteract the heat generated by exercise. These changes would not be possible without the concomitant increase in blood volume that accompanies aerobic training.

Data from animal studies indicate that exercise training induces an increase in coronary vascular transport capacity. This is a result of greater blood flow and capillary exchange capacity. The changes are due to 1) a structural vascular adaptation, and 2) control of vascular resistance. In the animal model a change occurs in the cross-sectional area of the proximal coronary arteries and angiogenesis. Adaptations in coronary vascular control induced by training include altered coronary responses to vasoactive chemicals, changes in vasoregulation at the endothelial level, and alterations at the cellular level in calcium kinetics of both the endothelial and vascular smooth muscle cells.

The sympathetic nervous system plays an important role during exercise as well. Sympathetic stimulation leads to systemic venoconstriction, which improves venous return; it also leads to vasoconstriction of vascular beds not participating in exercise. This vasoconstriction serves to limit flow to these beds to the amount needed for baseline function. If vasoconstriction did not occur, flow to these beds would increase as a result of the increase in cardiac output. Sympathetic stimulation leads to an increase in heart rate and contractility that underlies the increase in cardiac output (6).

Static Exercise

Resistance exercise, such as weight lifting, is used by athletes to gain strength and skeletal muscle mass. This static exercise causes significant increases in blood pressure, heart rate, myocardial contractility, and cardiac output. Static exercise is characterized by a pressure load to the heart, as opposed to dynamic isotonic exercise which involves a volume load to the heart. Physical training with static exercise leads to concentric left ventricular hypertrophy, whereas training with dynamic exercise leads to eccentric hypertrophy. The magnitude of cardiac hypertrophy is less with static exercise than with dynamic exercise.

Peripheral cardiovascular adaptation can occur in response to static exercise training. Some researchers believe that these adaptations can include modest decreases in resting blood pressure and smaller increases in blood pressure during a given workload. These responses are greater when the training involves frequent repetitions of moderate weight, rather than when training involves fewer repetitions of larger weight (3–5).

During isotonic exercise, the heart must provide a greater output to support the needs of the working muscle. Cardiovascular adaptation in exercise integrates functional changes in the peripheral circulation, the heart, and the sympathetic nervous system to allow the cardiac output to rise to levels four to five times that present at rest. Dynamic exercise leads to microvascular autoregulation of working muscles, which promotes blood flow to these beds. *Vasodilation* facilitates the increased cardiac output while not causing excessive afterload to the left ventricle. A second peripheral vascular response to exercise is *venoconstriction,* which directly leads to an increased gradient for venous return to the heart. In addition to the impact of venoconstriction, venous return is augmented by increased lower extremity muscle activity and by contraction of abdominal muscles.

End diastolic left ventricular diameter is increased in competitive athletes who perform dynamic or aerobic sports, but not in athletes who only perform strength training or anaerobic sports. This is explained by the different volume load on the heart. In sports with high dynamic and low static demands, wall thickness is usually proportional to the size of the internal diameter so that relative wall thickness is not different from that of nonathletes. This is called *eccentric hypertrophy.* In athletes who concentrate on strength, there is an increase in wall thickness without internal diameter change called *concentric hypertrophy,* and the changes in cardiac output and stroke volume are minimal (7).

These cardiovascular changes occur during isotonic exercise. Isometric exercise such as the hand grip maneuver leads to somewhat different changes. In this circumstance, the arterial pressure (afterload) is substantially elevated, such that the ejection fraction is not increased to the extent that it is in dynamic exercise. Also, because isometric exercise generally involves a smaller in-

crease in overall metabolic demand than does isotonic exercise, the changes in cardiac output and heart rate are less pronounced.

PHYSICAL EXAMINATIONS OF ATHLETES

In athletes, electrocardiographic, radiographic, and echocardiographic changes can occur that should be differentiated from pathologic states (8). Physical examination of the athletic heart is characterized by sinus bradycardia and sinus arrhythmia, as well as an occasional junctional bradycardia. Auscultation often reveals systolic ejection murmurs in the aortic area, and Valsalva maneuvers usually decrease the intensity of these murmurs. ECG abnormalities include left ventricular hypertrophy by voltage criteria, first-degree atrioventricular block, Mobitz type I second-degree block, and junctional bradycardia. Repolarization abnormalities are common and often normalize with exercise. Systemic blood pressure at rest differs little between trained athletes and normal individuals, but typically is lower in athletes for the same workload. The carotid pulses are hyperdynamic. A third heart sound is frequently present; a fourth heart sound is less common.

SUMMARY

The cardiovascular response to exercise occurs at multiple levels. Neurogenic regulation, structural change, cellular functions, and mechanical efficiency are all affected by physical training. The net result of the changes allows athletes to have greater maximal aerobic capacity and to perform submaximal work at lower levels of oxygen consumption and cardiovascular stress. These physiologic adaptations are accompanied by variations seen during physical examination and electrocardiography variations that should be recognized as changes of the athletic heart, rather than as abnormalities.

REFERENCES

1 Braunwald E. Contraction of the normal heart. In: Braunwald E et al., eds. Heart disease. 4th ed. Philadelphia: WB Saunders, 1992:370–382.

2 Smith V-E, Zile MR. Relaxation and diastolic properties of the heart. In: Fozzard HA et al., eds. The heart and cardiovascular system. 2nd ed. New York: Raven, 1991:1353–1368.

3 Kjaer M, Secher NH. Neural influences on cardiovascular and endocrine responses to static exercise in humans. Sports Med 1992;13:303–319.

4 Laughlin MH, McAllister RM. Exercise training-induced coronary vascular adaptation. J Appl Physiol 1992;73:2209–2225.

5 Longhurst JC, Stebbins CL. The isometric athlete. Cardiol Clin 1992;10:281–294.

6 Cox MH. Exercise training programs and cardiorespiratory adaptation. Clin Sports Med 1991; 10:19–32.

7 Fagard RH. Impact of different sports and training on cardiac structure and function. Cardiol Clin 1992;10:241–256.

8 Bryan G, Ward A, Rippe JM. Athletic heart syndrome. Clin Sports Med 1992;11:259–272.

Chapter 14
Sudden Cardiac Death

Brent S. E. Rich

Sudden cardiac death (SCD) is defined as a non-traumatic, nonviolent, unexpected event resulting from sudden cardiac arrest within 6 hours of previously witnessed usual state of normal health (1). Media attention leads to societal anxiety and creates the impression that this is a common occurrence. Fortunately, this is a relatively rare event, though several well-known athletes have succumbed to early demise.

INCIDENCE OF SCD

Exact statistics regarding the incidence of SCD are unknown. In 1992, Ades (2) estimated 4 cases per year per 1 million young athletes. For the 25 million competitive athletes in the United States this translates to 100 cases yearly. In the age group of 30 and under, the National Federation of State High School Associations (NFHSA) estimates 10 to 25 deaths per year (3). Exercise-related death in men ages 25 to 75 years in a Seattle study was calculated to be 1 per every 18,000 participants (4). Though the total number of yearly SCD events appears to be low, cardiac death still represents the leading cause of nontraumatic death in sport.

EXERCISE AND SCD

During exercise, physiologic changes are induced in the hemodynamic and electrical systems of the heart. Stimulation of sympathetic activity during exercise can produce changes in rhythm, myocardial contractility, myocardial tension, and myocardial oxygen uptake. All of these changes can promote cardiac arrhythmias leading to ventricular

fibrillation, which is believed to be the terminal rhythm prior to death (5). If the heart is affected by coronary artery disease, cardiomyopathy, aberrant coronary arteries, myocarditis, or conduction system abnormalities, the threshold for ventricular fibrillation may be lowered.

ETIOLOGY OF SCD

Statistically, different disease entities are responsible for SCD in two basic age groups: young athletes (age 30 and under) and mature athletes (over 30 years old).

Young Athletes (Age 30 and Under)
Congenital cardiovascular disease resulting in structural changes in the heart is the primary cause of disease in the young person who dies from SCD. SCD accounts for 19% of all deaths in the age group from 1 to 13 years; it accounts for 30% of deaths in those 14 to 21 years old (6). No sex preference has been found, though a 4:1 male to female ratio is reported (6). McCaffrey (7) reviewed seven different SCD studies, which revealed the following etiologic causes: hypertrophic cardiomyopathy (24%), coronary artery abnormalities (18%), coronary artery disease (14%), myocarditis (12%), Marfan's syndrome (4%), mitral valve prolapse (4%), and dysrhythmias (2%).

Hypertrophic Cardiomyopathy (HCM) Hypertrophic cardiomyopathy (HCM) is believed to have an autosomal dominant genetic link, leading to morphologic changes that become clinically significant in young adulthood. SCD due to HCM often occurs without premonitory symptoms. Because there is a familial predisposition, a thorough family history should be obtained, and echocardiography should be considered in first-degree relatives identified with the disorder (7). HCM is rare in the general population (0.1% to 0.2%) but has been estimated to account for up to 50% of SCD in those under age 30 years (8,9).

Echocardiographic diagnostic criteria of HCM include left ventricular free wall thickness ≥15 mm and asymmetric septal hypertrophy. Biopsy shows marked ventricular muscle cellular disarray. Physical exam findings suggestive of HCM include a systolic murmur heard best at the lower left sternal border that increases with a Valsalva maneuver, or decreases with squatting and increases on returning to a standing position (10). Electrocardiogram evidence of left ventricular hypertrophy may be present, and the chest x-ray may reveal cardiomegaly, but these are nonspecific findings. Because HCM varies in individual athletes, criteria for medical disqualification should be based on guidelines from the 26th Bethesda Conference (11) and the expertise of a knowledgeable cardiologist.

Congenital Coronary Artery Anomalies   Coronary artery anomalies include the left main artery arising from the right Valsalva's sinus, both left main and right coronary arteries originating from the right or left sinus, a single coronary artery, coronary hypoplasia, or the pulmonary artery as the origin of a coronary artery (3). The mechanism of death is myocardial ischemia due to hypoperfusion of the myocardium. SCD may be the first manifested symptom, as documented in the deaths of certain elite athletes.

Myocarditis   Sudden death secondary to ventricular arrhythmia may be linked to myocarditis, of which coxsackie B virus accounts for over 50% of cases (12). Though this is a difficult diagnosis to make, clinical suspicion should be aroused with an athlete who is unable to perform at his or her previous level following a recent viral illness.

Marfan's Syndrome   Aortic dissection may be the cause of SCD in the athlete with Marfan's syndrome. This genetically transmitted disease affects connective tissue and may lead to weakness of the vessel wall and eventual rupture of the aorta. Rare sporadic cases of Marfan's syndrome occur without a family history (13). Prominent athletes dying from Marfan's syndrome have typically been in sports such as volleyball or basketball, which emphasize height. The Marfan's patient may be affected in several ways, including tall stature, arm span exceeding height, pectus excavatum, kyphoscoliosis, lenticular dislocation, mitral valve prolapse, and aortic dilatation. Echocardiographic evaluation is recommended every 6 months (14). The patient with Marfan's may participate in some sports, according to established guidelines (see Chapter 20).

Aortic Stenosis   The severity of valvular aortic stenosis determines whether the athlete may participate in competitive sports (15). Aortic stenosis is a risk factor for SCD, though not a frequent cause. Physical exam reveals a harsh systolic ejection murmur that increases on squatting and decreases with Valsalva maneuver.

Mitral Valve Prolapse   Five percent of the general population have mitral valve prolapse (MVP), and a majority of athletes will demonstrate trivial amounts of documented valvular regurgitation (8,16). The prevalence of this condition makes identifying the pathologic case from the normal variant a daunting task. When a physician identifies an athlete with classic findings of MVP, such a systolic click followed by a late systolic murmur, the immediate question arises as to what extent to pursue cardiac evaluation.

MVP's association with SCD in a small number of athletes engaged in vigorous exercise suggests that a subset of individuals have a more serious valvular anomaly (17). Echocardiographers have attempted to define characteristics of the valves in MVP that would suggest a greater risk of clinical problems. In addition, a high degree of regurgitant flow more commonly occurs in patients who experience more clinical problems. Continued research on objective changes in MVP may in the future help better define the patient at greater risk.

Currently, clinicians should perform more extensive cardiac evaluations and postpone clearance for sports participation in those athletes with significant symptoms. These typically are dizziness, syncope, palpitations, and/or shortness of breath (12). Athletes with a positive family history of SCD who have MVP should also be considered for more extensive workup. Physical findings that would alert the clinician include a murmur suggestive of significant mitral valve regurgitation, body habitus consistent with Marfan's syndrome, or a question as to whether the murmur represents HCM. Electrogradiographic findings of significant supraventricular or ventricular arrhythmias, or marked resting changes, also merit comprehensive evaluation. The majority of athletes who have none of these findings should receive full clearance for sports participation and are a low risk for SCD.

Other Wolff-Parkinson-White syndrome, idiopathic long QT syndrome, idiopathic concentric left ventricular hypertrophy, and cocaine and anabolic steroid use have also been linked to SCD in the young athlete.

Mature Athletes (Over Age 30)

Atherosclerotic Coronary Artery Disease By far the most common cause of SCD in the mature athlete is atherosclerotic coronary artery disease. Modifiable risk factors include smoking, inactivity, hypertension, hypercholesterolemia, diabetes, and obesity. Male sex and positive family history are nonmodifiable factors. Strategies to modify risk factors are crucial to prevent unexpected death.

SCREENING FOR SCD

Screening methods for SCD have been investigated, but no clear-cut cost-effective method has emerged. Different approaches have been suggested, including physical exam alone or coupled with screening echocardiography and ECG. Epstein and Maron (17) have concluded that to identify one athlete under age 35 years who will die from SCD, 200,000 athletes would have to be screened and 1000 would have to have cardiovascular disease.

The most effective mechanism of identifying an athlete with the potential for SCD is to ask appropriate historical questions that may lead to further investigation. The following questions have been recommended (10,18):

- Have you ever passed out during or after exercise?

- Have you ever been dizzy during or after exercise?
- Have you ever had chest pain during or after exercise?
- Do you tire more quickly than your friends during exercise?
- Have you ever had high blood pressure?
- Have you ever been told you have a heart murmur?
- Have you ever felt a racing of your heart or skipped heart beats?
- Has anyone in your family died of heart problems before the age of 50?
- Have you had a recent viral infection?
- Do you currently or have you recently used any drugs (i.e., anabolic steroids or cocaine)?
- Has a physician ever denied you sports participation for a cardiac reason?

CARDIAC EXAMINATION OF THE ATHLETE

The preparticipation screening physical examination is most often normal, but should include resting blood pressure, pulse, palpation of radial and femoral pulses, and auscultation of the heart. Careful assessment of the first and second heart sounds, extra sounds in systole and diastole, and the quality, location, pitch, and intensity of systolic or diastolic murmurs occasionally detects cardiac problems.

Determining when to perform a more thorough evaluation or refer to a cardiologist may pose a dilemma for the primary care physician, but the following factors have been suggested (10):

- New onset systolic murmur greater than 3 over 6 in intensity.
- Diastolic murmur.
- SCD in a first-degree relative.
- Exercise-induced or unexplained syncope, fatigue, dyspnea, or chest pain.
- New onset rhythm abnormalities.
- First-degree relative with HCM, Marfan's syndrome, or unexplained cardiomyopathy.
- Significant family history of coronary artery disease.
- Prolonged recovery from a viral or systemic disease.

- Exercise prescription for a sedentary individual with two or more cardiac risk factors.

SUMMARY

Though SCD is an uncommon entity, the sports medicine practitioner must be familiar with the major causes. Cases must be evaluated individually, using the 26th Bethesda Conference guidelines (11) and referral to experts as necessary. Emergency access should be well planned and practiced in an effort to minimize sudden cardiac death.

REFERENCES

1 Maron BJ, Epstein SE, Roberts WC. Causes of sudden death in competitive athletes. J Am Coll Cardiol 1986;7:204–214.

2 Ades PA. Preventing sudden death. Physician Sports Med 1992;20:75–89.

3 Van Camp SP. Sudden death. Clin Sports Med 1992;11:273–289.

4 Siscovick DS, Weiss NS, Fletcher RH, Lasky T. The incidence of primary cardiac arrest during vigorous exercise. N Engl J Med 1984;311:874–877.

5 Amsterdam EA, Laslett L, Holly R. Exercise and sudden death. Cardiol Clin 1987;5:337–343.

6 Oppenheim EB. Sudden cardiac death: what primary care providers need to know. Res Staff Physician 1989;35:97–102.

7 McCaffrey FM, Braden DS, Strong WB. Sudden cardiac death in young athletes. A review. Am J Dis Child 1991;145:177–183.

8 Maron BJ, Isner JM, McKenna WJ. 26th Bethesda conference: recommendations for determining eligibility for competition in athletes with cardiovascular abnormalities. Task force 3: hypertrophic cardiomyopathy, myocarditis, and other myo-

pericardial diseases and mitral valve prolapse. Med Sci Sports Exerc 1994;26(suppl 10):S261–S267.

9 Maron BJ, Roberts WC, McAllister HA, et al. Sudden death in young athletes. Circulation 1980;62:218–229.

10 Rich BS. Sudden death screening. Med Clin North Am 1994;78:267–288.

11 Maron BJ, Mitchell JH, Raven PB, eds. American College of Sports Medicine, American College of Cardiology. 26th Bethesda Conference. Medicine and Science in Sports and Exercise 26(suppl 10), 1994.

12 Bresler MJ. Acute pericarditis and myocarditis. Emerg Med 1992;24:35–36,39–42,51.

13 Pyeritz RE. The Marfan syndrome. Am Fam Physician 1986;34:83–94.

14 Graham TP Jr, Bricker JT, James FW, Strong WB. 26th Bethesda conference: recommendations for determining eligibility for competition in athletes with cardiovascular abnormalities. Task Force 1: congenital heart disease. Med Sci Sports Exerc 1994;26(suppl 10):S246–S253.

15 Cheitlin MD, Douglas PS, Parmley WW. 26th Bethesda conference: recommendations for determining eligibility for competition in athletes with cardiovascular abnormalities. Task Force 2: acquired valvular heart disease. Med Sci Sports Exerc 1994;26(suppl 10):S254–S260.

16 Corrado D, Thiene G, Nava A, et al. Sudden death in young competitve athletes: clinicopathologic correlation in 22 cases. Am J Med 1990;89:588–596.

17 Epstein SE, Maron BJ. Sudden death and the competitive athlete: perspectives on preparticipation screening studies. J Am Coll Cardiol 1986;7:220–230.

18 Lombardo J, Nelson M, Smith D. Preparticipation Physical Evaluation. American Academy of Family Practice, American Academy of Pediatrics, American Medical Society for Sports Medicine, American Orthopaedic Society for Sports Medicine, American Osteopathic Academy of Sports Medicine, 1992.

Chapter 15
Cardiomyopathies in Athletes

Henry W. B. Smith III

The cardiomyopathies are a group of diseases that primarily affect the ventricular myocardium. Three pathophysiologic categories, based on alterations in ventricular function and structure, have been described as dilated, hypertrophic, and restrictive. The etiology is often unknown (primary or idiopathic); however, specific causes (secondary) related to metabolic, infiltrative, toxic, and genetic disorders are recognized (1,2). Both the left and right ventricles are usually involved, but focal involvement of either ventricle can occur.

The identification of cardiomyopathy in athletes is important because of the potential for cardiovascular collapse during competition. Fortunately, sudden death during athletic competition is rare; however, when it occurs, cardiomyopathy is one of the most common causes (3–5). Idiopathic cardiomyopathy is rarely an antemortem diagnosis in athletes because most are asymptomatic (or do not recognize symptoms as such), and widespread preparticipation screening is not cost effective (6,7). Table 15-1 lists the most common myocardial diseases associated with sudden death in young athletes (3–5).

HYPERTROPHIC CARDIOMYOPATHY

Hypertrophic cardiomyopathy occurs in up to 0.2% of the population (2). It is genetically transmitted as an autosomal dominant trait, with variable expression and penetrance in over half the cases. Spontaneous mutations are responsible for the remaining cases. Single defects on several different chromosomes may result in the phenotypic expression of hypertrophic cardiomyopathy. Myocardial disarray is the distinctive feature noted on

histologic evaluation (Fig 15-1). Genetic testing may become useful in preclinical detection (8).

Since overt symptoms may be absent, many are diagnosed as part of a screening process when a family member is identified with the disease. Others are diagnosed from clinical signs and symptoms or during echocardiographic evaluation for sometimes unrelated problems (9). The diagnosis is based on the documentation of inappropriate left ventricular hypertrophy (LVH) (in absence of hypertension, aortic stenosis, and other causes) on echocardiography. The echocardiographic hallmarks of the disease are

- Asymmetrical septal hypertrophy (ASH), where the ventricular septum is 1.3 to 1.5 times thicker than the posterior wall and at least 15 mm in absolute thickness (Fig 15-2)
- Systolic anterior motion (SAM) of the anterior mitral leaflet
- Small left ventricular cavity
- Normal or increased systolic contractility

Table 15-1 Myocardial Disease Associated with Risk of Sudden Death in Athletes

1 Idiopathic hypertrophic cardiomyopathy
2 Idiopathic concentric left ventricular hypertrophy
3 Right ventricular cardiomyopathy
4 Other
   Sarcoidosis
   Myocarditis (viral, other)
   Restrictive cardiomyopathy
   Idiopathic cardiomyopathy

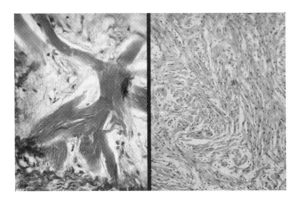

Figure 15-1. Myocardial disarray. (Courtesy of Gower Medical Publishing Ltd.)

A left ventricular outflow gradient may occur and is related to the degree of SAM (1).

Diastolic dysfunction due to the hypertrophied and stiff left ventricle causes dyspnea, which is the most common complaint in symptomatic patients. Other symptoms can include anginal quality chest pain, fatigue, palpitations, presyncope, and syncope. The physical examination may be normal. Most patients have an S_4 gallop rhythm and a left parasternal systolic murmur. An increase in murmur intensity with Valsalva's maneuver or standing is pathognomonic in patients with outflow obstruction. The ECG is rarely normal, with usual findings that include ST-segment and T-wave abnormality, evidence of LVH, and occasionally prominent Q waves.

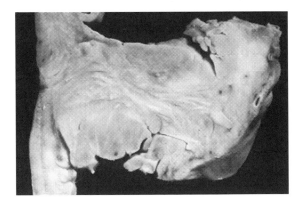

Figure 15-2. Massive septal hypertrophy associated with hypertrophic cardiomyopathy. (Courtesy of Gower Medical Publishing Ltd.)

Hypertrophic cardiomyopathy is the most common cause of sudden death in young athletes (under 35 years old), accounting for up to 50% of cases in most series (3–5,10). The mechanism of death is most likely arrhythmic and may be potentiated by hemodynamic and electrical alterations caused by physical and emotional stress, dehydration, and electrolyte shifts. Some athletes with hypertrophic cardiomyopathy are able to train and compete at very high levels of performance on the amateur and professional level (11). Unfortunately, there is no proven method of risk stratification to identify those athletes at particular risk for sudden death. Therefore, athletes with the diagnosis should be excluded from all competitive sports with the exception of some very low-intensity activities (12).

IDIOPATHIC CONCENTRIC LEFT VENTRICULAR HYPERTROPHY

Idiopathic concentric LVH is associated with sudden death in athletes. Pathologic series document this entity and separate it from hypertrophic cardiomyopathy because

- Hypertrophy is concentric (Fig 15-3)
- Myocardial disarray is absent
- Genetic transmission has not been documented in first-degree relatives (3,4,13)

The degree of LVH exceeds the usual physiologic increase in ventricular muscle mass that results from athletic training. The etiology is unknown, and Maron (4) has postulated that this condition could be a variant of hypertrophic cardiomyopathy or a physiologic response to undetected severe hypertension. No specific clinical or diagnostic features have been identified.

A potential hazard is the erroneous diagnosis of pathologic hypertrophy (hypertrophic cardiomyopathy or idiopathic concentric LVH) in a well-trained athlete with physiologic hypertrophy ("athlete's heart") (14–16). Both isotonic and isometric conditioning cause adaptive cardiac structural changes—usually varying degrees of mild LVH and chamber enlargement. It is rare for the

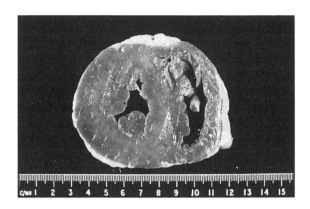

Figure 15-3. Concentric enlargement of the left ventricle. (Courtesy of Medi-Cine Ltd.)

left ventricular wall thickness to exceed 13 mm when measured by echocardiography, even in the highly trained elite athlete. The upper limit of physiologic hypertrophy is 16 mm (15). Therefore, an athlete with a left ventricular wall thickness greater than 16 mm and a normal or small cavity is likely to have hypertrophic cardiomyopathy.

An athlete with a left ventricular wall thickness between 14 and 16 mm is in an indeterminate zone, where hypertrophic cardiomyopathy and possibly idiopathic LVH cannot be totally excluded, if other explanations (such as hypertension) are not obvious. In these circumstances, additional clinical data may be helpful in making a distinction between physiologic and pathologic hypertrophy. A familial pattern of transmission and echocardiographic evidence of diastolic dysfunction would support the diagnosis of pathologic hypertrophy (17). Finally, a period of deconditioning causes a reduction in left ventricular wall thickness in physiologic hypertrophy, but not in hypertrophic cardiomyopathy (18).

IDIOPATHIC RIGHT VENTRICULAR CARDIOMYOPATHY

Idiopathic right ventricular cardiomyopathy (arrhythmogenic right ventricular dysplasia) is a myocardial disease of unknown cause associated with fibro-fatty replacement of myocardium. The disease is rare (incidence unknown), but is reported

to be a relatively common cause of death among competitive athletes in some regions of Italy (5). Clinical features include

- Right ventricular enlargement and hypocontractility on echocardiography
- Precordial T-wave inversions on ECG
- Left bundle branch block–type ventricular tachycardia (on ECG, Holter monitor, or exercise testing)
- Family history with autosomal dominant inheritance (30% of cases) (19,20).

Athletes with the disease should not participate in competitive sports (12).

OTHER MYOCARDIAL DISEASES IN ATHLETES

Dilated and restrictive cardiomyopathies are uncommonly reported as causes of sudden death in athletes. The incidence in an athletic population is suspected to be quite low because symptoms probably limit participation.

Sarcoidosis is an uncommon problem with a predilection for African Americans. Myocardial sarcoidosis may cause sudden death during exertion as the initial manifestation of disease (21).

Myocarditis due to infectious or toxic causes (such as illicit cocaine use) can result in cardiovascular collapse, presumed secondary to fatal arrhythmia (22,23).

SUMMARY

Cardiomyopathies are uncommon in an athletic population (6,7). When they occur, athletic performance may be adversely affected, and there is potential for sudden cardiovascular collapse. Preparticipation screening is not cost effective, but symptoms of chest pain, excessive dyspnea, fatigue, palpitations, and near-syncope or syncope should stimulate further cardiac evaluation. This may include a detailed history and physical, electrocardiography, echocardiography, and stress testing. The echocardiogram is the most sensitive tool for identifying cardiomyopathy in athletes. In general, the diagnosis of cardiomyopathy excludes the athlete from participation in most competitive sports (12). It is therefore imperative that the diagnosis be made with as much accuracy as possible to avoid overdiagnosis and needless disqualification from sports.

REFERENCES

1 Wynne J, Braunwald E. The cardiomyopathies and myocarditides: toxic, chemical, and physical damage to the heart. In: Braunwald E, ed. Heart disease, a textbook of cardiovascular medicine. Vol. 2. Philadelphia: WB Saunders, 1992:1394–1450.

2 Codd MB, Sugrue DD, Gersh BJ, Melton LJ. Epidemiology of idiopathic dilated and hypertrophic cardiomyopathy. Circulation 1989;80:564–568.

3 Hillis WS, McIntyre PD, Maclean J, et al. Sudden death in sport. Br J Med 1994;309:657–660.

4 Maron BJ, Epstein SE, Roberts WC. Causes of sudden death in competitive athletes. J Am Coll Cardiol 1986;7:204–214.

5 Corrado D, Thiene G, Nava A, et al. Sudden death in young competitive athletes: clinicopathologic correlations in 22 cases. Am J Med 1990;89:585–596.

6 Lewis JF, Maron BJ, Diggs JA, et al. Preparticipation echocardiographic screening for cardiovascular disease in a large, predominantly black population of collegiate athletes. Am J Cardiol 1989;64:1029–1033.

7 Maron BJ, Bodison SA, Wesley YE, et al. Results of screening a large group of intercollegiate competitive athletes for cardiovascular disease. J Am Coll Cardiol 1987;10:1214–1221.

8 Rosenzweig A, Watkins H, Hwang DS, et al. Preclinical diagnosis of familial hypertrophic cardiomyopathy of genetic analysis of blood lymphocytes. N Engl J Med 1991;325:1753–1760.

9 Maron BJ, Peterson EE, Maron MS, Peterson JE. Prevalence of hypertrophic cardiomyopathy in an outpatient population referred for echocardiographic study. Am J Cardiol 1994;73:577–580.

10 Burke AP, Farb A, Virmani R. Causes of sudden death in athletes. Cardiol Clin 1992;10:303–317.

11 Maron BJ, Klues HG. Surviving competitive athletics with hypertrophic cardiomyopathy. Am J Cardiol 1994;73:1098–1104.

12 Maron BJ, Isner JM, McKenna WJ. Task force 3: hypertrophic cardiomyopathy, myocarditis, and other myopericardial diseases, and mitral valve prolapse. J Am Coll Cardiol 1994;24:880–885.

13 Burke AP, Farb A, Virmani R, et al. Sports-related and non-sports-related sudden death in young adults. Am Heart J 1991;121:568–575.

14 Maron BJ. Structural features of the athlete heart as defined by echocardiography. J Am Coll Cardiol 1986;7:190–203.

15 Pelliccia A, Maron BJ, Spataro A, et al. The upper limit of physiologic cardiac hypertrophy in highly trained elite athletes. N Engl J Med 1991;324:295–301.

16 Huston TP, Puffer JC, Rodney WM. The athletic heart syndrome. N Engl J Med 1985;313:24–32.

17 Lewis JF, Spirito P, Pelliccia A, Maron BJ. Usefulness of Doppler echocardiographic assessment of diastolic filling in distinguishing "athlete's heart" from hypertrophic cardiomyopathy. Br Heart J 1992;68:296–300.

18 Maron BJ, Pelliccia A, Spataro A, Granata M. Reduction in left ventricular wall thickness after deconditioning in highly trained Olympic athletes. Br Heart J 1993;69:125–128.

19 McKenna WJ, Thiena G, Nava A, et al. Diagnosis of arrhythmogenic right ventricular dysplasia/cardiomyopathy. Br Heart J 1994;71:215–218.

20 Thiene G, Nava A, Corrado D, et al. Right ventricular cardiomyopathy and sudden death in young people. N Engl J Med 1988;318:129–133.

21 Roberts WC, McAllister HA, Ferrans VJ. Sarcoidosis of the heart: a clinicopathologic study of 35 necropsy patients and review of 78 previously described necropsy patients. Am J Med 1977;63:86–108.

22 Lecomte D, Fornes P, Fouret P, Nicholas G. Isolated myocardial fibrosis as a cause of sudden cardiac death and its possible relation to myocarditis. J Forensic Sci 1993;38:617–621.

23 Kloner RA, Hale S, Alker K, Rezkalla S. The effect of acute and chronic cocaine use on the heart. Circulation 1992;85:407–419.

Chapter 16
Hypertension in Athletes

Thomas R. Sachtleben
Karl B. Fields

Systemic hypertension is the most common cardiovascular disease seen worldwide and is also the most common cardiovascular condition found in competitive athletes (1). Demographic studies suggest that the prevalence of hypertension among adults ranges as high as 25% in certain countries, including the United States (2). Certain populations appear at higher risk, including men, older individuals, African-Americans, and some Asian populations. The chance of any individual developing hypertension also relates to clustering of other cardiovascular risk factors, such as hyperlipidemia, glucose intolerance, obesity, hyperinsulinemia, insulin resistance, hyperuricemia, and left ventricular hypertrophy.

BLOOD PRESSURE

Blood pressure is a product of cardiac output times total peripheral resistance, an equation that suggests that either a high cardiac output or increased arterial resistance leads to hypertension. In most individuals, increased vascular resistance is likely to be the primary process.

In general, blood pressure readings can be classified into six categories: normal blood pressure, high normal blood pressure, and mild, moderate, severe, and very severe hypertension ([3] Table 16-1). In each of these categories the hemodynamics differ so that cardiovascular function varies proportionally to the blood pressure and is most affected with true hypertension.

Hypertension is typically defined as systolic blood pressure in excess of 140 mm Hg, or diastolic higher than 90 mm Hg. However, for children and adolescents blood pressure should be compared to age-adjusted tables, with hypertensive individuals identified as those with levels greater than two standard deviations above the normative value in their age group ([4] Table 16-2).

Blood Pressure and Exercise

Exercise affects the blood pressure differently in each of the six categories of blood pressure.

Normal Blood Pressures Individuals with normal blood pressure have an increased cardiac output and a lower total peripheral resistance during exercise. This allows them to maintain a normal blood pressure throughout activity. In individuals with high normal blood pressure, the cardiac output remains normal, but hemodynamic function is suboptimal. Total peripheral resistance is at a normal level, but does not fall to the same extent that it does in normotensive individuals. For this reason these individuals experience a higher blood pressure level for a given activity. Compensatory changes in peripheral resistance disappear as an individual develops hypertension.

Hypertensive Blood Pressures For patients with documented hypertension, only those with mild hypertension have normal cardiac output during exercise. With ongoing activity, they develop higher cardiac output, but rather than a decline, they show an increased total peripheral resistance. Once an individual demonstrates moderate hypertension, cardiac output in exercise actually drops below the level expected, and the peripheral resistance increases steadily. This increasing afterload ultimately leads to left ventricular hypertrophy. By the time severe hypertension is present, many individuals also show signs of diastolic dysfunction. This implies that the myocardium cannot relax adequately or fill efficiently in the dia-

Table 16-1   Classification of Hypertension

	Systolic (mm Hg)	Diastolic (mm Hg)
Normal	<130	<85
High normal	130–139	85–89
Hypertension		
Stage 1 (mild)	140–159	90–99
Stage 2 (moderate)	160–179	100–109
Stage 3 (severe)	180–209	110–119
Stage 4 (very severe)	≥210	≥120

NOTE: For adults aged 18 and older. This categorization applies to individuals who are not taking antihypertensives and are not acutely ill. When systolic and diastolic pressures fall into different categories, the higher category should be selected to classify the athlete's blood pressure status.
SOURCE: Adapted from the Fifth Report of the Joint National Committee on Detection, Evaluation, and Treatment of High Blood Pressure. National Institutes of Health, NIH Publication no. 93-1088, 1993.

stolic phase of cardiac contraction. Those with very severe hypertension can no longer increase their cardiac output in response to exercise. They generally have marked left ventricular hypertrophy and poor cardiac contractility. This may lead them to develop congestive heart failure with vigorous exercise or stress (5,6).

PHYSIOLOGIC CONSEQUENCES OF HYPERTENSION

The key consequences of the physiologic changes of hypertension are major end organ damage. Statistical data have found that both hypertensive

men and women face an increased risk ratio ranging from 2.0 to 4.0 for commonly associated complications such as coronary artery disease, stroke, peripheral artery disease, and cardiac failure. This is particularly significant for coronary artery disease because of the high prevalence of myocardial infarction in many Western nations. Hypertension predisposes to unrecognized myocardial infarctions so that these serious events initially go unrecognized in 35% of the men and 45% of women with hypertension (2).

Risk Factors
Combining hypertension with other cardiac risks factors increases the risk on a logarithmic scale,

Table 16-2   Classification of Hypertension in Children (6 to 15 years old)

	High Normal 90–94th Percentile (mm Hg)	Significant 95–99th Percentile (mm Hg)	Severe >99th Percentile (mm Hg)
Children 6–9 years			
Systolic blood pressure	114–121	122–129	≥130
Diastolic blood pressure	74–77	78–85	≥86
Children 10–12 years			
Systolic blood pressure	122–125	126–133	≥134
Diastolic blood pressure	78–81	82–89	≥90
Children 13–15 years			
Systolic blood pressure	130–135	136–143	≥144
Diastolic blood pressure	80–85	86–91	≥92

SOURCE: Adapted from the Report of the Second Task Force on Blood Pressure Control in Children, 1987. Pediatrics 1987;79:1–25.

rather than linearly. For example, individuals with hypertension and a combination of risk factors—diabetes, cigarette smoking, physical inactivity, left ventricular hypertrophy, and hyperlipidemia—may be at 5- to 10-times greater risk for myocardial infarction than individuals with none of these risk factors. The same gradation of risk is seen for stroke, and is expected to exist for other cardiovascular complications. Evidence continues to mount that obesity, particularly with an emphasis on abdominal adiposity, promotes hypertension so that the majority of cases in men and women of early onset hypertension can be attributed to excess body fat (2).

Symptoms

Unfortunately, individuals who develop hypertension generally experience few symptoms. When the disease becomes advanced, individuals may note fatigue, particularly with exertion, and ultimately may develop early symptoms of congestive heart failure. The association of hypertension with headaches is variable, and certainly this symptom cannot reliably predict the relative blood pressure level. On the other hand, hypertensive individuals do develop physical findings that include narrowing of the retinal arteries, which can be observed on funduscopic evaluation. In addition, the heart may reveal an S_4 gallop sound and late in the disease may show signs of enlargement. Associated vascular disease may cause bruits that can be heard over the carotids, renal, or femoral arteries.

Evaluation

Diagnostic evaluation of the hypertensive patient first centers around confirming the actual diagnosis, which requires more than a single measurement of blood pressure. The blood pressure should be measured after the patient has relaxed and is in a comfortable position. Blood pressures typically are collected seated from the left arm, but can be measured in multiple positions should questions arise. Blood pressures in the upper extremity should be compared to blood pressures in the lower extremity to rule out the possibility of coarctation of the aorta. Similarly, a comparison of both arms helps eliminate the possibility that the elevation seen is caused by a local constriction of the vessel.

Initial evaluation of a newly diagnosed hypertensive patient, at minimum, consists of an ECG. Evidence of left ventricular hypertrophy on the ECG correlates with a much higher risk of all the pathologic complications of hypertension and of overall morbidity and mortality. This type of finding would prompt more aggressive intervention. Laboratory workup should follow, and include testing for elevated lipids, glucose, uric acid, kidney function, electrolytes, and hemoglobin levels. A urinalysis should be obtained to look for signs of proteinuria and/or hematuria. A chest radiograph can be utilized to demonstrate anatomical enlargement of the heart. When enlargement of the heart is suspected, either from ECG or chest radiograph, an echocardiogram is indicated to confirm the presence of true cardiac enlargement and to determine how this enlargement affects the various chambers of the heart.

Because 90% to 95% of hypertensive patients in primary care have essential hypertension, a similar or smaller percentage would be expected in athletes. However, abnormalities of history, examination, or objective tests can point to a need to assess the patient for secondary causes of hypertension, such as renal artery stenosis, renal parenchymal disease, pheochromocytoma, Cushing's disease, coarctation of the aorta, and hyperaldosteronism (7). The history should also probe for other potential causes of increased blood pressure, particularly use of vasoconstrictor medication usage, illicit drugs (such as cocaine or amphetamines), androgens or growth hormone, and excessive alcohol intake. Erythropoietin causes increased blood pressure in one-third of end-stage kidney patients (3), but whether erythropoietin causes the same response in athletes is unknown.

SPECIAL CONSIDERATIONS IN ATHLETES

Dramatic elevations in blood pressure occur particularly during static (isometric) exercise, but even during dynamic exercise increased stroke volumes and heart rates lead to a subsequent rise in mean arterial pressure in normotensive athletes. Stroke volume, heart rate, and cardiac output all proportionately increase with higher workloads. Heart rate increases to maximal levels and stroke volume increases above rest by approximately 24%. The product of HR × SV leads to a cardiovascular output of about 2.3 times resting level (8).

In normotensive individuals, the body compensates for the hemodynamic changes so that small decreases in diastolic pressures occur due to decreased total peripheral resistance. Similarly, systolic pressures also decrease with prolonged exercise due to arteriole dilation. Athletes with any degree of hypertension have an increased total peripheral resistance (TPR) during dynamic exercise, and these same compensatory falls in blood pressure do not occur.

Dynamic Exercise

Significant reductions in resting blood pressures are observed as a result of exercise training over time. Dynamic training has been shown to reduce resting systolic pressures an average of 11 mm Hg, and diastolic pressures an average of 9 mm Hg (9). Numerous studies have pointed to a beneficial effect of aerobic exercise on blood pressure levels; experimentally, decreased arterial stiffness occurs in association with higher maximum oxygen consumption rates ($\dot{V}o_2$max) (10). Dynamic exercise also affects cardiac architecture so that a significant increase in left ventricular diameter and lumen size occurs (eccentric hypertrophy) (11). An associated increase in left ventricular mass is present in the conditioned individual, but after the training stimulus is withdrawn, these cardiovascular effects return to baseline levels after as little as 2 months.

Static Exercise

During isometric exercise bouts of high-intensity training, systolic blood pressures often rise one-and-a-half to twofold. Systolic pressures over 300 mm Hg have been recorded in weight lifters due to the enormous increases in intrathoracic pressure associated with Valsalva's maneuver (12). Other factors that augment these dramatic blood pressure elevations are increased peripheral resistance and heart rates. Whether these intermittent marked blood pressure elevations pose any immediate or long-term risk is unknown.

Concentric left ventricular hypertrophy can ultimately result from the thickened left ventricular walls caused by repetitive static exercise (11). However, left ventricular diastolic function is spared (13), and stroke volume changes from continued resistance training have been equivocal (14). This remains true for normotensive individuals, as well as for adolescent athletes who have a higher resting cardiac output. Cardiac morphologic changes may be more prevalent in African-American athletes.

Because dynamic and isotonic exercise programs appear to lower blood pressures, studies have examined the long-term effects of isometric exercise training in athletes. Data to date do not point to harm from the substantial elevations in blood pressure seen during static exercise, although case reports of subarachnoid hemorrhage in weight lifters has certainly raised this question (15). Higher resting blood pressures do not result from chronic resistance training (9); rather, training of this type has been shown to lower resting blood pressures (14).

Environmental Factors

Exercising in the heat is particularly dangerous for hypertensive athletes, as core temperatures can rise unexpectedly. During exercise, hypertensive athletes do not shunt blood to the skin as effectively as normotensive athletes. Vigorous activity in a hot, humid environment can also lead to free-water loss and hypokalemia, which is especially dangerous for hypertensive athletes.

Screening Older Athletes

Athletes over 35 years of age have a greater risk of coronary artery disease, and since hypertension accounts for approximately 35% of atherosclerotic cardiovascular events (2), older hypertensive athletes require special screening. These individuals should be considered candidates for exercise tolerance testing, and in many cases may warrant an echocardiogram. In athletes undergoing exercise tolerance testing for any reason, an exercise systolic blood pressure that exceeds 225 to 240 mm Hg (17–19) should prompt more careful assessment, as this may well precede the development of hypertension. Similarly, any rise in diastolic pressure is unexpected on exercise testing and suggests that peripheral resistance is elevated. Echocardiogram findings of concentric hypertrophy in adults also suggest higher risk and may warrant hypertensive treatment at lower than standard levels.

TREATMENT STRATEGIES IN THE ATHLETE

Due to dramatic increases in blood pressure during exercise, hypertensive athletes should be adequately treated before participating in high intensity physical activity. They should have their blood pressure rechecked periodically throughout the season as well. Clearance for participation varies with the level of hypertension and with any associated complications. General guidelines are as follows:

- **Stages 1 and 2 hypertension.** Athletes should be *allowed* to play if there is no evidence of end organ damage, including heart disease.
- **Stages 3 and 4 hypertension.** Athletes should be *restricted* from play until blood pressure is controlled. This should be strictly enforced for athletes participating in sports with a strong isometric component (wrestling, weightlifting, gymnastics, etc.).
- **Hypertension with complications or associated cardiac conditions.** Generally, the type and severity of the associated conditions determines the ability to participate (1).

Nonpharmocologic Therapy

Athletes with hypertension should be appropriately counseled regarding nonpharmacologic methods of reducing blood pressure. These include dietary changes, particularly to reduce salt; more consistent aerobic exercise (supplemental aerobic training for athletes in strength sports); reduction of body fat; avoidance of offending medications, drugs, or alcohol; and smoking cessation. One key advantage of nonpharmacologic therapies for athletes with all stages of hypertension is that a good response allows participation without the risk of medication side effects. However, athletes with higher stages of hypertension (stages 2 to 4) often require concomitant use of antihypertensive medications.

Weight   Body composition alterations should be emphasized, especially in athletes with a high body mass index (BMI > 30 kg/m²). Obesity increases both preload and afterload on the heart, creating a hypertensive effect in these individuals. Reducing an athlete's percentage of body fat is the most effective nonpharmacologic strategy for blood pressure reduction. A 10 kg weight loss can reduce systolic blood pressure an average of 15 mm Hg, and diastolic blood pressure an average of 10 mm Hg (9).

Diet   Altering the diets of athletes is often an unpopular but effective method for reducing blood pressure. Decreasing dietary sodium intake to 2.3 g (6 g NaCl) per day is particularly effective in lowering blood pressure in African-American athletes. Increasing potassium intake is also effective, since hypokalemia may increase blood pressure and induce ventricular ectopy. High dietary potassium may also be protective against the development of hypertension and may reduce the subsequent risk of stroke. Supplementing diets with elemental calcium may also help reduce blood pressure in some athletes, particularly those with an inadequate dietary intake (20). Although caffeine has been found to rapidly raise blood pressure, its avoidance is unnecessary due to the swift development of tolerance. Alcohol, on the other hand, has a direct influence on hypertension, and consumption should be restricted to 1 ounce of alcohol per day (2 beers).

Exercise   The incorporation of high-intensity exercise into the daily lifestyle of all calibers of athletes has been proven beneficial for reducing hypertension. Prospectively, athletes who exercise regularly have a lower risk of developing hypertension. As noted, hypertensive athletes may lower their systolic and diastolic blood pressure with regular aerobic exercise training, with the most dramatic reductions occurring in those athletes with high normal and stage 1 hypertension. The enhancement of work capacity through vigorous aerobic training influences the magnitude of the blood pressure reduction.

The most effective method of lowering blood pressure through exercise therapy is incorporating 20 to 60 minute exercise sessions 3 to 5 times per week (9). The level of intensity should be dictated by maximum heart rate predictions. Young athletes should start training at an intensity level of

65% to 70% of their maximum heart rate (MHR). Older and less fit patients should begin at 55% to 60% of their MHR. It has been demonstrated that moderate intensity exercise (55% to 70% MHR) more effectively lowers blood pressure than higher intensity (80% to 85%) exercise. (9) In fact, higher intensity exercise may actually increase resting blood pressures. Hypertensive athletes should also avoid intense resistance training with heavy weights and low repetitions, as this is associated with large increases in blood pressure.

Pharmacologic Therapy

There are numerous pharmacotherapeutic options when a decision is made to prescribe antihypertensive medication for athletes. Several items should be considered before choosing an antihypertensive, including whether or not the drug is banned from competition, and whether it will have a harmful effect on the athlete's performance.

In general, classes of drugs that work by reducing TPR have less effect on exercise performance. With the exception of beta-blockers and diuretics, all classes of antihypertensives permit normal exercise capacity. In about 50% of patients, single-drug therapy controls hypertension. For those individuals who fail on a starting dose of medication from one of the following drug classes, therapeutic options include increased dosage, switching to a drug from another class, or using a combination of medicines from two classes.

ACE Inhibitors   ACE inhibitors (ACEIs) are the drug of choice for many athletes because of the low incidence of side effects. ACEIs effectively reduce TPR by indirectly blocking the vasoconstriction caused by angiotensin II. They have been shown to blunt the amplified blood pressure response during exercise, and reduce hypertension without an associated decrease in $\dot{V}o_2$max (7). Secondary to the potassium-sparing effect of ACEIs, care must be taken to avoid hyperkalemia, especially when these are taken concomitantly with nonsteroidal anti-inflammatory drugs.

Alpha₁-Receptor Blockers   Alpha$_1$-receptor blockers act by reducing TPR through a competitive blockade of postsynaptic smooth muscle receptors in arterioles. They are often used as first-line agents because of their low incidence of side effects and because they do not adversely affect concomitant diseases. Athletes should be cautioned about the possibility of an orthostatic hypotensive response to initial dosing. Alpha$_1$-receptor blockers, like ACEIs, are long-acting agents and can be conveniently dosed once daily.

Beta-Blockers   Although they are subject to International Olympic Committee (IOC) regulation, beta-blockers are popular antihypertensive drugs primarily due to their effectiveness in reducing blood pressure and their relatively low cost. They are listed in a U.S. National Institutes of Health (NIH) report as one of two preferred classes of antihypertensives for initial treatment (3). Drugs within this class do differ, and they are often classified according to whether they possess intrinsic sympathomimetic activity. Beta-blockers affect cardiac output by reducing myocardial contractility and lowering the heart rate. Cardioselective agents (those that are relatively specific to cardiac beta$_1$-receptors) can be used safely in athletes. However, noncardioselective agents are contraindicated in athletes, as they increase perceived exertion and dramatically reduce maximal aerobic capacity.

Beta-blockers have metabolic side effects that can make them a poor choice for athletes. Their use is associated with an increased incidence of hyperkalemia, clinical depression, and hyperthermia. Noncardioselective agents block glycogenolysis, which may lead to hypoglycemic episodes during prolonged or intense exercise. In addition, beta-blockers negatively influence lipoprotein status and increase triglyceride levels. Due to their effect on pulmonary beta receptors, beta-blockers are contraindicated in athletes with asthma.

Labetalol is a combined alpha- and beta-blocker and is often preferred to other beta-blockers in hypertensive athletes. It is a very effective agent in reducing blood pressure at rest and during exercise, primarily due to a decrease in peripheral resistance. Although labetalol does not alter $\dot{V}o_2$max (21), cardiac index (cardiac output indexed to body surface area) decreases approximately 10% to 15% at rest and during exercise after 1 year of therapy. This effect gradually returns to baseline over 5 years due to increases in stroke volume (22).

Thus, it appears a combined alpha and beta blockade promotes normalization of central hemodynamics, as compared to beta-blockers alone.

Diuretics Diuretics are also listed as a preferred initial choice for antihypertensive therapy by NIH (3). Their use is regulated by the IOC because diuretics can serve as a masking agent for anabolic steroids. Although they are effective, low-cost medications for controlling hypertension, diuretics' side effects make them a less ideal choice for athletes. Hypokalemia, hyponatremia, and hyperuricemia are all potentially troublesome metabolic effects. Hypokalemia in particular raises concerns about potential arrhythmias in athletes who are participating in stressful athletic contests. These metabolic effects can be minimized by careful monitoring and by utilizing low-dose diuretics either alone or in combination with a different class of drug. As a therapeutic class, they may be especially effective for African-American athletes whose hypertension is more salt sensitive.

While good hydration minimizes excessive loss, diuretics primarily work by reducing intravascular volume. This is usually undesirable in athletes as it is associated with a decrease in cardiac output. Hemodynamic changes occur during the first month of therapy, and short-term use has been noted to reduce exercise capacity and endurance. These negative effects are maximal in endurance athletes who have greater fluid loss from activity and in any athlete exercising during unfavorable climatic conditions (23). Dehydration and greater risk of heat illness are concerns for athletes using these products for treatment.

Calcium Channel Blockers Calcium channel blockers are effective antihypertensives, and are usually classified according to their mechanism of action. Verapamil and diltiazem lower blood pressure through negative chronotropic and inotropic effects on the heart and a lesser effect on peripheral resistance. The dihydropyridines, such as nifedipine and amlodipine, are primarily peripheral vasodilators, and therefore are excellent at reducing TPR. These agents are popular among athletes because of their low side-effect profile and their lack of effect on maximal aerobic capacity. The use of calcium channel blockers allows normal hemodynamics, both at rest and during exercise. They

may be the preferred agent in treating African-American athletes.

There has been a concern over potential deleterious cardiac effects associated with the use of short-acting forms of certain calcium channel blockers (24). Much of this concern centers around recent studies that have suggested an associated higher morbidity and mortality among cardiac patients treated with the shorter-acting dihydropyridines. Studies to date have not implicated the longer-acting forms, and no recommendations suggest dismissing calcium channel blockers from the treatment alternatives. However, since there are numerous long-acting calcium channel blocker preparations and other effective alternatives for athletes, initial therapy with short-acting calcium channel blockers should probably be avoided while current prospective investigations are ongoing.

Central Alpha Antagonists Central alpha antagonists act on alpha$_2$-receptors in the central nervous system to block central sympathetic stimulation. Although they reduce both heart rate and TPR at rest, they provide a normal hemodynamic response to most levels of exercise. For intense exercise, further studies are needed to confirm the efficacy of central alpha antagonists in the athletic population. In addition, they are associated with a high side-effect profile, and are not recommended as first-line therapy.

Angiotensin II Receptor Blockers Angiotensin II receptor blockers are a recent addition to the pharmacologic treatment options of hypertension and provide a safe and effective alternative for treatment. They work by inhibiting the renin–angiotensin system at a different point in the pathway than the ACEIs. One advantage is that they are less likely to induce cough than ACEIs. They appear equally efficacious to ACEIs in clinical trials, but their use in athletes is not yet established.

SUMMARY

Systemic hypertension is the most common cardiovascular condition in athletes and warrants careful assessment. The great majority of athletes with elevated blood pressures have essential hypertension. If evaluation does not point to secondary causes,

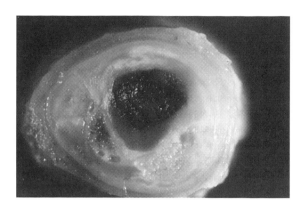

Figure 17-1. A completely occluded coronary artery noted at autopsy. (Courtesy of Mercke Sharp & Dohme.)

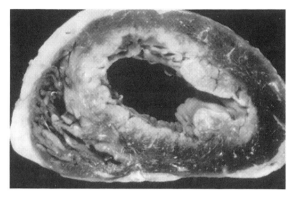

Figure 17-2. Myocardial infarction involving left ventricular wall. (Courtesy of Gower Medical Publishing Ltd.)

SYMPTOMS AND SIGNS OF CORONARY ARTERY DISEASE

Coronary atherosclerotic heart disease is the most common cause of exercise-related sudden cardiac death in adults over 30 years. As the most common disease in Western societies, it must be suspected in all adult subjects planning to take part in athletic endeavors.

If suspected, symptoms of coronary artery disease may be easily recognized. Typical symptoms include classic angina (a pressure-type pain in the chest) or similar discomfort in the neck, jaws, shoulders, arms, and back precipitated by exercise or excitement that disappears with cessation of activity, relief of tension, or the use of coronary dilating drugs such as nitroglycerin. Rapid onset of tiredness or shortness of breath, out of proportion to the physical activity, that is relieved with cessation of activity could also be related to coronary artery disease.

Ischemia of the myocardium decreases contractility and can lead to symptoms other than the typical anginal discomfort, such as shortness of breath or unusual fatigue. Cardiac arrhythmias often produce dizziness or syncope. Ischemia can produce the arrhythmias, or conversely the arrhythmias may be a result of exercise-induced ischemia, with both tachycardia and bradycardia occurring in association with coronary artery spasm, as described by Prinzmetal. A history of irregular heart activity of all types, even without symptoms, should be noted and appropriately investigated and treated, if necessary.

Physical findings may be totally absent even with advanced coronary disease. Findings of a significantly increasing or decreasing blood pressure during exercise, particularly when associated with angina-like pain, suggest significant coronary artery disease. Rapid heart rhythms, which may be regular or irregular, and rather sudden bradyarrhythmias with or without chest discomfort during or after exercise may be related to ischemia of the conduction system or a neurohumoral mechanism. Change in the quality of cardiac sounds after exercise, such as a decreased S_1, development of an S_3 or S_4 gallop and systolic murmurs indicating mitral regurgitation, may be due to myocardial ischemia. The murmur results from decreased muscular support of the mitral valve and changes in ventricular contractility that are characteristic of exercise-related changes in coronary occlusive disease.

EVALUATION

Considering the prevalence of coronary artery disease, preventing exercise-related sudden cardiac death hinges upon careful screening and assessment of subjects prior to their participation in physically demanding activity. Preparticipation medical evaluation has been discussed in previous chapters. With respect to coronary disease, inquiring about commonly known risk factors such as hyperlipidemia, hypertension, use of tobacco (specifically smoking), diabetes mellitus, and inactivity is very important. In addition, a family history of coronary artery disease, unexplained sudden death, or symptoms or physical findings that suggest either intracranial arterial disease or peripheral vascular disease may indicate a greater likelihood for coronary artery disease.

If coronary artery disease is known, good blood pressure control is an important prerequisite before exercise. Blood pressures consistently over 140/90 mm Hg, elevated diastolic pressure greater than 100 and systolic greater than 200, should be controlled before an athlete participates in events, even though this may be tolerated in the absence of coronary or other vascular problems.

Presence of a total cholesterol >200 mg/dL (5.2 mmol/L), LDL >130 mg/dL (3.4 mmol/L), HDL <35 mg/dL (0.9 mmol/L), total cholesterol/HDL ratio of >4.5, and triglycerides >250 mg/dL (2.85 mmol/L) may be correlated with an increased likelihood of coronary artery disease. In the presence of coronary disease, lipid levels should be controlled to a total cholesterol of less than 180 mg/dL (4.64 mmol/L), LDL less than 100 mg/dL (2.6 mmol/L), and HDL above 40 mg/dL (1.07 mmol/L). Deviation from these goals does not imply that the individual should eliminate physical activity, but continuation of lipid abnormalities may be associated with progression of atherosclerosis and an increased likelihood of exercise-related cardiac events. To lessen morbidity, all individuals and certainly the serious exercise participant should be willing to control lipids and other risk factors.

Recent studies by Blair et al. (6) demonstrate that, even without evidence of coronary disease, poor conditioning (as indicated by a maximum graded exercise test of less than 7 METs) is associated with a significantly higher frequency of cardiovascular events than with even moderate conditioning. For example, data show that subjects who have either work or recreational activity levels approaching 8400 kJ/week are far less likely to have significant coronary disease (7). Poor fitness levels and inactivity both appear to increase the risk of cardiac events.

Careful control of diabetes to avoid both hypoglycemic and hyperglycemic events is absolutely essential in individuals of any age who participate in athletic events. This is particularly true for those with coronary artery disease; with profuse sweating and/or polyuria, hypoglycemia and loss of body fluids may cause a drop in blood pressure and precipitate coronary events. A common-sense approach to evaluating subjects with diabetes or other major and minor cardiac risk factors will help lessen the risk of exercise-related sudden cardiac events.

Diagnostic Evaluation

The diagnostic studies most valuable in subjects with known coronary disease are those that test physical tolerance and cardiac function during an exercise activity that equals or exceeds the exercise level anticipated in training or competition. The graded exercise test with electrocardiographic and blood pressure monitoring alone, or preceded and followed by echocardiography, has been our most valuable method of assessment. The graded exercise test provides information regarding a subject's blood pressure, pulse rate, and electrocardiographic changes associated with increasing levels of exercise. Adding the pre- and postexercise echocardiogram detects the effect of exercise on myocardial contractility. Hypocontractility or other changes in the ventricular wall following exercise are highly suggestive of decreased myocardial blood flow and can forewarn that cardiac events may take place during training or competition. A resting two-dimensional echocardiogram alone may be all that is required to assess the magnitude of the effect of coronary artery disease on left ventricular function by determining left ventricular wall motion abnormalities, left ventricular ejection fraction, and chamber size. Radionuclear studies to evaluate myocardial perfusion may be helpful in determining the cause of myocardial contractile abnormalities. In all graded exercise tests, valuable information related to maximum exercise, pulse rate, and rate of perceived exertion allows the subjects to monitor themselves, and potentially prevent the arrhythmias or ischemia that may precipitate cardiac events.

With the availability of good noninvasive studies where the exercise level approximates or exceeds the subject's training regimen or competitive demands, one can usually obtain all the information needed to determine the risk of exercise-induced cardiac events. Invasive studies such as cardiac catheterization, coronary arteriography, and left ventriculograms are not usually necessary to determine whether a subject can participate in an athletic event.

SPECIAL CONSIDERATIONS IN ATHLETES WITH CORONARY ARTERY DISEASE

By using risk factor stratification in subjects with known coronary disease, one can predict whether certain cardiac events are more likely during training and competition. With this information, the physician can advise the potential athlete at which level he or she should perform and the types of sporting events in which competition probably would be safe.

Risk Stratifications

Subjects with coronary artery disease can be stratified into those who have low, intermediate, and high risk. For the purpose of this discussion, low risk subjects have a mildly increased likelihood of having sudden cardiac events with exercise; those with intermediate or greater risk have a significantly increased risk of exercise-induced cardiac events.

Low Risk   Althletes would fall into the low risk category if they have the following:

- Absence of exercise-induced ischemia or angina on graded exercise testing.
- Absence of complex ventricular arrhythmias during exercise.
- An exercise tolerance on the treadmill or ergometer of greater than 10 METs if less than 50 years of age; greater than 9 METs from age 50 to 59 years; greater than 8 METs from age 60 to 69 years; and greater than 7 METs if age 70 years and above (8).

- Echocardiographic or noninvasive finding of normal left ventricular systolic function with ejection fractions of >50%.
- If catheterization has been performed, subjects should have no significant coronary luminal diameter narrowing (<60% blockage) that is uncorrected by myocardial revascularization by intracoronary intervention or surgical procedures.

Intermediate Risk   Althletes have intermediate risk, with significant increase in risk of sudden events, with any of the following:

- Evidence of myocardial ischemia by electrocardiographic or symptomatic changes with exercise.
- Evidence of complex ventricular arrhythmias associated with exercise.
- Impaired left ventricular function with ejection fractions of less than 45%.
- Untreated stenotic coronary artery obstruction of >60% lumen diameter.

Medications and Risk Evaluation   Because individuals with coronary disease who participate in athletic events usually take medication, the exercise evaluation should be performed while these patients are on their usual medication regimen. Thus, a more accurate blood pressure and pulse rate associated with various levels of exercise can be determined, particularly in the presence of beta-blockers and calcium channel blocking medications. However, the athlete should be tested *off* these medications if the drugs are prohibited in the events in which he or she wishes to participate. For example, because of the medication's effect in decreasing tremors and catecholamine response, beta-blockers are prohibited in a number of competitive sports such as archery and riflery.

Athletic Competition

Clearly, individuals with coronary artery disease who participate in athletic competition are at higher risk than those who do not. However, with careful evaluation and testing, they should be able to compete in certain events. In the 26th Bethesda Conference, Mitchell and co-workers (9) looked at the types of competitive sporting events and classified them as to their degree of static and dynamic activity. They concluded that the patients with low risk coronary disease could safely participate in sporting events with low dynamics and low-to-moderate static activities. Such sports include golf, riflery, lawn bowls, bowling, billiards, archery, horseback riding, and curling. In addition, many patients in cardiac rehabilitation programs and other individuals with documented coronary disease have competed in distance running events (ranging from 5 km to marathons) after careful evaluation and extensive training. Such athletes should, however, consider that their risk of sudden events is greater than that of the normal person their age, and they must be carefully instructed as to warning signs and symptoms. Exercise should be limited to a predetermined safe heart-rate range.

For those individuals with intermediate risk (with substantially increased risk of having cardiac events), the physician must judge the severity of the risk when determining whether they can participate in events other than golf, bowling, and billiards. Competitive running can precipitate ventricular arrhythmias. But again, even those with decreased ventricular function can participate in noncompetitive walking, running, and other aerobic events if their exercise evaluation and echocardiogram indicate that the exercise level of the event does not cause any difficulty with myocardial function.

Counseling Athletes

Regardless of the individual's fitness level, physicians, instructors, and trainers must be aware that these participants remain at higher risk. The objective measurements gained by the electrocardiogram and blood pressure cuff best determine the safe levels of exercise, because competitive individuals tend to minimize symptoms and their rate of perceived exertion during exercise testing, and denial of symptoms may be more prevalent during competition. At-risk athletic participants should be warned of the symptoms of myocardial ischemia and ventricular dysfunction, and be told to stop or markedly decrease their exercise level when these occur. Repeated instruction to observe

all signs and symptoms of problems cannot be overemphasized—subjects with coronary disease need to be told repeatedly that the absence of ischemic or arrhythmic events on exercise testing and the presence of good left ventricular function does not preclude sudden cardiac events.

The physician must discuss with the participant the magnitude of the risk, and together they must decide whether he or she should compete. Many competitive athletes insist on participating, regardless of medical advice. For this reason, physicians should provide written documentation of their recommendations for participants with coronary artery disease. Written instructions can eliminate any confusion about what has been discussed in regard to training and competition. Safe exercise heart rate ranges, duration of competition at high levels, and fluid recommendations can all be included. Both participants and physicians should sign the document.

Recovery Reevaluation

When individuals with coronary artery disease have an event such as unstable angina, myocardial infarction, nonsustained arrhythmias, or even a sudden death event from which they recover, they must be reevaluated completely and their risk level reclassified following their recovery. The athlete's individual physician, who must be aware of the complications and the severity of the disease process, decides how long the athlete will need to refrain from competition following coronary artery bypass surgery and myocardial infarction. Currently, patients are discharged 4 to 5 days after coronary bypass surgery and approximately 5 to 6 days after myocardial infarction. After leaving the hospital, they gradually resume daily activities over the next 2 to 3 weeks. However, even the gradual increasing exercise is at a much lower level than that experienced by those training for competitive events. Depending on the circumstances, training should be delayed for 6 to 12 weeks. Exercise testing is an excellent method for determining an athlete's ability to start training for the competitive arena after a major coronary event.

After any new coronary event, a complete reevaluation that includes a graded exercise test is essential, and it must be performed while the athlete is taking the prescribed medications used during competition (even if they are the same as taken during the previous tests). Repeating the previous instructions or giving new written instructions— as well as emphasizing the significance of a new exercise-induced coronary event—should be a part of the physician's counseling, as the likelihood of subsequent events may be higher than before.

REFERENCES

1 Thompson PD, Funk EJ, Carleton RA, Sturner WQ. Incidence of death during jogging in Rhode Island from 1975 through 1980. JAMA 1982;247:2535–2538.
2 Davies MJ. Anatomic features in victims of sudden coronary death. Coronary artery pathology. Circulation 1992;85(suppl):119–124.
3 Little WC. Angiographic assessment of the culprit coronary artery lesion before acute myocardial infarction. Am J Cardiol 1990;66:44G–47G.
4 Pollock ML, Dawson GA, Miller HS Jr, et al. Physiologic responses of men 49 to 65 years of age to endurance training. J Am Geriatr Soc 1976;24:97–104.
5 American College of Sports Medicine. Guidelines for exercise testing and prescription. 4th ed. Philadelphia: Lea & Febiger, 1991:8.
6 Blair SN, Kohl HW, Paffenbarger RS Jr, et al. Physical fitness and all-cause mortality. A prospective study of healthy men and women. JAMA 1989;262:2395–2401.
7 Paffenbarger RS Jr, Hyde RT, Wing AL, Hsieh CC. Physical activity, all-cause mortality, and longevity of college alumni. N Engl J Med 1986;314:605–613.
8 Thompson PD, Klocke FJ, Levine BD, Van Camp SP. 26th Bethesda Conference: recommendations for determining eligibility for competition in athletes with cardiovascular abnormalities. Task force 5: coronary artery disease. J Am Coll Cardiol 1994;24:888–892.
9 Mitchell JH, Haskell WL, Raven PB. Classification of sports. J Am Coll Cardiol 1994;24:864–866.

Chapter 18
Arrhythmias

Karl Lee Barkley II

Sudden death on the playing field, in the athletic arena, or due to physical exertion is not a new phenomenon and has received much attention due to the untimely deaths of prominent athletes at the elite and professional level (1). The mechanism of sudden death in many athletes is undoubtedly due to malignant arrhythmias (usually ventricular) even though the underlying condition that precipitates the lethal arrhythmia may be structural (hypertrophic obstructive cardiomyopathy, congenital anomalies of the coronary arteries, right ventricular dysplasia, etc.).

The athlete with symptoms of an arrhythmia (e.g., syncope or near syncope) presents a special challenge for the team physician who must correctly identify the arrhythmia, uncover any underlying cardiac conditions, and advise the athlete on prerequisites for safe return to play or competition. The workup and decision making in complex cases is best approached with the assistance of a cardiology consultant. Additional guidelines come from recently published standards for the management of athletes with arrhythmias (2).

APPROACH TO ARRHYTHMIAS IN ATHLETES

Electrocardiographic Changes in Athletes

For evaluation of an athlete with a suspected arrhythmia, the team physician needs to have a working knowledge of some of the commonly seen electrocardiographic changes associated with the well-trained athlete. "Athlete's heart" syndrome has various electrocardiographic changes as well as structural alterations (3–8). A partial summation of some of the electrocardiographic changes found with greater frequency in the trained ath-

lete, as compared to the normal population, can be found in Table 18-1. Some of these changes (bradycardia and heart blocks) have been postulated to be associated with the increased vagal tone found in the trained athlete. Although the absolute frequencies of some of these electrocardiographic changes are low (e.g., atrial fibrillation), a significantly higher frequency of these conditions has been demonstrated in the athletic population compared with matched controls (3,5).

Symptoms and Historical Features of Arrhythmias in Athletes

Symptoms that suggest arrhythmias are found in Table 18-2. Syncope is one symptom that requires an explanation in the athlete. There may be an obvious reason for the syncopal episode, such as a recent illness, heat stress, or a vasovagal episode. Continued athletic participation is possible in these cases, but it is incumbent on the physician to demonstrate the absence of pathology. Syncope may be the prime warning sign for the risk of sudden death or the existence of underlying heart problems that can produce life threatening arrhythmias (e.g., hypertrophic obstructive cardiomyopathy). Subtle symptoms of arrhythmias may often be overlooked; the team physician must use clinical suspicion to detect conditions with vague symptoms of dizziness, anxiety, fleeting discomfort, or weakness during exercise. These nonspecific symptoms may or may not initially suggest the presence of an arrhythmia.

A relevant history should include previous episodes or symptoms, recent drug use (legal as well as "recreational"), eating disorders, and history of congenital heart disease or previous cardiac sur-

Table 18-1   Electrocardiographic Changes in Athletes Versus Normal Controls

ST segment changes
T wave changes
QRS changes
QT prolongation
Sinus bradycardia (as low as 25 beats/minute)
Sinus arrhythmia
Nodal rhythm
Wandering atrial pacemaker
Heart block (first, second, and third degree)
Atrial fibrillation
Accelerated idioventricular rhythm
PACs and PVCs*
Ventricular preexcitation (WPW syndrome)*

*It is unclear as to whether there is higher incidence in athletes versus the general population.

gery. Family history of sudden death, arrhythmias, or congenital cardiac conditions (hypertrophic cardiomyopathy, long QT syndrome, etc.) are important historical factors to uncover (9). The presence or absence of certain features may direct the individual workup and suggest the need for cardiology consultation.

Workup and Evaluation of the Athlete with Suspected Arrhythmia

Presenting symptoms, historical circumstances, and physical findings direct the extent of the evaluation. An unacclimatized athlete with no prior symptoms who experiences brief syncope while competing in a hot climate may need nothing

Table 18-2   Symptoms of Arrhythmias in Athletes

Syncope or near syncope
Palpitations
Dizziness or light-headedness
Easy fatigue
Anxiety
Chest pain or discomfort
Weakness
Pallor
Seizures

more than a good history, a physical examination, observation, and perhaps an electrocardiogram (ECG). This case may suggest simple heat syncope. The athlete with new exercise-related syncope and no suggestive circumstances needs more extensive evaluation—a history, physical examination, and an ECG are considered the minimum evaluation (10). Demonstration of an arrhythmia demands a more thorough evaluation to exclude structural heart disease, assess the severity of the arrhythmia, and evaluate the response of the arrhythmia to exercise (10).

Following the history, physical examination, and ECG, additional tools for evaluating the suspected or known arrhythmia include 24-hour Holter monitoring, event monitoring, echocardiogram, chest x-ray, signal-averaged ECG, metabolic assessment, cardiac catheterization, and electrophysiologic assessment (2,9,10). During monitoring, an attempt should be made to have the athlete duplicate the particular athletic activity or exertional circumstances associated with his or her symptoms. Any symptomatic arrhythmia requires referral to and evaluation by a cardiologist before the athlete can be cleared to compete (9). Repeated evaluation to assess the response of the arrhythmia to therapy is also indicated.

MANAGEMENT PRINCIPLES OF SPECIFIC ARRHYTHMIAS

An underlying principle in evaluation and then clearance of an athlete involves establishing whether this athlete has structural heart disease associated with the arrhythmia in question. Prognosis and management decisions are, as a rule, more complicated for arrhythmias associated with structural heart disease. Despite control of the arrhythmia, the presence of structural heart disease alone may preclude full athletic participation, depending on the nature of the lesion. Evaluation of the structural lesion or condition needs to be complete, and in some cases the team physician may need to suggest an alternative sport that does not place the same dynamic demand on the athlete's heart. Comprehensive recommendations for specific management of arrhythmias in athletes have

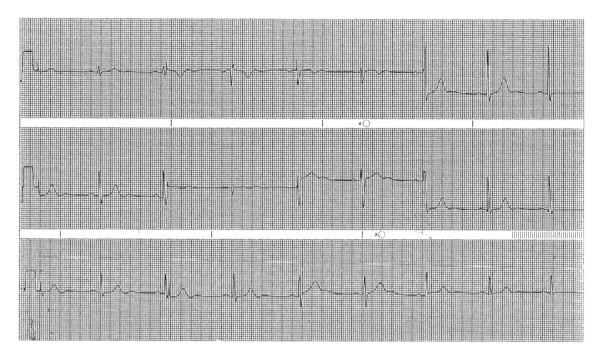

Figure 18-1.   61-year-old male marathoner running with bradycardia (HR49) typical of athletes.

been advanced by Task Force Six on arrhythmias at the 26th Bethesda Conference (2).

Sinus Node Disturbance

Athletes with a sinus node disturbance arrhythmia and no symptoms may participate in all activities and sports provided that the condition is not worsened with exercise and the heart is structurally normal (9). Sinus bradycardia (<60 beats/minute) and sinus tachycardia (>100 beats/minute) generally require no further evaluation if they occur in expected circumstances. Additionally, sinus arrhythmia (variable R-R interval) and wandering atrial pacemaker are seen commonly in athletes; in the absence of symptoms they require no restriction of activity (2) (Fig 18-1).

Athletes with syncope or other symptoms suggestive of arrhythmia should not participate until an explanation is found. Bradycardic conditions, sinus pauses, sick sinus syndrome, and inappropriate sinus tachycardia that are symptomatic should be treated with the assistance of a cardiologist. If asymptomatic for 3 to 6 months, the athlete may return to sports after reevaluation by the physician

(2,9,10). Some change in the intensity level of an activity or of the sport itself may be indicated in such cases. Classification of sports in terms of intensity helps direct safe participation, and physicians should use established standards that list sports by the degree of static and dynamic demand (2). Pacemaker patients need consultation with a cardiologist prior to sports participation, and contact sports are usually prohibited.

Premature Atrial Complexes (PACs)

The simplest form of supraventricular arrhythmia is the isolated premature atrial complex (PAC). Athletes with PACs can participate in all competitive sports (2,9,10). Evidence of Wolff-Parkinson-White syndrome, atrial flutter, and atrial fibrillation are treated differently and warrant evaluation by a cardiologist.

Atrial Flutter   Atrial flutter is an uncommon chronic arrhythmia and structural heart disease that needs to be excluded by an echocardiogram. In the absence of structural heart disease, the ventricular rate in atrial flutter must be controlled with drug therapy before the athlete is allowed to

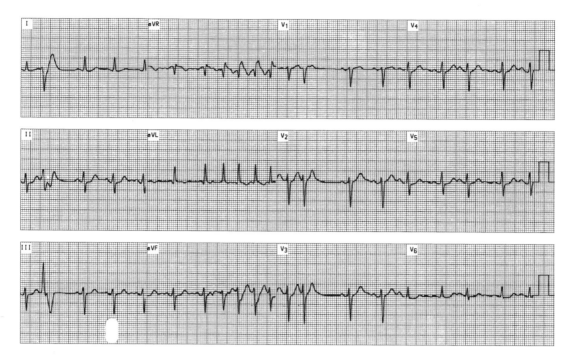

Figure 18-2.   58-year-old male marathon runner screened for positive cardiac risk factors. ETT revealed ST depression. Five minutes into exercise, the patient developed trigeminy which resolved. Three minutes into recovery, the patient developed a 6-beat run of atrial fibrillation with a heart rate of 180. Cardiac catheterization revealed triple-vessel disease.

compete in low-intensity sports. Generally, participation in all competitive sports is allowed after a 3- to 6-month period free of atrial flutter events (2,10). The athlete must be aware that rapid ventricular rates can still result. Atrial flutter in the presence of structural heart disease should limit participation of the athlete to low-intensity sports only after a 6-month period free of recurrence (2).

Atrial Fibrillation   Atrial fibrillation is found in the athletic population more often than in the general population. The physician should search for the underlying causes (e.g., thyrotoxicosis) but usually will not find structural heart disease. In the athletic population, alcohol and illicit drugs (cocaine) are also possible causes. Recommendations for athletes with atrial fibrillation without structural heart disease state that the ventricular heart rate response to exercise needs to reach the expected rate of sinus tachycardia for the athlete to compete in all competitive sports (2), with or without treatment. In the presence of structural heart

disease, the restriction is similar and takes second priority to recommendations pertaining to the structural lesion in question (Fig 18-2). Athletes requiring anticoagulation should not participate in contact sports or sports with danger of bodily collision because of the risk of bleeding complications (2,10).

Supraventricular Tachycardia (ST)

Athletes with supraventricular tachycardia (ST) whose episodes are prevented by therapy may participate in all sports (9). However, individual athletes with significant symptoms or structural heart disease need to be adequately treated and should not participate in competitive sports for 6 months (Fig 18-3). After the arrhythmia-free observation period, the athlete may pursue participation in low-intensity competitive sports (2,9,10). Athletes who undergo successful ablation of a concealed or accessory pathway may participate in all sports after 3 to 6 months without episodes. Follow-up elec-

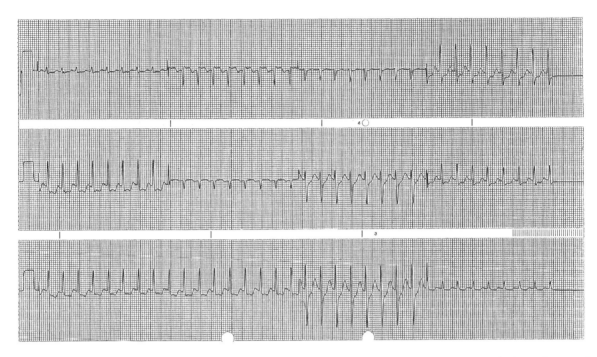

Figure 18-3. 50-year-old female water aerobics instructor who complained of fluttering in her chest and dizziness. She developed symptoms and supraventricular tachycardia with a rate of 196 and ST depression 5 minutes into the recovery phase following ETT. Rhythm and symptoms suppressed with Verapamil.

trophysiologic testing confirms adequate suppression of the arrhythmia (2).

Ventricular Preexcitation or Wolff-Parkinson-White Syndrome

A physician should have the most concern for preexcitation syndromes when they are associated with atrial flutter or fibrillation with a rapid response via an accessory pathway (Fig 18-4). Further evaluation via esophageal pacing or intracardiac electrophysiologic studies helps assess this risk. Ablation of the accessory pathway followed by 3 to 6 months of no spontaneous recurrence of tachycardia allows these athletes full participation in competitive activities (2).

Individuals greater than 20 years of age who are free of structural heart disease, palpitations, and tachycardia can participate in all competitive sports after appropriate workup (to include ECG, 24-hour Holter monitor worn during athletic activity, exercise stress test, and echocardiogram). Younger athletes have higher risk, however, and for this reason may need further evaluation before they are allowed participation in sports of greater intensity (2).

Premature Ventricular Complexes (PVCs)

Premature ventricular complexes (PVCs) occur spontaneously or are precipitated by stress, caffeine, other stimulants, sleep deprivation, or

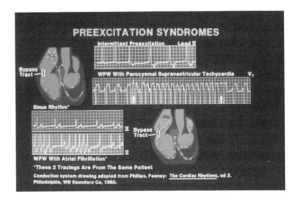

Figure 18-4. Wolff-Parkinson-White syndrome. (Courtesy of ICI Americas Inc.)

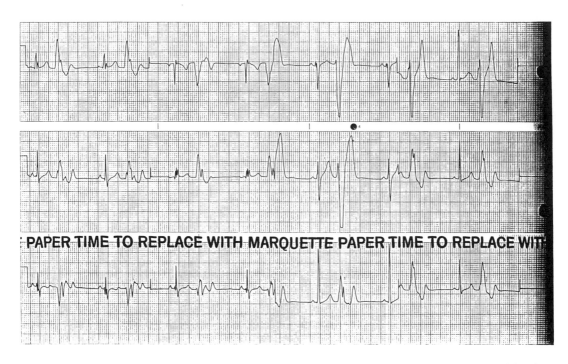

Figure 18-5. 16-year-old male guard on a basketball team who had bigeminy on preparticipation examination. ECG shows frequent PVCs with bigeminy.

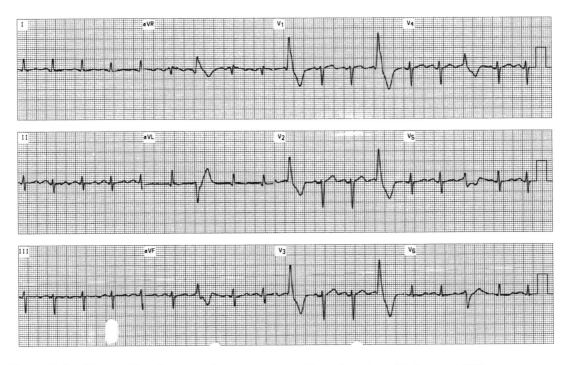

Figure 18-6. 58-year-old male runner's stress test, revealing trigeminy with frequent PVCs.

alcoholic beverages. An extremely common rhythm variant, PVCs have little prognostic significance in the individual with a healthy heart. Therefore, in the absence of symptoms, structural heart disease, coronary artery disease, or myocardial disease, athletes may participate in all competitive activities (2,9). Restriction to low-intensity sports is mandated when PVC worsens with exercise or when structural heart disease is present (9) (Figs 18-5, 18-6).

Ventricular Tachycardia

Ventricular tachycardia is defined as three or more PVCs in a row, and denotes a potentially serious arrhythmia. This includes nonsustained and monomorphic as well as sustained and polymorphic forms. Workup needs to be comprehensive and may necessitate a cardiac catheterization and electrophysiologic study. An athlete with ventricular tachycardia should not participate in competitive sports for at least 6 months following their last episode (2). If after 6 months there are no clinical episodes and the arrhythmia is not inducible, the athlete without structural heart disease may participate in all competitive sports. Athletes with structural heart disease should be limited to low-intensity sports as long as they have had no recurrences (2). An exception may be made for athletes with 8- to 10-beat salvos of nonsustained monomorphic ventricular tachycardia and rates less than 150 beats per minute (junctional tachycardia) if the arrhythmia is not worsened by exercise. Again, this implies a nonlethal arrhythmia only in the asymptomatic athlete without intrinsic heart disease (2,9).

Heart Block

First Degree and Type 1 Second Degree (Wenckebach) First degree heart block is defined by a PR interval in excess of 0.20 seconds. Second degree Wenckebach rhythm disturbance refers to a progressively prolonged PR interval until transmission of one ventricular complex is blocked. If these athletes are asymptomatic, without structural heart disease, and there is no worsening of block with exercise or during recovery, they may participate in all competitive sports (2,9) (Fig 18-7).

Type 2 Second Degree and Third Degree (Acquired and Congenital) Type 2 second-degree block is an incomplete conduction disturbance that typically occurs below the His bundle and carries a more serious prognosis than Wenckebach. In this condition, drop beats occur at a specific interval. Third-degree heart block represents a complete impasse of conduction through the AV barrier so that no P waves are transmitted to the ventricles. In both cases, the athlete should be treated with permanent pacing before any competitive activity is allowed. The presence of a pacemaker excludes the athlete from sports with risk of bodily collision (2,9).

Athletes with congenital third-degree heart block may participate in all competitive sports if

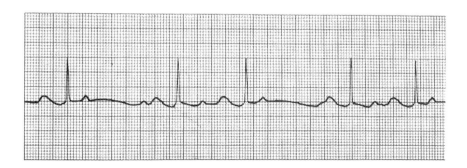

Figure 18-7.   Wenckebach phenomenon with unusually long PR prolongation. The strip displays four brief Wenckebach periods; most of these consist merely of two lengthening PR intervals followed by a dropped beat. (Reproduced by permission from Walraven G. Basic arrhythmias. 4th ed. Upper Saddle River, NJ: Prentice-Hall, 1992.)

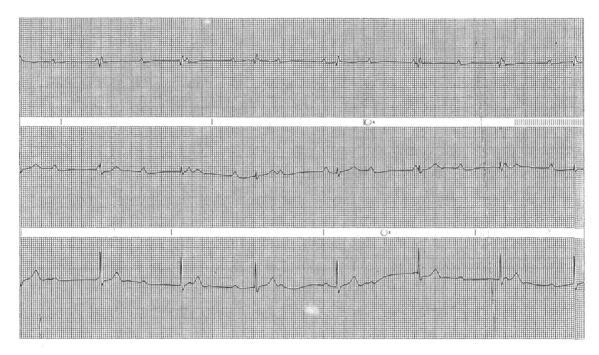

Figure 18-8.   76-year-old male senior Olympics competitor in a routine follow-up after a bout of viral pericarditis. ECG shows complete heart block.

certain conditions are met (Figs 18-8, 18-9). There must be no history of symptoms, an absence of structural heart disease, narrow QRS complex, and ventricular rates at rest of greater than 40 to 50 beats per minute. An appropriate increase in rate usually occurs as a response to exertion. Occasional PVCs are allowed, as long as ventricular tachycardia is not present. If symptoms are present or rates do not meet the criteria above, the athlete is a candidate for a pacemaker (2).

Complete Right or Left Bundle Branch Block

Complete right bundle branch block (RBBB) develops after impedance of the electrical impulse that travels down the right branch of the His bundle. Complete left bundle branch block (LBBB) represents the same phenomenon, affecting the left branch of the His bundle. In both conditions, the QRS complex widens to 0.12 second or more. Evaluation should include ECG, 24-hour Holter monitor, exercise test, and echocardiogram. Athletes may participate in all competitive sports, as-

suming no ventricular arrhythmias, no AV block with exercise, and no symptoms with exercise (2). In younger patients with LBBB, electrophysiologic studies should be considered.

Congenital Long QT Interval Syndrome

Congenital long QT interval syndrome is defined as a corrected QT interval greater than 450 milliseconds. A prolonged QT interval places the athlete at risk of the "R on T" phenomenon, in which a premature ventricular complex fires during a vulnerable phase of the recovery interval to initiate ventricular tachycardia. There is usually a positive family history associated. This excludes QT prolongation secondary to drugs or electrolyte imbalance. Persons with this syndrome should be excluded from competitive sports because of the risk of sudden death (2,9).

Commotio Cordis

Commotio cordis refers to cardiac concussion, usually from blunt trauma, and is a functional injury analogous to a cerebral concussion. In effect,

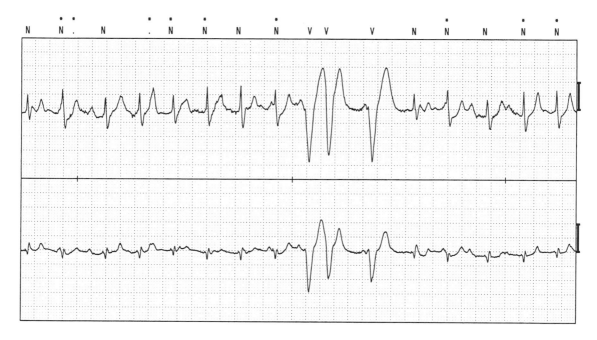

Figure 18-9. Same patient as seen in Figure 18-8. Holter monitor with exercise shows a 3-beat run of ventricular tachycardia.

there is no morphologic or structural injury, and it is a distinctly different entity from cardiac contusion. The effects of this type of injury can include sudden death despite a timely attempt at conventional resuscitation. The mechanism of death is postulated to be ventricular dysrhythmia. The event seems to be more common in children, and in some cases chest protection failed to prevent the lethal arrhythmia (11,12).

The typical scenario involves a child at play who is struck in the precordial region by a projectile such as a baseball, hockey puck, cricket ball, or lacrosse ball. The force of the blow is not noted to be unusual. The victim often becomes unconscious immediately or shortly following the impact. Resuscitative efforts are typically futile, despite being administered within the first 3 minutes in most cases (13).

Historically, the precordial thump has not been recommended for children in treatment of arrest because of the possibility of converting a benign rhythm to a malignant form. Because the mechanism of death in commotio cordis is believed to be ventricular fibrillation, at least one author has suggested that the precordial thump be considered as initial treatment when this clinical condition is suspected (11). Future research needs to be done regarding this question, and also in the matter of adequate chest protection for young athletes.

SUMMARY

Athletes with certain arrhythmias may participate fully in sports, but the presence of symptoms or structural heart disease places them in a high risk category. Individuals with a worse prognosis require careful assessment and usually need a comprehensive evaluation before returning to sport. Cardiology consultation and advanced diagnostic monitoring techniques assist in the determination of sports participation for more complicated cases. Knowledge continues to evolve about unusual conditions such as long QT interval, arrhythmogenic right ventricular dysplasia, and commotio cordis. Until more data emerge, the most comprehensive guidelines regarding sports participation of athletes with arrhythmias are detailed in proceedings from the 26th Bethesda Conference.

REFERENCES

1 Maron BJ. Sudden death in young athletes. Lessons from the Hank Gathers affair. N Engl J Med 1993;329:55–57.

2 Maron BJ, Mitchell JH. 26th Bethesda Conference. Recommendations for determining eligibility for competition in athletes with cardiovascular abnormalities. J Am Coll Cardiol 1994;24:844–899.

3 Huston TP, Puffer JC, Rodney WM. The athletic heart syndrome. N Engl J Med 1985;313:24–32.

4 Oakley GDG. The athletic heart. Cardiol Clin 1987;5:319–329.

5 Zehender M, Meinertz T, Keul J, Just H. ECG variants and cardiac arrhythmias in athletes: clinical relevance and prognostic importance. Am Heart J 1990;119:1378–1391.

6 Alpert JS, Pape LA, Ward A, Rippe JM. Athletic heart syndrome. Physician Sports Med 1989;17:103–107.

7 Zeppilli P. The athlete's heart: differentiation of training effects form organic heart disease. Practical Cardiol 1988;14:61–84.

8 Dailey SM, Oberman A. The athletic heart. Heart Dis Stroke 1993;2:53–58.

9 American Academy of Pediatrics. Committee on sports medicine and fitness. Cardiac dysrhythmias and sports. Pediatrics 1995;95:786–788.

10 Van Camp SP. Exercise related arrhythmias. Lecture at AAFP conference. Sports medicine: an in depth review. Dallas, Texas: February 15, 1995.

11 Abrunzo TJ. Commotio cordis. The single, most common cause of traumatic death in youth baseball. Am J Dis Child 1991;145:1279–1282.

12 Kaplan JA, Karofsky PS, Volturo GA. Commotio cordis in two amateur ice hockey players despite the use of commercial chest protectors:case reports. J Trauma 1993;34:151–153.

13 Maron BJ, Poliac LC, Kaplan JA, Mueller FO. Blunt impact to the chest leading to sudden death from cardiac arrest during sports activities. N Engl J Med 1995;333:337–342.

Chapter 19
Congenital Heart Disease

John M. MacKnight
Bryan W. Smith

Primary care and sports medicine physicians commonly encounter patients with congenital heart disease. Exercise recommendations must take into account the present and future functional state of the cardiovascular system, the demands placed on it by various activities, and the acute and chronic effects of the interaction between the two. Similarly, individual recommendations must consider the sport type and its specific requirements, intensity, duration, risk of injury, as well as the presence of anticoagulation.

ATRIAL SEPTAL DEFECT (ASD)

A persistent communication between the left and right atria, atrial septal defect (ASD) results from incomplete closure of the interatrial septum, usually near the foramen ovale. These are typically isolated anomalies that account for 10% to 15% of congenital heart disease cases (1). The long-term effects of an ASD are determined by the magnitude and duration of left to right shunting and the pulmonary vascular resistance (2).

Most ASDs go unrecognized for years or decades and cause no symptoms (2). When an individual is symptomatic, dyspnea and fatigue are the earliest and most frequent complaints. The classic auscultative finding is fixed splitting of S_2. A split S_1 with a loud tricuspid component, a grade II to III pulmonic midsystolic murmur, and a tricuspid mid-diastolic flow murmur may be heard.

Athletes with small defects and no pulmonary hypertension can participate in all competitive sports (3). Athletes with significant pulmonary hypertension, or a right to left shunt, or both can only participate in Class IA sports such as billiards, bowling, golf, or riflery (3,4). Patients with marked pulmonary hypertension, a large right to left shunt, and cyanosis (Eisenmenger's syndrome) are excluded from competitive sports (3).

If surgical repair is performed, patients should undergo a thorough evaluation of cardiac function and performance. Surgical repair after age 5 fails to normalize ventricular filling and relaxation, resulting in a subnormal ventricular response to exercise in 77% of patients (5). In addition, heart rate responses may be abnormal secondary to compensatory inhibition or sinus node damage during surgery. Six months after repair, athletes without evidence of pulmonary hypertension, symptomatic arrhythmias, or myocardial dysfunction may participate in all sports (3). Symptomatic athletes require an individualized exercise plan.

VENTRICULAR SEPTAL DEFECT (VSD)

Ventricular septal defects (VSDs) account for 30% of all congenital cardiac defects, with nearly 80% occurring as isolated lesions (1). Although as many as 50% of small to moderate VSDs spontaneously close by age 20, large defects rarely close (1,2). With shunting, there is a compensatory increase in left ventricular (LV) output that may lead to LV volume overload and congestive heart failure (1). Similarly, with high pulmonary volumes, pulmonary hypertension may develop and, if severe, may lead to a reversal in shunt flow direction (Eisenmenger's syndrome) and compromise of gas exchange (1).

With small defects and minimal shunting, patients are usually asymptomatic with a normal resting cardiac output. However, with exercise or increased shunting, impaired cardiac output and fatigue may occur (6). Physical examination reveals a distinctive harsh, holosystolic murmur best heard along the third and fourth left interspace and widely transmitted throughout the precordium.

Athletes with small or moderate VSDs by clinical features, normal heart size, and normal pulmonary artery pressures may participate in all competitive sports (3). Questions regarding the size or physiology of the VSD should be addressed via echocardiography or cardiac catheterization. Selected athletes with large VSDs may participate in low-intensity competitive sports (Class IA) (3).

Successful repair should result in the absence of symptoms, absence of significant cardiomegaly or arrhythmias, and normal pulmonary artery pressures. A small residual defect with evidence of a murmur may be present. Six months following repair, athletes with no residual defect or a small defect and no pulmonary hypertension, myocardial dysfunction, or arrhythmia are unrestricted in athletic participation (3). Those with a moderate or large residual defect can participate in low-intensity (Class IA) competitive sports but should have definitive repair performed (3). Athletes with residual cardiomegaly, myocardial dysfunction, or questionable pulmonary hypertension may require an exercise test or cardiac catheterization before clearance for athletic participation. Patients with persistent, severe pulmonary hypertension may not participate in competitive sports; those with significant arrhythmias, mild to moderate pulmonary hypertension, or ventricular dysfunction require individualized exercise prescription (3).

PATENT DUCTUS ARTERIOSUS (PDA)

Patent ductus arteriosus (PDA) is an abnormal persistence of the normal fetal vascular channel between the pulmonary artery and the aorta. It arises in 1 in 2000 live births and is associated with maternal rubella, birth at high altitude, and prematurity (2). The degree of left to right shunting is determined by the size of the communication, the pulmonary vascular resistance, and the functional

capability of the volume-loaded left ventricle (2). Most PDAs are small, have minimal shunting, are asymptomatic, and cause no long-term effects. Larger defects may result in LV enlargement, cardiomegaly, and heart failure symptoms. Physical examination reveals a continuous murmur that peaks around S_2 and is maximal in the first or second left intercostal space. Patients with larger PDAs may develop a widened pulse pressure.

Athletes with small defects can participate in all competitive sports. As defect size increases, exercise and the resulting peripheral vasodilation may induce a differential cyanosis as the shunt direction is reversed from right to left. Those with a moderate to large PDA must undergo surgical correction prior to unrestricted participation. Those with persistent right to left shunting and severe pulmonary hypertension (Eisenmenger's syndrome) are restricted completely from sports participation (3). Following repair, no restrictions are necessary for asymptomatic individuals with no evidence of pulmonary hypertension or cardiac enlargement (3). Athletes with residual pulmonary hypertension should be restricted from athletic participation.

CONGENITAL AORTIC STENOSIS (AS)

Congenital aortic stenosis (AS) occurs in approximately 2% of the population and is most commonly due to a bicuspid valve formation. Similar LV outflow obstruction may also be caused by subaortic or supravalvular etiologies. The pathophysiology arises from impaired LV outflow and compensatory hypertrophy of the interventricular septum, and LV free wall occurs over time. LV function then deteriorates, and patients may develop significant myocardial ischemia from the increased pressure workload of the heart (7). Patients subsequently develop angina, inappropriate diaphoresis, and congestive heart failure.

In a collaborative study of children with heart disease, AS was the most common cause of sudden unexpected death, accounting for 18% of total mortality with almost 20% of AS-associated death occurring during sports (8). Sudden death risk is even greater in adults and is more likely to occur with severe stenosis, severe LV hypertrophy, exertional syncope, chest pain, dyspnea, or LV strain on ECG (9).

An aortic ejection sound is characteristic of valvular stenosis and is most prominent at the cardiac apex. A midsystolic, harsh murmur is maximally heard in the right second intercostal space, radiating into the neck. The second heart sound, which is usually single, may be normal or paradoxically split. Occasionally, a systolic thrill maximal in the second intercostal space is found. Chest x-ray may show poststenotic dilatation of the aorta and a calcified aortic valve.

Prior to exercise prescription, an assessment of the severity of aortic stenosis is required. A peak systolic transvalvular pressure gradient at rest ≤20 mm Hg by Doppler or cardiac catheterization characterizes mild stenosis, 21 to 49 mm Hg characterizes moderate stenosis, and ≥50 mm Hg characterizes severe stenosis (9). In addition, patients with fatigue, light-headedness, dizziness, chest pain, syncope, or pallor on exertion may require a more extensive evaluation with cardiac catheterization and exercise testing.

Untreated athletes with mild AS can participate in all sports if they have a normal ECG and exercise tolerance, and no history of exercise-associated chest pain, syncope, or arrhythmia with symptoms (3). Athletes with moderate AS demonstrating mild or no LV hypertrophy by echocardiography, no LV strain on ECG, a normal exercise test, and absence of exercise-associated symptoms can participate in low-static or low-to-moderate dynamic exercises and moderate-static or low-dynamic exercises (Classes IA, IB, and IIA) such as baseball, volleyball, archery, or diving, along with Class IA sports (3–5). Athletes with severe AS should not participate in competitive sports (10).

When surgical repair is performed, hypertrophy may regress and exercise capacity may improve (11). However, patients may have residual outflow obstruction, aortic valve insufficiency, ventricular arrhythmias, or LV dysfunction (12). Following surgical repair, a thorough reevaluation, which may include exercise stress testing or cardiac catheterization, is required to assess for residual stenosis or regurgitation. Athletes with mild, moderate, or severe residual stenosis should be managed as outlined above. Those with aortic regurgitation should follow exercise recommendations for regurgitant lesions.

PULMONIC STENOSIS (PS)

Pulmonic valve stenosis generally presents as an isolated and uncomplicated anomaly resulting from valvular, subvalvular (infundibular), or rarely, supravalvular pathology. It accounts for approximately 10% of all congenital heart disease. Significant right ventricular (RV) pressure overload can occur, leading to RV hypertrophy and potentially subsequently resulting in RV failure (1).

Symptoms most commonly include exercise-induced dyspnea and fatigue. Patients may also experience giddiness, light-headedness, chest pain, or syncope, and are at increased risk for exercise-associated arrhythmias. Physical exam reveals jugular venous distention with giant A waves. The RV impulse extends up to the left third intercostal space. A midsystolic murmur and thrill are maximal in the second left interspace with radiation upward to the left. There may be a pulmonic ejection click, and the pulmonic component of S_2 is delayed and soft.

In untreated PS, athletes with a peak systolic gradient less than 50 mm Hg and normal RV function can participate in all competitive sports if asymptomatic and followed on an annual basis (3). Those with gradients greater than 50 mm Hg can participate in Class IA activities but should be referred for definitive treatment (3).

Balloon valvuloplasty is now the preferred reparative method in children. Those patients who have adequate relief of obstruction and normal RV function are unrestricted for athletic participation. Those undergoing valvuloplasty should resume athletic participation 1 month after their procedure, and those who require operative repair should begin 3 months afterward (3). Athletes with persistent peak systolic gradients greater than 50 mm Hg should participate in only Class IA activities (3). Patients with severe pulmonary incompetence with marked RV enlargement should be restricted from physical activity.

COARCTATION OF THE AORTA

Coarctation of the aorta is a vascular obstructive lesion typically located near the aortic origin of the ductus arteriosus. Severe systemic hypertension proximal to the obstruction greatly increases the risk of stroke, congestive heart failure, aortic rupture and dissection, and endocarditis (13). Ischemia and progressive myocardial dysfunction may occur if the LV load is not addressed (7).

Symptoms generally arise in early infancy or at 20 to 30 years of age and can include headache, spontaneous epistaxis, and leg fatigue. Physical examination may reveal disparity in arm, chest, and shoulder girdle development and in upper and lower extremity pulses and blood pressures. The aortic component of S_2 is typically accentuated. A medium-pitched systolic murmur with a blowing quality is classic, and a low-pitched continuous murmur of collateral circulation may be heard over the posterior chest wall. Chest x-ray may reveal characteristic rib notching as a result of increased intercostal artery pressures and flow.

Untreated patients with a mild coarctation and absence of large collateral vessels or severe aortic root dilatation, a normal exercise test, a pressure gradient between upper and lower limbs less than 20 mm Hg at rest, and a peak systolic blood pressure with exercise less than 230 mm Hg can engage in all competitive sports (3). Those with a systolic arm/leg gradient greater than 20 mm Hg or systolic blood pressure greater than 230 mm Hg may engage only in low-intensity competitive sports (Class IA) until treated (3).

The majority of patients undergo surgical repair or balloon arterioplasty during childhood. After repair, however, patients may continue to have exaggerated blood pressure and LV contractility responses to exercise (10). Participation in sports 6 months after repair is permitted for athletes with less than 20 mm Hg arm/leg blood pressure gradient at rest and a normal peak systolic blood pressure during rest and exercise (3). During the first postoperative year, patients should refrain from high-intensity static exercise and collision sports (3). After 1 year, asymptomatic individuals with normal blood pressures at rest and exercise may participate in all sports except power-lifting. Athletes with significant aortic root dilatation, wall thinning, or aneurysm formation should be restricted to low-intensity competitive sports (Class IA) (14).

TETRALOGY OF FALLOT (TOF)

Tetralogy of Fallot (TOF) consists of a VSD, RV outflow obstruction, RV hypertrophy, and an overriding aorta. It accounts for 10% of congenital heart disease cases and also represents the largest proportion of adults with cyanotic congenital heart disease (2). The pathophysiology of TOF is related to the degree of RV outflow tract obstruction and the systemic vascular resistance. With strenuous isotonic exertion, muscle arterioles dilate, causing a decrease in systemic vascular resistance and an increase in right to left shunting (7). Myocardial ischemia and systemic acidosis can result. Alternatively, high-intensity isometric exercise increases systemic vascular resistance and decreases right to left shunting; in the face of a fixed pulmonary obstruction, this causes a decrease in systemic flow, syncope, or, infrequently, death (15). Progressive RV dilatation causes 50% of patients to demonstrate a vital capacity less than 80% of predicted, a reduced respiratory reserve, and a low exercise capacity (16). A majority of patients also develop ectopy with exercise, including complex ventricular arrhythmias (16).

Patients most commonly complain of dyspnea on exertion; squatting for relief of symptoms, although rarely seen in adults, is considered diagnostic in children (2). A physical exam may frequently reveal clubbing. An RV impulse and systolic thrill can be palpable at the left midsternal border. A harsh midsystolic murmur may be heard in the same location with a single S_2 of aortic origin. Chest x-ray reveals a normal-sized, boot-shaped heart with a prominent RV and concavity of the RV outflow tract.

Most patients require surgical repair. Long-standing cyanosis or volume overload may cause residual LV dysfunction. A persistent reduction in work performance is directly related to the degree of residual disease (17). Sudden death correlates with the presence of exercise-induced ventricular arrhythmias (1).

Because repaired subjects often have diminished exercise performance despite excellent hemodynamics, exercise testing should be performed prior to sports participation (18). Patients with prominent symptoms or cardiomegaly should undergo echocardiography or cardiac catheterization as well. Those athletes with an excellent postoperative result, normal or near-normal right heart pressures, mild RV volume overload, no significant right to left shunt, and no rhythm disturbances may participate in all competitive sports (3). Patients with marked pulmonary regurgitation, RV hypertension (peak systolic RV pressure >50% of systemic pressure), or rhythm disturbances should participate in only low-intensity competitive sports (Class IA) (3).

TRANSPOSITION OF THE GREAT VESSELS (TGV)

Transposition of the great vessels (TGV) accounts for 5% to 8% of congenital heart cases (2). There are two basic forms: the classic noncommunicating type and the rare congenitally corrected type. Physical examination may reveal a forceful or hyperdynamic RV lift, an audible sound of pulmonic valve closure, or a pulmonic stenosis murmur. Chest x-ray may reveal an "egg-on-side" appearance of the heart due to the position of the pulmonary artery.

Most patients undergo surgical repair at an early age. Older procedures such as the Mustard or Senning repair have been replaced by the more anatomically correct arterial switch. Patients who have undergone a more dated repair may have an altered physiologic response to exercise because the right ventricle remains the systemic pump. Nevertheless, many long-term survivors may be asymptomatic with daily activities (13).

For the athlete with a Mustard or Senning repair, high-intensity isometric or dynamic sports are not recommended because of concerns about RV reserve and the unclear effects of RV hypertrophy and dilatation (19). Prior to participation, all postoperative patients should undergo a comprehensive evaluation including echocardiogram, Holter monitoring, and exercise testing. Cardiac catheterization may be necessary if hemodynamic status is unclear. Mustard or Senning patients with no significant cardiac enlargement, no history of atrial or ventricular arrhythmias, no history of syncope, and a normal exercise test may engage in low-to-moderate static, low-dynamic competitive sports (Classes IA and IIA) (3,4). Patients with any of these abnormalities must have an individualized exercise prescription.

Current recommendations for patients who have undergone an arterial switch procedure allow full participation 6 months after surgery if there is a normal heart size, no residual defects, normal ventricular function, a normal exercise test, and absence of arrhythmias with symptoms (3). High static sports associated with extreme isometric effort such as weightlifting, gymnastics, wrestling, and cycling (Classes IIIA, IIIB, and IIIC) should be discouraged because of the possibility of producing or worsening aortic regurgitation (3–5). Athletes with more than mild hemodynamic abnormalities or ventricular dysfunction but a normal exercise test may participate in low-to-moderate static/low-dynamic competitive sports (Classes IA, IB, IC, and IIA) (3). Patients with congenitally corrected TGV without other cardiac abnormalities and no evidence of cardiomegaly or arrhythmia may participate in all activities (3). Periodic reevaluation is necessary to follow for the development of arrhythmias, progressive RV deterioration, or systemic AV (tricuspid) valve regurgitation.

EBSTEIN'S ANOMALY

Ebstein's anomaly is a congenital malformation in which the tricuspid valve leaflets fail to attach normally to the tricuspid annulus, displacing the valve orifice into the right ventricle. Mean age of diagnosis is in the midteens and may be heralded by dyspnea, palpitations, cyanosis, and angina-like chest pain. Fifty to eighty percent of patients experience intermittent or persistent cyanosis, which tends to be progressive (2). Long-standing tricuspid valve dysfunction may lead to RV failure (2). Physical exam may reveal a systolic thrill and murmur of tricuspid regurgitation, wide splitting of the first and second heart sounds, prominent third and fourth heart sounds, and a pulsatile liver.

Athletes with mild disease, no cyanosis, and no arrhythmias may participate in all sports. Those with moderate tricuspid regurgitation and no evidence of arrhythmia may participate in low-intensity competitive sports (Class IA) (3). Athletes with severe uncorrected Ebstein's anomaly are precluded from any sports participation; however, following repair, those with only mild tricuspid regurgitation and absence of arrhythmias may participate in Class IA activities.

REFERENCES

1 Perrault H, Drblik SP. Exercise after surgical repair of congenital cardiac lesions. Sports Med 1989;7:18–31.
2 Perloff JK. The clinical recognition of congenital heart disease. 3rd ed. Philadelphia: WB Saunders, 1987.
3 Graham TP, Bricker JT, James FW, Strong WB. 26th Bethesda Conference. Revised eligibility recommendations for competitive athletes with cardiovascular abnormalities. Task Force 1: congenital heart disease. J Am Coll Cardiol 1994;24:867–873.
4 Mitchell JH, Haskell WL, Raven PB. 26th Bethesda Conference. Classification of sports. J Am Coll Cardiol 1994;24:864–866.
5 Reybrouck T, Bisschop A, Dumoulin M, van der Hauwaert LG. Cardiorespiratory exercise capacity after surgical closure of atrial septal defect is influenced by the age at surgery. Am Heart J 1991;122:1073–1078.
6 Jablonsky G, Hilton JD, Liu PP, et al. Rest and exercise ventricular function in adults with congenital ventricular septal defects. Am J Cardiol 1983;51:293–298.
7 Freed MD. Recreational and sports recommendations for the child with heart disease. Pediatr Clin North Am 1984;31:1307–1320.
8 Lambert EC, Menon VA, Wagner HR, et al. Sudden unexpected death from cardiovascular disease in children. A cooperative international study. Am J Cardiol 1974;34:89–96.
9 Doyle EF, Arumugham P, Lara E, et al. Sudden death in young patients with congenital aortic stenosis. Pediatrics 1974;53:481–489.
10 Braunwald E. Heart disease: a textbook of cardiovascular medicine. 4th ed. Philadelphia: WB Saunders, 1992
11 Cullen S, Celermajer DS, Deanfield JE. Exercise in congenital heart disease. Cardiol Young 1991;1:129–135.
12 Beekman RH. Exercise recommendations for adolescents after surgery for congenital heart disease. Pediatrician 1986;13:210–219.
13 Koster NK. Physical activity and congenital heart disease. Nurs Clin North Am 1994;29:345–356.
14 Pelech AN, Kartodihardjo W, Balfe JA, et al. Exercise in children before and after coarctectomy: hemodynamic, echocardiographic, and biochemical assessment. Am Heart J 1986;112:1263–1270.
15 Deanfield JE, McKenna WJ, Hallidie-Smith KA. Detection of late arrhythmia and conduction disturbance after correction of tetralogy of Fallot. Br Heart J 1980;44:248–253.
16 Rowe SA, Zahka KG, Manolio TA, et al. Lung function and pulmonary regurgitation limit exercise capacity in postoperative tetralogy of Fallot. J Am Coll Cardiol 1991;17:461–466.
17 Wessel HA, Cunningham WJ, Paul MH, et al. Exercise performance after tetralogy of Fallot intracardiac repair. J Thorac Cardiovasc Surg 1980;80:582–593.
18 Goldberg B, Fripp RR, Lister G, et al. Effect of physical training on exercise performance of children following surgical repair of congenital heart disease. Pediatrics 1981;68:691–699.
19 Graham TP Jr. Hemodynamic residua and sequelae following intraatrial repair of transposition of the great arteries: a review. Pediatr Cardiol 1982;2:203–213.

Chapter 20
Marfan's Syndrome

Bryan W. Smith
John M. MacKnight

Marfan's syndrome is an autosomal dominant, heritable disorder of connective tissue. For more than 100 years since Antoine Bernard-Jean Marfan, a French pediatrician, reported arachnodactyly and scoliosis in a 5 year old, the diagnosis of this multisystem disorder has been elusive due to the clinical variability both among and within families (1,2). For some, the diagnosis is made postmortem following sudden death. Aortic dissection and rupture along with severe aortic regurgitation account for the majority of deaths in adolescents and adults with Marfan's syndrome (3). In athletes, Maron et al. (4) have reported that approximately 6% to 7% of sudden death events in young athletes are due to aortic rupture secondary to Marfan's syndrome.

EPIDEMIOLOGY AND GENETICS

The prevalence of Marfan's syndrome is estimated to be 1 in 10,000 (5). There is no racial or ethnic predilection, and males and females are equally affected (6). The syndrome does not skip generations, but at least 25% to 35% of the cases occur sporadically with the absence of a family history (2,5). The mutation may occur more frequently with advanced parental age (5).

The genetic defect has been located on the long arm of chromosome 15 that encodes for a glycoprotein called fibrillin, which is widely distributed in elastic tissues (2). There are multiple mutations, 14 identified so far. Unfortunately, the mutations appear to be unique by family, which limits the usefulness of routine genetic screening (2).

Clinical Manifestations

Multiple variations can be seen in a variety of organ systems in dealing with Marfan's syndrome (Table 20-1, Fig 20-1). Even though a family may have a unique mutation, the clinical features may vary due to the pleiotropic effect of the mutation. The most commonly affected organ systems are the musculoskeletal, cardiovascular, and ocular. Many of the common clinical manifestations worsen with growth, such as pectus deformities and scoliosis, which can delay diagnosis until adolescence or early adulthood.

Cardiovascular Manifestations

Numerous cardiovascular manifestations have been documented in individuals with Marfan's syndrome (see Table 20-1). Prior to the advent of echocardiography, such abnormalities were estimated to occur in 40% to 60% of patients (7). Now, it is well established that more than 95% of those with Marfan's syndrome have cardiovascular abnormalities. For optimal management, these abnormalities need to be identified prior to serious or life-threatening complications. The structural defects that lead to complications such as congestive heart failure, endocarditis, and dysrhythmias involve either a redundant mitral valve, a dilated aortic root, or not uncommonly both abnormalities.

The mitral valve can have multiple abnormalities that lead to mitral valve prolapse and to moderate or severe mitral regurgitation in greater than 25% of cases (8). Abnormal chordae tendineae at the origin of the posterior leaflet and increased annular distensibility are believed responsible for mitral valve prolapse (9). The altered architecture results in uniform billowing of the leaflets as seen on echocardiography (9). Pini et al. (9) noted this finding on every Marfan's patient with mitral valve prolapse, compared with 50% of

Table 20-1 Manifestations of Marfan's Syndrome

Skeletal
  Anterior chest deformity
  Arachnodactyly
  Scoliosis
  Thoracic lordosis
  Tall stature
  High arched palate
  Congenital flexion contracture
  Hypermobile joints
Ocular
  Superior lens dislocation*
  Flat cornea
  Elongated globe
  Retinal detachment
  Myopia
Pulmonary
  Spontaneous pneumothorax
  Apical bleb

Cardiovascular
  Ascending aorta dilatation*
  Aortic dissection*
  Aortic regurgitation
  Mitral regurgitation 2° to MVP
  Calcification of mitral annulus
  Mitral valve prolapse
  Abdominal aortic aneurysm
  Dysrhythmia
  Endocarditis
Skin and Integument
  Striae distensae
  Inguinal hernia
Central Nervous System
  Dural ectasia*
  Sacral meningocele
  Dilated cisterna magna
Learning Disabilities
Hyperactivity With or Without ADD

*Major manifestations listed in decreasing specificity.
SOURCE: Pyeritz RE, McKusick VA. The Marfan's syndrome: diagnosis and management [review]. N Engl J Med 1979;300:772–777.

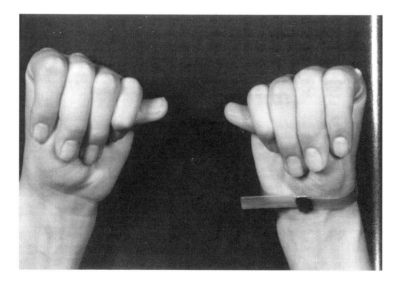

Figure 20-1. The "thumb sign" in Marfan's syndrome. The thumbs protrude from the clenched fists of a 24-year-old man who presented with congestive heart failure due to severe chronic aortic regurgitation and left ventricular dysfunction. Arachnodactyly ("spider finger") and loose joints account for the ability to position the fingers this way. The patient also had other skeletal features of Marfan's syndrome, including pectus excavatum and a high arched palate. (Reprinted by permission of the *New England Journal of Medicine,* from Falk RH. Images in clinical medicine: the "thumb sign" in Marfan's syndrome. N Engl J Med 1995;333:430. Copyright 1995 Massachusetts Medical Society. All rights reserved.)

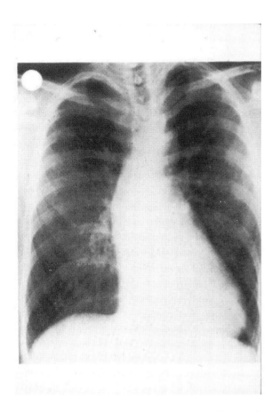

Figure 20-2. Posteroanterior chest radiograph of an 18-year-old male swimmer with Marfan's syndrome. (Reprinted with permission from the American College of Cardiology, from Maron BJ, Epstein SE, Roberts WC. Causes of death in competitive athletes. J Am Coll Cardiol 1986;7:204–214.)

non-Marfan's patients with mitral valve prolapse. Other factors involved in the development of mitral regurgitation are calcification of the annuli, rupture of the chordae tendineae, and papillary muscle dysfunction (10). Around the time of adolescence to early adulthood, palpitations and dysrhythmias become noticeable. The more redundant the mitral valve, the more prevalent ventricular and supraventricular dysrhythmias become (8).

Aortic root and sinus dilation may be present at the time of birth, whereas dilatation of the ascending aorta usually does not begin until the child is older (11) (Fig 20-2). The rate of dilatation is unpredictable, but any enlargement beyond the time of long bone epiphyseal closure should be ascribed

to pathologic dilatation (8). Throughout childhood, Marfan's patients have aortic root diameters at the upper limit of normal or larger (11). When the Valsalva's sinuses have dilated such that the cusps fail to coapt in diastole, aortic regurgitation occurs. This is usually seen in adulthood. The aortic root must dilate to 50 to 55 mm to have audible aortic regurgitation. Prophylactic surgical repair of the aortic root is usually recommended when the root diameter reaches 55 mm (5,8,12,13).

The most dramatic cardiovascular manifestation is aortic dissection, which occurs in about two-thirds of cases (14). This was thought to be due to cystic medial necrosis, but now it is believed to be the result of separation and fragmentation of elastic components of the aorta (15). With dilatation, there is an increase in the longitudinal wall stress that results in a transverse tear of the aortic intima (13). Dissection and eventual aortic rupture do not occur in the absence of a tear. The predisposing factor for the tear is that the aorta lacks the usual amount of distensibility due to the elastic architectural deficiency (7,16).

The usual location for aortic dissection is just distal to the origin of the coronary arteries. Other sites in the aorta have been documented, such as the aortic arch, descending aorta, and abdominal aorta. The greater the degree of aortic dilatation, the greater the risk of dissection (8).

DIAGNOSIS

Due to the intrafamilial clinical variability, the definitive diagnosis is difficult to establish. Diagnosis becomes more problematic when no family history exists. There are several disorders of connective tissue that mimic Marfan's syndrome, such as homocystinuria, familial mitral valve prolapse syndrome, Ehlers-Danlos syndrome, congenital contractual syndrome, and Stickler's syndrome (17,18). Table 20-2 outlines the criteria for diagnosis of Marfan's syndrome. Urine amino acid analysis in the absence of pyridoxine supplementation should be performed to rule out homocystinuria (17). Conclusive diagnosis usually requires confirmation by several subspecialists working in conjunction with the primary care physician (7).

Table 20-2 Diagnostic Criteria for Marfan's Syndrome

Negative Family History (Primary Relative)
Skeletal involvement
Involvement of two other organ systems
At least one major manifestation
Absence of homocystinuria

Positive Family History (Primary Relative)
Involvement of two organ systems
At least one major manifestation (depends on family phenotype)
Absence of homocystinuria

SOURCE: Beighton P, de Paepe A, Danks D, et al. International nosology of heritable disorders of connective tissue, Berlin, 1986. Am J Med Genet 1988;29:581–594.

Marfan's syndrome remains a clinical diagnosis because of variable expressions of the multiple, identified mutation of the fibrillin gene. Recent molecular research questions the current diagnostic criteria for Marfan's syndrome and the risk for life-threatening cardiovascular malformations. Pereira et al. (2) suggest that a major manifestation should be required for diagnosis in all cases, with molecular analysis being utilized in cases of atypical disease.

A four-year, prospective study to develop a Marfan's screening protocol for athletes was conducted at the University of California at Los Angeles. Otis et al. (19) evaluated females taller than 5'10" and males taller than 6'4", using echocardiography and slit-lamp examination if any of the following criteria were positive:

- Arm span greater than height
- Moderate kyphoscoliosis
- Heart murmur or midsystolic click
- Family history of Marfan's syndrome or sudden death before 40 years
- Pectus deformity
- Decreased upper body length to lower body length ratio

No cases of Marfan's syndrome were identified from the more than 1000 athletes who participated. Arm span and body ratio, which are commonly employed as crude clinical screens, were not discriminating (19,20). Mellion (21) has suggested that individuals with two of the six above-mentioned criteria be sent for echocardiography and slit-lamp eye evaluation, but there are no data to validate the usefulness of this practice.

MANAGEMENT

Considering the many potential manifestations of Marfan's syndrome, a multidisciplinary approach to management is usually optimal. Musculoskeletal manifestations such as a pectus deformity or scoliosis are common in childhood and adolescence, and they may require surgical intervention if either cardiopulmonary compromise or progressive spinal curvature beyond 45° occurs.

Ocular screening should be conducted annually. Rarely is lens surgery necessary for the typical upwardly dislocated lens seen in 60% to 80% of patients (22,23). Dislocated lenses should not disqualify one from athletic participation, but contact sports should be restricted because of the increased risk of retinal detachment (22).

Prompt cardiovascular management is critical, as this is the cause of death in over 95% of cases. Gerry et al. (8) state that the cornerstones of management are early diagnosis, physical activity restriction, reduction of hemodynamic stress on the ascending aorta, and early prophylactic surgery prior to dissection or heart failure. An annual evaluation should be a minimal requirement. This evaluation should include a complete cardiac examination and echocardiography. Either MRI or transesophageal echocardiography should be done to evaluate or monitor aortic dissection (24). Endocarditis prophylaxis should be instituted for any mitral or aortic valve defects.

In children, mitral regurgitation may be a more significant problem than aortic root dilatation. If mitral regurgitation is severe, mitral valve repair may be necessary, although the long-term results are not known. Mitral valve repair obviates the need for anticoagulation. This can allow the child to engage in mild to moderate physical activity. Competitive sports as well as activities with the danger of bodily collision should be avoided (8,25). Depending on the situation, restriction from all physical education activities may be required.

More frequent examination is needed as the aortic diameter increases. Quarterly monitoring of the aorta once the root has reached 50 mm is suggested, because the risk for dissection significantly increases at this point (26,27). Recent research has confirmed that prophylactic beta-blocker therapy slows the rate of aortic dilatation (28,29). Once the aortic root diameter has reached 55 to 60 mm, surgical evaluation for aortoplasty, graft repair, and/or aortic valve replacement is advised (5,8,12,13). Anticoagulants may be required, depending on the procedure performed.

In terms of athletic participation, the 26th Bethesda Conference was convened in 1994 to present recommendations for competitive athletes with cardiovascular abnormalities. Several recommendations were posed for individuals with Marfan's syndrome. Athletes should not participate in sports that risk bodily collision (30). Individuals with aortic regurgitation and aortic dilatation should not participate in competitive sports (25). Athletes with aortic root dilatation can participate in competitive sports such as golf, bowling, and billiards (30,31). Athletes without a family history of sudden death and no evidence of mitral regurgitation or aortic root dilatation may participate in sports such as archery, golf, bowling, and billiards (30,31). Brisk walking for aerobic exercise is acceptable. Serial 6-month echocardiographic evaluation is required for continued sports participation (30).

SUMMARY

Marfan's syndrome is a complex, connective tissue disease with life-threatening cardiovascular manifestations. The sports medicine physician needs to be aware of the clinical features and have a high degree of suspicion when evaluating athletes for participation. Although diagnostic and monitoring techniques continue to emerge, until more is known, significant restriction of sports participation continues to be the norm.

REFERENCES

1 Manusov EG, Martucci E. The Marfan's syndrome: an underdiagnosed killer. Arch Fam Med 1994;3:822–826.

2 Pereira L, Levran O, Ramirez F, et al. A molecular approach to the stratification of cardiovascular risk in families with Marfan's syndrome. N Engl J Med 1994;331:148–153.

3 Pyeritz RE, Francke U. The Second International Symposium on the Marfan's syndrome. Am J Med Genet 1993;47:127–135.

4 Maron BJ, Shirani J, Mueller FO, et al. Cardiovascular causes of "athletic field" deaths: analysis of sudden death in 84 competitive athletes. Circulation 1993;88:1–50.

5 Pyeritz RE. The Marfan's syndrome. Am Fam Physician 1986;34:83–94.

6 Cantwell JD. Marfan's syndrome: detection and management. Physician Sports Med 1986;14:51–55.

7 Pyeritz RE, McKusick VA. The Marfan's syndrome: diagnosis and management [review]. N Engl J Med 1979;300:772–777.

8 Gerry JL Jr, Morris L, Pyeritz RE. Clinical management of the cardiovascular complications of the Marfan's syndrome. J LA State Med Soc 1991;143:43–51.

9 Pini R, Roman MJ, Kramer-Fox R, Devereux RB. Mitral valve dimensions and motion in Marfan patients with and without mitral valve prolapse. Comparison to primary mitral valve prolapse and normal subjects. Circulation 1989;80:915–924.

10 Roberts WC, Honig HS. The spectrum of cardiovascular disease in the Marfan's syndrome: a clinico-morphologic study of 18 necropsy patients and comparison to 151 previously reported necropsy patients [review]. Am Heart J 1982;104:115–135.

11 El Habbal MH. Cardiovascular manifestations of Marfan's syndrome in the young. Am Heart J 1992;123:752–757.

12 Gott VL, Pyeritz RE, Cameron DE, et al. Composite graft repair of Marfan aneurysm of the ascending aorta: results in 100 patients. Ann Thorac Surg 1991;52:38–45.

13 Robicsek F, Thubrikar MJ. Hemodynamic considerations regarding the mechanism and prevention of aortic dissection. Ann Thorac Surg 1994;58:1247–1253.

14 Marsalese DL, Moodie DS, Vacante M, et al. Marfan's syndrome: natural history and long-term follow-up of cardiovascular involvement. J Am Coll Cardiol 1989;14:422–428.

15 McDonald GR, Schaff HV, Pyeritz RE, et al. Surgical management of patients with the Marfan's syndrome and dilatation of the ascending aorta. J Thorac Cardiovasc Surg 1981;81:180–186.

16 Hirata K, Triposkiadis F, Sparks E, et al. The Marfan's syndrome: abnormal aortic elastic properties. J Am Coll Cardiol 1991;18:57–63.

17 Beighton P, de Paepe A, Danks D, et al. Interna-

tional nosology of heritable disorders of connective tissue, Berlin, 1986. Am J Med Genet 1988;29:581–594.

18 Cohen PR, Schneiderman P. Clinical manifestations of the Marfan's syndrome. Int J Dermatol 1989;28:291–299.

19 Otis CL, Child JS, Perloff JK, Malotte K. Protocol for screening athletes for Marfan's syndrome: report of four-years' experience. Med Sci Sports Exerc 1993;25(suppl):S180.

20 Magid D, Pyeritz RE, Fishman EK. Musculoskeletal manifestations of the Marfan's syndrome: radiological features. *AJR Am J Roentgenol* 1990;155:99–104.

21 Mellion MB. Diagnosing Marfan's syndrome. Heart Dis Stroke 1994;3:241–245.

22 Maumenee IH. The eye in the Marfan's syndrome. Trans Am Ophthalmol Soc 1981;79:684–742.

23 Cross HE, Jensen AD. Ocular manifestations in the Marfan's syndrome and homocystinuria. Am J Ophthalmol 1973;75:405–420.

24 Nienaber CA, von Kodolitsch Y, Brockhoff CJ, et al. Comparison of conventional and transesophageal echocardiography with magnetic resonance imaging for anatomical mapping of thoracic aortic dissection. A dual noninvasive imaging study with anatomical and/or angiographic validation. Int J Card Imaging 1994;10:1–14.

25 Cheitlin MD, Douglas PS, Parmley WW. 26th Bethesda conference: Recommendations for determining eligibility for competition in athletes with

cardiovascular abnormalities. Task Force 2: acquired valvular heart disease. Med Sci Sports Exerc 1994;26(suppl):S254–260.

26 Child JS, Perloff JK, Kaplan S. The heart of the matter: cardiovascular involvement in Marfan's syndrome [editorial]. J Am Coll Cardiol 1989;14:429–431.

27 Pyeritz RE. Predictors of dissection of the ascending aorta in Marfan's syndrome. Circulation 1991;86:II–351.

28 Shores J, Berger KR, Murphy EA, Pyeritz RE. Progression of aortic dilatation and the benefit of long-term beta-adrenergic blockade in Marfan's syndrome. N Engl J Med 1994;330:1335–1341.

29 Tahernia AC. Cardiovascular anomalies in Marfan's syndrome: the role of echocardiography and beta-blockers. South Med J 1993;86:305–310.

30 Graham TP Jr, Bricker JT, James FW, Strong WB. 26th Bethesda conference: recommendations for determining eligibility for competition in athletes with cardiovascular abnormalities. Task Force 1: congenital heart disease. Med Sci Sports Exerc 1994;26(suppl):S246–S253.

31 Mitchell JH, Haskell WL, Raven PB. Classification of sports. Med Sci Sports Exerc 1994;26(suppl):S242–S245.

32 Falk RH. Images in clinical medicine: the "thumb sign" in Marfan's syndrome. N Engl J Med 1995;333:430.

33 Maron BJ, Epstein SE, Roberts WC. Causes of death in competitive athletes. J Am Coll Cardiol 1986;7:204–214.

Chapter 21
Special Techniques for Evaluation of Cardiac Problems

David Andrew Tate

As discussed in preceding chapters, routine screening of recreational, competitive, or even professional athletes does not generally include highly specialized diagnostic techniques. The low incidence of cardiac events in athletes together with the expense and inadequate specificity of such studies renders them impractical for broad-based screening programs. Nevertheless, in any population of athletes there are a number in whom the initial history and physical examination (or possibly the electrocardiogram [ECG] or chest x-ray) suggest a possible cardiac abnormality. In addition, there are patients with known cardiovascular disorders who wish to participate in sports activities. To advise such patients appropriately, physicians treating athletes require a working knowledge of specialized diagnostic techniques.

ECHOCARDIOGRAPHY

Although primary arrhythmic events or coronary spasm occurs occasionally in athletes, the vast majority of sudden cardiac death and other lesser events occur secondary to underlying structural heart disease or coronary artery disease. The presence of structural heart disease is particularly high in athletes suffering cardiac death before the age of 30, in whom hypertrophic cardiomyopathy is the most common abnormality (1). Echocardiography is the most accurate noninvasive method to assess cardiac structure and, in conjunction with Doppler, provides a great deal of information about cardiac function.

Echocardiography uses ultrasound beams of 2 to 10 megahertz to examine cardiac structures. These beams are emitted from a transducer on the surface of the chest and are reflected when they strike an interface between two tissues of different acoustical impedance. The reflected beam is detected by the transducer, and the signals are processed to provide an image.

- **M-Mode Echocardiography** In the case of M-mode echocardiography, the image has been referred to as an "ice pick–like" view of the heart, in that it detects structures in a one-dimensional linear array. This information, however, is displayed on a strip chart recorder, which thereby adds the temporal dimension.
- **2-D Echocardiography** In two-dimensional (2-D) echocardiography, the ultrasonic beam moves rapidly over a wedge-shaped sector, and the data are processed to allow a two-dimensional or planar image to be constructed.
- **Doppler Echocardiography** Doppler echocardiography allows blood flow within the heart to be analyzed and provides a great deal of pathophysiologic information, particularly with respect to stenotic and regurgitant valves.

The principle underlying the Doppler examination is that the frequency of an ultrasonic beam is altered when it is reflected from a moving target, in this case, the red blood cell. When blood flows toward the transducer, the frequency increases; when it flows away, the frequency decreases. The change in frequency is proportional to the velocity of the target object, thus permitting an assessment of both the direction and velocity of blood flow. Doppler information is usually obtained in three formats (continuous wave, pulsed wave, and color flow) and provides a wealth of information including the presence and magnitude of valvular regur-

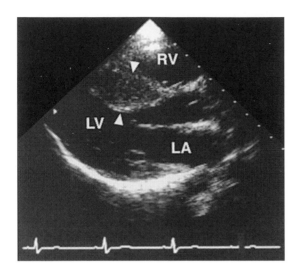

Figure 21-1. Echocardiographic parasternal long axis view in a woman with hypertrophic cardiomyopathy and pronounced asymmetric septal hypertrophy. The interventricular septum (arrows) measures 24 mm at end-diastole.

gitation, the velocity of flow across stenotic valves, the presence of abnormal communication between chambers, and a variety of secondary calculations such as transvalvular gradients and estimates of pulmonary artery pressure.

Applications

Echocardiography is the clinical gold standard for the evaluation of left ventricular hypertrophy and hypertrophic cardiomyopathy (Fig 21-1). When assessment of the patient raises the possibility of these diagnoses, echocardiography becomes part of the standard workup. This includes, for example, patients with presyncope, syncope, dyspnea, angina, or a family history of sudden death.

An echocardiogram should also be considered in patients whose physical exam reveals a midsystolic crescendo–decrescendo murmur, a fourth heart sound, a left ventricular heave, a bisferiens carotid pulse, or a prominent a-wave in the jugular venous pulse. Finally, patients whose ECGs reveal left ventricular hypertrophy, ST segment or T wave abnormalities, or Q waves should undergo echocardiography. Because hypertrophic cardio-

myopathy is usually genetically transmitted, relatives of patients carrying this diagnosis should also be examined.

Hypertrophic cardiomyopathy is a relatively common postmortem diagnosis in young athletes who have died suddenly. In one study of 29 such cases, 14 were found to have hypertrophic cardiomyopathy and another 4 were ascribed to "idiopathic" left ventricular hypertrophy (1). Ventricular septal thickness ranged from 15 to 30 mm with a mean of 20 mm in these patients, well above the usual upper limit of normal by echocardiography of 12 mm. Thus, the majority of such patients are at least potentially identifiable antemortem, and the echocardiographic findings are usually not equivocal. The marked degree of hypertrophy present in these patients is also reflected in the recommendations of the 26th Bethesda Conference on Cardiovascular Abnormalities in the Athlete (2). This panel recommended that competitive sports be prohibited in patients with ventricular wall thickness greater than or equal to 20 mm. Prohibition from competitive sports was also recommended when echocardiography indicated significant obstruction to left ventricular outflow under basal conditions.

A second area in which echocardiography may be useful is in the diagnosis of aortic root dilation. In young patients without hypertension, abnormalities are usually due to connective tissue changes, and may or may not be associated with other features of Marfan's syndrome. While far less common as a cause of sudden death than hypertrophic cardiomyopathy, aortic rupture was the underlying cause in 3 of 29 reported cases of sudden death in young athletes (1). Echocardiography may identify not only aortic root dilatation but also aortic insufficiency and mitral valve prolapse, which are frequently associated.

There are a large number of other conditions in which echocardiography is helpful in either establishing a diagnosis or assessing the hemodynamic significance and consequent risk of a cardiac abnormality. These include a wide variety of congenital anomalies (atrial septal defect, ventricular septal defect, pulmonic stenosis, aortic stenosis, etc.), mitral valve prolapse, right ventricular dysplasia, and occasionally congenital coronary anomalies.

These specific diagnoses are discussed in other chapters.

EXERCISE STRESS TESTING

Exercise treadmill testing (ETT) is the test most often used in the diagnosis and evaluation of ischemic heart disease. The test begins with a baseline heart rate, blood pressure, and ECG. Exercise is then performed in a standard incremental fashion according to a variety of protocols. The supervising physician monitors heart rate, blood pressure, symptoms, and the ECG. Usually the test is symptom-limited, meaning the patient exercises as long as possible until it is necessary to stop due to chest discomfort, shortness of breath, dizziness, leg fatigue, or generalized fatigue. The physician may also stop the test due to a decline in systolic blood pressure, development of ventricular arrhythmias,

or clear-cut ECG positivity. The symptom-limited aspect of the test allows it to be used as a general assessment of exercise tolerance, in addition to an assessment of ischemic heart disease.

An electrocardiographically positive test is one in which there is flat or downsloping ST segment depression of greater than 0.1 millivolts lasting 0.08 seconds (as measured from the J-point) (Fig 21-2). A test in which the heart rate does not reach 85% maximal predicted heart rate for the patient's age and sex is considered nondiagnostic. Thus, a negative test is defined as one with no anginal chest pain or ischemic ECG changes in a patient reaching 85% of the maximal predicted heart rate. Other possible results of a treadmill test are "equivocal," when the findings are borderline, or "positive with decreased specificity" when ST segment changes occur but could be due to other factors such as left ventricular hypertrophy, drug effect (particularly digoxin), or other baseline ECG abnormalities.

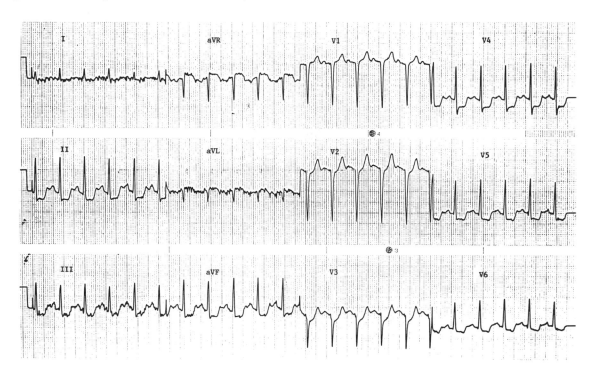

Figure 21-2. 12-lead ECG at peak exercise in a middle-aged man with exertional chest pain subsequently shown at catheterization to have 3-vessel coronary artery disease. There is 3 to 4 mm of horizontal ST segment depression in leads II, aVF, and V4. There is 1 to 3 mm of down-sloping ST segment depression in leads III, V5, and V6.

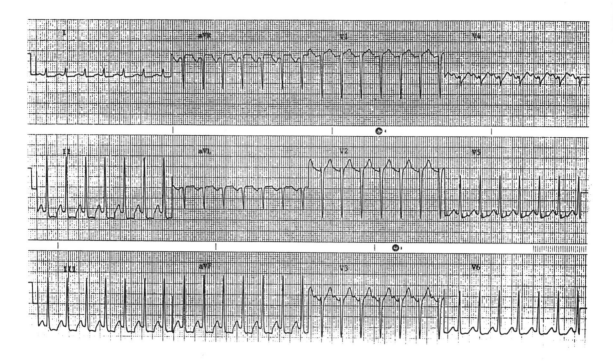

Figure 21-3. False-positive treadmill test in a 43-year-old woman with chest pain subsequently shown at catheterization to have no hemodynamically significant coronary artery disease. There is horizontal ST segment depression noted in leads II, III, aVF, and V6. In this case, the false positivity may be due to left ventricular hypertrophy as suggested by the prominent voltage.

Screening Athletes

Intuitively, exercise stress testing seems ideally suited to evaluation of the athlete. Exercise testing replicates the physical exertion of sporting activities, and, in athletes over 35 years of age, the most common cause of sudden death is coronary artery disease (1). In fact, however, exercise testing of the athlete is fraught with problems. Most importantly, exercise treadmill testing, like any test, does not have 100% specificity or sensitivity. Such limitations of specificity become particularly problematic in a study population, such as asymptomatic athletes, in whom the disease prevalence is low. False-positive tests and equivocal tests are common (Fig 21-3).

The magnitude of this problem is described by Bayesian theory and is documented in multiple studies. Patterson and Horowitz (3) demonstrated that whereas a positive test in a 55-year-old male with typical angina is associated with a greater than 90% probability of disease, the same test result in a

45-year-old asymptomatic male without risk factors is associated with a less than 10% probability of disease. Epstein, Maron, Spirito, and Bonow (4,5) have looked specifically at the problem of exercise testing in the asymptomatic athlete. In a study of 75 young asymptomatic athletes, 9% were found to have positive treadmill tests (4). A screening strategy incorporating such testing would therefore entail considerable expense, effort, and anxiety in following up the large number of false-positive studies.

An analysis of the Seattle Heart Watch Study suggests that even in older patients the benefit of treadmill screening seems doubtful (5–7). In this group of over 2000 men without heart disease, the annual incidence of sudden cardiac death was approximately 0.05%. Risk factor analysis and exercise testing identified 1% of this population as having an 18-fold greater risk of angina, myocardial infarction, or death relative to the rest of the group. If one assumes that a subgroup with an 18-

fold sudden death risk can be identified, it would require screening 10,000 subjects to identify 100 (1%) in a high risk group, only one of whom would be expected to experience sudden death. Ironically, as Epstein and Maron (5) point out, the remaining 9900 subjects not identified as high risk would include four of the five subjects ultimately experiencing sudden death.

These and other studies (8,9) have cast considerable doubt on the utility of exercise treadmill testing as a routine screening strategy. In selected patients and patient subsets, however, exercise testing is appropriate either as a screening study in selected high-risk or symptomatic patients, or for exercise prescriptions in patients with established coronary disease. As Bayes' theorem predicts, a positive test in high risk or symptomatic patients much more often represents a "true positive" finding that directs the physician to do further evaluation.

OTHER FUNCTIONAL TESTS FOR ISCHEMIA

In recent years, a variety of other so-called functional tests for ischemia have come into common use. These include exercise thallium studies, thallium studies utilizing pharmacologic stress, stress radionuclide ventriculography, and stress echocardiography. In general, these diagnostic procedures, though not as extensively studied as treadmill testing, would be expected to have many of the same problems as discussed above. Indeed, while these modalities gain sensitivity by combining an imaging modality with electrocardiographic monitoring, additional problems with specificity may develop. In addition, these tests are much more expensive than routine treadmill testing, compounding the cost of any screening program. Nevertheless, there are selected subjects in whom these tests are indicated, and a brief description of them is therefore provided here.

Thallium Studies

Thallium 201 (^{201}Tl) is a potassium analog and is the most commonly used radiopharmaceutical in the evaluation of myocardial perfusion. Following intravenous injection, thallium 201 accumulates in

viable myocardial cells in proportion to myocardial blood flow. Thus, it is particularly useful in conjunction with exercise testing in the evaluation of ischemic heart disease. In this setting, thallium is injected at peak exercise, and the patient is then immediately imaged with a gamma camera. Myocardial segments supplied by stenotic coronary arteries take up less thallium and appear as relative thallium defects or poor uptake. Over the next several hours, the thallium redistributes and washes out of myocardial segments with normal perfusion. Thus, defects that improve over time suggest ischemia, whereas defects that persist suggest nonviable myocardium, such as prior infarction. Thallium is also commonly administered in conjunction with pharmacologic vasodilators such as dipyridamole or adenosine. This allows evaluation for ischemia in patients unable to exercise, and obviously has little role in the evaluation of the athlete.

Radionuclide Ventriculography

The other commonly used nuclear cardiac study is radionuclide ventriculography. This technique does not evaluate myocardial perfusion directly but rather examines global and segmental myocardial function. Technetium 99 (^{99}Tc) is injected and labels the patient's own red blood cells. Cardiac images are then acquired for multiple cardiac cycles timed, or "gated," by the ECG. The data acquisition from multiple images is then combined and displayed in an endless cine-loop format. From these images, one can determine volumes and ejection fractions for both the left and right ventricles, examine global and segmental left ventricular function, and assess diastolic function by examining left ventricular peak filling rate. By comparing the left ventricular global and segmental contractions during supine exercise on a bicycle ergometer with those at rest, radionuclide ventriculography can be used as a functional test for myocardial ischemia. An ischemic response to stress is typically accompanied by a focal wall motion abnormality and an ejection fraction that either declines or fails to rise.

Stress Echocardiography

Stress echocardiography is another means of functional testing for ischemia. In the normal left ventricle, echocardiography reveals systolic thickening of all segments of the left ventricular wall. When myocardial ischemia is induced by exercise or pharmacologic stressors, however, the ischemic segment does not thicken normally. In recent years, there have been a number of technical advances, including digital technology, the utilization of continuous loop 2-D images, and split-screen simultaneous display of resting and exercise images. With these advances, stress-induced wall motion abnormalities may be reliably identified.

TESTS OF CARDIAC RHYTHM

In rare circumstances, specific testing of cardiac rhythm is necessary. As discussed above, most cardiac disease in the athlete is due to underlying structural heart disease and/or coronary artery disease. These are the usual substrates underlying electrical abnormalities, and evaluation of the underlying substrate is usually the most fruitful diagnostic approach. Occasionally, however, diagnostic techniques that specifically evaluate disorders of cardiac rhythm are utilized. These tests include Holter monitors, event recorders, signal-averaged electrocardiography, invasive electrophysiologic study, and tilt table testing.

The Holter Monitor
A variety of ECG monitoring systems are available, all of which have certain advantages and disadvantages. All monitoring approaches are limited by the fact that clinical arrhythmias are, by their nature, episodic. The most commonly used long-term ECG recording system is the Holter monitor. Holter monitors are generally worn for 24 to 48 hours and record a continuous two-channel ECG on magnetic tape. A variety of automated systems are used to scan and quantitate arrhythmic events, and selected tracings are printed out for interpretation by the physician. The patient provides a diary of events and symptoms so that clinical correlation can be made with any arrhythmia detected.

Holter monitors have the advantage of at least potentially recording every heartbeat during the monitoring period. However, the study is only as good as the scanning, analysis, and interpretation of the recording. In addition, Holter monitors are obviously of limited utility in the evaluation of infrequent events. Finally, it must be noted that a wide array of rhythms may be seen in normal, healthy persons and should not necessarily be considered abnormalities. Premature ventricular complexes, premature atrial complexes, sinus bradycardia, sinus arrhythmia, and Wenckebach second-degree AV block, for example, are often seen on 24-hour tracings from normal individuals.

Event Recorders
The problems presented by infrequent events and the incidental detection of nonclinical arrhythmias are solved in part by a variety of event recorders presently available. Some of these systems are worn like a Holter monitor but only record when the patient identifies a symptom and triggers the recording. Other systems require the patient to attach wrist or finger electrodes when a symptom is experienced, and the tracing is then recorded on tape and/or transmitted by telephone to a medical facility. Although these systems allow evaluation of infrequent symptoms and decrease the detection of extraneous rhythms, they require more responsibility and participation on the part of the patient and, obviously, are of limited utility in patients who are frankly syncopal. Finally, these systems do not detect asymptomatic arrhythmias, some of which may have diagnostic or prognostic significance.

Invasive Electrophysiologic Study
Invasive electrophysiologic (EP) studies are rarely required in the evaluation of the athlete. In these procedures, multipolar electrode catheters are placed, usually through the venous system, into various intracardiac sites. These catheters are then used to obtain local intracardiac electrograms and to deliver paced beats or programmed extrastimuli. Thus, arrhythmias may be induced and analyzed in a detailed fashion.

The information obtained with EP study is considerable and can be tailored by clinical circumstances. Sinus node function may be evaluated by determining sinus node recovery time and sinoatrial conduction time. Atrioventricular block or conduction delay can be assessed by determining the site of block or delay and by determining atrioventricular (A-V) and His-ventricular (H-V) intervals. Supraventricular arrhythmias can be stimulated, and the presence of accessory pathways or dual pathways in the A-V node can be documented. Ventricular tachycardia may be induced in susceptible patients, and the effect of drug therapy on these arrhythmias may be assessed.

The potential advantage of invasive electrophysiologic study is that it allows very sophisticated evaluation of arrhythmias, even when the spontaneous clinical arrhythmias are infrequent. However, the decision to proceed with EP study, and the ultimate interpretation of the study, should include careful attention to the clinical setting and the presence of underlying heart disease. For example, induction of ventricular tachycardia in a patient with syncope and prior myocardial infarction identifies a high-risk patient warranting therapy. In contrast, the induction of nonsustained, polymorphic ventricular tachycardia in a patient with equivocal symptoms and no structural heart disease may be of little clinical relevance and may in fact be misleading.

In evaluating syncope by EP study, the diagnostic yield is approximately 70% in patients with structural heart disease and 12% in patients without structural heart disease (10). Thus, EP studies should generally only be considered in patients with clear symptoms that remain undiagnosed following a thorough noninvasive evaluation.

Signal-Averaged Electrocardiography

Signal-averaged electrocardiography is rarely required in the athlete, but is discussed briefly here for completeness and because of growing clinical interest in the test. Signal-averaging is a technique whereby several hundred cardiac cycles are recorded from body surface electrodes and then filtered and averaged by computer. The averaging cancels random electrical potentials such as those in skeletal muscle and allows detection of electrical potentials of a few microvolts generated by the sinus node, the A-V node, the His bundle, the bundle branches, and areas of conduction delay in the ventricle. The most common clinical application of signal-averaged electrocardiography has been to detect late potentials in the terminal portion of the QRS complex and ST segment, which are believed to represent delayed, fragmented conduction in the ventricle (11). These occur most commonly in patients following myocardial infarction and appear to be an independent risk factor for the subsequent occurrence of ventricular tachycardia or sudden death (12,13).

Tilt-Table Testing

Tilt-table testing is an evolving diagnostic technique used to evaluate patients suspected of having neurally mediated or neurocardiogenic syncope. The exact pathophysiologic mechanisms of this disorder are still being elucidated, but the major features are becoming reasonably clear. The inciting event in neurally mediated syncope appears to be rapid, excessive venous pooling. In susceptible patients, there is a sudden increase in left ventricular contractility and activation of cardiopulmonary mechanoreceptors, most notably left ventricular C fibers. These events then trigger a paradoxic heart rate and/or blood pressure response. In some patients, there is a prominent cardioinhibitory component. In others, the vasodepressor response is the sole or major feature. In addition, there is evidence that some of these patients have altered cerebrovascular autoregulation (14,15). Thus, in recognition of the complex, multifaceted pathophysiology of this disorder and the relatively limited role played by parasympathetic outflow (16), the terms "neurally-mediated syncope" or "neurocardiogenic syncope" are now generally preferred over the older term "vasovagal syncope."

Tilt-table testing is a provocative diagnostic strategy used to reproduce the symptoms of syncope or near-syncope, and/or hypotension, bradycardia, or asystole. Patients are placed in the supine position on a standard tilt table with footboard, and an intravenous line, an electrocardiographic monitor, and a sphygmomanometer are put in place. In some institutions and circumstances, other monitoring modalities are included, such as electroencephalography, Doppler transcranial blood flow monitors, or heart rate variability monitors. After approximately 15 minutes of equilibration, the patient is gradually elevated to an upright position, usually to an angle between 60° and 80°. Patients are then observed for a period of 30 to 60 minutes. In many institutions, adjunctive isoproterenol is administered intravenously during the protocol. Isoproterenol increases left ventricular contractility, which, in the presence of orthostatic stress, may promote neurally mediated syncope.

The sensitivity and specificity of tilt-table testing varies widely according to which protocol is used (tilt angle, tilt duration, use of adjunctive isoproterenol) and which group of patients is studied. The technique has been applied most commonly in patients with recurrent syncope that has remained undiagnosed after an extensive workup, which often may have included a negative electrophysiologic study. In numerous studies of patients with syncope and negative electrophysiologic studies, tilt-table testing without isoproterenol has provoked a hypotensive response in 27% to 67% of patients, compared with approximately 10% in controls without syncope (17). When isoproterenol is used, positive tilt-table tests have been obtained in 87% of such patients, compared with 11% in both control patients and patients with positive electrophysiologic studies (18).

Evaluating Athletes   Tilt-table testing is occasionally useful in the evaluation of athletes with exercise-induced syncope. Other diagnoses such as hypertrophic cardiomyopathy, valvular disease, coronary artery disease, coronary anomalies, and exercise-induced arrhythmias should be excluded first, but recent studies suggest that some athletes may be prone to neurocardiogenic syncope. Stegemann et al. (19) have shown that rigorous endurance training alters blood pressure regulation in a manner that increases exercise tolerance but decreases orthostatic tolerance (19). In one small study of seven endurance-trained athletes, all experienced syncope during tilt-table testing (20). In a larger study of 24 athletes with recurrent exertional syncope and a negative extensive evaluation, Grubb et al. (21) demonstrated that 19 (79%) of the participants had a positive tilt-table test. Seventeen of these patients were treated and rendered symptom-free at a mean follow-up of 23 months.

The remaining two patients declined therapy and had persistent symptoms.

SUMMARY

A number of special techniques exist for evaluation of an athlete with possible cardiac disease. In all but rare circumstances, noninvasive testing provides adequate information for the young athlete's physician to assess the risks of sports participation. ETT, other functional tests for ischemia, and cardiac catheterization may all be needed in evaluating patients with suspected coronary artery disease. Holter monitors and specialized event recorders are standard in the assessment of rhythm disturbances. EP studies and signal-averaged ECGs should be reserved for the diagnostic dilemma and for patients with a high likelihood of serious arrhythmias. Finally, tilt-table testing is being studied as a way to identify patients with true neurogenic syncope after other cardiac disorders have been carefully excluded.

REFERENCES

1 Maron BJ, Epstein SE, Roberts WC. Causes of sudden death in competitive athletes. J Am Coll Cardiol 1986;7:204–214.
2 Maron BJ, Gaffney FA, Jeresaty RM, et al. Task Force III: hypertrophic cardiomyopathy, other myopericardial diseases and mitral valve prolapse. J Am Coll Cardiol 1985;6:215–217.
3 Patterson RE, Horowitz SF. Importance of epidemiology and biostatistics in deciding clinical strategies for using diagnostic tests: a simplified approach using examples from coronary artery disease. J Am Coll Cardiol 1989;13:1653–1655.
4 Spirito P, Maron BJ, Bonow RO, Epstein SE. Prevalence and significance of an abnormal S-T segment response to exercise in a young athletic population. Am J Cardiol 1983;51:1663–1666.
5 Epstein SE, Maron BJ. Sudden death and the competitive athlete: perspectives on preparticipation screening studies. J Am Coll Cardiol 1986;7:220–230.
6 Bruce RA, DeRouen TA, Hossack KF. Value of maximal exercise tests in risk assessment of primary coronary heart disease events in healthy men. Five years' experience of the Seattle Heart Watch study. Am J Cardiol 1980;46:371–378.

7 Bruce RA, DeRouen TA, Blake B. Maximal exercise predictors of coronary heart disease events among asymptomatic men in Seattle Heart Watch. Circulation 1977;56(suppl):III–15. Abstract.

8 McHenry PL, O'Donnell JO, Morris SN, Jordan JJ. The abnormal exercise electrocardiogram in apparently healthy men: a predictor of angina pectoris as an initial coronary event during long-term follow-up. Circulation 1984;70:547–551.

9 Siscovick DS, Ekeland LG, Johnson JL, et al. Sensitivity of exercise electrocardiography for acute cardiac events during moderate and strenuous physical activity. Arch Int Med 1991;151:325–330.

10 Zipes DP. Genesis of cardiac arrhythmias: electrophysiological considerations. In: Braunwald E, ed. Heart disease: a textbook of cardiovascular medicine. Philadelphia: WB Saunders, 1992:588–627.

11 Mehta D, McKenna WJ, Ward DE, et al. Significance of signal-averaged electrocardiography in relation to endomyocardial biopsy and ventricular stimulation studies in patients with ventricular tachycardia without clinically apparent heart disease. J Am Coll Cardiol 1989;14:372–379.

12 Kuchar DL, Thornburn CW, Sammel NL. Prediction of serious arrhythmic events after myocardial infarction: signal-averaged electrocardiogram, Holter monitoring and radionuclide ventriculography. J Am Coll Cardiol 1987;9:531–538.

13 Gomes JA, Winters SL, Martinson M, et al. The prognostic significance of quantitative signal-averaged variables relative to clinical variables, site of myocardial infarction, ejection fraction and ventricular premature beats: a prospective study. J Am Coll Cardiol 1989;13:377–384.

14 Grubb BP, Gerard G, Roush K, et al. Cerebral vasoconstriction during head upright tilt induced syncope: a paradoxic and unexpected finding. Circulation 1991;84:1157–1164.

15 Janosik D, Gomez C, Njemaze P, et al. Abnormalities in cerebral blood flow autoregulation during tilt-induced neurocardiogenic syncope. PACE 1992;15:592.

16 Rea R, Thames M. Neural control mechanisms and vasovagal syncope. PACE 1993;4:587–595.

17 Kapoor WN. Hypotension and syncope. In: Braunwald E, ed. Heart disease: a textbook of cardiovascular medicine. Philadelphia: WB Saunders, 1992:875–886.

18 Almquist A, Goldenberg IF, Milstein S, et al. Provocation of bradycardia and hypotension by isoproterenol and upright posture in patients with unexplained syncope. N Engl J Med 1989;320:346–351.

19 Stegemann J, Busert A, Brock D. Influence of fitness on the blood pressure control system in man. Aerospace Med 1974;45:45–48.

20 Ebert TJ, Denahan T. Hemodynamic responses of high-fit runners during head upright tilt testing to syncope. Proceedings of the American Autonomic Society Annual Scientific Session 1993, Nashville, TN. Abstract.

21 Grubb BP, Temesy-Armos P, Samoil D, et al. Tilt-table testing in the evaluation and management of athletes with recurrent exercise-induced syncope. Med Sci Sports Exerc 1993;25:24–28.

Chapter 22
Pulmonary Problems in Athletes

Karl B. Fields
Curtis D. Reimer

LUNG STRUCTURE AND DEFENSE

The lungs are a complex organ system that functions to provide oxygen for all bodily activities. Because the lungs constantly derive inhaled gas from the environment, they need an effective defense system to avoid injury and infection. Three key components of the airways protective system are the nasopharynx, ciliated cells, and the alveolar exchange zone. The unique anatomy of the airways allows the high minute ventilation necessary for sports participation while preventing damage to the respiratory tree.

The Nasopharnx
The nasopharynx deals with foreign substances in a variety of ways. Particles deposited in distal nasal epithelium are removed mechanically by sneezing. Particles deposited in proximal nasal surfaces are swept posteriorly by ciliated cells lined with a mucus layer, and they subsequently are expectorated or swallowed. Most debris is removed or is neutralized by reflex closure of the glottis, by cough, or by antibody secretion. This system functions well as the lower respiratory tract generally remains sterile despite its location adjacent to the oropharynx, which is colonized by numerous microorganisms.

Ciliated Cells
Ciliated pseudostratified columnar epithelium represents 80% of the cells in the central airways and forms the primary defense barrier. These cells help remove particles through a complex action. Each cell has approximately 200 cilia that beat at 1000 times per minute in a coordinated, wave-like motion. A slower backstroke and a more rapid forward stroke lead to forward propulsion of material toward the oropharynx. Cilia are immersed in a liquid film that helps coordinate their motion. The mucus-secreting cells in the trachea and bronchi provide this material, which has an outer viscous layer that helps trap particles.

The Alveolar Exchange Zone
The alveolar zone is the area of dynamic exchange between inspired air and circulating blood. The interface is formed by permeable membranes that allow gas exchange between the capillary beds and the alveolar sacs. This region contains two types of cells that serve as the final defense barrier against foreign substances. Type 1 (flattened alveolar cells) and type 2 (rounded cells) produce substances such as surfactant, fibronectin, and immunoglobulin, which along with alveolar macrophages, lymphocytes, and a few polymorphonuclear cells allow the alveoli to dispose of foreign material (1).

LUNG FUNCTION IN SPORTS

Excellent lung function allows maximal performance in sports requiring high aerobic demand. For example, during a 1 hour competition an elite distance runner exchanges an amount of air equal to that ventilated by a sedentary individual in 24 hours (2). However, certain strength-related sports do not require high $\dot{V}O_2$max levels for the athlete to perform at elite levels. In addition, athletes with chronic lung disease have succeeded in sports like basketball, swimming, and soccer. The lung function needs to be adequate to meet the demands of the sport, but in most cases this can be less than maximal ventilatory capacity.

In regard to sports participation and chronic lung disease, asthma is the best understood condition. The reversibility of the physiologic effects of asthma means that treatment can allow full participation for most athletes in almost all sports. This chapter reviews asthma as well as chronic obstructive lung disease, restrictive lung disease, and immune lung disease with attention to what is known regarding these diverse entities and sports performance. Each of these processes may cause limitations of pulmonary function that may restrict full athletic activity.

ASTHMA

Overview

Asthma was recognized as a problem during sports performance even in ancient times. For example, Aretaeus wrote in the second century, "If from any running, gymnastic exercises, or any other work, the breathing becomes difficult, it is called asthma . . . " (3). Galen, a contemporary of Aretaeus, imperfectly understood the role of "pneuma," which he felt was a life-giving force in the air that was brought into the lungs and transferred to the heart (4). However, he did note that an increased respiratory rate occurred with exercise, and that under certain conditions such as marching in the colder air of Gaul, soldiers developed more breathing difficulties.

Ancient physicians in the first and second century A.D. already had a clinical understanding of different respiratory conditions and had wide experience with using medicines to lessen breathing difficulty and to suppress cough. Ephedra (ma huang), a substance still used in asthma treatment, first emerged in China as a treatment for respiratory problems in the reign of the Red Emperor, Shen Nung, who tested herbs on himself and compiled the *Pen-tsao* treatise circa 2800 B.C. (5). This and other herbal medications were brought to ancient Greece and became part of the standard treatment regimens in Western medicine.

Just as in ancient times, the key symptom of an asthma attack in an athlete is shortness of breath during or after exercise. Other typical symptoms include persistent cough (e.g., figure skater's cough, 1500-meter hack), chest pain, or dizziness with exertion. Cough may be the only marker in a number of athletes having problems with exercise-induced asthma (EIA). Preparticipation testing shows that individuals who complain of persistent cough after exercise have a greater than an 80% chance of testing positive for EIA (6). In young athletes, chest pain often accompanies bronchospasm. In pediatric age groups, chest pain occurs more commonly from EIA than from cardiac causes, as demonstrated by a study showing that 72.7% of athletes referred to pediatric cardiology for evaluation of chest pain in fact had bronchospasm (7).

For years physicians noted the association of asthma attacks with certain environmental conditions, and laboratory testing confirmed the clinical observations that dry air, cold air, and air with irritants or antigens reproduce bronchospasm. However, at normal respiratory rates most of these factors do not produce symptoms; a high minute ventilation, such as occurs during exercise, was a necessary cofactor to produce the clinical response. Airway responsiveness and hyperactivity remain imperfectly understood processes, but appear to be mediated by leukotrienes, histamine, neutrophil chemotactic factor, or similar chemical mediators. Recent studies indicate that airway rewarming after cooling causes a vasodilation that releases these chemicals and may trigger bronchospasm, more so than airway drying (8).

Clinical Presentations of Asthma

In general, physicians find that asthma patients fall into three broad categories: atopic individuals who cough with exercise, true asthmatics, and classic EIA patients. Each of these three categories has unique characteristics. The advantage of identifying the type of patient being treated lies in different management strategies for each category.

Atopic Asthma   Atopic patients with asthma problems demonstrate a seasonal variation in symptoms. Time of year is more important than temperature or humidity. Atopic patients typically experience problems only when certain antigens such as particular pollens are present in the environment. At other times of the year, these patients tolerate the same exercise level without any decline in pulmonary function. These patients may occasionally wheeze without an exercise stimulus, particularly when they have respiratory infections or the antigen load in the atmosphere is extremely high. However, the typical atopic athlete requires exercise plus antigens to precipitate bronchospasm.

One marker for the atopic patient at risk for asthma is allergic rhinitis. About half of the individuals with a history of hay fever will at some point develop EIA. In addition to allergic rhinitis or respiratory symptoms, allergic patients frequently have other complaints that develop during exertion. These include generalized skin itching, watery eyes, hives, and rarely anaphylaxis. Atopic patients may also find that ingestion of certain foods precipitates their symptoms.

True Asthma True asthmatics experience symptoms in all seasons and almost always show falls in peak flow with sustained aerobic exercise. Effort in asthmatics further stresses a system in which chronic inflammation plays a significant role in symptoms. Bronchoscopic studies show that low-grade inflammatory change never completely resolves from the airways in chronic lung conditions. Exercise affects some of the inflammatory cells in the airway; these cells then release the chemical mediators that initiate the cascade of events that leads to bronchospasm. For this reason, attempts to stop inhaled corticosteroid therapy in stable mild asthmatics generally fail (9).

True asthmatics potentially have more severe attacks than individuals with only exercise-induced symptoms. The rare fatal asthmatic attacks that occur in association with exercise occur in true asthmatics and often involve excessive mucus production and mucus plugging of airways. Fortunately, because of more experience with the symptoms, true asthmatics usually recognize sooner that they are wheezing and seek appropriate intervention. These individuals are often sensitive to many of the same irritants that trigger other types of asthma and are more prone to attacks from emotional stimuli. This has been a relatively frequent problem for certain athletes who, experiencing competitive anxiety, may hyperventilate and actually trigger a true asthmatic attack.

Classic EIA Classic EIA patients find that cold temperatures are a major precipitator of symptoms. Dry air may be equally provocative, and the combination is worse than either alone. Because cold, dry air conditions predominate in winter sports, EIA commonly occurs in this setting. One study of long-term Arctic residents suggests that prolonged exposure to cold air may act as an airway toxin, causing the type of airway insult that ultimately leads to bronchospastic problems (10). Conversely, inhalation of hot, humid air blocks the early phase of bronchoconstriction.

High minute ventilation rapidly dries and cools the airway, thus explaining why the level of aerobic exertion also influences the likelihood of EIA. This correlates with certain sports being extremely provocative of symptoms. Examples of sports considered most to be asthmogenic are long-distance running, cross-country skiing, ice skating, soccer, rugby, wrestling, and other sports with continuous activity. One study of cross-country skiers found that 79% were troubled by asthma symptoms or bronchial hyper-responsiveness (11).

Sports like swimming may actually attract asthmatics, who experience fewer symptoms because the exercise takes place in an environment with moist, heated air. However, recent reports note that the chlorine content in pools may set up a chemical irritant that triggers bronchospasm in susceptible individuals, even when the content in the pool is at safe standard levels for recreational swimming (12).

Screening Tests to Confirm the EIA Diagnosis

The most practical way to make a diagnosis of EIA is a clinical trial with an inhaled bronchodilator. When the history fits the diagnosis, a treatment trial poses little risk and allows the athletes to judge for themselves whether they benefit from a bronchodilator. The response of the patient to medication is particularly important, as a normal screening test does not preclude a diagnosis of EIA. Often a baseline peak expiratory flow rate (PEFR) may be in the normal range, but a significant improvement (15%) in baseline PEFR on a return visit following treatment proves that the athlete was experiencing a decline in pulmonary function during the initial evaluation. This type of objective measure provides as much information as an exercise challenge.

Despite the value of a clinical trial, useful information about the athlete can be obtained from a standard exercise challenge. For example the magnitude of decline in peak flow helps classify the severity of asthma. Athletes who drop 20% or less usually have mild asthma; 20% to 50%, moderate EIA; and greater than 50%, severe EIA. Additionally, the timing of the drop in peak flow may indicate whether the individual has a late-phase reaction that would be more likely to respond to anti-inflammatory medications. For example, continued monitoring may demonstrate a significant delayed bronchospasm in the athlete who begins to show a drop only after 15 to 20 minutes.

The exercise challenge consists of vigorous activity for 6 to 12 minutes, utilizing free running, cycling, a step test, or a treadmill. PEFR measurements are taken before exercise and at 1, 3, 6, 10, 15, and 20 minutes after exercise. PEFR should drop by 15% to be positive; a drop of 10% is considered borderline. The decline in PEFR usually occurs 8 to 10 minutes after exercise. Two advantages of peak flow meter testing are low cost and ease of administration. Peak flows can easily be obtained on the track, beside a playing field, or in a gymnasium. This allows testing to take place in the environment in which the athlete becomes symptomatic. This has obvious advantages for higher detection rates in individuals who may be sensitive to a provocative agent unique to the playing locale.

The standard exercise screen done with standard pulmonary functions generates even more information and is a more sensitive test for asthma. In this situation, the positive result is a drop in forced expiratory volume (FEV1) of 15% or greater. Despite the ease of use of peak flow meters, development of more portable pulmonary function test equipment allows this to be done in the field as well. Because standard pulmonary function tests pick up more cases of asthma and provide a better screen for small and medium-sized airway disease, they offer advantages when cost is not a drawback.

Additional testing with chest radiographs and blood work rarely makes the diagnosis of asthma. Chest radiographs typically show hyperinflation, which is consistent but not specific with the diagnosis. Similarly, blood testing may show an increase in eosinophil or a serum radioallergosor-

bent test (RAST) may document allergy to inhalants, but these alone do not confirm the diagnosis of asthma. Eosinophilic inflammation of airways, however, is a characteristic feature of asthma so that a post-exercise sputum stain demonstrating eosinophils strongly suggests the diagnosis (13). The nasal smear for eosinophil (a positive test should note greater than 3 to 5 eosinophil per HPF) is a presumptive test for allergic rhinitis, and when coupled with pulmonary symptoms indicates probable asthma.

Screening confirms that EIA is an extremely common condition in athletes. Exercise challenge tests identified 11.2% of the U.S. Olympic athletes to have EIA on testing in 1984 (14,15), and similar numbers were found in 1988. Screening of a group of young and older adolescents with free running yielded a rate of 17% having EIA (16). These tests are consistent with estimates based on pooled results that suggest that younger athletes have rates in excess of 20%. Studies typically utilized only one exercise challenge, and since EIA occurs more frequently with certain environmental conditions, repeat testing would be expected to yield higher results. In addition, most screens for EIA did not incorporate laboratory or radiographic findings, which may have helped confirm the diagnosis in borderline cases. Only 50% of athletes were aware that they had EIA before the screening, indicating that EIA frequently remains undiagnosed.

Treatment of EIA: Goals of the International Consensus Report on Asthma

The World Health Organization and various national health programs have published standards of care for the patient with asthma. A major emphasis is returning responsibility for management of the disease back to the patient. Another focus of newer guidelines is to direct treatment more toward causal factors in asthma and less toward bronchospasm. Anti-inflammatory agents serve as maintenance medicines for all but the mildest forms of asthma.

For the athlete, asthma may cause a twin burden. Coaches or teammates who fail to recognize symptoms may label the asthmatic patient as lazy. Sometimes the athletes themselves lose self-esteem and begin attributing poor performances to lack of desire rather than to poor pulmonary function. Having objective measures of lung function on a daily basis allows athletes to better appreciate the relationship of performance to respiratory status and allows them to supplement medications accordingly.

Six key goals published as a part of the International Asthma Management Project are directed at improving the quality of life and ability of asthma patients to pursue activity. This panel of experts recommends the following (17):

1 Educate patients to develop a partnership in asthma management.
2 Assess and monitor asthma severity with objective measures of lung function.
3 Avoid or control asthma triggers.
4 Establish medication plans for chronic management.
5 Establish plans for managing exacerbations.
6 Provide regular follow-up care.

These goals apply to all patients and imply that any patient who has more than a rare asthma episode should use a peak flow meter to monitor severity of their disease. Having developed an objective measure of disease severity, the patient should have an established plan of treatment built upon the concept of a green zone, yellow zone, and red zone.

The zones give the asthma patient a guideline as to how to adjust medication to lung function. The red zone indicates that the patient needs to stop all but essential activities, because the PEFR is less than 50% of the patient's established maximum level. This type of flare requires maximal medical treatment and a visit to the doctor. Unless the patient responds dramatically to other medicines, they often need an oral corticosteroid (which are subject to International Olympic Committee [IOC] regulation). The yellow zone correlates with a PEFR of 50% to 80% of maximum. This represents a time for caution but pulmonary function may improve into the green zone with the use of high doses of inhaled medications and limited activity. A green zone measurement is a PEFR greater than 80% of maximum. This indicates nor-

mal lung function or at most mild airway obstruction. The athlete can pursue all activities with use of a pre-exercise bronchodilator and continuation of any standard medications (17).

Questions often arise about the athlete continuing training while PEFR measures remain in the yellow zone. Some athletes have tolerated poor asthma control for years and typically work out with moderate airway obstruction. For sports with significant aerobic demand this is not advisable. In general, the only activities that do not have the potential for worsening a moderate asthma attack are ones in which the $\dot{V}O_2max$ requirement is low. These include weightlifting, shooting drills for basketball, passing drills in American football, or any form of drills, skill training, or strength training in a sport that allows complete recovery between activities.

Treatment of Asthma Patients Based on the Clinical Features of Their Illness

Pharmacologic treatment of all types of asthma patients focuses first on reduction of inflammation and second on treating the consequences of this process, such as bronchospasm.

Atopic Asthma Once a clinician identifies a patient as primarily in the atopic class, treatment centers around prevention. Treatment should begin with the earliest symptoms or at the beginning of a high risk season. An inhaled corticosteroid and, for selected patients, a nasal corticosteroid are first-line therapy for most adults. Patient tolerance is good and 80% to 90% respond well. Nedocromil or cromolyn sodium are generally the first drugs used in younger patients, although relative efficacy compared with inhaled steroids has not been established.

Antihistamines have a limited role in atopic individuals with asthma, although some patients find them necessary. Terfenadine, astemizole, loratidine, and ketotifen (not approved in the United States) are among a limited number of antihistamines thought to produce bronchodilation. Most athletes experience side effects with antihistamines, although these are not as common with newer agents. For example, drowsiness can be troublesome, and airway drying can worsen other asthma symptoms.

A bronchodilator helps the atopic patient most during acute flares and before workouts and competitions. Their use can be directed by peak flow measures so that at stable periods some atopic athletes do not need routine pre-exercise bronchodilators. Inhaled albuterol is listed as the drug of choice, but probably has similar efficacy to other beta agonists such as terbutaline, pirbuterol, and salbutamol. The IOC permits inhaled beta agonists, but not oral beta agonists, with notification of the National Sporting Organization or IOC.

True Asthma   True asthmatic patients require more consistent and aggressive therapy than other individuals with periodic wheezing. The goal is reduction of chronic inflammatory changes to prevent the secondary problems of asthma, which include significant bronchospasm with exercise. Adult patients even with mild asthma should use maintenance inhaled corticosteroids as first-line treatment unless they have intolerable side effects (18). For pediatric age groups nedocromil (age 12 or older) or cromolyn sodium may be tried first. Patients not completely controlled with anti-inflammatory agents should take beta agonists on schedule, routinely before exercise, and otherwise as needed for exacerbations. Long-duration beta agonists, such as salmeterol, provide a helpful alternative. In one study, salmeterol (inhaler permitted by the IOC with notification) twice daily gave superior results to albuterol four times daily (19). However, long-acting beta agonists primarily benefit severe asthmatics or athletes who consistently have difficulty in timing the use of short-acting beta agonists. An additional use of salmeterol is for longer competitions, such as marathons or triathlons.

Other options in the true asthmatic include a trial of ipratropium in refractory cases. Ipratropium and other anticholinergic medications are not standard medications but can be tried as supplemental therapy to block bronchospasm. Nasal anti-inflammatory preparations should be supplemented in the asthmatic who also experiences allergic rhinitis. Patients with significant asthma require early antibiotic intervention when sputum or nasal secretions become purulent in appearance. Theophylline has limited use in the treatment of most asthmatic athletes due to its side effects and the need for serum levels. Theophylline may have particular benefits to the patient troubled by nocturnal symptoms, but necessitates good monitoring. Short bursts of an oral corticosteroid (prohibited by the IOC) for 3 to 7 days may help asthmatics whose peak flows drop significantly with infection or extremely high pollen counts. (Athletes should check IOC restrictions on all theophylline products because many of them contain banned substances.)

Classic EIA   Classic EIA patients often respond well to environmental manipulation, for example, running with a mask in cool air or using a humidifier in an indoor workout area. Another training modification involves a slower, longer warmup period to attempt to enter the "refractory phase" of asthma. This unexplained physiologic phenomenon represents the period in which the athlete is unlikely to develop EIA symptoms in response to a given exercise challenge. When patients require medication, most respond well to beta agonists, but the timing must be individualized for the sport and the patient. For example, one runner may get an adequate response using an inhaler 30 minutes before competition, whereas another needs two doses spaced 20 to 30 minutes apart, with the last dose 15 minutes before competition. Ice hockey competitors may wish to supplement the beta agonist at each period break. Different sports performance responses guide the therapeutic approach to each patient.

Nedocromil or cromolyn sodium may be considered alternative drugs of choice for pretreatment of classic exercise-induced asthma patients, but generally are somewhat less efficacious than beta agonists. However, the addition of nedocromil or cromolyn sodium 15 minutes after beta agonist use improves the response of difficult patients when compared with monotherapy (8,20).

New Treatments   New treatment strategies continue to emerge for all clinical types of asthma. Using anti-inflammatory medications on a regular basis decreases the tendency of the lungs to develop bronchospasm and lessens the frequency of asthma attacks, so as to decrease the dose of beta agonists (21). Trials suggest that this benefits a number of EIA patients who have a late phase response, even when the early bronchoconstriction is blocked. Other trends in therapy include use of H$_2$ blockers for patients in whom reflux triggers asthma attacks. Another clinical strategy is to increase the anti-inflammatory dose for 4 to 6 weeks after respiratory infections. Allergic immunotherapy helps specific individuals, but its use remains limited because of inconsistent response. Any athlete whose asthma symptoms have flared after using nonsteroidal anti-inflammatory drugs or aspirin should avoid these medications.

Causes for Treatment Failure

The athlete who does not improve with standard therapy requires reassessment before changing medications. Many factors influence therapeutic response, including suboptimal dosing, empty canisters, mistiming of medication use, and poor inhaler technique. Education lessens these problems, and athletes who have difficulty using a particular product may benefit from a spacer device, a breath actuated inhaler, or a powdered inhaler not dependent on propellants. Impediments such as occult infection (particularly sinusitis), presence of high pollen counts, or levels of air pollution may also interfere with therapy. When no obvious reason for poor response to therapy is found, the physician should consider the possibility of misdiagnosis or of secondary gain from the illness. Some athletes don't want to continue a sport, but are pressured by a parent or coach. In these situations, asthma allows the athlete a face-saving way to stop an unwanted activity. New medications for asthma, not adequately studied in athletes, include inhaled furosemide, inhaled heparin, and oral leukotriene antagonists.

Asthma Summary

EIA is a common condition treated by sports physicians and can be diagnosed by history, response to medication, or an exercise challenge with, before, and after measures of pulmonary function. Clinical symptoms, while nonspecific, usually include shortness of breath, coughing, or chest pain. Wheezing is rarely noticed. Three clinical groups often develop problems during exercise: atopic, true asthmatic, and classic EIA patients. The primary focus of therapy is control of inflammation with use of supplemental bronchodilators as

needed. New guidelines suggest that the athlete should play an active role in managing his or her illness and should adjust training based on objective measures such as peak expiratory flow rates. The goal of treatment is to return all asthma patients to full activity and to encourage them to participate in appropriate sports activity.

CHRONIC OBSTRUCTIVE PULMONARY DISEASE (COPD)

Chronic obstructive pulmonary disease (COPD) falls into two major categories: chronic bronchitis and emphysema. Patients in both groups experience a variety of the manifestations of asthma. Unlike COPD, asthma by definition causes reversible obstruction to airflow. In COPD physiologic testing shows chronic obstruction to airflow secondary to either bronchitic or emphysematous changes, and these changes are only partly reversible. *Chronic bronchitis* is diagnosed by a history of recurrent cough with mucus production for at least 3 months of the year for 2 years. *Emphysema* is defined by distention of air spaces distal to the terminal bronchioles.

Chronic Bronchitis

Chronic bronchitis subsets are classified by the character of sputum production. The simple mucoid type differs from chronic purulent mucoid types that often have an association with bronchiectasis. A common condition in most Western nations, the prevalence of chronic bronchitis is 20% in adult males (22). Smoking seems to be the primary etiologic factor, with occupational and environmental changes additive. Perhaps because males smoke more, men are more frequently affected than women.

Pathologic changes in chronic bronchitis include hyperplasia of mucus-producing glands in the bronchiolar wall and the small airways, fibrosis, mucus plugging, inflammatory changes, and damage to ciliated cells. FEV1 may remain normal until late in disease, but progressive airway narrowing and decreased airway flow with high airway resistance occur in advanced stages. Even in early smokers small airway resistance increases, so that while overall pulmonary function seems good, irreversible change is underway. The high airway resistance leads to pulmonary artery hypertension at rest and with exercise. Clinically, patients with chronic bronchitis often are described as "blue bloaters" because they become cyanotic and retain CO_2 without showing much distress.

Emphysema

Emphysema patients undergo a series of pathologic changes that affect their ability to increase ventilatory capacity. These changes occur in the airways, alveoli, and chest wall. Airway caliber narrows and becomes less compliant after damages from the chronic inflammatory process on the epithelial lining. The favorable balance point for elastic recoil is shifted so that the chest wall no longer assists in exhalation. This particularly becomes true after the chest cavity expands; outward recoil of the chest wall is increased at the same time that inward recoil is diminished. The collapsibility of small airways increases as elastic tissue breaks down. This further decreases the effectiveness of elastic recoil as well as leaving areas of dead space within the lung that are not ventilated. Essentially, the respiratory system can be compared with a hyperinflated inner tube, stretched and distorted from its original shape.

Patients with emphysema differ from chronic bronchitis patients in a number of ways. They often appear in distress, using accessory respiratory muscles, leaning forward and pursing their lips with each expiration. They compensate for the mechanical breakdown of lung structure by increasing their ventilatory rate. Cough and sputum production are not prominent. Often they show weight loss and have a poor ability to handle respiratory infection. These patients are often labeled as "pink puffers" because they do not tolerate hypoxia or hypercarbia as do the chronic bronchitis patients. Prognosis for them is poor if some stress upsets the delicate balance and tips them into acute respiratory failure (22).

Exercise and the COPD Patient

The physiologic changes in the respiratory system make significant COPD incompatible with most high-level athletic activities. Nevertheless, a number of COPD patients, particularly with mild disease, are returning to adult sports activities because of the physical benefits. The degree of impairment determines the level of sports activity that a given COPD patient can pursue. Studies of smokers demonstrate that they cannot regain lost capacity, but cessation of smoking allows them to parallel the same physiologic decline curve of nonsmokers. In addition, a number of active adults who have not been smokers have developed COPD, probably related to other factors such as occupational exposure, genetic predisposition, air pollution, recurrent pulmonary infections, and the physiologic decline of aging.

To advise the COPD patient who wishes to exercise, the physician must estimate what physiologic limits exist for a given individual. For example, the resting minute ventilation of 5 to 7 liter air/minute may be doubled in a patient with COPD. Only 1% to 2% of oxygen consumption is used to support the work of breathing in the average individual, but the COPD patient often uses 10%. As this increased cost of respiratory effort exists, the physician must estimate how much pulmonary reserve can be devoted to physical activity (23). Three findings that preclude physical activity are cor pulmonale (which is associated with syncope during exercise), resting hypercapnia, or dyspnea at rest. These changes generally correlate with an FEV1 of less than 25%. Dyspnea on mild exertion generally indicates an FEV1 of less than 50% and is about the minimal level of function at which the patient can tolerate most physical activities. The physician can time the onset of dyspnea at a measured workload such as an exercise treadmill test to determine an exercise prescription for a given patient. In any, case an exercise treadmill test seems appropriate for most COPD patients because of a high risk of concomitant coronary artery disease in any who have been smokers.

Fortunately, a number of physical changes in COPD patients have a certain element of reversibility. For example, the inspiratory pressure measurement correlates with the isometric strength of respiratory muscles. This is typically reduced by 15% to 30% in COPD, but muscle strength does respond to training (24). This allows an increase in dynamic respiratory muscle function so that a maximum ventilatory volume (MVV) measured at onset of an exercise program may increase with effective training. In addition, as most COPD patients have some asthmatic component to their symptoms, reversal of any bronchospasm that occurs with activity may improve performance (25).

Treatment of COPD in the Athletic Patient

Treatment of COPD in an athletic individual requires careful monitoring. For example, the physician may need objective evidence that the COPD patient does not develop oxygen desaturation with more vigorous activity. All nonpulmonary factors need to be addressed to allow treatment of any other medical illnesses or orthopedic problems that might also affect exercise capacity. Smoking cessation is a mandatory aspect of treatment. In addition, early antibiotic treatment of any significant respiratory infection (even though many are viral) may prevent deterioration of respiratory status. Supplemental high calorie foods may help balance the excess calorie demands in the COPD patient who begins an exercise program.

Medications for treatment of COPD are the same as those for asthma. However, theophylline plays a more important role, as the primary effect of this drug is to improve respiratory muscle function as opposed to bronchodilation (23). Beta agonists remain a better choice when a significant component of bronchospasm is present. Ipatropium has established benefits in COPD patients who respond less well to beta agonists and other medications. Oral and inhaled corticosteroids are helpful in acute flares, although no clear recommendations exist for their ongoing use in COPD (also, note IOC provisions on their use in oral and inhaled forms). Recent studies suggest that inflammatory change is constantly present in COPD patients, and for this reason many clinicians use inhaled corticosteroids as a part of long-term maintenance therapy (25). Trials using digoxin or calcium channel blockers in advanced COPD have not shown any improvement in exercise capacity (26,27). For the chronically hypoxic patient, continuous oxygen is the only therapeutic measure shown to improve outcomes as well as allow the patient to continue some level of physical activity.

Benefits of Exercise to the COPD Patient and Exercise Recommendations

Documented short-term benefits of exercise for COPD patients have emerged in recent years. The most important of these are as follows (23):

- Increased endurance
- Improved maximal performance
- Reduced hospitalizations
- Enhanced ability to walk
- Improved activity in daily life

Unfortunately, no long-term studies exist to document a continued benefit of exercise therapy. Failure of studies to show consistently that exercise improves pulmonary function tests has limited the widespread use of exercise treatment in COPD. Currently, the primary reason for therapy is the physical performance improvements noted above and beneficial psychological effects among COPD patients who improve their fitness.

Recommendations should emphasize the positive outcomes from studies. Advise the patient that respiratory muscle weakness can be strengthened. Walking capacity and work ability can improve if the exercise training starts at both low intensity and short duration. The training regimen must be moderate and not worsen pulmonary symptoms. Once started, exercise must be continued or reversal of benefits will ensue quickly. Recovery time for COPD patients is prolonged, so maximal exercise frequency is only three times weekly, and exercise time per session must increase gradually. For example, a program might start for only 10 minutes per session, with session times increasing 2 minutes per month until a total time of 20 to 40 minutes is reached. Walking, swimming, cycling, and other aerobic activities can be alternated with strength exercise for a balanced, all-around approach to fitness. Upper extremity activity is difficult for many patients because the exercise may recruit accessory respiratory muscles and lead to rapid fatigue. Although many sports activities remain out of reach of the COPD patient, current thinking advises physical activity within the limits of exercise capacity with the goal of improving quality of life, even if the effect on longevity is unknown.

RESTRICTIVE LUNG DISEASE

Sarcoidosis

Sarcoidosis is the most common restrictive lung disease to affect athletes. Even though the lung findings resemble those of interstitial pulmonary fibrosis (IPF) and occupational lung disease, this syndrome differs in that changes are diffuse and involve multiple organ systems. Worldwide distribution and prevalence in all races suggest that this disease does not relate to exposure to a single toxin or to a specific genetic trait. Women typically are affected more often than men. Racial prevalence is inconsistent: blacks are at a much higher risk than whites in the United States, but in Europe blacks are at a lower risk. Marked variations in frequency of sarcoidosis occur within the same geographic areas, with the disease 20-fold more common in Sweden than in Poland. Some areas such as New Zealand or Southeast Asia report few cases of sarcoidosis. The epidemiology becomes more confused by occurrence of family clusters, community outbreaks, spouses who are both affected, and twins with the disease. This variable pattern points to a multifactorial etiology. Apparently a genetically susceptible individual has an exaggerated cellular immune response to an unknown antigen, which leads to complex pathologic and immune changes consistent with sarcoidosis.

Pathology   Pathologic changes establish the diagnosis. Noncaseating granulomas are considered a pathognomonic feature. Before the formation of these granulomas, T lymphocytes and mononuclear phagocytic cells infiltrate involved organs. This cellular migration is accompanied by changes in immune system function. Examples of this are that tissues show an exaggerated response of helper T lymphocyte cells; a nonspecific increase in gamma globulins may reflect nonspecific stimulation of B cells by T cells; and decreased cellular immune response leads to anergy on skin testing. The organs typically affected are the lungs and lymph nodes in 90% of cases. Skin, eyes, upper respiratory tract, liver, spleen, and bone marrow are involved in 25% of cases. Also, 5% or fewer show infiltration of cardiac, musculoskeletal, renal, endocrine, exocrine, central nervous, and gastrointestinal systems (28).

Clinically three presentations of sarcoidosis account for most of the 90% of cases with pulmonary involvement. About 20% are asymptomatic patients less than 40 years old who have the disease diagnosed based on incidental chest radiograph findings. Another 20% of cases develop vague constitutional symptoms, which include fever, fatigue, weight loss, anorexia, cough, dyspnea, and occasionally chest pain. Although the majority of these individuals have a mild illness, up to 25% may ultimately develop more severe symptoms. Unfortunately, 60% of patients have insidious but progressive respiratory symptoms, and the disease can be advanced before they seek care or receive a correct diagnosis. Most of this latter group experience a gradual increase in respiratory problems which usually become chronic; 10% of these patients also develop symptoms of other organ involvement (28).

Diagnosis   Diagnostic confirmation requires a combination of clinical, radiologic, and pathologic changes, with leading differential diagnostic candidates being idiopathic pulmonary fibrosis, tuberculosis, lymphoma, fungal infection, and HIV-associated pulmonary infections. Attempts to use the Kveim-Stilzbach skin test for diagnosis have not proven this to be reliable. Chest radiographs are helpful, as 90% of all cases have an abnormal chest picture at some point. Radiographic abnormalities are permanent in 50% of patients, and 5% to 15% of cases develop progressive fibrosis (28). Typical chest radiographs are classified as

Type 1: increased hilar nodes
Type 2: bilateral increase in hilar nodes plus diffuse parenchymal changes (Fig 22-1)
Type 3: diffuse parenchymal changes without hilar adenopathy

In spite of a standard classification system, the radiographic appearance can mimic most pulmonary problems and remains one of the most variable features of the disease. Partly because of this, most cases are confirmed on transbronchial biopsy during bronchoscopy or from tissue obtained from the skin or a lymph node.

Other diagnostic tests include standard laboratory panels, which reveal nonspecific findings. For example, complete blood profiles may show lym-

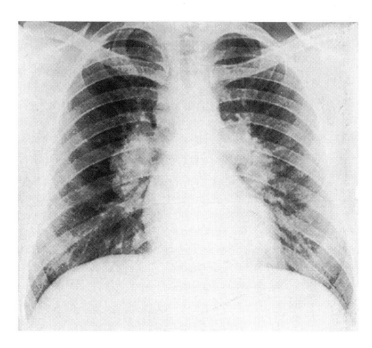

Figure 22-1.   Hilar adenopathy consistent with sarcoidosis. (Reproduced by permission from Squire LF, Colaiace WM, Strutynsky N, et al. Chest, abdomen, bone and the total patient. Exercises in diagnostic radiology, combined 2nd ed. vols. 1, 2, 3, 4. Philadelphia: WB Saunders, 1982:28.)

phocytopenia, eosinophilia, and elevated liver function tests. Calcium levels are only rarely elevated. Erythrocyte-sedimentation rates and C-reactive protein levels sometime increase, as is the case with gamma globulins. Pulmonary function tests help distinguish the symptoms from conditions such as asthma by typically showing classic restrictive findings with decreases in total lung capacity, vital capacity, and residual volume along with a decreased diffusion capacity.

Special Presentations That May Influence Sports Participation   Pulmonary problems obviously have the potential for affecting sports participation. Sarcoidosis may trigger bronchospasm. At least one death has occurred from this during a marathon race (29). A number of other clinical changes in sarcoidosis can also affect the athlete. Splenomegaly, which occurs in 5% to 10% of patients, should preclude participation in contact or collision sports. Löfgren's syndrome, a complex of erythema nodosum, hilar adenopathy, and joint symptoms, has occurred in athletes who presented

with joint pain (30). Failure to diagnose and treat this condition appropriately delays the resolution of joint swelling and the return to sports. A serious but rare complication of sarcoidosis is granulomatous infiltration of the cardiac conduction system, which can lead to serious arrhythmias.

Idiopathic Pulmonary Fibrosis (IPF)

Idiopathic pulmonary fibrosis (IPF) resembles sarcoidosis and most commonly these patients come to medical care at about age 50 years because of a nonproductive cough and shortness of breath. Often the initial chest radiograph shows reticulonodular patterns in lower lung fields, and pulmonary function tests show a restrictive pattern. Several known factors that may precipitate problems include occupational and environmental inhalants, drugs, and radiation. In addition, family clusters are common (e.g., several miners in the same family), but whether this reflects a genetic predisposition to pathologic change or a reaction to a common toxin has not been determined. In 33%

of cases, a viral illness precedes onset of symptoms, which usually show slow progression but can steadily worsen to chronic respiratory failure. This is a diverse class of disorders that lead to restrictive lung disease with an unknown etiology. Pathology may also show noncaseating granulomas, but does not show other organ system involvement as seen in sarcoidosis.

Physical examination progresses through three stages, which parallel the findings on chest radiograph.

- **Physical exam stages**
  Stage 1: normal
  Stage 2: rales ≫ tachypnea ≫ cyanosis and clubbing
  Stage 3: cor pulmonale with RVH and right-sided S_3 heart sounds
- **Radiologic exam stages**
  Stage 1: diffuse reticulonodular changes in lung fields
  Stage 2: ground glass appearance to lung fields; sometimes nodules that coalesce into larger size masses
  Stage 3: lung fields diminished in size; honeycombing may appear

Laboratory testing shows nonspecific changes such as an increased erythrocyte sedimentation rate, positive cryoglobulins, increased immunoglobulins, and low titer changes in rheumatoid factor, antinuclear antigens, and complement levels. Pulmonary function tests gradually evolve into the classic findings of restrictive lung disease. A key diagnostic feature is reduction in carbon monoxide diffusion (DLCO) of 30% to 50% (31).

Treatment of Sarcoidosis and Interstitial Pulmonary Fibrosis

Aggressive intervention early in the course of the disease is required to interrupt the progressive pathologic sequence before irreversible damage occurs. Generally this requires immunosuppressive therapy. An example of a treatment protocol for IPF or sarcoidosis is (31):

1 Begin with prednisone, 1 milligram per 1 kilogram body weight per day for a total of 8 to 12 weeks; if clinically responsive, patients may undergo progressive weaning over 6 to 12 months as long as improvement continues.
2 In unresponsive patients, reduce prednisone to 0.25 milligram per 1 kilogram body weight per day and add cyclophosphamide at 1 mg/kg/day as long as white blood cell counts do not drop by 50% or more. Azathioprine can be used as an alternative.
3 Continuous O_2 therapy is useful in patients with significant hypoxia.

While athletes might begin some light training during a period of medication weaning, the goal is to get the patient into remission and then resume active sport based on a new exercise prescription. During an active course of disease continuous, exercise poses significant risk. Sarcoidosis patients often run a milder course than IPF patients; 50% may show residual changes on chest radiographs or pulmonary function tests, but only 20% develop progressive disease to the extent that they cannot return to exercise. Exercise limitations in sarcoidosis and IPF relate to the DLCO impairment in that not enough oxygen exchange occurs for vigorous exercise (32). These are not straightforward cases, and primary care physicians should use pulmonary consultants and others to help manage these individuals and to prescribe new therapies as more information evolves.

PULMONARY CONDITIONS RELATED TO THE IMMUNE SYSTEM OR COLLAGEN VASCULAR DISEASE

A wide variety of processes and diseases can lead to pulmonary infiltrates. Only a few of these affect athletes, and all of these processes are relatively rare. Among these pulmonary diseases are hypersensitivity pneumonias, eosinophilic pneumonias, environmental lung disease, and collagen vascular disease. No direct association of these processes with sports participation has been made, although a few potentially could be worsened by aspects of training.

Hypersensitivity Pneumonias

Hypersensitivity pneumonias occur after exposure to a specific toxin. Clinically, three presentations differ, based on the amount of antigen exposure. Acute processes lead to fever, chills, cough, and shortness of breath within 6 to 8 hours of an exposure. Subacute processes develop over a few weeks, with progressive pulmonary symptoms that ultimately can lead to respiratory failure. Chronic hypersensitivity pneumonias arise from continuous, low-dose antigen exposure, leading to a slowly progressive pulmonary syndrome.

The most common known causes for these pneumonias are moldy hay, silage and grain, pet birds, foods, and chemicals and heating, cooling, or humidification systems. Chemicals used in pools or to clean wrestling mats, ventilation systems in athletic dormitories, and indoor workout arenas have been implicated in respiratory problems in athletes. The high minute ventilation of athletes in swimming pools, indoor tracks, or wrestling gymnasiums leads to greater antigen loads among participants than those experienced by inactive individuals. Avoidance of the causative agent resolves these processes.

Eosinophilic Pneumonias

Eosinophilic pneumonias resemble any of the hypersensitivity pneumonias except that eosinophilia is a feature. Two types warrant some mention because of possible occurrence in athletes: tropical eosinophilia and drug-induced eosinophilic pneumonia.

Athletes travel to competitions from all over the world, so the sports physician may see some athletes who come from areas with common endemic parasites. Examples of parasites that cause tropical eosinophilia are filaria (the most common cause), ascaris, ancylostoma, strongyloides, and wuchereria.

Drug-induced eosinophilic pneumonias occur from many medications such as penicillin, sulfonamide, nitrofurantoin, tricyclics, and isoniazid. These medications are particularly confusing when they are prescribed for a pulmonary process—the question arises as to whether the original infection is worsening or whether a drug reaction is taking place. Withdrawing the offending medication and treating with a short course of corticosteroid medication (subject to IOC regulation) usually resolves the process.

Environmental Lung Disease

Environmental lung disease follows exposure to dusts, chemicals, and organic and inorganic substances. Millions of cases worldwide are attributed to asbestos, coal dust, cotton dusts, silica, and similar substances. Solubility of the chemicals and particle size of various substances determine the type of pulmonary injury that arises from repeated exposures. These pose no excess risk to athletes, but two types of chemicals have been suggested as problematic for athletes. These include the common chemicals that cause urban air pollution, as athletes have been found to have increased respiratory infections following competitions in cities with high levels of smog. Similarly, indoor arenas with poor ventilation and those that allow cigarette smoking have been linked to increased respiratory symptoms among competitors.

Collagen Vascular Disease

Certain collagen vascular diseases affect younger individuals, including athletes; most of these diseases have pulmonary effects. Systemic lupus erythematosus is one of the most common and can cause pleurisy, pleural effusions, autoimmune pneumonitis (as well as increased risk for secondary bacterial pneumonias), and rarely pulmonary fibrosis or hemorrhage. Ankylosing spondylitis limits maximal pulmonary effort primarily through restriction of full chest expansion. Rheumatoid arthritis affects 1% of the world population with a 3:1 predilection for women. Lung effects, though, are more common in men and include pleuritis and pulmonary fibrosis. Systemic sclerosis (scleroderma) causes diffuse interstitial fibrosis and ultimately may lead to pulmonary hypertension (31).

SUMMARY

Excellent pulmonary function remains a prerequisite for success in many sports with high aerobic demand. A unique anatomy allows the lung to avoid injury or infection even when subjected to prolonged periods of training at extremely high minute ventilation. For many sports with less aerobic demand, mild to moderate respiratory impairment does not preclude participation. In addition, many patients with chronic lung disease have begun exercise programs to try to improve their quality of life.

This chapter reviews the approach to treating asthma, the most common pulmonary problem of athletes, as well as strategies for dealing with the most common chronic diseases of the lungs and some of the rare conditions that affect the pulmonary system. In each of these conditions, appropriate therapy offers the patient a chance to return to some level of exercise or, in the best of cases, to competitive sports.

REFERENCES

1 Levison ME. Pneumonia, including necrotizing pulmonary infections (lung abscess). In: Isselbacher KJ, Braunwald E, Wilson JD, et al., eds. Harrison's principles of internal medicine. 13th ed. New York: McGraw-Hill, 1994:1184–1186.

2 Costill D. Inside running: basics of sports physiology. Indianapolis, IN: Benchmark Press, 1986:46–47.

3 Adams F. The extant works of Aretaeus the Cappadocian. London: Sydenham Society, 1856:316.

4 Scarborough J. Roman medicine. Ithaca, NY: Cornell UP, 1969:119.

5 Lyons AS, Petrucelli RJ. Medicine: an illustrated history. Ancient China. New York: Harry N. Abrams, 1978:124–130.

6 Frobase JF, Kyle JM, Hanna SD, et al. Sensitivity of post-exercise cough in predicting exercise-induced bronchospasm in young athletes. Med Sci Sports Exerc 1992;4(suppl):854. Abstract.

7 Wiens L, et al. Chest pain in otherwise healthy children and adolescents is frequently caused by exercise-induced asthma. Pediatrics 1992;90:350–353.

8 McFadden ER Jr., Gilbert IS. Exercise-induced asthma. N Engl J Med 1994;330:1362–1367.

9 van Grunsven PM, et al. Treatment of mild asthma with inhaled corticosteroids: is discontinuation of therapy possible? Fam Med 1996;28:46–51.

10 Schaefer O, et al. Respiratory function impairment and cardiopulmonary consequences in long-time residents of the Canadian Arctic. Can Med Assoc J 1980;123:997–1004.

11 Larsson K, et al. High prevalence of asthma in cross country skiers. Br Med J 1993;307:1326–1329.

12 Drobnic F, et al. Assessment of chlorine exposure in swimmers during training. Med Sci Sports Exerc 1996;28:271–274.

13 Bousquet J, et al. Eosinophilic inflammation in asthma. N Engl J Med 1990;323:1033–1039.

14 Voy RO. The U.S. Olympic Committee experience with exercise-induced bronchospasm. Med Sci Sports Exerc 1986;18:328–330.

15 Katz RM. Coping with exercise-induced asthma in sports. Physician Sports Med 1987;15:101–108.

16 Fields KB. Three common medical problems in sports. In: Richmond JC, Shahady EJ, eds. Sports medicine for primary care. Boston: Blackwell Science, 1996:541–554.

17 U.S. Dept of Health and Human Services. International consensus report on diagnosis and management of asthma. Publication 92-3091, 1992:1–68.

18 Haahtela T, et al. Comparison of a β2-agonist, terbutaline, with an inhaled corticosteroid, budesonide, in newly detected asthma. N Engl J Med 1991;325:388–392.

19 Pearlman DS, et al. A comparison of salmeterol with albuterol in the treatment of mild-to-moderate asthma. N Engl J Med 1992;327:1420–1425.

20 Anderson SD. Drugs and the control of exercise-induced asthma. Eur Respir J 1993;6:1090–1092.

21 Henriksen JM, Dahl R. Effects of inhaled budesonide alone and in combination with low-dose terbutaline in children with exercise-induced asthma. Am Rev Respir Dis 1983;128:993–997.

22 Ingram RH Jr. Chronic bronchitis, emphysema, and airways obstruction. In: Isselbacher KJ, Braunwald E, Wilson JD, et al., eds. Harrison's principles of internal medicine. 13th ed. New York: McGraw-Hill, 1994:1197–1206.

23 Barker AF. Exercise and pulmonary disease. In: Goldberg L, Elliot DL, eds. Exercise for prevention and treatment of illness. Philadelphia: FA Davis, 1994:271–288.

24 Belman MJ, King RR. Pulmonary profiling in exercise. Clin Sports Med 1984;3:119–136.

25 Kerstjens HAM, et al. A comparison of bronchodilator therapy with or without inhaled corticosteroid therapy for obstructive airways disease. N Engl J Med 1992;327:1413–1419.

26 Brown SF, et al. Effects of verapamil on pulmonary hemodynamics during hypoxemia, at rest, and during exercise in patients with chronic obstructive pulmonary disease. Thorax 1983;38:840–844.

27 Brown SF, et al. Effects of digoxin on exercise capacity and right ventricular function during exercise in chronic airflow obstruction. Chest 1984;85:187–191.

28 Crystal RG. Sarcoidosis. In: Isselbacher KJ, Braun-

wald E, Wilson JD, et al., eds. Harrison's principles of internal medicine. 13th ed. New York: McGraw-Hill, 1994:1679–1684.

29 Parsons MA, et al. An "unavoidable" death in the people's marathon. Br J Sports Med 1984;18:38–39.

30 Green GA, Maltz BA. Bilateral ankle pain in an aerobic dancer. Med Sci Sports Exerc 1992;24:1316–1320.

31 Reynolds HY. Interstitial lung diseases. In: Isselbacher KJ, Braunwald E, Wilson JD, et al., eds. Harrison's principles of internal medicine. 13th ed. New York: McGraw-Hill, 1994:1206–1211.

32 Keogh BA, et al. Importance of the lower respiratory tract in oxygen transfer. Exercise testing in patients with interstitial and destructive lung disease. Am Rev Respir Dis 1984;129:S76–S80.

Chapter 23
Gastroenterology and Sport

David Hughes

Gastrointestinal disease affects nearly all individuals at some stage. Many conditions are mild and transient with little or no long-term sequelae. Other gastrointestinal conditions have serious consequences for individuals, causing long-standing morbidity and significantly affecting their quality of life. Some gastrointestinal disease processes have special significance for the athletic population because the disease or the treatment regimen affects the ability of the individual to exercise. Exercise itself can affect the disease process. This chapter details several gastrointestinal conditions and analyzes the particular relevance that they hold for the active individual.

GASTRITIS AND PEPTIC DISEASE

Peptic disease (PD) refers to pathologic processes that result in injury to the mucosal lining of the upper gastrointestinal tract as a result of the actions of pepsin and acid. Pepsin and acid not only cause injuries themselves, but also act synergistically with other agents to cause damage. There is a broad spectrum of physical injury that may occur in PD. Some mild forms of mucosal injury are detectable only by biopsy. Erythema, erosions, and frank ulceration are other macroscopic forms of PD. Symptoms correlate poorly with the severity of lesions so that patients with severe dyspepsia may have a visibly normal mucosa, while patients with endoscopic evidence of severe ulceration may be asymptomatic (1).

Gastritis is a common peptic injury with different diagnostic interpretations by the clinician and the pathologist. To the endoscopist, gastritis may refer to mucosal thinning, erythema, or erosions.

To the pathologist, gastritis refers to inflammatory cells within the gastric mucosa and may be subdivided into acute, chronic, erosive, and nonerosive.

Population Demographics and Prevalence

PD (including gastritis and ulcers) affects 10% to 15% of males and 4% to 15% of females in Western societies. The incidence of acute gastric ulcer in Western countries, estimated at 0.4 to 0.5 per 1000, is approximately one-fourth as common as duodenal ulcers. In some countries (Peru, Norway, Japan), duodenal ulcer is more common than gastric ulcer. Nonerosive gastritis may be a variant of the aging process, with over 50% of the population over 50 years of age having superficial antral and fundic gland gastritis (2).

Pathophysiology or Infectious Agents

PD is thought to result from an imbalance between those factors that protect the mucosal lining and those factors that are harmful to it. Thus, injury occurs not only when harmful factors are present in excess, but also when protective factors are deficient and harmful factors are at "normal" levels. Acid and pepsin are almost always implicated in PD. A pH of 1 to 2 enhances the activity of pepsin. Acid also acts synergistically with other harmful agents such as nonsteroidal anti-inflammatory drugs (NSAIDs) and bile acids. Alcohol is able to damage the mucosal lining with or without the presence of acid. Physiologic (e.g., major surgery) and psychological stress predisposes the mucosa to injury as does corticosteroid ingestion and smoking. Various dietary components have been implicated in the past, but these tend to vary from individual to individual in terms of their tendency to aggravate the PD.

Prostaglandins, particularly the E and I series, protect the gastric and duodenal mucosa. These prostaglandins stimulate mucosal blood flow and enhance secretion of bicarbonate and mucus. NSAIDs inhibit prostaglandins and through this mechanism predispose the mucosa to injury. The risk of injury from NSAIDs increases with high and frequent doses of the drugs, use of more than one NSAID, use with corticosteroids, and a previous history of PD.

Helicobacter pylori Evidence emerged in the early 1980s of an infectious origin of gastritis and PD. *Helicobacter pylori* has now been confirmed as a major cause of upper gastrointestinal pathology, with 40% of the population in Western countries infected. This bacterium causes chronic active gastritis, which is a prerequisite for duodenal ulcer and gastric ulcer in the absence of other precipitating factors such as NSAID ingestion. *H. pylori* infection precedes most ulcer disease, and eradication of *H. pylori* leads to more rapid and effective ulcer healing with decreased rates of recurrence. Evidence now supports a link between *H. pylori* infection and gastric carcinoma such that patients infected with *H. pylori* have a three- to sixfold increased risk (3).

Common Symptoms and Atypical Presentations

Abdominal pain is the most common symptom of PD, although some patients may be asymptomatic. The pain classically begins in the epigastric region and lessens after food or antacid ingestion. The pain is often burning in nature and may radiate to the back, although this may also indicate perforation with involvement of the pancreas. Other symptoms include nausea and vomiting and a sense of fullness or abdominal distension. Many patients, however, present with nonspecific, poorly localized abdominal pain, which may arise from various gastrointestinal or even cardiac causes. Gastric ulcer, whether benign or malignant, often causes weight loss.

Unusual presentations in PD may indicate a complication. Hematemesis as a result of ulcer hemorrhage is usually recognized as serious by the patient and the physician, and it prompts immedi-ate attention. More commonly, however, bleeding ulcers cause persistent or intermittent melena or fatigue from a hypochromic, microcytic anemia. Similarly, a perforation of the stomach or duodenum, with loss of contents into the peritoneum—with the signs of pallor, sweating, abdominal rigidity, generalized acute tenderness, and rebound—develops quickly into a surgical emergency. Chronic perforation into another hollow viscus may lead to more subtle and wide-ranging symptoms, and thus may delay diagnosis.

The presentation of abdominal pain with repeated vomiting in a patient with a background of PD suggests gastric outlet obstruction. However, in cases of partial obstruction, vomiting may not be a feature, and anorexia, weight loss, and constipation may be the primary complaints. Despite a declining trend for overall mortality from PD, awareness of PD complications is important, as the mortality from each of these three complications continues to be 5% to 20%.

Physical Findings

The physical examination in uncomplicated PD is often completely normal or may only show some mild epigastric tenderness. If PD is suspected, the physician must check for signs associated with complications, including melena on rectal examination, pallor, clinically significant weight loss, succussion splash, and visible peristalsis.

Diagnostic Evaluation

The patient with mild, uncomplicated PD probably does not warrant investigation for the first occurrence. If the patient responds well to first-line therapy and the symptoms settle with no evidence of recurrence or complication, a "wait and see" approach may be adopted. If symptoms persist or there is a suspicion of complications, then further investigation is warranted.

Hemoccult testing for blood in the stool, a full blood picture, and ferritin are relatively inexpensive first-line tests that can indicate whether anemia or iron deficiency is present. If pain radiates through to the back, a serum amylase is recommended to exclude pancreatic involvement. Upper gastrointestinal barium studies may ascertain the presence of ulcerative lesions. Upper gastrointestinal endoscopy is the gold standard to definitively diagnose the nature and severity of mucosal lesions. Endoscopy also allows biopsies to be taken to exclude neoplastic change within the lesions.

All patients with PD should be screened for *H. pylori* infection. Most commonly, *H. pylori* is diagnosed by antral biopsy during endoscopy. Serology can detect *H. pylori* infection in untreated individuals, but it is not an accurate assessment of eradication therapy because titers remain elevated for up to a year following eradication. The C-urea breath test relies on the ability of *H. pylori* to split urea (ingested radiolabeled urea for the purposes of this test), after which the CO_2 is measured in the breath. This test is accurate but not yet widely available.

Special Considerations in Athletes

Incidence of PD increases with age, thus the younger athletic population is at less risk than the average adult population. Similarly, smoking and excessive alcohol intake, which are known risk factors for PD, are less common among the athletic population than the general population. On the other hand, ingestion of NSAIDs is quite prevalent in the athletic community, and athletes often self-medicate and increase doses of their medication without first checking with their physician. A history of NSAID ingestion should be sought with any athlete presenting with dyspepsia.

No data compare the prevalence of dyspepsia in the athletic community with that in the general population, but several studies do document a high incidence of upper gastrointestinal symptoms during actual exercise. Studies report symptoms of dyspepsia in approximately 10% of recreational runners, and these symptoms increase with the severity of exertion and among more inexperienced runners (4). One study reported endoscopic findings in marathon runners who suffered abdominal pain during the marathon and had occult fecal blood loss after the marathon. The endoscopic findings were of oozing mucosal lesions at the gastric antrum. The lesions were consistent with local ischemia and resolved quickly after cessation of exercise (5). It is postulated that these transient bleeding gastric lesions were caused by

mucosal hypoperfusion during the marathon. Other studies have shown an 80% reduction in visceral perfusion during maximal exertion (6).

A common presenting complaint among the athletic population is fatigue or underperformance. If the athlete is taking NSAIDs, one must check the stool for occult blood loss, even in the absence of dyspeptic symptoms. A low ferritin with true anemia may cause a loss of stamina and merits concern. Depletion of iron stores or hypochromic microcytic anemia, in conjunction with occult fecal blood loss, requires full investigation to exclude peptic ulcer.

GASTROESOPHAGEAL REFLUX DISEASE

Gastroesophageal reflux disease (GERD) is a syndrome that encompasses all the symptomatology and pathology associated with reflux of gastric contents into the lower esophagus. Some reflux of gastric contents occurs normally as a physiologic process in asymptomatic individuals. This process is benign and should not be considered part of the GERD syndrome. The presenting symptomatology varies enormously, and there is little correlation between subjective symptoms and objective findings.

Population Demographics and Prevalence

In Western societies, over 50% of the population will at some stage experience the symptoms of heartburn and regurgitation, and approximately 10% of the adult population suffer daily symptoms of heartburn. The growing recognition that GERD can produce atypical symptoms indicates a considerably higher prevalence than previously estimated. An association with GERD has been noted in up to 50% of patients with noncardiac chest pain, 78% of patients with chronic hoarseness, and 82% of patients with asthma (7).

Pathophysiology and Infectious Agents

Many factors contribute to the development of GERD. The lower esophageal sphincter (LES) provides the major antireflux barrier, and any compromise of normal LES function renders the individual more susceptible to GERD. The nature and volume of gastric contents also influence the likelihood of GERD. Efficiency of esophageal clearance determines the length of time of esophageal exposure to reflux material and hence the extent and severity of any damage. Delayed gastric emptying may feature in the etiology of GERD by allowing greater volumes of acid–pepsin mixtures to remain in the stomach for longer periods of time.

A positive pressure gradient between the abdomen and the thorax would cause continuous reflux if no barrier existed at the gastroesophageal junction. The LES consists of 2 to 4 cm of asymmetrically thickened smooth muscle. LES pressure is maintained in the resting position but relaxes with swallowing, esophageal distension, or vagal stimulation. The resting pressure tends to vary from moment to moment, especially in the postprandial period. Frequent, regular relaxations of LES pressure allow a small amount of "physiologic reflux" in asymptomatic individuals. With pathologic reflux, other factors such as increased gastric pressure or a decreased resting LES pressure allow the excessive reflux, even though most reflux occurs during the period of physiologic relaxation. There is debate as to whether the lower resting LES pressure seen in individuals with GERD is primary or secondary to the inflammation-caused injury.

Efficient esophageal acid clearance minimizes contact time between acidic reflux material and the distal esophagus. Effective acid clearance depends on both effective peristalsis and normal salivation. Peristalsis removes the bulk of the volume from the distal esophagus, and saliva neutralizes any remaining acidic residue. Esophageal clearance times are two to three times longer in individuals with GERD. The amplitude of peristaltic contraction is lower in GERD patients than in controls, and GERD patients also have an increased proportion of failed peristaltic contractions with hypotensive foci in the distal esophagus (8).

The nature of gastric contents is an important factor in GERD. Acid causes protein denaturation in the esophagus and allows back-diffusion of hydrogen ions into the deeper layers of the esophagus. Pepsin digests esophageal intercellular substance, causing shedding of epithelial cells. Bile salts from the duodenum, if refluxed into the esophagus, cause dissolution of lipids in the epithelial cell membrane and make the mucosa more permeable to hydrogen ion back-diffusion.

Delayed gastric emptying may be due to systemic diseases such as hypothyroidism and diabetes, or to mechanical gastric outlet obstruction from PD. The delay predisposes the patient to increased gastric volumes, particularly in the postprandial period, and the resultant elevation in gastric pressure increases the likelihood of reflux. Some foods and medications aggravate GERD. These substances are thought to exert their effect by decreasing LES pressure (Table 23-1).

Complications of GERD include strictures, Barrett's esophagus, esophageal ulcers and bleeding, and pulmonary manifestations. Strictures usually develop in the lower third of the esophagus and occur in up to 11% of GERD patients. Symptoms such as dysphagia with solids occur after the esophageal lumen is less than 12 mm in diameter. Some

Table 23-1   Substances Decreasing LES Pressure

Foods	Medications	Other
Caffeine	Anticholinergics	Cigarette smoking
Fat	Theophylline	
Chocolate	Progesterone	
Alcohol	Calcium channel blockers	
Peppermint	Diazepam	
	β2 adrenergic agonists	
	α adrenergic antagonists	

patients with severe esophagitis will develop esophageal ulcers, which may penetrate as deep as the muscular layers. A biopsy of these ulcers is needed to exclude malignancy, particularly if they occur in a region of Barrett's epithelium. Occasionally the ulcer may perforate a major vessel, causing significant bleeding.

Approximately 10% of patients with GERD will develop Barrett's esophagus, where the normal squamous epithelium is replaced by metaplastic columnar epithelium as a result of chronic esophagitis. Barrett's esophagus is associated with esophageal ulcer and stricture, but more importantly it is known to progress to adenocarcinoma in 3% to 9% of cases (1). Although it is difficult to prove, GERD may also play a role in the etiology of pulmonary diseases such as asthma, laryngitis, hoarseness, bronchitis, and aspiration pneumonia. Most but not all people with these conditions suffer symptoms of GERD.

Common Symptoms and Atypical Presentations

The majority of symptomatic individuals who have GERD never seek treatment, perhaps because they perceive their symptoms as "normal." Some who have persistent, significant symptoms delay care unless they develop a complication.

Heartburn, the most common symptom of GERD, is described as a retrosternal burning that radiates upward, occurring usually within 3 hours of a meal (particularly a large or fatty meal). The burning sensation worsens with recumbency or bending forward and usually lessens within 5 minutes of antacid ingestion. Regurgitation is experienced as nocturnal reflux of sour and bitter material into the mouth. It is exacerbated and relieved by the same factors as heartburn.

Dysphagia, when due to inflammation and edema in the distal esophagus, responds to conservative medical therapy; but when due to an esophageal stricture dysphagia requires more aggressive therapy. Odynophagia, or painful swallowing, often accompanies severe esophagitis. Waterbrash refers to the sudden filling of the mouth with clear, salty fluid. This fluid is not reflux material, but rather is a hypersecretion of saliva in response to GERD (9).

GERD mimics cardiac, pulmonary, and other gastrointestinal diseases. GERD causes angina-like chest pain, possibly from irritation of elongated rete pegs that protrude into the esophagus. In individuals with proven coronary artery disease, esophageal acid perfusion has in fact caused ischemic changes on ECG (1).

Hemorrhage from esophagitis may cause anemia or frank hematemesis as does PD. Pulmonary symptoms are sometimes the only manifestations of GERD, either from aspiration or neurally mediated vagal stimulation that triggers symptoms of recurrent cough, wheeze, and hoarseness.

Physical Findings

The diagnosis of GERD can usually be made through a careful history, sometimes supported by a trial of antacids. Physical examination often contributes little to the diagnosis in this condition. If there is slow bleeding due to esophagitis, the patient may have signs of pallor, tachycardia, tachypnea, and hyperdynamic apex beat. In cases where there is associated PD, epigastric tenderness may be a feature.

Diagnostic Evaluation

Assessment of Mucosa   Once there is suspicion of mucosal injury to the esophagus, a number of diagnostic options are available. Single-contrast barium studies have low accuracy in the diagnosis of GERD. Double-contrast barium studies, though capable of demonstrating small malignancies and some cases of esophagitis, fail to adequately dilate the gastroesophageal junction in approximately 30% of patients and may miss some pathology. Sensitivity with double-contrast barium improves for severe esophagitis and erosions as opposed to mild esophagitis (7).

Upper gastrointestinal endoscopy provides direct visualization of the whole esophagus and as a result has a high sensitivity and specificity. Endoscopy also allows biopsy of the esophagus to determine the grade of esophagitis and to exclude malignancy. Nevertheless, many patients with typical symptoms of GERD and excessive acid exposure on ambulatory pH monitoring have normal macroscopic and histologic findings on endoscopy.

Assessment of Exposure to Acid   The Bernstein, or acid perfusion, test involves the alternate infusion of normal saline and hydrochloric acid through a nasogastric tube that has been passed to the midesophagus. The test is considered positive when the patient's symptoms have been produced twice by the HCl and relieved twice by the infusion of normal saline. Sensitivity and specificity of this test is about 80%.

The standard acid reflux test requires a pH monitor to be placed 5 cm above the gastroesophageal junction. Intra-abdominal pressure is increased via a series of maneuvers, both before and after a gastric infusion of hydrochloric acid. A drop in pH to less than 4.0 on three occasions is considered positive. Sensitivity and specificity is about 80% (1).

A gastroesophageal scintiscan involves the infusion of a radiolabeled sulfur colloid into the stomach. Reflux is then measured on a scanner while intra-abdominal pressure is increased using an abdominal cuff. Sensitivity and specificity is believed to be about 90%.

Ambulatory pH monitoring is the gold standard for measuring acid reflux. A pH monitor is positioned 5 cm above the gastroesophageal junction, and pH is measured over a 24-hour period in relation to meals, body position, activity, and sleep. Reflux is considered to be present any time the pH drops below 4.0. This test is excellent for assessing patients with reflux symptoms but negative endoscopies, and it also assesses the relationship between reflux and pulmonary symptoms. It will not detect "alkaline reflux" of bile salts, but otherwise has a sensitivity and specificity of 96% (7).

Assessment of Esophageal Motility   Esophageal manometry is not a reliable means of determining the presence or absence of significant reflux. However, in the patient with proven GERD manometry is a useful means of determining whether abnormal peristalsis and/or a hypotensive lower esophageal sphincter are contributing to the disease. Manometry is particularly useful in the patient being considered for antireflux surgery. If peristalsis is weak, any surgery to tighten the gastroesophageal junction may result in profound dysphagia.

Special Considerations in Athletes

Symptoms of GERD are commonly reported by athletes. As noted above, approximately 10% of recreational runners experienced heartburn while running. Marathon runners have found that heartburn was more prevalent during hard runs rather than easy runs, which suggests that the likelihood of reflux occurring during exercise relates to the intensity of that exercise.

Effects on gastric emptying may account for some of the upper gastrointestinal tract symptoms experienced by athletes. Trained individuals at rest have faster gastric emptying rates than sedentary individuals. Furthermore, submaximal levels of exercise have been shown to increase the rate of gastric emptying relative to the resting state. This may be due to the mechanical effect of abdominal muscle contraction. As the intensity of training increases, the rate of gastric emptying decreases, probably due to decreased visceral blood flow and the effects of circulating catecholamines and endogenous opioids on gastric motility.

In a study that continuously monitored esophageal pH during a 1-hour run that followed a low-fat meal, a high incidence of gastroesophageal reflux was found in runners. The timing of lowest pH was demonstrated to coincide with subjective reporting of reflux symptoms (10). In another study, reflux was demonstrated in athletes during weight training and running, but not during cycling (11). The same study showed that the reflux occurring during running and weight training was worse if the exercise took place in the postprandial period. The mechanisms postulated for gastroesophageal reflux in runners include air swallowing, mechanical disturbance of gastric contents, decreased gastric emptying, and transient relaxations in the lower esophageal sphincter.

When treating athletes with symptoms of GERD, the physician needs to be aware of the special risks pertaining to the exercising population. Symptoms of GERD mimic angina pectoris, and some authors feel that GERD may have a causal link to myocardial ischemia in susceptible individuals (12). When dealing with an athlete who experiences symptoms of GERD during exercise, the physician should conduct the history and examination with the possibility of angina in mind. Any suggestion of a cardiac component to the athlete's symptoms necessitates follow-up investigation, including an exercise stress ECG.

Athletes should not use NSAIDs in the presence of GERD, because these medications may trigger complications such as esophageal ulceration and bleeding. For "tired" athletes with GERD, the physician should suspect gastrointestinal blood loss and evaluate fully.

Strategies for Treatment of PD and GERD in the Athlete

The treatment strategies for PD and GERD are similar, as a reduction of gastric acid production and the resultant elevation in gastric pH relieve the symptoms of both conditions.

Nonpharmacologic Treatment Strategies Dietary treatment of PD and GERD in the athlete involves avoidance of alcohol and caffeine, both of which can irritate the gastric mucosa and stimulate acid secretion. No other specific dietary manipulation has proven beneficial, although individuals may wish to skip foods that they have identified as sources of aggravation.

Nonpharmacologic treatment strategies in GERD include various lifestyle modifications. Numerous physiologic studies have indicated that elevating the head of the bed, ceasing smoking, decreasing fat in the diet, and avoiding recumbency for 3 hours following a meal can reduce acid reflux (7). The patient with exercise-related reflux should abstain from exercising in the postprandial period as this exacerbates symptoms.

Smoking and excessive dietary fat intake are less common in the athletic population than in the wider community. Among other effects on gastric function, smoking interferes with the action of H_2-receptor antagonists, inhibits pancreatic bicarbonate secretion, decreases mucosal blood flow, and inhibits mucosal prostaglandin production. If the athlete has either of these two risk factors, counseling toward a reduction of these risk factors is likely to improve not only the symptoms of PD and GERD but also the individual's general health and exercise performance.

Many athletes experience significant mental and physical stress in their quest for excellence, and chronic stress related to frustration is significantly and independently associated with the onset and relapse of PD. If athletes suffering from PD appear to be troubled by psychological stress, they should receive advice on stress management from the physician or a properly trained psychotherapist.

Pharmacologic Treatment Strategies *Antacids* Taking antacids alleviates symptoms of PD and GERD by increasing the pH of the gastric contents and by deactivating pepsin. Antacids possibly also increase lower esophageal sphincter pressure, thereby decreasing the volume of refluxed material in GERD patients. Side effects of antacids include cramping and constipation with aluminum-containing products, and diarrhea with magnesium-containing compounds. These side effects can affect performance, so antacids should be avoided prior to competition. The majority of antacids contain both magnesium and aluminum components and minimally affect gastrointestinal motility, but they do decrease the bioavailability of iron, tetracyclines, and indomethacin. Thus, an alternative to antacids should be considered in athletes concomitantly taking those medications.

H_2-Receptor Antagonists H_2-receptor antagonists (H_2RAs) competitively inhibit the interaction of histamine with H_2 receptors, located on the surface of parietal cells in the gastric mucosa. Stimulation of the receptors causes activation of H^+,K^+-ATPase, which in turn leads to the secretion of HCl by the parietal cells. The H_2RAs, which are highly selective, bind minimally to H_1 or other receptors or to H_2 receptors in pulmonary or cardiac tissues. The H_2RAs cause few side effects. No literature reports detrimental effects on exercise performance or drug interactions with medications commonly used by athletes. H_2RAs decrease episodes of reflux in runners and decrease symptoms of nausea in marathon runners. It is difficult to be certain about the long-term effects of regular ingestion of these medications, but it seems prudent to recommend that athletes suffering reflux symptoms during exercise use H_2RAs prophylactically after proper investigation.

Proton Pump Inhibitors   The ultimate mediator of gastric acid secretion is the H^+,K^+-ATPase (proton pump) on the parietal cell membrane. Inthe late 1980s a proton pump inhibitor, omeprazole, was released, and it demonstrated a profound ability to suppress the secretion of acid. Daily production of acid falls by 95% and does not regain pretreatment levels until 5 days after withdrawal of therapy. While side effects from omeprazole seem to be minimal at present, there is some concern over the possible effects of prolonged suppression of acid secretion. Patients on omeprazole often develop a relative hypergastrinemia; there are concerns that long-term omeprozole use might cause trophic or metaplastic changes in the gastric mucosa. To date, omeprazole has not caused mucosal proliferation. Additionally, no reports of adverse effects on exercise performance have arisen (13).

Prokinetic Agents   In conjunction with acid-suppression therapy, prokinetic agents have a role in the treatment of GERD by reducing the duration of acid exposure in the lower esophagus. Metoclopramide relaxes the pylorus and duodenum, increases antral contractions, and increases tone in the lower esophageal sphincter. These effects combine to increase the rate of gastric emptying and decrease the tendency to reflux. Combined therapy with cimetidine and metoclopramide improves the healing of esophagitis in comparison to cimetidine alone (7). Unfortunately, metoclopramide's side effects include dizziness, drowsiness, and occasionally, extrapyramidal effects, thus making its use in athletes problematic.

Cisapride, a second prokinetic agent, treats esophagitis as effectively as standard doses of H_2RAs; in combination with H_2RAs, cisapride is more effective than single-agent therapy. Cisapride, unlike metoclopramide, increases colonic motility and can cause diarrhea; athletes experiencing this side effect may need alternative treatment.

Antibacterial Therapies   In the athlete with proven *H. pylori* infection, antibacterial therapy eradicates PD. Numerous different drug combinations are used, and the following are examples of two popular treatment options.

1. **Bismuth triple therapy.** Bismuth subcitrate, one tablet four times daily, plus tetracycline, 500 mg four times daily, plus metronidazole, 400 mg three times daily, for 2 weeks.
2. **Proton pump inhibitor triple therapy.** Omeprazole, 20 mg twice daily, plus amoxycillin, 500 mg three times daily, plus metronidazole, 400 mg three times daily, for 2 weeks. The proton pump inhibitor triple therapy causes fewer side effects and ensures rapid healing at the same time as eradication. Metronidazole commonly has the side effects of headache, nausea, and dry mouth, any of which could be detrimental to an athlete's performance.

Return to Competition or Training

The athlete with PD or GERD can often continue to train and compete. Symptoms of exercise-induced reflux may interfere with running performance, but the introduction of acid-suppressive therapy usually results in immediate relief with no effect on performance. If the athlete has gastrointestinal bleeding and/or anemia as a result of PD, training should be ceased until the bleeding is controlled; training should then remain moderate until the blood profile returns to normal.

INFLAMMATORY BOWEL DISEASE

Inflammatory bowel disease (IBD) refers to a group of chronic inflammatory gastrointestinal conditions of unknown etiology. The diseases have no pathognomonic features or specific diagnostic tests and thus remain diagnoses of exclusion. Typical features are sufficiently characteristic to allow IBD to be divided broadly into two major disease groups: ulcerative colitis (UC) and Crohn's disease (14).

Population Demographics and Prevalence

The incidence of IBD varies widely in different population groups. Asian, Middle Eastern, and Mediterranean countries have a relatively low incidence, whereas European countries, the United States, Canada, Australia, and New Zealand have a significantly higher incidence. In these latter countries, the annual incidence of UC is 5 to 8 per

100,000, with a prevalence of 70 to 150 per 100,000 (15). Crohn's disease has an annual incidence in Europe and North America of 2 to 4 per 100,000 and a prevalence of 20 to 40 per 100,000 (14).

The peak incidence of both diseases occurs between the ages of 15 to 35 years (14), which is the age grouping of the bulk of athletes seen in a general sports medicine clinic. The sports physician should thus be aware of the possibility of IBD in any athlete presenting with the relevant symptoms.

Patients with IBD tend to be nonsmokers and to have a family history of IBD, atopy, or celiac disease (15). Women tend to be affected by Crohn's disease twice as often as men; there is no gender difference in the incidence of UC (16).

Pathophysiology or Infectious Agents

Because the causes of IBD remain obscure, the fundamental questions as to pathogenesis can be summarized as follows: Does this chronic, recurring inflammation of the gastrointestinal tract reflect an appropriate response to a persisting or recurring abnormal stimulus, such as a causative agent or a structural abnormality in the intestine? Or is it an abnormally prolonged response to a normal stimulus, such as immunologic dysfunction (17)?

Genetic factors may play a role in the etiology of IBD, as evidenced by an increased prevalence of IBD (about 10%) among first-degree relatives of affected individuals. Recently, studies comparing monozygotic versus dizygotic twins reported a very high concordance rate among monozygotic twins with Crohn's disease, and a lesser extent with UC (18).

A high prevalence of ileitis and colitis occurs among patients with ankylosing spondylitis and other HLA-B27-positive arthropathies. Transgenic rats expressing HLA-B27 also develop intestinal inflammation and arthritis (17). Symptoms of an inflammatory arthropathy should be explored in an athlete presenting with a history suggestive of IBD; conversely, the athlete with a seronegative arthropathy should be questioned about associated symptoms of gastrointestinal disturbance (Fig 23-1).

An infectious cause may trigger IBD, as pathologic changes in Crohn's disease resemble those of mycobacterial diseases. *Mycobacterium tuberculosis* has been isolated from the tissues of some Crohn's

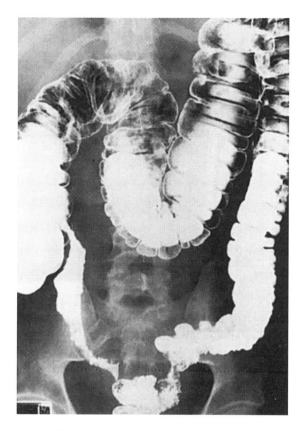

Figure 23-1. A predominantly lower-limb arthritis is seen in association with inflammatory bowel disease. This barium enema shows typical Crohn's disease with a narrowed terminal ileum (string sign) and a skip lesion in the sigmoid colon. The arthritis may move from one joint to another. (Reproduced by permission from Shipley M. Rheumatic diseases. Baltimore: Williams & Wilkins, 1985:86.)

disease patients, but attempts to consistently isolate an infective agent in ulcerative colitis or Crohn's disease have failed (17).

A "physiologic" inflammatory response is present at all times in the lamina propria of the intestine and colon. This state of immune readiness results from the huge antigenic load presented through the lumen of the gastrointestinal tract. One theory suggests that the intestinal inflammation in IBD represents an exaggerated and unrestrained activation of the mucosal immune system as a result of impaired regulating mechanisms (17).

UC inflames the mucosa in the rectum (95%) and colon, with gross pathologic changes of ulcer, hyperemia, and hemorrhage. The inflammation is continuous with no intervening areas of normal mucosa and extends proximally from the rectum for a variable distance. The mucosal damage with loss of surface epithelium results in multiple ulcerations but does not usually involve the deeper layers of the bowel beneath the submucosa.

Crohn's disease, in contrast to UC, typically involves all layers of the intestine, developing in a patchy distribution anywhere in the gastrointestinal tract. The primary site is often the small intestine, particularly the terminal ileum, although Crohn's colitis is also common. Rarely, Crohn's disease affects the esophagus or stomach (1). In chronic disease, the bowel thickens and the lumen narrows enough that stenosis may lead to varying degrees of obstruction. Unlike UC, the mucosa often looks normal, although advanced cases have a classic "cobblestone" appearance.

Common Symptoms and Atypical Presentations

The main symptoms of UC are abdominal pain and bloody stool. If the disease is confined to the rectum, the stool may be formed, but if the disease involves much of the colon, patients have frequent, liquid stools containing blood and/or pus. The diarrhea arises from poor absorption of water and electrolytes by the damaged mucosa, and can cause dehydration, anemia, fever, and weight loss. When the disease is limited to the rectum, different symptoms predominate, such as constipation and tenesmus. Abdominal distension may occur as a result of toxic dilatation of the colon.

Crohn's disease typically presents with right lower quadrant pain and diarrhea, but rarely leads to blood in the stool. Fatigability, weight loss, and severe anorectal complications such as fistulas, fissures, and perirectal abscess (65% of cases [19]) are frequent disease manifestations, as is intestinal obstruction (20% to 30% of patients [14]).

Extraintestinal manifestations of IBD occur in association with both ulcerative colitis and Crohn's disease (Fig 23-2). Joint manifestations affect approximately 25% of IBD patients and are of two main types. The first type of manifestation is a non-

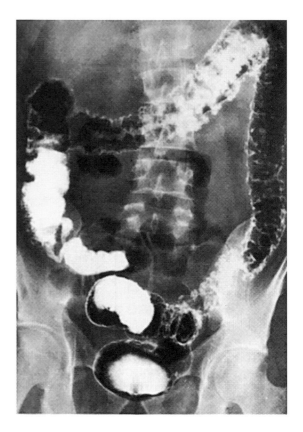

Figure 23-2.   Peripheral arthritis occurs with ulcerative colitis (UC), here typically involving the rectum and colon in continuity (i.e., no skip lesions). With both Crohn's disease and UC, the peripheral arthritis and bowel lesions show parallel activity. In UC, a successful total colectomy will usually abolish the arthritis. (Reproduced by permission from Shipley M. Rheumatic diseases. Baltimore: Williams & Wilkins, 1985:86.)

deforming arthritis, which is polyarticular and often migratory in nature, that affects the knees, ankles, and wrists. Disease activity mirrors that of the bowel disease. Serologic tests for arthritis (rheumatoid factor, antinuclear antibody, LE factor) are negative. The second form of joint disease is ankylosing spondylitis, a central arthritis often presenting as lower back pain and stiffness. There may be associated sacroiliitis or enthesopathy. The symptoms of ankylosing spondylitis are unrelated to the activity of the IBD; they may antecede the IBD by years, as well as persist after remission of the

IBD. Ankylosing spondylitis has a strong association with HLA-B27, whether or not IBD is present.

Skin manifestations occur in approximately 15% of IBD patients and include erythema nodosum, pyoderma gangrenosa, and aphthous ulcers. The severity of the skin conditions correlates with the activity of the bowel disease.

Ocular manifestations occur in 5% of IBD patients and include episcleritis, uveitis, and recurrent iritis. The ocular symptoms are associated with a more severe expression of the disease, and their activity parallels that of the bowel disease. Ocular disease will often resolve dramatically following colectomy.

Approximately 4% of patients develop hepatic or biliary complications, particularly sclerosing cholangitis, which is characterized by high serum alkaline phosphatase. Less commonly, cirrhosis, chronic active hepatitis, and rarely, bile duct carcinoma may occur.

Physical Findings

Patients with IBD are often thin and undernourished; anemia from chronic disease or from blood loss may cause pallor. Ill patients may have tachycardia and fever; in UC, patients may have generalized tenderness of the abdomen; a right lower quadrant mass is classic in Crohn's disease. Rectal examination in UC reveals bloody stool or frank blood, whereas Crohn's disease will often reveal anorectal disease. A tender, distended abdomen is suggestive of toxic megacolon, but it also occurs with obstruction, perforation, and other problems. The physician should look for extraintestinal manifestations of the disease, as they may help indicate which IBD is more likely.

Diagnostic Evaluation

A full blood count, liver function tests, serum electrolytes, ESR, C-reactive protein, and serum iron, folate, and B_{12} are reasonable investigations in the patient with IBD. Anemia may be present due to blood loss, chronic disease, or deficiency of folate or vitamin B_{12}. B_{12} deficiency may relate to chronic terminal ileitis in Crohn's disease. With significant diarrhea, electrolyte deficiencies such as hypokalemia may arise; hypocalcemia indicates malabsorption of vitamin D due to extensive mucosal involvement. Hypoalbuminemia can occur as a result of amino acid malabsorption or a protein-losing enteropathy. Elevation of alkaline phosphatase occurs with sclerosing cholangitis.

Stools should be examined for leukocytes, ova, and parasites, then cultured for bacterial pathogens and tested for *Clostridium difficile* titer. Fecal leukocytes help differentiate inflammatory conditions of the colon from irritable bowel syndrome or noncolonic diarrhea. Amebiasis may be diagnosed by the presence of ova and parasites in the stool. Bacterial pathogens may be identified by stool culture. *Campylobacter jejuni* iliocolitis may present with fever, abdominal pain, and bloody diarrhea with mucus, and the radiologic, endoscopic, and histologic features very closely resemble those of UC. The disease should resolve spontaneously within a few days; otherwise, it should respond to a course of erythromycin. *C. difficile* testing identifies antibiotic-associated pseudomembranous colitis, which also may be confused with UC (although *C. difficile* may at times exacerbate preexisting UC).

Plain radiograph of the abdomen is usually normal in mild to moderate IBD. Double-contrast barium studies can detect a granular appearance in the mucosa of even early UC. Loss of haustration, ulcerations, pseudopolyps, and shortening of the bowel are findings of more advanced disease. Radiographs in Crohn's disease show narrowing of the bowel, fistulas, involvement of the terminal ileum, skip lesions in the colon, mucosal ulcerations, and linear fissures. The upper gastrointestinal tract series, small bowel series, and barium enema all are useful in the evaluation of a patient with suspected Crohn's disease.

Sigmoidoscopy provides direct visualization of the rectum and distal colon. In UC the mucosal surface is irregular, granular, and friable; it bleeds easily when it is touched, or spontaneously in more advanced disease. Pseudopolyps may be seen in cases of chronic UC. The rectum in Crohn's disease is normal, or when there is rectal involvement, the mucosa may mimic that of UC or show linear ulcerations or fissures.

Rectal biopsy should be taken at sigmoidoscopy from a site 8 to 10 cm from the anal margin to look for latent disease in macroscopically normal mu cosa. Histologic features help to distinguish UC from Crohn's disease, but true differentiation usually relies on a combination of histology, radiology, and colonoscopy. Colonoscopy allows multiple biopsies to be taken at several different locations in the bowel to help confirm an IBD diagnosis and to assess the extent and severity of the disease.

Scanning of radiolabeled white cells may reveal areas of increased disease activity. These scans are not diagnostic of Crohn's disease, but can demonstrate areas of inflammation and thereby lend weight to the clinical diagnosis. This test is particularly useful in cases where Crohn's disease is limited to the small intestine.

Special Considerations in Athletes

There is very little written in the literature with regards IBD in athletes. Given that the cause or causes of IBD remain unknown, the effects of exercise are speculative. No evidence has emerged for an increased risk of IBD in athletes.

Certain facts in the athlete may confound the diagnosis such as the bloody diarrhea that follows gruelling endurance events, particularly marathons and ultramarathons. While exercise may not predispose an individual to developing IBD, this type of endurance stress could exacerbate the condition in an individual with preexisting disease, whose mucosal surface is fragile and bleeds easily. Running causes repetitive mechanical trauma to the bowel, and in an individual with UC this may be sufficient to cause bleeding and exacerbation of the inflammatory process. The physician must therefore resist the temptation to dismiss the presentation of bloody diarrhea as "runner's trots" and a thorough history and examination should be performed to evaluate the risk of IBD.

An ill athlete with IBD with dehydration, anemia, electrolyte disturbance, and hypocalcemia obviously could not exercise fully. In assessing an athlete with gastrointestinal symptoms, IBD and some of the complications warrant further consideration.

During high intensity exercise, physiologic shunting causes visceral blood flow to be reduced by as much as 80%, enough to produce relative ischemia in the bowel. This hemodynamic change may contribute to the symptoms of abdominal pain and the gastrointestinal blood loss that follows exercise. This exercise-induced stress potentially worsens findings in IBD.

Treatment Strategies in the Athlete

Management of IBD requires accurate diagnosis and staging of the disease's severity. Nutritional support helps stabilize weight and protects young athletes from growth retardation. In cases of severe IBD, a reassessment of the athlete's goals and a discussion of the advisability of certain sports may be required.

Medical treatment of IBD aims to resolve acute episodes and maintain remission. Medications vary and some contravene laws of athletic competition. Sulfasalazine and corticosteroids are the backbone of medical therapy in IBD.

Sulfasalazine Sulfasalazine is composed of 5-aminosalicylic acid (5-ASA) and sulfapyridine, with the 5-ASA as the active chemical. This drug is permitted under IOC guidelines for use during training and competition. Side effects include nausea and dyspepsia from the 5-ASA portion, folate deficiency due to competition for absorption, and (rarely) bone marrow suppression from the sulfur portion (1). Sulfasalazine is the first-line drug in maintenance therapy for ulcerative colitis and many cases of Crohn's disease. While sulfasalazine effectively induces and maintains remission, many patients are intolerant of the sulfapyridine portion. Recently, mesalamine and other 5-ASA derivatives without the sulfapyridine portion have demonstrated efficacy in the treatment of UC and Crohn's disease while producing fewer side effects than sulfasalazine. Mesalamine acts locally in a suppository form for proctitis or as an enema for colitis; the efficacy of oral therapy remains under study (20).

Corticosteroids Corticosteroids have had primary use in the treatment of UC and Crohn's disease, but widespread side effects have relegated use of these drugs to severe cases or those resistant to sulfasalazine and mesalamine. Use of oral corticosteroids is not permitted under IOC guidelines, and patients with disease severe enough to require maintenance rarely reach elite level. When an athlete with mild IBD has an acute flare, the benefits of oral corticosteroids must be balanced by the need to report steroid usage and receive a waiver from athletic governing bodies.

Other Drugs   Metronidazole is commonly used in the treatment of IBD for intercurrent infections; the drug is believed to modulate immune reactions and improve wound healing (21). Paresthesias occur in 50% of patients (taking 1000 mg/day) at a mean time of 6.5 months (22). This limits long-term use and would likely impair athletic performance.

NSAIDs, in spite of their activity against inflammation, exacerbate IBD and should be avoided. Athletes with IBD should try other methods of injury treatment.

The athlete with a significant flare up of IBD is likely to have symptoms (diarrhea, fecal urgency, cramping abdominal pain, fatigue, etc.) that make exercise more arduous. Prudent advice suggests a graduated return to activity during times of remission so that activity does not aggravate the disease through mechanical irritation and other effects.

RUNNER'S DIARRHEA

Exercise-induced lower intestinal symptoms such as cramping, urge to defecate, and diarrhea commonly affect running athletes. Many theories postulate a cause for the increased lower intestinal motility. At rest, trained athletes have increased parasympathetic tone, and during exercise, catecholamine levels rise. Both of these factors decrease intestinal transit times. Increased food intake and higher levels of dietary fiber in the athletic population also increase intestinal motility, but this does not explain the higher incidence of diarrhea in runners as opposed to cyclists. During exercise, reduced visceral blood flow may affect symptoms, as they worsen with exercise. However, Rehrer et al. (23) think that this reflects the fluid status of the patient.

Physiologic diarrhea of the athlete remains a diagnosis of exclusion. Infectious diarrhea may be due to bacterial, viral, or parasitic agents, all of which should be eliminated as causal factors.

Common Symptoms and Atypical Presentations

With physiologic, exercise-induced diarrhea, the athlete is well at rest, but diarrhea occurs with higher intensity running and even more so at times of suboptimal hydration. Onset is usually gradual, but is reproducible with exercise. The athlete may describe abdominal cramping or a recurrent "stitch" while running. Submaximal running, cycling, and swimming do not commonly cause diarrhea. The signs and symptoms of infectious diarrhea are absent.

The patient history should exclude medications such as antibiotics and magnesium-containing compounds that may increase motility. Concurrent medical conditions such as IBD, diabetes, irritable bowel disease, and celiac disease preclude a confident diagnosis of physiologic, exercise-induced diarrhea.

Physical Findings

Examination fails to show chronic changes such as weight loss or signs of specific deficiencies such as koilonychia (iron), glossitis (B_{12}), or bruising (vitamin K). No fever, abdominal tenderness, abnormal rectal findings, or masses should be noted. As this is a physiologic change, examination must be normal.

Diagnostic Evaluation

The majority of cases of diarrhea are acute, mild, and self-limiting and require no investigation. Bloody diarrhea requires stool microscopy and culture, and sometimes sigmoidoscopy or colonoscopy. Hospitalization should be considered in cases of severe dehydration, systemic toxicity, or severe abdominal pain. Physiologic diarrhea does not lead to hospitalization.

Special Considerations in Athletes

Athletes do have special risks that require differentiation for runner's diarrhea. A vigorous travel schedule exposes athletes to increased risk of "traveler's diarrhea" from various infective organisms. Unusual foods or local water may cause increased intestinal motility in sensitive individuals, even in the absence of any infectious agent. The physiologic effects of running on the gastrointestinal tract may increase with training changes. Psychological stresses also commonly affect the life of an elite athlete, particularly in the period leading up to an important competition. These stresses may also manifest themselves as increased intestinal motility and "nervous diarrhea."

The athlete with true runner's diarrhea is unlikely to suffer dehydration and electrolyte disturbance. With mild diarrhea, there still may be some need to suggest fluids to avoid electrolyte disturbance. If deficient in K^+ the athlete may feel weak, have decreased exercise tolerance, and exhibit poor coordination. Thermoregulatory mechanisms may also be disordered, posing risks in contact or endurance events staged in hot or humid conditions.

Because weight-loss strategies are used by athletes competing in events with weight classifications or where points are scored on aesthetic criteria, the physician should consider the possibility of laxative abuse in such athletes.

Treatment Strategies in the Athlete

Preventative measures may help lessen the problem of diarrhea in the athlete. Traveling teams need safe water; if there is any doubt about the suitability of drinking water, the athletes should be advised to drink only from sealed drink containers. Supplies of bottled mineral water should be used for both drinking and brushing teeth. Athletes should not have ice in their drinks as the ice will invariably be frozen local water. The physician must also advise the athletes as to which foods pose the least threat of infection. In general, meats should be well cooked, and salads washed in local water should be avoided.

For the athlete with purely exercise-induced diarrhea, precompetition caffeine should be discouraged as this is a known gastrointestinal stimulant (24). Use of cathartics is certainly to be discouraged. Precompetition and intracompetition hydration should be given high priority in an athlete prone to exercise-induced diarrhea.

Antidiarrheal agents should be prescribed with caution. Anticholinergic medications will decrease gut motility, but they may also cause unpleasant symptoms such as a dry mouth. These agents can also reduce the sweating response and make the athlete more vulnerable to heat illness. Weak antispasmodics such as loperamide and diphenoxylate are recommended only when other measures fail.

GASTROINTESTINAL BLOOD LOSS IN SPORT

Population Demographics

Gastrointestinal bleeding can be classified into acute or chronic bleeding, and be further subdivided into upper or lower gastrointestinal bleeding. Upper gastrointestinal bleeding affects 50 to 150 per 100,000 in Western countries, and the risk of bleeding tends to increase with age. Eighty percent of acute upper gastrointestinal bleeds will resolve spontaneously (25). Most patients with upper gastrointestinal lesions caused by aspirin or other NSAIDs do well, as these lesions heal quickly.

Lower gastrointestinal bleeding also increases with age, as many of the underlying conditions such as neoplasm, diverticulitis, and ischemic enteritis are more common in the elderly. Patients often complain of secondary symptoms, and the bleeding itself may go unnoticed.

Pathophysiology

Bleeding occurs throughout the gastrointestinal tract and is often associated with other medical conditions. Inflammation and erosions of the upper gastrointestinal tract, PD, and portal hypertension all predispose a patient to upper gastrointestinal bleeding. The number of associated medical conditions directly increases the risk of mortality in acute gastrointestinal bleeding. Ingestion of aspirin or other NSAIDs compromises the gastric mucosa via inhibition of prostaglandins and alters platelet function, thus preventing normal clotting.

Hemorrhoids, diverticular disease, and neoplasms, among many other disease processes, may cause lower gastrointestinal bleeding in a wide variety of differing age groups. Not only do lesions of the lower gastrointestinal tract produce bleeding distally, but lesions of the *upper* gastrointestinal tract may manifest as rectal bleeding.

Common Symptoms and Atypical Presentations

The clinical picture varies greatly, even in patients with the same hemoglobin level. Patients with a large, acute bleed show hemodynamic compromise, with active bleeding, dizziness, weakness, and breathlessness. On the other hand, a more subtle, chronic bleed leads to reduced exercise tolerance, vague nausea, or long-standing fatigue. A careful history reviews medications ingested, abdominal symptoms, change in stool color, and exercise tolerance.

Physical Findings

Patients with acute bleeds have pallor, cool extremities, rapid thready pulse, and postural hypotension. Examination may not reveal the site of the lesion, but signs of liver disease or an abdominal mass on palpation may be useful. In cases of subtle bleeds, rectal examination may be the only part of the exam to give a positive result. Fresh blood or melena on the glove, palpation of a carcinoma, or visualization of hemorrhoids or fissures can point to a diagnosis.

Diagnostic Evaluation

A full blood count helps differentiate chronic and acute bleeds. Serum electrolytes, creatinine, and coagulation studies should be performed when an acute bleed is suspected. Full blood profiles help identify significant coexisting disease. Stool samples should be tested for occult blood.

Barium studies may reveal the site of a bleed, but endoscopy is better for detection and evaluation of gastrointestinal bleeds. Treatment of esophageal varices differs significantly from that for a bleeding peptic ulcer or a Mallory-Weiss tear and is guided by accurate identification. Proctosigmoidoscopy is the initial investigation of choice in cases of lower gastrointestinal bleeding; colonoscopy follows if no cause is identified. In cases where the site of bleeding remains obscure, radionuclide scanning or selective arteriography may be indicated.

Special Considerations in Athletes

Many studies of gastrointestinal bleeding in athletes use occult stool blood tests. A study of ultra-marathon runners by Baska et al. (26) revealed over 80% of runners having traces of blood in their postrace stool, as opposed to 3% in the prerace sample. Postrace endoscopic studies by Schwartz et al. (5) demonstrated lesions of the gastric mucosa consistent with local ischemia and also showed these lesions to heal rapidly. Mechanical trauma to the gut during running has also been postulated as a cause for bleeding. The so-called "cecal slap syndrome" is believed by some to account for a proportion of hemoccult-positive runners. Ingestion of NSAIDs may contribute to gastrointestinal bleeding in athletes and should be discontinued in those with known problems.

No specific anemias are known to be more prevalent in the athletic community than in the general population. However, the athlete who has preexisting anemia from other causes may be at special risk during a significant gastrointestinal bleed, as he or she will have less reserve to allow compensation mechanisms to take effect.

Treatment Strategies in the Athlete

Prevention of gastrointestinal bleeding in at-risk athletes has been effectively demonstrated by Baska et al. (26), who gave cimetidine to half the participants in an ultramarathon race. The rate of gastrointestinal bleeding was significantly lower in the cimetidine group than in controls. This provides the basis for prophylactic H_2RA usage prior to races in athletes with a tendency to gastrointestinal bleeding during exercise, as long as any underlying gastrointestinal pathology has been excluded. To avoid gastrointestinal ischemia, good prerace and intrarace hydration helps athletes lessen the shunting of blood from viscera during exercise.

In the athlete who has suffered a significant bleed, a return to sport should only be permitted after the cause of the bleed has been positively identified and treated. Any resulting anemia should also be corrected before maximal activity.

ANORECTAL DISEASE

Fissure in Ano

Approximately 10% of visits and 30% of procedures in colorectal clinics are for treatment of anal

tis. Investigations should include serum ferritin, serum iron, and iron-binding capacity. The gold standard for confirmation of diagnosis is liver biopsy. Treatment is aimed at preventing the sequelae of iron overload by regular phlebotomy.

Special Considerations in the Athlete

In the patient with systemic manifestations of hemochromatosis, a thorough medical assessment is required before clearance to compete is given. A full workup by a cardiologist is mandatory to exclude CHF or dangerous arrhythmias. The athlete should have a fasting blood glucose test. If the athlete is affected by arthropathy, exercise programs should be tailored so that further damage is not caused to the affected joints.

SUMMARY

A wide variety of gastrointestinal diseases can potentially affect athletes and their sports performance. Some conditions, such as GERD and runner's diarrhea, have a specific association with exercise. In the vast majority of conditions, effective therapy and modifications to the exercise regimen allow the continued participation in sport.

REFERENCES

1 Eastwood GL, Avunduk C. Manual of gastroenterology. 2nd ed. Boston: Little, Brown, 1994.
2 Johnson DA, Cattau EL Jr. Evaluation and management of gastric ulcer. In: Chobanian SJ, Van Ness MM, eds. Manual of clinical problems in gastroenterology. Boston: Little, Brown, 1988:43–46.
3 Axon ATR. *Helicobacter pylori*. In: Pounder RE, ed. Recent advances in gastroenterology. London: Churchill Livingstone, 1992:27–48.
4 Sullivan SN. The gastrointestinal symptoms of running [letter]. N Engl J Med 1981;304:915.
5 Schwartz AE, Vanaganus A, Kamel PL. Endoscopy to evaluate gastrointestinal bleeding in marathon runners. Ann Intern Med 1990;113:632–634.
6 Clausen JP. Effect of physical training on cardiovascular adjustments to exercise in man. Physiol Rev 1977;57:779–815.
7 DeVault KR, Castell DO. Current diagnosis and treatment of gastroesophageal reflux disease. Mayo Clin Proc 1994;69:867–876.
8 Hollaway RH, Dent J. Lower esophageal sphincter

dysfunction in gastroesophageal reflux disease. Gastroenterol Clin North Am 1990;19:517–535.
9 Goff JS. Reflux esophagitis: diagnosing the problem. Mod Med Aust 1990;Jan:41–43
10 Krauss BB, Sinclair JW, Castell DO. Gastroesophageal reflux in runners. Ann Intern Med 1990;112:429–433.
11 Clark CS, Kraus D, Sinclair J, Castell D. Vigorous exercise induces gastroesophageal reflux (GER). Gastroenterology 1988;94:A612.
12 Mellow MH, Simpson AG, Watt L, et al. Esophageal acid perfusion in coronary artery disease. Gastroenterology 1983;85:306–312.
13 Brunton LL. Agents for control of gastric acidity and treatment of peptic ulcers. In: Gilman AG, Rall WR, Nies AS, Taylor P. The pharmacological basis of therapeutics. New York: Pergamon Press, 1991:897–913.
14 Glickman RM. Inflammatory bowel disease. In: Isselbacher KJ, Braunwald E, Wilson JD, et al., eds. Harrison's principles of internal medicine. 13th ed. New York: McGraw-Hill, 1994:1738–1752.
15 Mayberry JF, Rhodes J, Williams GT. Ulcerative colitis. Med Int 1994;22:8:314–320.
16 Andrews J, Goulston K. Inflammatory bowel disease—its history, current status and outlook. Med J Aust 1994;160:219–223.
17 Podolsky DK. Inflammatory bowel disease. N Engl J Med 1991;325:13:928–937.
18 Tysk C, Lindberg E, Jarnerot G, Floderus-Myrhed B. Ulcerative colitis and Crohn's disease in an unselected population of monozygotic and dizygotic twins: a study of hereditability and the influence of smoking. Gut 1988;29:990–996.
19 Pokorny CS. Inflammatory bowel disease: diagnosis and treatment. Mod Med Aust 1994;Nov: 48–62.
20 Geier DL, Miner PB Jr. New therapeutic agents in the treatment of inflammatory bowel disease. Am J Med 1992;93:199–208.
21 Hanauer SB. Inflammatory bowel disease revisited: newer drugs. Scand J Gastroenterol 1990; 25(suppl 175):97–106.
22 Brandt LJ, Bernstein LH, Boley SJ, Frank MS. Metronidazole therapy for perineal Crohn's disease; a follow up study. Gastroenterology 1982;83:383–387.
23 Rehrer NJ, Janssen ME, et al. Fluid intake and gastrointestinal problems in runners competing in a 25 km race and a marathon. Int J Sports Med 1989;10(suppl):S22–S25.
24 Green GA. Gastrointestinal disorders in the athlete. Clin Sports Med 1992;11,2:453–470.
25 Jones M. Upper gastrointestinal bleeding. In: Manual of clinical problems in gastroenterology. Boston: Little, Brown, 1988:37–40.
26 Baska RS, Moses FM, et al. Gastrointestinal bleed-

ing during an ultramarathon. Dig Dis Sci 1990;35:276–279.

27 Abcarian H, Alexander-Williams J, Christiansen J, et al. Benign anorectal disease: definition, characterization and analysis of treatment. Am J Gastroenterol 1994;89,8:S182–S193.

28 Johanson JF. Epidemiology of hemorrhoids. In: Everhart J, ed. Digestive diseases in the United States. National Institutes of Health and National Center for Health Statistics. Washington, DC: USGPO, 1994.

29 Kinney TB, Deluca SA. Idiopathic hemochromatosis. Am Fam Physician 1991;44:873–875.

Chapter 24
Ears, Eyes, Nose, and Throat Problems

Wade A. Lillegard
Janus D. Butcher

EAR PROBLEMS: HEARING LOSS

Aerobic Exercise and Hearing

Approximately 4% of Americans suffer from noise-induced hearing loss (1). This hearing loss may result either from acute acoustic trauma or, more commonly, from cumulative noise exposure. In athletes, the hemodynamic changes associated with exercise can result in inner ear vasoconstriction that can cause a temporary hearing loss (2). Thus, exercising in noisy environments may augment the hearing loss caused by excessive noise exposure. In support of this, Vittitow et al. (3) have shown that the noise-induced temporary threshold shift in the 3 to 6 kHz range is significantly greater for individuals aerobically exercising with music, compared to those merely listening to music. There is, however, no evidence that chronic exercise leads to permanent hearing loss. In fact, fit individuals demonstrate a smaller degree of hearing loss than unfit individuals when exposed to either noise or a combination of noise and exercise (4). These associations indicate that exercise-augmented hearing loss is likely due to a combination of metabolic and vascular changes in the cochlea during exercise.

Athletes used to exercising in loud environments should be cautioned regarding their increased risk of hearing loss. Exposure to noise levels greater than 85 dB (decibels) for 8 hours may cause hearing loss; noise in aerobic classes, for example, ranges from 87 dB during warmup to 93 to 96 dB during peak exercise (5). Hearing protection is advised when exposed to loud noise sources (85 dB) such as music, automobile traffic, or airports.

Hearing Loss and Acoustic Trauma

Hearing loss in athletes can result either from direct trauma to the outside of the ear or from indirect trauma to the inner ear. Blunt trauma to the external ear can generate sufficient force to rupture the pars tensa of the tympanic membrane. This can occur in any contact sport but is more common in boxing and wrestling (6). A penetrating trauma can occur from a jet of water from water skiing. Athletes will complain of acute ear pain and loss of hearing.

Vertigo and tinnitus, if present, are generally transient. Physical examination may reveal a bloody discharge from the external canal, and there is generally a visible perforation at the anterior inferior aspect of the pars tensa. Most perforations heal spontaneously, but close follow-up is imperative. An audiogram should be performed soon after the injury to document the degree of hearing loss and to evaluate potential inner ear damage. With direct trauma injuries (i.e., water jet injuries) prophylactic antibiotic ear drops should be used. All patients should be followed until the perforation is completely healed, at which time another audiogram should be performed. If hearing loss persists, the patient should be referred to an otolaryngologist for evaluation and treatment of possible ossicle chain injury (7).

Sudden hearing loss, with or without vestibular symptoms, can also occur in athletes secondary to a sudden increase in the inner ear pressure. Increased intrathoracic or intra-abdominal pressure causes an increase in cerebral spinal fluid pressure, which can disrupt the cochleovestibular apparatus (8). This type of inner ear injury has been described in a gymnast and a weightlifter (9), but could potentially affect any athlete. Affected athletes should be evaluated with an audiogram and referred to an otolaryngologist for further evaluation.

Barotrauma

Deep water diving imposes significant stresses to the ear: for each 10 meters of descent, water pressure increases one atmosphere and gas volume decreases proportionately (10). This pressure can cause hearing loss, tinnitus, vertigo, or any combination of these. Indeed, approximately 60% of professional divers in Australia demonstrate a significant sensorineural hearing loss (11). Depths as shallow as 8 feet can cause middle or inner ear barotrauma (12).

Barotitis Externa

A negative pressure can develop between the tympanic membrane (TM) and ear plugs or a cerumen impaction that causes the TM to bulge outward. The blood vessels of the TM and external canal then dilate, causing edema, hemorrhagic bullae, and possible TM rupture. There may be a temporary conductive hearing loss. Treatment involves avoidance of diving until the lesions heal. For prophylactic purposes, athletes should fill the ear canal with water prior to diving or place the edge of the face mask under the edge of the hood during diving (10).

Barotitis Media

Eustachian tube dysfunction can transform the middle ear into a closed space. The increased pressure from diving will cause the TM to retract into this closed space, resulting in hemorrhage and possible rupture. Physical examination will reveal a normal-appearing external canal and a retracted and possibly bloody or perforated TM. There may be fluid in the middle ear, and any hearing loss will be conductive and transient. Avoidance of diving until the injury resolves is the only treatment necessary. Prevention is afforded by not allowing individuals with eustachian-type dysfunction to dive.

Barotrauma Auris Internae

Inner ear barotrauma is less common than external or middle ear trauma but is potentially much more serious. Divers who cannot equalize ear pressures via a Valsalva maneuver maintain a negative middle ear pressure, forcing a pressure differential between the inner and middle ear compartments. When inner ear hemorrhage, intracochlear membrane tears, or a fistula of the round or oval windows occurs, almost always there is a history of difficulty equalizing ear pressure during the dive (13). Patients experience a fullness in the ear(s) and a mild to profound hearing loss, which may be accompanied by vertigo, dizziness, or tinnitus. Vertigo and dizziness resolve spontaneously in hours to weeks, but tinnitus resolution is variable.

With isolated inner ear barotrauma, the physical examination is often unremarkable. The external and middle ears appear normal, and hearing loss ranges from mild to severe. The Romberg test may be positive if vestibular dysfunction is present.

Any diver suspected of having inner ear dysfunction should receive audiometry and be referred to an otolaryngologist for detailed evaluation and treatment. Divers with documented inner ear barotrauma are generally instructed to permanently discontinue diving. There is recent evidence, however, that cochleovestibular function does not further deteriorate if divers are properly reinstructed on how to maximize eustachian tube dysfunction (14). This is done by a jaw thrust or yawning maneuver at the surface, descent feet first down an anchor line, while continuously equalizing pressure (via Valsalva maneuver) for the first 20 feet.

Balance Disorders

Maintenance of balance is a complicated process involving input from multiple sensory structures, including the eyes, the otolith/cochlea apparatus, and peripheral proprioceptors. Balance disorders from an abnormality of any of these systems are relatively common in the general population, accounting for 7 million U.S. emergency room visits each year (15). In the athletic population, balance dysfunction is primarily due to otolith/cochlea trauma and is especially prevalent in high-impact aerobics. The repetitive jarring trauma of this activity causes damage to both the vestibular and cochlear apparatus, leading to vertigo, tinnitus, disequilibrium, and partial hearing loss (16). These symptoms affect 20% to 25% of individuals who regularly participate in high-impact aerobics; they are most prominent in individuals who participate frequently (e.g., aerobic instructors) (16).

Physical examination should differentiate cervical versus vestibular causes of vertigo. In particular, examination should reveal nystagmus solicited by the Bárány-Nylan maneuver, a test that uses a rotation chair to spin the patient at a predetermined rate (17). Peripheral etiologies (i.e., vestibular or cochlear) can be differentiated from central nervous system lesions by the character of nystagmus: peripheral lesions show a 2 to 40 second latency of onset, fatigability, habituation, severe intensity of vertigo, and poor reproducibility. Further evaluation should include a formal audiologic assessment, electronystagmography, and caloric testing, which are best performed by an otolaryngologist.

The best treatment is education and prevention. Decreasing the noise levels in the workout area and substituting low-impact activities significantly reduces the occurrence of symptoms. Common therapy for vestibular dysfunction that includes vertigo are medications such as meclozine or transdermal scopolamine (18). Other treatment options for established vestibular/cochlear disorders are being investigated, including vestibular habituation exercises, acupuncture, and medications such as acetazolamide (Diamox) or astemizole (Hismanal) (16,18).

EYE PROBLEMS

Vision and Sport

The visual system in athletes contributes 70% of the information reaching an athlete's brain and is the trigger for the first movement (19). Sports performance may be enhanced either through correcting abnormal visual acuity or through sports vision training for those with normal vision.

Crisp, clear vision enhances optimal performance, yet fewer than half of elite athletes have received a complete visual examination, and 10% to 30% of those fail the exam (20). Apparently, many undiagnosed athletes could benefit from corrective lenses; the risks and benefits of spectacles, rigid lenses, soft lenses, and extended-wear lenses must be assessed with respect to the athlete's particular sport. Spectacles slip, break, may not enhance peripheral vision, and can cause direct trauma to the eye when struck. For this reason, 94% of optometrists recommend contacts over spectacles for athletes (20); 85% recommend soft lenses; 5% recommend rigid lenses; and 21% recommend extended-wear contacts (20).

The main advantages of contacts are ease of wear, good central vision, and an approximately 15% improvement in peripheral awareness (21). Rigid gas permeable (RGP) lenses are less desirable than soft lenses because they are more likely to be dislodged, are less comfortable initially, and may scatter light rays causing a "flare" or "glare" (which is especially troublesome to athletes playing under night lights). Flare is rarely a problem with soft contacts (20). Athletes in contact or water sports should avoid rigid lenses because ejection is likely (unless goggles are worn). Disposable or frequent replacement lenses may be ideal for athletes who frequently lose lenses or have difficulty properly cleaning and caring for lenses.

Disposable lenses are frequently worn overnight, which poses a special problem for the water athlete. Overnight wear causes corneal hypoxia, acidosis, and epithelial compromise. This, in combination with water-borne organisms, predisposes to infectious keratitis (22). These athletes should be cautioned not to use extended-wear contacts. Contact-wearing athletes involved in water sports should be further advised to wear goggles whenever possible. If contacts must be worn without goggles, the risk of dislodgement can be minimized by 1) closing the eyes upon contact with water, 2) opening the eyes under water using a 5 to 7 mm "squint," and 3) pointing the nose in the intended direction of gaze (22). Contacts should be disinfected after water sports by using heat disinfection to kill amoebic cysts and fungi.

Protecting the eye from trauma is also an important aspect of sports care. Approved goggles, protective lenses, and other forms of eye guards should be used in high-velocity racket sports and other sporting situations in which they are indicated. Some advocate for their use in basketball, and they are being worn by many professional players. Further discussion of this issue can be found in the standard texts (23).

Sports Vision Training

Optimal sport-related visual processing is generally associated with exceptional eye–hand coordination. Performance in certain sports—such as baseball, cricket, hockey, or racket sports—can be enhanced either by maximizing the speed and efficiency of a normal visual system or by correcting deficits. In support of this, tennis and squash players (who require a rapid anticipatory response) have been shown to have shorter vision-evoked potential latencies than rowers (24). Approximately 35% of professional teams and 19% of Division 1A teams in the United States use visual training techniques, primarily for performance enhancement rather than to correct deficits (20).

A sports optometrist or ophthalmologist is necessary to evaluate an athlete's visual skills (visual acuity, eye movement, binocularity, accommodation, and stereopsis), visual cognitive skills (speed of recognition, span of recognition), and reaction. Identified deficits can be corrected through home visual training exercises (binocular strings, flip-cards, balloon strings), or through specialized training devices (tachistoscope, saccadic fixator) (25). Some athletes without visual deficits may benefit from visual enhancement exercises using these same techniques.

Glaucoma

Glaucoma refers to a persistent increase in intra-ocular pressure and is described as either open angle or closed angle. Angle closure glaucoma results from the acute closure of an already narrow anterior chamber angle. Open angle glaucoma is an idiopathic process, is associated with aging, accounts for over 90% of all glaucoma cases, and affects 1% to 5% of individuals over age 40 (26).

There are no symptoms initially with open angle glaucoma. As the disease progresses, the visual fields gradually constrict from out to in, with central vision spared. Untreated, this condition often progresses to complete blindness in 20 to 30 years. Acute angle closure glaucoma usually presents with severe pain and blurred vision associated with pupillary dilation (e.g., sitting in a darkened room).

Ophthalmoscopic visualization of the optic disk for marginal cupping and central visual field testing should be performed in suspected cases of glaucoma. The most reliable screening test is tonometry. All persons over the age of 40 should have screening tonometry and an ophthalmologic exam, which should be repeated every 3 to 5 years (18). This screening should be done annually if there is a family history of glaucoma.

The athlete with glaucoma presents unique challenges due to the effects of medications on performance and the restrictions on their use. Beta-agonist blocking agents (timolol [Timoptic], 1 drop, 0.25% to 0.5% twice a day; or betoxolol [Betoptic], 0.5%, 2 drops twice a day) are the most commonly used class of drugs. These drugs, however, are associated with reduced exercise performance and the potential to exacerbate reactive airways disease (27). In addition, the topical beta-blockers are banned by the U.S. National Collegiate Athletic Association (NCAA) for rifle competitions, and by the International Olympic Committee (IOC) for numerous events (28). Another commonly used medication, dipivefrin (Propine), 0.1%, is also banned by the IOC (28). Pilocarpine (0.25% to 10% solution), 1 drop four to six times per day, is a good alternative for many patients and is allowed by the NCAA and IOC (28). Surgical trabeculotomy may be considered in patients not responsive to medical therapy.

Photokeratoconjunctivitis (PKC)

Photokeratoconjunctivitis (snowblindness, or PKC) is caused by exposure to high-dose ultraviolet radiation (UVR) primarily in the "B" wavelength (UVB). High exposure for even 1 hour can cause damage to the superficial epithelium and underlying stroma in what amounts to a sunburn of the cornea. This injury is most common in athletes participating in environments with extreme ambient light conditions (e.g., high altitudes) or on highly reflective surfaces (snow, ice, and choppy water).

Clinically, there is a period of 2 to 12 hours after exposure when the patient is symptom free. This is followed by intense pain, hyperlacrimation, foreign body sensation, blepharospasm, and photophobia. Examination usually reveals erythema and conjunctival epithelial edema. In severe cases, corneal pitting may be observed with fluorescein application.

PKC generally heals completely over 2 to 7 days (29). Initial doses of topical analgesics are useful for examination purposes, but their subsequent use should be avoided. In cases with significant photophobia (suggestive of iritis), mydriatic-cycloplegic drops such as homatropine 5% (permitted by both the NCAA and IOC [28]) reduce the pain. Because of the intense pain associated with this injury, a short course of narcotic analgesics (banned by the IOC) should be considered. UVR protective lenses with side panels should be used to prevent further injury. In severe cases, compressive dressings with topical antibiotic ointment may be used for the first 24 hours. Essentially, all of these injuries are preventable, and athletes participating in high-intensity UVR environments should be counseled on the use of UVR-protective lenses, which transmit less than 10% UVB.

Keratoconjunctivitis Sicca (KCS)

Keratoconjunctivitis sicca (KCS) or "dry eye" results from abnormal tear production, abnormal tear delivery (tear duct occlusion), or abnormal tear content. KCS occurs with aging, hereditary conditions, autoimmune disorders, drug use, malnutrition, and excessive evaporation of tears (due to extreme environmental factors such as hot, dry, or windy conditions).

Patients usually complain of dry, red, and itching eyes, and in more severe cases complain of a foreign body sensation or photophobia. Outdoor athletes commonly develop KCS by exposure to severe environmental conditions without proper protective eyewear. Some medications predispose individuals to problems, and these include antihistamines, tricyclic antidepressants, diuretics, and anticholinergics.

Physical examination may reveal an injected conjunctiva although routine ophthalmoscopic exam is often completely normal. Slit-lamp evaluation often demonstrates a decrease in the fluid meniscus along the lower lid (normal is 0.3 mm), as well as corneal surface irregularities. Specific testing, such as the Schirmer test (which measures fluid migration along a piece of filter paper placed in the lower lid) may be helpful, but are generally best performed by an ophthalmologist.

Treatment for environmentally induced KCS involves moistening with artificial tears and the use of protective lenses to reduce evaporation of tears. In persistent cases, an evaluation for systemic illnesses such as allergies, AIDS, and Sjögren's syndrome should be considered.

Pterygia and Pinguiculae

A pterygium is a vascularized triangular band of conjunctival and subconjunctival tissue along the medial sclera and intrapalpebral fissure (Fig 24-1). This forms through elastoid degeneration of the substantia propria and is associated with frequent or continuous exposure to ultraviolet light. The condition is often seen in tennis players, lifeguards, golfers, and other outdoor athletes. Pterygium is the most common conjunctival lesion and is often bilateral. A pinguiculum is a yellow elevated nodule on the conjunctival surface that develops by a similar process of elastoid degeneration.

Treatment of pterygium is only necessary if the membrane encroaches on the cornea and affects vision. Surgical excision is the usual approach; however, recurrence is very common. These recurrences are more aggressive than the primary lesions, so postsurgical adjunctive therapy with ei-

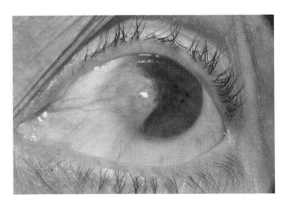

Figure 24-1. A pterygium extending across a portion of the cornea. (Courtesy of Brad Pearman, MD.)

ther beta radiation or topical mitomycin-C (0.01% to 0.02% for 5 to 14 days) is often used (30). Pinguicula are generally treated with excision and rarely recur.

Due to their association with UVR exposure, these lesions are preventable through the use of UVR-protective lenses in high-light environments. The use of hats, caps, and wraparound glasses or side panels is advised to further limit exposure.

NOSE AND THROAT PROGRAMS

Rhinitis Medicamentosa

Prolonged use of local nasal decongestants can lead to a "mucosal dependence," whereby termination of use leads to increased nasal stuffiness (rhinitis medicamentosa). This is due either to rebound vasodilation after the vasoconstrictor effect of the drug has disappeared or to mucosal hypoxia and edema (31). To prevent such occurrence, oxymetazoline (Afrin), a commonly used decongestant (not restricted by the NCAA or IOC [28]), is recommended for no more than 3 contiguous days. A recent study showed no rebound effect after 10 days of continuous use in 8 subjects, but rebound congestion occurred in all subjects at 30 days (31).

Treatment of established rhinitis medicamentosa requires tapering of the nasal decongestants and controlling the rebound swelling with steroids. As the patient decreases the frequency of decongestant use, a 1-week oral steroid taper is given. On the fourth day of the taper, dexamethasone nasal spray, 2 squirts four times daily, is started. After 1 week, the nasal decongestant and oral steroids should be stopped, and the patient kept on the nasal steroid spray for 2 to 3 more weeks. The NCAA does not restrict oral or topical steroid use; the IOC bans oral corticosteroid use, but generally allows the use of topical steroids with appropriate notification at the time of competition (28).

Nasal Polyps

Nasal polyps are not a disease, but a physical finding with an ill-defined pathophysiology. They are present in approximately 1% to 2% of the adult population with a peak prevalence between 20 and 60 years of age (32). One-third of patients with polyps have associated bronchospasm (33) and 8% have the triad of asthma, nasal polyps, and aspirin hypersensitivity (34). Allergies are no more common in patients with polyps than in the normal population (35).

Patients may present with either isolated nasal disease or nasal disease associated with panrespiratory disease. Predisposing factors include anatomic abnormalities of the middle meatus, chronic sinusitis, and late onset asthma. Almost all patients with nasal polyps have some degree of sinus opacity on radiographs, but infectious sinusitis is present in only 15% (36).

Nasal speculum examination reveals a bulging, pale, fluid-filled mucosal swelling. Sinus opacity and/or tenderness should be assessed, and the lungs should be auscultated for evidence of wheezing. Further evaluation may include exercise pulmonary function testing for associated bronchospasm.

Treatment options include topical corticosteroids, which can help prevent surgery in up to 50% of cases, or surgery for those refractory to topical intranasal therapy (22). Two betamethasone drops (0.1%), or two sprays of beclomethasone or flunisolide in each nostril twice a day for 1 month, is the first line of treatment; these drugs are allowed by both the IOC and NCAA. Failure of medical treatment warrants computerized tomography to evaluate the sinuses and middle meatus, followed by a possible referral for surgery.

Nasal polyps per se have no impact on athletic performance but may be a marker for exercise-limiting reactive airway disease. Because of the association with aspirin, hypersensitive athletes with nasal polyps should exercise caution in the use of aspirin and nonsteroidal anti-inflammatory drugs (which may cross-react with aspirin).

Epistaxis

The nose has a very generous blood supply to warm and humidify air as it enters the upper airways. In contact sports like wrestling and rugby, injury to the nose resulting in epistaxis is relatively common. The bleeding can be profuse following seemingly minor trauma. Epistaxis usually occurs after injury to Kiesselbach's plexus on the anterior nasal septum. Associated factors that predispose athletes to nasal mucosal friability include allergic rhinitis, sinusitis, dry ambient conditions, and a deviated nasal septum.

Often the bleeding resolves without aggressive treatment. The patient should sit with the head tilted slightly forward to allow the blood to drain from the anterior nares. Applying direct pressure by firmly squeezing the nares for 10 to 15 minutes stops the majority of cases. Nasal decongestants such as oxymetazoline (Afrin) and ephedrine (banned by the IOC [28]) can help to slow bleeding. If these measures fail, an attempt to identify the source of the bleed should be made. Cauterization of the bleeding site with silver nitrate sticks is usually effective. On occasion, anterior packing may be necessary. Using a nasal speculum, a long strip of ¼ inch (0.05 cm) gauze, treated with antibiotic ointment, should be inserted with a bayonet forceps. Alternatively, Merocel (Merocel Corporation, Mystic, CT), a compressed sponge that expands when wet, can be used. Merocel should be treated with an antibiotic ointment before insertion to prevent the development of a secondary infection or toxic shock syndrome (37).

Approximately 5% of epistaxis originates posteriorly in the nasal cavity. These tend to bleed profusely and frequently require packing to stop the bleeding. Posterior packing is technically more difficult than anterior packing and usually requires an otolaryngologist to effect adequate hemostasis (37). Nasal occlusive balloons are somewhat easier to use, but are associated with the complications of pressure necrosis and eustachian tube dysfunction.

Obstructive Sleep Apnea (OSA), Snoring, and Tonsillar Enlargement

The sports medicine practitioner should consider the possibility of obstructive sleep apnea (OSA) in patients who report undue fatigue, either related or not related to exercise.

OSA can occur in any age group, but is most commonly encountered in the older, relatively sedentary individual. The prevalence of OSA is esti-

mated to be 0.2% to 8.5% in men, and is 8 to 10 times lower in women (38,39). The fundamental abnormality in OSA is a periodic collapse of the pharyngeal airway during sleep (39). This results in asphyxia, which triggers an increasing respiratory effort against the collapsed airway until the individual awakens.

Clinical sequelae relate to both the apnea (recurrent hypoxia and hypercapnea) and the interrupted sleep. Cumulative asphyxia may lead to polycythemia, hypertension, arrhythmias, pulmonary hypertension, right-sided heart failure, left ventricular dysfunction, or sudden death. Poor sleep causes daytime fatigue, irritability, memory impairment, and depression. Predisposing factors include obesity, hypothyroidism, hypertension, and alcohol or sedative use. Snoring is present in virtually all patients with OSA (40), but it is also common in normal adults (20% of adults and 60% of men >40 years old [39]). For this reason, excessive snoring should be considered a marker for the development of OSA, but is not pathognomonic.

Signs and symptoms increase insidiously over the years, marked by excessive daytime sleepiness and fatigue (40). Family members may relate loud, irregular snoring with periods of absent breathing and restless sleep. Impaired concentration, judgment, and memory, as well as irritability and depression, become apparent as the disease progresses. Affected patients often, but not always, are obese and have a short, thick neck.

Physical examination in suspected cases should be directed toward the causes and sequelae of OSA. The nares should be inspected for nasal polyps, deviated septum, or chronic rhinitis; the oropharynx should be inspected for tonsillar hypertrophy or macroglossia. Evaluation should assess whether hypertension, cardiac arrhythmias, pulmonary hypertension, and cor pulmonale are present. An electrocardiogram and a chest roentgenogram may show evidence of cor pulmonale or left ventricular hypertrophy. Polysomnography, performed in a sleep laboratory, is the most definitive test to differentiate obstructive sleep apnea from simple excess snoring (40).

Treatment involves correcting any underlying disorder: treatment of hypothyroidism or chronic rhinitis, avoidance of alcohol or sedatives, weight reduction, and sleeping in the lateral decubitus position. Adenoidectomy or tonsillectomy may be necessary. Most patients require additional treatment, such as nasal CPAP (continuous positive airway pressure), upper airway surgical revision, and/or oral appliances.

REFERENCES

1 National Institute of Health. Noise and hearing loss. NIH Consensus Development Conference Consensus Statement. Bethesda, MD, 1990:22–24.

2 Axelsson A, Vertes D, Miller J. Immediate noise effects on cochlear vasculature in the guinea pig. Acta Otolaryngol (Stockh) 1980;91:237–246.

3 Vittitow M, Windmill I, Yates J. Effect of simultaneous exercise and noise exposure. J Am Acad Audiol 1994;5:343–348.

4 Manson J, Alessio HM, Cristell M, Hutchinson KM. Does cardiovascular health mediate hearing ability? Med Sci Sports Exerc 1994;26:866–871.

5 Mirbod SM, Lanphere C, Fujita S. Noise in aerobic facilities [letter]. Ind Health 1994;32:49–55.

6 Strunk CL. Ear injuries in sports. Texas Med 1986;82:32–36.

7 Rybak LP, Johnson DW. Tympanic membrane perforations from water sports: treatment and outcome. Otolaryngol Head Neck Surg 1983;91:659–662.

8 Goodhill V. Sudden deafness and round window ruptures. Laryngoscope 1971;81:1462–1474.

9 Katsarkas A, Baxter JD. Cochlear and vestibular dysfunction resulting from physical exertion or environmental pressure changes. J Otolaryngol 1976;5:25–32.

10 Molvaer OI, Natrud E. Ear damage due to diving. Acta Otolaryngol Suppl (Stockh) 1979;360:187–189.

11 Edmonds C, Freeman P. Hearing loss in Australian divers. Med J Aust 1985;143:446–448.

12 Schuknecht HF, Gacek RR. Surgery on only-hearing ears. Trans Am Acad Ophthalmol Otolaryngol 1973;77:257–266.

13 Parell GJ, Becker GD. Conservative management of inner ear barotrauma resulting from scuba diving. Otolaryngol Head Neck Surg 1985;93:393–397.

14 Parell GJ, Becker GD. Inner ear barotrauma in scuba divers: a long-term follow-up after continued diving. Arch Otolaryngol Head Neck Surg 1993;119:455–457.

15 Jenkins H, Furman J, Honrvbia V, Linthicum F, et al. Disequilibrium of aging. Otolaryngol Head Neck Surg 1989;100:272–282.

16 Weintraub MI. Vestibulopathy induced by high impact aerobics. A new syndrome: discussion of 30 cases. J Sports Med Phys Fitness 1994;34:56–63.

17 Ballenger JJ, ed. Diseases of the nose, throat, ear, head, and neck. 14th ed. Philadelphia: Lea & Febiger, 1991:1020.

18 Goroll AH, May LA, Gordon AG. Primary care medicine. 3rd ed. Philadelphia: JB Lippincott, 1995.

19 Weiskrantz L. Behavioural analysis of the monkey's visual nervous system. Proc R Soc Lond B Biol Sci 1972;182:427–455.

20 Zieman B, Reichow A, Coffey B. Optometric trends in sports vision: knowledge, utilization, and practitioner role expansion potential. J Am Optom Assoc 1993;64:490–501.

21 Benjamin W. Visual optics of contact lenses. In: Bennett E, Weissman B, ed. Clinical contact lens practice. Philadelphia: JB Lippincott, 1991:Chapter 14.

22 Legerton JA. Prescribing for water sports. Optom Clin 1993;3:91–110.

23 Shingleton B, Hersh P, Kenyon K. Eye trauma. St. Louis: Mosby Year Book, 1991.

24 Delpont E, Dolisi C, Suisse G, et al. Visual evoked potentials: differences related to physical activity. Int J Sports Med 1991;12:293–298.

25 Kirscher DW. Sports vision training procedures. Optom Clin 1993;3:171–182.

26 Tielsch J. The epidemiology of primary open angle glaucoma. Ophthal Clin North Am 1991;4:649–657.

27 Eichner E. Ergolytic drugs in medicine and sports. Am J Med 1993;94:205–211.

28 Fuentes R, Rosenberg J, Davis A. Athletic drug reference '95. Research Triangle Park, NC: Clean Data, 1995.

29 Friedlander J, Lowe N. Exposure to radiation from the sun. In: Auerbach P, ed. Wilderness medicine: Management of wilderness and environmental emergencies. 3rd ed. St. Louis: Mosby, 1995:291–311.

30 Frucht-Pery J, Ilsar M. The use of low-dose mitomycin C for prevention of recurrent pterygium. Ophthalmology 1994;101:759–762.

31 Graf P, Juto JE. Decongestion effect and rebound swelling of the nasal mucosa during 4-week use of oxymetazoline. ORL J Otorhinolaryngol Relat Spec 1994;56:157–160.

32 Hosemann W, Gode U, Wagner W. Epidemiology, pathophysiology of nasal polyposis, and spectrum of endonasal sinus surgery. Am J Otolaryngol 1994;15:85–98.

33 Maloney J, Collins J. Nasal polyps, nasal polypectomy, asthma and aspirin sensitivity. J Laryngol Otol 1977;91:837–846.

34 Samter M, Lederer F. Nasal polyps: their relationship to allergy, particularly to bronchial asthma. Med Clin North Am 1958;42:175–179.

35 Drake-Lee AB. Medical treatment of nasal polyps. Rhinology 1994;32:1–4.

36 Dawes P, Bates G, Watson D, et al. The role of bacterial infection of the maxillary sinus in nasal polyps. Clin Otolaryngol 1989;14:447–450.

37 Josephson GD, Godley FA, Stierna P. Practical management of epistaxis. Med Clin North Am 1991;75:1311–1320.

38 Partinen M, Telakivi T. Epidemiology of obstructive sleep apnea syndrome. Am Sleep Disord Assoc Sleep Res Soc 1992;15:S1–S4.

39 Wiegand L, Zwillich CW. Obstructive sleep apnea. Dis Mon 1994;40:197–252.

40 Brown LK. Sleep apnea syndromes: Overview and diagnostic approach. Mt Sinai J Med 1994;61:99–112.

Chapter 25
Dental Problems in Athletes

John P. Fricker

In a review of problems presented to the polyclinic at the Barcelona Olympic Games (1992), oral problems were noted as the second most common complaint after general medical problems and were more common than trauma or orthopedic conditions (1). Oral problems accounted for 12.5% of total visits to the clinic. Of the 174 teams that participated, 99 (57%) reported oral problems. The number of people seen at the clinic ranged from one person on day 2, to a high of 41 visits on day 17. There was a mean of 30 visits a day for days 11 to 20 of the games. The majority of dental problems followed pre-Olympic treatment interventions with the most frequent complaint being a broken, loose, or lost filling. Other common complaints included pulpitis, pericoronitis, and dental caries.

Dental problems must be recognized as significant in limiting an athlete's performance, so the sports physician requires a basic understanding of the more common dental complaints. This chapter is limited to a description of toothache, related pain, and oral medicine. For a review of dental trauma, the reader is referred to Bloomfield et al. (1995) (2).

CARIES AND RELATED INFECTIONS

Dental Caries

Dental caries should be thought of as an infectious disease that results in demineralization of tooth structure (Fig 25-1). Microorganisms produce acid (from carbohydrates), which in turn demineralizes the inorganic tooth components within the tooth structure at the infected site. Caries is a disease with delayed expression—repeated bacterial attacks are required to demineralize the enamel to a point where the surface cavitates. If a caries-conducive environment continues, the lesion advances through the enamel into the buffer dentine. The rate of demineralization increases into the dentine, leading to greater cavitation of the enamel. Once the dentinal tubules are exposed, they provide a pathway for bacteria and toxins to the pulp to produce pulpitis. Dental caries are a major cause of discomfort and are the major cause of tooth loss prior to age 35 years.

Dental plaque is an organic nitrogenous mass firmly attached to tooth structure. It is composed primarily of bacteria, with extracellular dextrans, salivary glycoproteins, and food debris. *Streptococcus mutans* predominates in *smooth surface* caries because these organisms carry an ability to adhere to the tooth surface. *Lactobacillus* is the predominant bacteria in *pit and fissure* caries.

Lactic acid is produced by these bacteria within dental plaque; thus, demineralization of enamel is a result of both the concentration of acid at the tooth surface and the amount of time the enamel is exposed to low pH conditions.

Sucrose is the most caries-conducive carbohydrate, and the percentage of *S. mutans* in dental plaque increases with frequent ingestion of sucrose. Thus, a controlled diet and good oral hygiene reduce the incidence of plaque and the duration of enamel exposure to lactic acid.

Once caries has resulted in cavitation of enamel, a restorative filling of the deficient tooth structure is required. Materials such as amalgam, composite resin, and glass ionomer cements are used to restore masticatory function once the decayed tooth structure is removed.

Increasing the resistance of enamel to acid at-

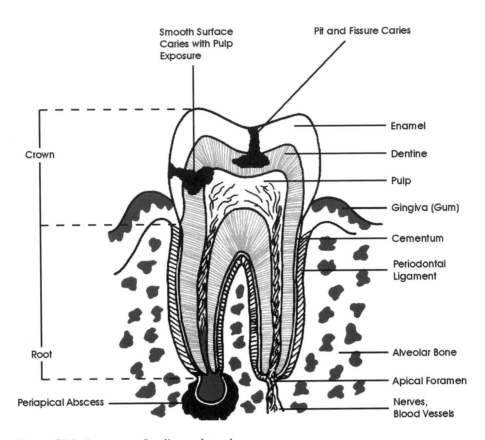

Figure 25-1. Anatomy of a diseased tooth.

tack is possible with the use of fluorides. Fluoride ions incorporated into tooth enamel alter the structure of hydroxyapatite and decrease enamel solubility. Fluoride added to reticulated water supplies has been found to be the most effective public health measure against dental caries. This can be supplemented with fluoride toothpastes and topical applications from dental practitioners.

Pulpitis

As caries spreads to the pulp chamber, microorganisms can produce an acute pulpitis. Pulpitis pain is severe, and the patient often cannot localize it to a particular tooth. Such a severe throbbing pain is typically precipitated by extremes in temperature. However, in some cases the pain may be relieved by cold fluids held over the offending tooth. Pulpitis may persist for several days and usually stops quite suddenly, implying necrosis of the pulp.

Acute pulpitis may also follow the restorative filling of a tooth, either immediately or after an in-

terval of several years. Often this is iatrogenic, as a result of cavity preparation with rotary instruments or the potential toxic effect of materials used for treatment or restoration. Placing poorly sealed restorations over residual bacteria also results in pulpitis.

A careful history of recent fillings and their relationship to the pain is essential, but if the pain is diffuse and many teeth are heavily filled, it is often very difficult to identify the tooth that is causing the pain.

Cracked Tooth Syndrome (CTS)

A cracked tooth syndrome (CTS) results from an incomplete fracture of a vital (alive) posterior tooth, involving dentine and possibly the pulp (3). The patient usually complains of a sharp pain on biting and is able to accurately localize the offending tooth. In this respect, CTS differs from pulpitis, where localization is difficult. When a patient presents with pain in an unfilled or lightly filled tooth, CTS should be suspected. Treatment is aimed at supporting the remaining crown of the affected tooth, usually by applying a full cover crown.

Acute Periapical Abscess

An acute periapical abscess may follow acute pulpitis and necrosis. Most often a periapical abscess develops in connection with a tooth in which the pulp has asymptomatically necrosed following caries, trauma, or restorative treatment. Pain can be very severe when the acute inflammatory process is held within bone.

The affected tooth becomes mobile and is very sensitive to percussion. Suppuration occurs early, and if pus extends outside the bone, it forms an abscess cavity within the attached gingiva adjacent to the apex of the root of the tooth. This is called a dentoalveolar abscess.

A radiographic survey reveals an area of radiolucency at the apex of the root. Treatment consists of drainage via the root canal and root canal therapy. Antibiotics are useful to reduce the infection and associated symptoms until treatment from a dentist is available.

Periodontal Disease

Periodontal disease is a collective term embracing pathologic states of cementum gingiva, periodontal ligament, and alveolar bone. Inflammatory destruction of these tissues results in mobility of teeth and tooth loss. The multifactorial etiology of periodontal disease involves an interaction between the periodontal microflora and the defense mechanisms of the host (4). The primary etiologic agent is subgingival microorganisms derived from dental plaque. These produce lytic enzymes, metabolic end products, and antigenic components that are potentially harmful or initiate damage to the periodontium. Periodontal disease is the major cause of tooth loss over the age of 35 years.

Subgingival plaque contains anaerobic microorganisms, including

- *Actinobacillus actinomycetemcomitans*
- *Eikenella corrodens*
- *Fusobacterium nucleatum*
- *Porphyromonas gingivalis*
- *Treponema* species and spirochetes

Thus, periodontal disease is an infection of the oral cavity exerting its effect on the periodontium. The control of this disease is by antimicrobial agents and by mechanical removal of microorganisms.

When considering the use of antimicrobial agents, one must consider the patient's general health, with particular emphasis on any factor that may adversely effect immunocompetency. Periodontal bacteria trigger inflammatory host responses that lead to tissue destruction. The neutrophil/antibody/complement axis is critical for protection against periodontal disease. Abnormalities in this axis often lead to increased susceptibility to periodontal disease, and there is significant variability in host susceptibility to this disease.

Early periodontal disease may go unrecognized as it is often asymptomatic. However, it is readily confirmed with radiographs to assess bone loss and with clinical examination. As bone loss continues, there is increased tooth mobility, gingival erythema, and pain associated with gingival exudate. If bone loss is allowed to continue, the tooth is eventually lost.

PROBLEMS RELATED TO TOOTH GROWTH/EXTRACTION

Impacted Teeth

An impacted tooth is an unerupted tooth that is prevented from completely erupting due to lack of space from surrounding bone or teeth. The most commonly impacted tooth is the lower third molar or wisdom tooth. Pain from an impacted tooth is diffuse and dull, and may occur spontaneously or on biting. Pain may radiate to adjacent teeth or surrounding structures such as the temporomandibular joint or middle ear.

Unerupted lower third molars may weaken the mandible at the angle of the jaw and contribute to jaw fractures in this area. Less commonly, the maxillary canines may be impacted in the palate, causing symptoms of pain in the premaxillary region of the palate or adjacent teeth. Treatment is by surgical removal of the offending tooth.

Acute Postextraction Osteitis (Dry Socket)

Acute postextraction osteitis, or dry socket, is a complication of tooth extraction that occurs after

3% to 4% of routine extractions (5). It is characterized by severe pain, halitosis (bad breath), breakdown of the blood clot, and exposure of alveolar bone in the tooth socket. Severe throbbing pain usually starts after 48 hours and peaks after an additional 48 hours. The incidence of dry socket is higher in females than males, and may be related to the use of oral contraceptives, which produce an increased fibrolytic activity that predisposes the patient to the development of dry socket. Lower molars are the most frequent locations; mandibular third molars (wisdom teeth) are most common site of problems, at approximately 20%.

Clinical examination reveals an empty (hence dry) socket with accumulated food debris. Dry socket is usually self-limiting; however, it can be potentially serious in individuals who have had radiotherapy of the jaws or who are immunocompromised. Systemic antibiotics are indicated if there is malaise or lymphadenopathy, and metronidazole is the drug of choice, given orally at 400 mg three times per day for 5 days. Metronidazole should be avoided during pregnancy.

Acute Pericoronitis

Acute pericoronitis results from inflammation around the crown of a tooth and is most frequently related to an erupting lower third molar (wisdom tooth). Acute pain, swelling, trismus (muscle spasm), and tender submandibular and or upper cervical lymph glands are common. Oral examination reveals considerable inflammation, with swelling and maceration of the gum around the affected tooth. The tooth may not be visible but is palpable, and pus can be expressed from the overlying flap of gum tissue (operculum).

Fusobacteria and spirochetes are found at all stages of the disease process. These anaerobic organisms can cause severe infections with massive cellulitis. The drugs of choice are oral amoxicillin, 500 mg, three times per day for 7 days, or oral metronidazole, 400 mg, three times per day for 5 days.

Infective Endocarditis

Dental procedures commonly cause an asymptomatic transient bacteremia, usually of alpha hemolytic *Streptococcus viridans*, recognized as part of the normal flora of the oral cavity. Such procedures include gingival (gum) surgery, extraction oral surgery, endodontics (root canal therapy), and professional scaling and cleaning of teeth.

Antibiotic prophylaxis is required for those with a history of rheumatic fever, congenital heart disease, cardiac valve surgery, hemodialysis, previous endocarditis, or arterial or bypass surgery. Heart murmurs may be innocent (functional) or organic (resulting from cardiac abnormalities). Only organic murmurs require antibiotic prophylaxis. If emergency dental care is required (e.g., for a knocked-out tooth) and the status of the murmur is unknown, it is prudent to provide an antibiotic cover (6).

The standard regimen is amoxicillin, 3.0 g orally, 1 hour before the dental procedure, followed by 1.5 g, 6 hours after the initial dose. For those allergic to penicillin, 800 mg of erythromycin ethyl succinate, or oral erythromycin stearate, 1.0 g, 2 hours prior to the dental procedure followed by half the dose 6 hours later, should be prescribed.

Other patients at increased risk of cardiac anomalies predisposing to endocarditis include those with Down syndrome, Marfan's syndrome, and Ehlers-Danlos syndrome.

ORAL ULCERS AND LESIONS

Acute Necrotizing Ulcerative Gingivitis (ANUG)

Acute necrotizing ulcerative gingivitis (ANUG), also known as trench mouth or Vincent's gingivitis, is a fusospirochetal infection that usually affects only the gingival margins but occasionally is more extensive (7). The gingival margins are inflamed and the soft tissues between the teeth are ulcerated with pockets of gray necrotic tissue. Symptoms include pain, malaise, bad breath, and a metallic taste. The most important etiologic factor is poor oral hygiene. Other contributing factors are those that reduce the host's immune defenses, such as fatigue, stress, smoking, or overexertion.

Treatment is supportive and aimed at improvement in oral hygiene. Metronidazole may also be prescribed orally, 400 mg, 3 times per day for 7 days. If the condition does not respond to such therapy, the physician must immediately refer for investigation of underlying conditions such as blood dyscrasias.

Primary Herpetic Gingivostomatitis

Primary herpetic gingivostomatitis is a common form of herpes simplex virus type I. The peak incidence is in children aged from 2 to 4 years; however, an increasing number of young adults are also being affected. The incubation time is 3 to 7 days, and 50% of infections remain subclinical. Symptoms include fever, malaise, and severe local pain. This is followed within a few days by intense redness and swelling of the gums and by small vesicles distributed throughout the mouth. The vesicles soon rupture, leaving painful small ulcers surrounded by a red border.

Management includes supportive treatment with analgesics and topical anesthetics. Tetracycline—250 mg capsules, two at a time, emptied into a tumbler of water and used as a mouth rinse four times per day (*not* swallowed)—assists in controlling secondary infections. Recovery is usually within 1 week.

Denture Sore Mouth

Ill-fitting dentures, either full (replacing all teeth in a dental arch) or partial, may cause discomfort by rocking on the mucosa and causing ulceration. Pain may radiate to adjacent areas and occasionally present as temporomandibular joint pain. Where dentures are severely worn down so that the jaws overclose to maintain tooth contact, there is an inadequate lip seal at the corners of the mouth and the area is constantly moist. This provides an ideal environment for the opportunistic fungus *Candida albicans*. The lips become cracked and painful, resulting in angular cheilitis. A poorly fitting upper denture with full cover over the palate also provides an environment for *C. albicans* and results in a "denture sore mouth."

In both cases, the dentures require adjustment to maintain the correct vertical dimension for a lip seal and good palatal fit. Antifungal agents can be used topically over the lips in angular cheilitis and placed on the tissue-bearing surface in the denture sore mouth during waking hours. Dentures should never be worn during sleep.

Aphthous Ulcers

Recurrent aphthous ulcers (stomatitis, canker sores) are characterized by multiple or solitary painful ulcers of the oral mucosa. The lesions are covered by a pale gray membrane and surrounded by an erythematous halo. This condition affects 20% of the population (8), with a greater incidence among young adults and women.

No single etiologic factor has been found, although predisposing factors include heredity, autoimmune disorders, stress, hormonal changes (menstruation), and trauma. Antimucosal antibodies have been detected in some sufferers of recurrent aphthous ulcers. Nutritional deficiencies of iron and folic acid are common in patients with aphthous ulcers. Minor ulcers are less than 1 cm in diameter and heal spontaneously within 10 to 14 days without scarring. Major ulcers are larger than 1 cm in diameter; healing may take weeks and often results in scarring.

Topical gels containing lignocaine or corticosteroid, such as triamcinolone acetonide 0.1% as a proprietary paste (e.g., Kenalog in orabase), can provide local pain relief. Referral to a specialist is recommended when endocrine, dietary factors, or local dental trauma is involved.

Oral Cancer

Most oral malignancies are squamous cell carcinomas, and there has been a steady increase in incidence over the past 20 years. Younger patients and women are increasingly being affected. Alcohol and tobacco—especially in combination—are the primary etiologic agents.

Of particular concern is smokeless tobacco, which is now heavily marketed to a younger population. There is strong evidence that dry snuff causes oral cancer and can aggravate other systemic diseases. The continued use of smokeless tobacco leads to localized tissue changes such as leukoplakia, white wrinkled mucosa adjacent to where the tobacco is placed. Leukoplakia can become cancerous in up to 5% of cases (9).

Use of smokeless tobacco is widespread among high-profile professional baseball players in the United States and is to be condemned. Baseball players using smokeless tobacco have *60 times* the risk of developing leukoplakia compared with nonusers.

All health professionals involved in sport must take the responsibility of advising their athletes about the risks of tobacco and must learn to recognize early lesions. Early diagnosis is imperative as metastasis can arise in up to 30% of tobacco users, with lesions less than 2 cm wide.

Human Immunodeficiency Virus (HIV)

Acquired immunodeficiency syndrome (AIDS) is the most severe manifestation of a clinical spectrum of illness resulting from infection with the human immunodeficiency virus (HIV). The syndrome is defined by the development of serious opportunistic infections, neoplasms, or other life-threatening disorders resulting from progressive HIV-induced immunosuppression (10).

The immunocompromised patient is at risk of developing oral mucosal disorders that are rarely seen in immunocompetent persons. The most common complication is infection, especially with viruses, fungi, and mycobacteria. Herpes lesions and candidiasis predominate. Herpes simplex virus infections are frequent, persistent, and severe. Oral candidiasis is a criterion in most staging systems for HIV infections, and *C. albicans* is the most common species seen in oral lesions (11).

In association with HIV, oral candidiasis occurs in the following forms.

- Pseudomembranous: "thrush," yellow removable plaques that can occur on any mucosal surface
- Erythematous: red patches on any mucosal surface
- Angular cheilitis: cracks, fissures, or redness at the corners of the mouth

Persistent, frequent presentation of these lesions should alert the practitioner to decreased immunocompetency, and the athlete must be referred to the appropriate specialist for immediate management.

GLANDULAR, MUSCULAR, AND NEUROLOGIC PROBLEMS

Acute Maxillary Sinusitis

The maxillary sinus, or antrum, is an air-filled space lined by respiratory mucosa. The roots of the maxillary premolar and the molar teeth closely approximate the floor of the sinus. Diseases of the sinus may create symptoms that the patient interprets as being of dental origin; conversely, dental diseases may influence the health of the sinus. A periodontal or periapical abscess on a maxillary molar may produce a localized inflammatory response in the sinus.

A patient with symptomatic sinusitis may complain that maxillary posterior teeth are sensitive to percussion or biting pressure. Runners or jumpers with sinusitis experience toothache as their feet hit the ground. Pain is usually local, centers around the cheek, and radiates to the region above the ipsilateral eye. Other signs include a purulent postnasal drip and pyrexia.

The main causative organisms are Gram-positive cocci, so a broad-spectrum antibiotic such as co-trimoxazole or amoxicillin should be prescribed over 14 days. If the infection is of dental origin, metronidazole (400 mg, 3 times per day for 7 days) should be prescribed. Surgical procedures are kept to a minimum because of the risk of inducing osteomyelitis when bone is breached. Antral washout is indicated if there is a persistent collection within the antra that does not respond to antibiotics.

Temporomandibular Joint Dysfunction

The temporomandibular joints (TMJs) are non-weightbearing articulating joints between the mandibular condyles and the glenoid fossae of the temporal bones. The movement of the mandible is integrated by proprioceptive feedback from the muscles of mastication the periodontal ligaments of the teeth and the meniscus of the joint capsules. Bruxism (grinding of teeth during sleep) and malocclusion contribute to disharmony of the muscles, ligaments, and menisci within the joints. Recent tooth fillings with "high" spots cause avoiding actions in mandibular movements, and direct trauma to the TMJs can also produce dysfunction.

Forced opening of the mandible during surgical procedures such as intubation or removal of wisdom teeth has also been implicated as a contributing factor to TMJ pain. Systemic joint laxity may also be an etiologic factor (12).

Up to 50% of the general population may suffer from TMJ disorders at any one time, and they may present with any of the following symptoms:

- Pain in TMJs or the temporalis masseter or pterygoid muscles
- Clicking or locking of TMJs
- Limited movement of the jaw

Pain is usually worst in the mornings (after sleep) and is correlated with clenching and grinding of teeth during sleep, which may occur particularly when the individual is suffering from psychological stress. A transient joint inflammation results, and deviation on opening and closing produces a click.

Examination by a dentist is indicated to determine and correct any occlusal discrepancies in masticatory function. Explanation of the muscular nature of symptoms, along with reassurance, is necessary. Consideration should be given to lifestyle stresses where relevant, and their impact on symptoms.

Salivary Glands

Sialoliths (salivary calculus) commonly affect the submandibular gland. The duct is blocked to a greater or lesser extent so that as saliva forms it cannot escape. The gland swells, and as the pressure builds up there is pain. Gradually the saliva escapes, the swelling goes down, and the pain decreases. Radiographs supported by clinical palpation usually reveal the stone. Treatment is by surgical removal.

Trigeminal Neuralgia

Sufferers of trigeminal neuralgia experience brief episodes of severe, sharp, shooting pain over the distribution of the maxillary and mandibular divisions of the trigeminal nerve which last from seconds to 1 to 2 minutes. These pains can be triggered by innocuous stimuli such as washing, shaving, or tooth brushing. Demyelination may be involved, and vascular compression of trigeminal nerve rootlets has also been reported in association with trigeminal neuralgia.

Symptoms can usually be controlled with carbamazepine in divided oral doses; initial pain control requires 200 to 800 mg daily, and adequate maintenance therapy is 200 to 400 mg daily. Phenytoin (300 mg daily) is a second choice. Cryotherapy of affected nerves can provide relief with low morbidity, but recurrence on the order of 70% within 2 years has been reported (13).

CONCLUSION

Dental problems can limit the performance of an athlete, both directly and indirectly. Toothache and related pain need to be recognized for their debilitating effects and regular dental screening is recommended to avoid these problems.

REFERENCES

1 Soler Badia D, Batchelor PA, Sheiham A. The prevalence of oral health problems in participants of the 1992 Olympic Games in Barcelona. Int Dent J 1994;44:44–48.
2 Fricker JP, O'Neill L. Dental problems. In: Bloomfield J, Fricker PA, Fitch KD, eds. Science and medicine in sport, 2nd ed. Melbourne: Blackwell Science, 1995:339–347.
3 Ehrmann EH, Tyas MJ. Cracked tooth syndrome: diagnosis, treatment and correlation between symptoms and post-extraction finding. Aust Dent J 1990;35:105–112.
4 Liebana J, Castillo A. Physiopathology of primary periodontitis associated with plaque. Microbial and host factors. A review. Part 2. Aust Dent J 1994;39:310–315.
5 Fazakerley M, Field EA. Dry socket: a painful post-extraction complication. A review. Dent Update 1991;Jan/Feb:31–34.
6 Hall EH, Sherman RG, Emmons WW, Naylor GD. Antibacterial prophylaxis. Dent Clin North Am 1994;38:707–718.
7 Chapple ILC. Periodontal diseases in children and adolescents: classification, aetiology and management. Dental Update 1996;June:210–216.
8 Ship JA. Recurrent aphthous stomatitis. Oral Surg Oral Med Oral Pathol Oral Radiol 1996;81:141–147.
9 Van Der Waal I. The diagnosis and treatment of precancerous lesions. FDI World 1995;March/April:6–9.
10 McCullough MJ, Firth NA, Reade PC. Human immunodeficiency virus infection: a review of the mode of infection, pathogenesis, disease course and the general clinical manifestations. Aust Dent J 1997;42:30–37.
11 Lamster IB, Begg MD, Mitchell-Lewis D, et al. Oral manifestations of HIV infection in homosexual men and intravenous drug users. Oral Surg Oral Med Oral Pathol Oral Radiol 1994;78:163–174.
12 Buckingham RB, Braun T, Harinstain DA, et al. Temporomandibular joint dysfunction syndrome: a close association with systemic joint laxity (the hypermobile joint syndrome). Oral Surg Oral Med Oral Pathol 1991;72:514–519.
13 Barrett AP, Schiffter M. Trigeminal neuralgia. Aust Dent J 1993;38:198–203.

Chapter 26
Neurology

Kieran E. Fallon

This chapter reviews neurologic problems common to sports. Because neural tissue cannot regenerate, neurologic disease or injury has potentially catastrophic outcomes, and a thorough knowledge of them is required for the practicing sports physician.

HEAD INJURY AND CONCUSSION

In the United States alone, 250,000 concussions occur yearly in high school football. Controversy centers around the clinical definition of concussion, but clearly loss of consciousness is not mandatory for the brain to be concussed. A widely accepted description has come from the Committee of Head Injury Nomenclature of the Congress of Neurological Surgeons (1) in which concussion is defined as a clinical syndrome characterized by immediate and transient posttraumatic impairment of neural functions, such as alteration of consciousness, disturbance of vision, equilibrium, and so forth due to brain stem involvement. The three cardinal features of concussion are precipitation by mechanical trauma, transient impairment only of neurologic functioning, and an absence of structural damage.

A second problem involves classification of injury severity. Because of concerns about subtle intracranial hemorrhages masquerading as concussions and well-documented occurrences of catastrophic "second-impact injuries," conservative guidelines for managing concussion were published by the Colorado Medical Society using a clinical grading system (2):

- Grade 1 concussions: "confusion without amnesia, and no loss of consciousness." This is syn-

onymous with what is often referred to as a "bell ringer."
- Grade 2 concussion: "confusion with amnesia, no loss of consciousness."
- Grade 3 concussion: "loss of consciousness" that indicates a potentially serious intracranial injury.

Grade 1 Concussion Grade 1 concussion may be difficult to recognize as the player may be only momentarily stunned and may continue to play without seeking medical attention. Fellow players, the coach, or medical attendants may notice that the player is not playing appropriately. Clinically, this player has impairment of intellectual function and memory, and cannot process commands correctly; these individuals need close follow-up to detect the development of amnesia or postconcussive symptoms. If players remain symptom-free and without neurologic deficits, they can safely return to competition after 20 minutes of observation. A period of observation and repeat neurologic examinations may be the only treatment needed for these mild concussions when they are identified.

Grade 2 Concussion Grade 2 concussions cause a greater degree of neurologic dysfunction and do not clear momentarily. Many athletes may dismiss having their "brain scrambled" as a minor problem, and will not hesitate to return to play, but persistent symptoms of any nature warrant more cautious evaluation than mere sideline observation. A player exhibiting a grade 2 concussion should *not* be allowed to return to play until 1 week after all symptoms resolve, and should become a candidate for imaging studies if symptoms persist.

Grade 3 Concussion Any player recognized as having a grade 3 concussion, defined as loss of consciousness, must be taken from the field no matter how briefly he or she remains unconscious. In the unconscious player, attention to the principles of airway, breathing, and circulation is the first priority; the cervical spine must be stabilized prior to transport from the field. Once an examination to exclude cervical spine injury is performed, neurologic examination and monitoring commences. Grade 3 concussions should always be regarded as potentially severe injuries. In addition to clinical observation, these patients merit neuroradiologic imaging. Athletes should not be allowed to return to activity until 2 weeks after all symptoms resolve.

Postconcussion Observation

The follow-up of more severe concussions involves monitoring symptoms such as headache, dizziness, impaired memory, disorientation, poor concentration, nausea, and vomiting. Signs such as heart rate, blood pressure, level of consciousness, pupillary reactions, eye movements, and other aspects of neurologic functioning, both central and peripheral, must be checked at least every 15 minutes.

Concussion cannot progress to a more serious brain injury, but the early signs of structural brain injury differ little from concussion—a worsening of the patient's clinical condition indicates a search for a more serious lesion. The clinical features of concern that can indicate an increase in intracranial pressure include nausea and vomiting, increasing headache, progressive decrease in level of consciousness, gradual rise in blood pressure, gradual decrease in pulse rate, inequality in pupillary size, and nystagmus.

Should the player be in the care of a relative or friend for a period of observation following medical consultation, he or she should be informed of the following symptoms that need early medical review: increasing drowsiness or difficulty rousing the patient, repeated vomiting, increasing headache, irrational behavior or incoherence, convulsions, and abnormalities of neurologic functioning such as loss of power in a limb, visual disturbance, and so on. More serious concussions and situations in which reliable home care cannot be established merit hospital observation, even when emergent computed tomography (CT) evaluation is normal.

Following a concussion, medications and recreational drugs that may mask important symptoms are to be avoided. These include alcohol, sedatives, and strong analgesics. Heavy mental or physical activity should also be avoided, and athletes should always be medically reviewed prior to return to sport.

Clinical Tests

The best clinical guide to recovery from concussion is the resolution of symptoms that typically follow a blow to the head. These include headache, tiredness, poor concentration, and dizziness or lightheadedness. A more objective measure of recovery involves neuropsychological testing. The digital substitution test (3) is simple to administer and score, and it is recommended that a baseline study be performed on athletes prior to the sporting season in sports involving a high risk of head injury. Postconcussion neuropsychological testing is indicated in cases of concussion featuring loss of consciousness of more than 5 minutes, posttraumatic amnesia longer than 24 hours, posttraumatic convulsion, postconcussion symptoms persisting longer than 2 weeks, repeated concussions, and whenever uncertainty exists regarding full recovery in an athlete returning to sport.

The trend is for early use of neuroradiologic imaging for all grade 3 concussion patients and even for grade 2 concussion patients with worsening or persistent postconcussive symptoms. Unenhanced CT is considered the imaging method of choice for acute head injury (4). The advantages include increased availability, decreased time, and high sensitivity for picking up acute fractures and hemorrhages.

Although CT scans identify most contusions, magnetic resonance imaging (MRI) appears to have better sensitivity for detecting smaller contusions not evident on CT (4). An MRI scan may help to identify persons at risk for a second-impact catastrophe, although long-term clinical studies have not determined the significance of small abnormalities seen on MRI.

Focal Intracranial Pathology

In spite of improvements in helmets in some sports and rule changes to lessen head trauma, intracranial hemorrhage remains a serious cause of death in athletes. In sports such as American football, approximately 20% of players suffer head injuries each season, and deaths continue to occur (1). Between 1945 and 1984, head injuries led to 433 fatalities, most of these among high school athletes.

Prolonged unconsciousness, persistent or worsening mental state alteration, worsening postconcussion symptoms, and abnormalities on neurologic examination are all indications for urgent hospital admission and neurosurgical consultation. These findings should raise doubt about a diagnosis of concussion, as any of several types of intracranial injuries may be involved.

Epidural Hematoma   The epidural hematoma usually follows injury to the middle meningeal artery, which leads to a collection of blood under high pressure between the outermost covering of the brain, the dura mater, and the skull (Fig 26-1). The arterial damage commonly occurs from a frac-

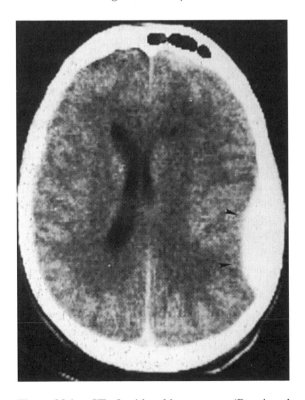

Figure 26-1.   CT of epidural hematoma. (Reprinted from Bloomfield J, Fricker PA, Fitch KD. Science and medicine in sport. 2nd ed. Oxford: Blackwell Science, 1995:320.)

ture of the temporal bone, which crosses the middle meningeal groove. As classically described, the athlete sustains a blow to the head, suffers a brief period of unconsciousness, and recovers rapidly (the lucid interval). After a period that may extend as long as several hours, he or she may develop a severe headache; his or her level of consciousness then rapidly deteriorates such that a comatose condition develops within 30 minutes. If left untreated, the athlete will die, but prompt surgery commonly leads to a normal neurologic outcome.

Subdural Hematoma   The subdural hematoma collects in the space between the dura mater and the arachnoid mater in the subdural space. The origin of the bleeding is often venous; therefore, symptoms may arise slowly, as in the case with the chronic subdural hematoma. The acute subdural hematoma, on the other hand, can have a rapid onset.

Chronic Subdural Hematoma   The chronic subdural hematoma may be seen in the athletic population, but it is more commonly encountered among the elderly who may have experienced a seemingly trivial head injury or among those who have fallen while intoxicated. The bleeding, from low-pressure vessels, collects slowly. Symptoms and signs typically arise 10 to 14 days following injury; initially they may be subtle, and they may progress slowly. The CT scan or MRI is the investigation of choice. Treatment is by surgical evacuation, and full recovery is expected unless underlying cortical injury has occurred.

Acute Subdural Hematoma   An acute hematoma occurs when blood collects in association with a relatively severe brain injury. The clinical course of the acute subdural hematoma can be rapid, and a lucid interval does not occur. The acute subdural hematoma is accompanied by significant mortality, and surgery is required within 12 hours of injury.

Intracerebral Bleeding   Intracerebral bleeding is less common than the previously mentioned lesions and usually accompanies significant brain injury. However, the increased use of MRI scans has revealed minor hemorrhages in a number of patients who had appeared to have sustained mild head injuries. The significance of these small bleeds remains undetermined, but at present they are generally handled in the same fashion as severe concussions, but with a 30-day waiting period before return to sport.

Subarachnoid Hemorrhage   Subarachnoid hemorrhage may occur following head trauma, but this mechanism is relatively infrequent. When this does occur, an AV malformation or other vascular anomaly may be an underlying factor.

Return to Play

One of the most vexing questions related to concussion involves the return of the althlete to play. Table 26-1, for example, may be taken as a general guide for return to contact sports. Different sports and sporting associations have their own specific guidelines. In amateur boxing, for example, various periods of exclusion are based on periods of unresponsiveness to normal stimuli or on the referee's decision to stop the contest after observation of blows delivered to an athlete's head. As a rule, in amateur boxing a boxer who receives a blow to the head and demonstrates a lack of normal responsiveness—whether knocked down or standing—is automatically placed on a 30-day restriction from sparring or competition (5).

Second-Impact Syndrome

Patients still displaying symptoms of concussion must not return to participation in sports. Second-impact syndrome, one of the most important sequelae of head injury, carries a high mortality—

prevention of this syndrome is one of the major aims of the return-to-sport criteria (6). Second-impact syndrome is usually precipitated when a minor head injury occurs in a patient who has residual symptoms following previous head trauma, but it also can occur when a blow to the trunk imparts an accelerative force to the head.

In the typical scenario, an athlete appears to be stunned momentarily, but returns to play in a slightly dazed state. After a short period, the athlete collapses and rapidly becomes comatose, with fixed dilated pupils and total unresponsiveness. Many die before reaching medical attention. This condition carries a mortality rate of 50%, and a morbidity approaching 100%.

The primary defect in second-impact syndrome is dysfunction of vascular autoregulation of the brain. Intracranial vasodilatation and vascular engorgement lead to increased intracranial pressure. Herniation of the uncus of the temporal lobe below the tentorium or of the cerebellar tonsils through the foramen magnum then occurs, leading to compromise of the brain stem. Development of this disorder is dramatic: the period between the injury and the symptoms of brain stem failure, such as respiratory failure and coma, is less than 5 minutes.

To have any hope of success, treatment must be immediate, with rapid intubation and hyperventilation. As soon as intravenous access is estab-

Table 26-1   Guidelines for Return to Football Play After Concussion*

Grade	First Concussion	Second Concussion	Third Concussion
1 (mild)	Return to play if asymptomatic for 1 week	Return to play in 2 weeks if asymptomatic	Terminate season. Return to play next year if asymptomatic
2 (moderate)	Return to play if asymptomatic for 1 week	Consider terminating season. 1 month minimum restriction; then return to play if asymptomatic for 1 week	Terminate season. Return to play next year if asymptomatic
3 (severe)	1 month minimum restriction; then return to play if asymptomatic for 1 week	Terminate season. Return to play next year if asymptomatic	

*Note minor differences from the Colorado Medical Society guidelines.
SOURCE: Cantu RC. Guidelines for return to contact sport after cerebral concussion. Physician Sports Med 1986;14:79.

lished, osmotic diuresis must be induced by agents such as intravenous mannitol. Corticosteroids have also been used, but their efficacy remains unproven. CT or MRI scans are required, and intracranial pressure monitoring should be commenced. Treatment is primarily medical, but decompressive craniotomy or craniectomy may be attempted.

Postconcussion Syndrome

Postconcussion syndrome generally follows a mild injury, and may comprise one or more symptoms. The most common symptoms are headaches, dizziness, tinnitus, diplopia, blurred vision, irritability, anxiety, depression, fatigue, sleep disturbance, poor appetite, poor memory, impaired concentration, and slowed reactions. Diffuse neuronal injury and more specific pathologies such as vestibular damage are thought to underlie these symptoms. The probability of persistence of symptoms and neuropsychological deficits is the same, whether a player is only dazed or has lost consciousness for up to an hour.

Controversy exists regarding the prognostic value of the period of posttraumatic amnesia and the likelihood of persistence of postconcussion symptoms. Electroencephalogram (EEG) findings and auditory brain stem responses have no predictive value, but frontal and temporal lesions found via MRI scan have prognostic value for memory and frontal lobe function deficits (7). Patients who are more mature and have higher levels of employment, education, occupation, and income can be predicted to return to work early; prior head injury, alcohol abuse, and multiple trauma indicate a poorer prognosis (8).

The incidence of postconcussion symptoms is difficult to determine, and many factors affect the estimates. Some reports suggest postconcussion syndrome is a frequent complication, and that 3 months after injury up to 79% of individuals may complain of persistent headaches and up to 60% have problems with memory (8). Neurologic examination is usually normal, but neuropsychological testing may reveal problems with attention, concentration, memory, or judgment. Resolution of symptoms occurs in most patients by 3 to 6 months after injury.

Treatment must be individualized depending on the patient's complaints. Analgesics, nonsteroidal anti-inflammatory drugs (NSAIDs), antidepressants, and muscle relaxants have been used for the muscle-contraction headache that commonly occurs as a component of this syndrome. Education and reassurance regarding the likely favorable outcome are important, as is psychological support and psychotropic medication when needed. Medications, however, primarily treat associated symptoms—the most efficacious method of treatment appears to be time.

Chronic Brain Injury

Boxing   The most serious consequence of repeated head injury is chronic brain damage. Professional boxers are at special risk; thus, chronic progressive traumatic encephalopathy, the most florid form, is termed *dementia pugilistica*. The incidence in professional boxers, which ranges between 9% and 25% (9), correlates with the number of fights and length of the boxing career. Pugilists involved in fewer than 20 to 30 professional bouts rarely exhibit clinical or subclinical evidence of brain injury. Amateur boxers appear at low risk, and studies have found little evidence of even minor psychological impairment in this group.

The spectrum of neurologic dysfunction in dementia pugilistica ranges from subclinical dysfunction demonstrable only on formal neuropsychological testing to full-blown dementia with cerebellar dysfunction and parkinsonian symptoms. Affected boxers are often referred to as being "punch drunk," and have a clinical syndrome that slowly progresses through three stages. Early affective changes and incoordination evolve into major psychiatric manifestations such as paranoid ideation and physical changes of dysarthria and tremor. The third stage is characterized by memory deficits, poor hearing, dysarthria, intention tremor, incoordination, and hyperreflexia along with worsening cortical functions. Progressive dementia coupled with personality changes suggests frontal lobe impairment.

Neuropathologic findings of neurofibrillary tangles in the absence of senile plaques suggest a different etiology from Alzheimer's disease. CT and MRI scans commonly reveal central and cortical atrophy and a cavum septum pellucidum (9). Neuropsychological tests usually demonstrate signs of brain dysfunction. All of these findings are irreversible, so the only effective management strategy is prevention.

Soccer   Evidence for a similar syndrome from heading the ball in soccer has recently caused concern. Thirty percent of former soccer players complain of headache, dizziness, irritability, and impaired memory. In one study, 32% (n = 37) of former players, who had played an average of 359 games, had some EEG abnormality; one-third demonstrated central cerebral atrophy on CT scan; and 81% showed neuropsychological impairment including problems in attention, concentration, memory, and judgment (10). However, despite these anatomic and functional abnormalities, the normal daily activities and social functioning of the former players appeared unaffected.

Prevention of this problem in soccer involves teaching correct heading technique: players should hold the head and neck rigid and immobile at the point of impact, and strengthen their neck muscles. In addition, balls should be coated so as to remain waterproof, and heavier, worn balls should be discarded.

EPILEPSY

Epilepsy is characterized by recurrent seizures, with or without convulsions, that arise from paroxysmal discharges of cortical and subcortical neurons. Approximately 2% of the general population has epilepsy, but up to 10% have had a seizure at least once. A single seizure does not necessarily lead to a diagnosis of epilepsy, but the recurrence rate after a first seizure is about 70%.

Epilepsy typically becomes apparent before the age of 20 and is a common disorder in the young active population. Most cases are idiopathic and are based on a clinical diagnosis; ancillary investigations are useful but not diagnostic. An eyewitness account of the seizure episode is invaluable in aiding diagnosis. The EEG and CT/MRI scan are primary tests, but difficult cases may require continuous video and EEG telemetry.

Table 26-2   Classification of Epileptic Seizures

1. Partial (focal, local) seizures
   A. Simple partial seizures
   B. Complex partial seizures (associated with alteration of consciousness)
   C. Partial seizures evolving to secondary generalized seizures
2. Generalized seizures
   A. Absence seizures
   B. Myoclonic seizures
   C. Clonic seizures
   D. Tonic seizures
   E. Tonic-clonic seizures
   F. Atonic seizures
3. Unclassified epileptic seizures

Classification

Classification of epilepsy is based on the characteristics of the seizure and depends on whether the seizure is focal or generalized and whether consciousness is lost (a complex seizure) (Table 26-2).

Partial Seizures   Simple partial seizures (focal/local epilepsy) cause no loss of consciousness, but jerking or twitching of a limb, disturbance of sensation with an unusual smell or visual distortion, or psychological symptoms may occur. The motor disturbance can spread from the primary area to ipsilateral body parts, a phenomenon known as the Jacksonian march. Complex partial seizures impair consciousness, either at onset of the seizure or following a simple partial seizure pattern. When partial seizures evolve into secondary generalized seizures, they are more often associated with structural brain lesions. MRI is the imaging modality of choice in the detection of these lesions.

Generalized Seizures   Generalized seizures have a number of subtypes. The differential diagnoses include migraine, fainting (vasovagal attacks) transient ischemic attacks, cardiogenic problems such as arrhythmias, and hysterical behavior. In the majority of cases no cause for epileptic seizures emerges, but head injury, birth trauma, tumors, stroke, toxic exposures, and infection all cause seizures in specific cases. Trigger factors that precipitate attacks include cessation of medication, fatigue, sleep deprivation, alcohol, illicit drugs, stress, hyperventilation, and photic stimuli.

Tonic-Clonic Seizures   Tonic-clonic are the most common generalized seizure. Structural brain lesions are rarely present, but genetic predisposition is a risk factor. These episodes occur without warning: the patient falls to the ground in the tonic phase, which is characterized by spasm of the limbs. This phase lasts about 10 seconds, after which a clonic phase of rhythmic jerking of the limbs occurs for 1 to 2 minutes or longer. A few minutes following the latter phase, the patient wakes. After a seizure, the patient may complain of postictal drowsiness, headache, and confusion, and may not feel completely normal for a number of days. Urinary and fecal incontinence may occur during seizures, and postictal paralysis (Todd's paresis) can last for variable periods.

Absence Seizure   The absence seizure generally occurs in children. Pathognomic features are sudden, momentary interruption of conscious activity, with or without spontaneous motor discharges such as myoclonic jerks of the upper limb. The patient typically stops in midactivity or sentence, stares blankly, and, after a few seconds, resumes activity without awareness of his or her seizure.

Status Epilepticus   Status epilepticus refers to prolonged or repetitive seizures without a period of recovery. This condition constitutes a medical emergency as prolonged tonic-clonic seizures can lead to respiratory collapse. There are no reports of status epilepticus triggered by exercise.

Management

Principles of epilepsy management include patient education on appropriate occupational, recreational, and sporting activities, avoidance of trigger factors, pharmacologic treatment, and, rarely, surgery. Pharmacologic agents successfully control recurrences of seizures, and monotherapy is desirable when efficacious. In general, the focal epilepsies are more difficult to treat; among the medications utilized are carbamazepine, phenytoin, sodium valproate, or the newer agent vigabatrin. Carbamazepine is the current drug of choice. Treatment of primary generalized seizures usually involves the use of sodium valproate, ethosuximide, phenytoin, clonazepam, or lamotrigine; sodium valproate is the currently preferred drug. Acute status epilepticus requires intravenous, or (less preferably) rec-

tal diazepam, clonazepam, midazolam, or paraldehyde to obtain rapid response.

The pharmacokinetics of anticonvulsant medication are not altered by regular exercise, but the side effects of these medications—particularly nystagmus, dysarthria, ataxia, confusion, drowsiness, and nausea—can affect sporting performance. Tolerance to the side effects can be effected by starting with low doses then gradually increasing the drug until stable therapeutic levels are achieved.

Associated with the use of these medications are the problems of compliance and regular monitoring of drug levels. Biochemical and hematologic parameters (in particular liver function tests) are checked at the initiation of treatment and when toxicity is suspected. In young females, an interaction between oral contraceptive pills and antiepileptic medications, particularly carbamazapine and phenytoin, decreases efficacy of the oral contraceptives. Specific restrictions regarding use in pregnancy exist because of the teratogenicity of antiepileptic agents.

As the risk of a second seizure is 70% to 80% in an adult who has had a single, unequivocal generalized seizure unaccompanied by precipitating factors, empirical treatment seems reasonable. A consultant neurologist can help with the decision to treat or not treat an isolated seizure.

Involvement of the Epileptic in Sports

In the past, physicians placed undue restrictions on sports participation by those affected by epilepsy. Epilepsy has no apparent effects on physiologic performance (except in the postictal phase). Medication side effects can hinder performance through their effects on higher motor functions such as coordination, but with careful medication choice, epileptics can safely perform the majority of sports. At minimum, these patients should maintain optimal fitness.

Maintenance of a regular exercise program improved seizure control in some studies (11). There is some evidence that the incidence of seizure during exercise declines, possibly because of endorphin release (12), although the cool-down period has a higher than normal risk. Overall, the sports accident risk for children with seizures appears unchanged. If sports worsen trigger factors—such as fatigue, sleep deprivation, physical and psychological stress, hyperventilation, hypoxia, hyperhydration, and subsequent hyponatremia, hyperthermia, and hypoglycemia—then potentially the seizure threshold could be lowered.

No firm guidelines exclude epileptic patients from any sport. Poorly controlled epileptics do have a higher risk of injury during sport, but their chances of drowning, falling, or suffering a worsening of epilepsy during exercise remain low. Common sense dictates that participation in high-risk sports such as aviation, skydiving, boxing, and scuba diving is contraindicated in those with regular seizures. In other situations, individual decisions require a coordinated assessment by the doctor and patient of the potential benefits and risks.

Assuming that the athlete has a genuine interest in competing, has no progressive neurologic disease, has a normal neurologic examination, takes all medications, and maintains therapeutic blood levels of his or her anticonvulsant, participation in collision or contact sports is not contraindicated. Participation in sports such as boxing and martial arts where heavy blows to the head may be encountered is not advisable, but no current evidence suggests that repetitive minor head traumas, such as heading the ball in soccer, have a detrimental effect on seizure frequency or control. Thus, sports such as rugby, soccer, and American football are allowed, except in those individuals with a clear history of recurrent seizures precipitated by head trauma.

For those with regular seizures, close supervision is mandatory during any involvement in aquatic sports such as swimming and diving. The relative risk of drowning is approximately four times greater for the epileptic, probably secondary to poor seizure control, noncompliance with medication, and lack of supervision.

Generally, participation in motor sports is subject to the attaining of a driver's license, and the regulations pertaining to this vary from country to country. Certification to use public roads can be seen as a reasonable clearance for motor sport.

When questions arise about the appropriateness of sports participation, rather than offer blanket advice or undue restrictions, the physician should consult with experts in the management of epilepsy, consider the liberalized sport recommendations, and carefully counsel the athlete.

HEADACHE IN SPORT

Sport-related headache is a complex diagnostic issue because considerable confusion exists regarding classification, variability in presentation, and features that would be consistent with migraine. A number of varieties of headache associated with exercise but without head trauma have been described. These headaches often display overlapping features.

Intrathoracic/Intracranial Pressure Headache

Headaches related to brief periods of activity during which an increase in intrathoracic and intracranial pressure occurs are typically seen in sports that involve Valsalva maneuvers, such as weightlifting. Such headaches may also occur in relation to coughing, sneezing, straining, bending forward, and sexual orgasm. The onset is rapid, with the peak of pain at the onset of or very early in the headache. The pain is often initially severe and is usually bilateral, but the distribution, although consistent in one individual, is variable in general. Severe pain lasts only a few minutes and may fade to a dull ache lasting up to 24 hours. There are no associated neurologic symptoms.

Physical examination findings are characteristically normal. As up to 5% of such patients may have organic disease at the base of the brain such as platybasia or basilar impression, investigation with CT or MRI scanning is appropriate (13). Should the results of the investigations prove normal, physical activity is not contraindicated.

Treatment of the athlete includes modification of activity to whatever degree is practical. Indomethacin, 25–50 mg with food three times a day, is effective, as is moderate dosage of other NSAIDs.

Vascular Headache

Vascular headaches after prolonged low-intensity exercise have been called "benign exertional headache," "effort headache," and "prolonged exertional headache." Long-distance running often precipitates this type of pain, which is variable in character and similar to exercise-related migraine, but less intense. The pain is often generalized or frontal and is rarely unilateral. Nausea, visual disturbance, and other neurologic symptoms mimic the pattern of typical migraine headache. These features suggests that physiologic changes may lie on the tension-vascular/common migraine/migraine continuum. Poor conditioning plays a role, but well-trained athletes may experience these at high altitudes. Dehydration, heat stress, hypoglycemia, and caffeine use are risk factors, as is a past history of tension-vascular headache.

The results of physical examination of these patients are usually normal, but transient neurologic deficits may be found. Attention to training and warmup, and avoidance of dehydration and excessive heat are important in prevention. NSAIDs are the standard treatment.

Acute Effort Migraine

The acute effort migraine is precipitated by short periods of vigorous activity such as sprinting. It has been described following such sports as netball, hockey, cycling, swimming, and weightlifting. It is commonly unilateral, severe, usually preceded by an aura, and accompanied by nausea and often vomiting and neck stiffness. Acute effort migraines typically are throbbing or pounding in character, and recovery may require hours or even a full night's sleep. A past or family history of migraine is often present. Treatment of the acute attack may include ergotamine preparations, oral or injected sumatriptan, analgesics, and antinauseants.

Weightlifter's Headache

"Weightlifter's headache" is thought to be caused by referred pain from ligaments and muscles in the neck. It is typically occipital, severe, and prolonged and responds to analgesics, anti-inflammatory medication, massage, and physiotherapy techniques.

Altitude Headache

Headache associated with exercise at high altitudes typically occurs at greater than 2500 m among those not acclimatized and is a component of acute mountain sickness. The onset may occur as early as 6 hours following initial exposure, and the headache is throbbing in nature, generalized, and improves over a few days if the altitude is not increased. More severe headache occurs as a component of high-altitude cerebral edema. Prevention is possible by gradual ascent and use of prophylactic acetazolamide. Descent is the most obvious form of treatment.

Walk Headache

"Walk headache" is uncommon but has been described as a manifestation of ischemic heart disease. The onset is related to exertion, and it is relieved by rest and antianginal medications.

Diver's Headache

Scuba divers suffer various types of headaches that are related to a multitude of factors, including excessive gripping of the mouthpiece, sinus barotrauma, and tight goggles. Headache related to external compression of the scalp may also occur following the wearing of tight headbands, masks, and helmets.

Intracranial Hemorrhage

The most common atraumatic cause of an intracranial bleed in the athletic population is subarachnoid hemorrhage, the majority of which are due to aneurysms. It is rarely a cause of death in athletes, it but may leave the patient with significant disability. The precipitating factor during sporting activity is an acute elevation of blood pressure, often associated with the Valsalva maneuver.

The classic presentation is one of explosive headache ("the worst headache I've ever had"), neck stiffness, photophobia, and collapse. Occasionally, however, the headache is quite mild. The athlete may simply be confused or, alternatively, may be found unconscious.

The CT scan is the investigation of choice, and in early cases the increased density characteristic of fresh blood may be seen in the basal cisterns or lateral ventricles. On diagnosis of the lesion, the site and anatomy of the aneurysm should be ascertained, usually by angiography. Surgical management of the aneurysm is commonly required.

Headache Originating in the Cervical Spine

Pain originating from the cervical spine is not necessarily felt in the neck: it may present as a headache that is usually suboccipital and unilateral, but at times bilateral. The upper three cervical nerve roots converge with cells in the spinal cord that are associated with trigeminal fibers, and this connection explains the distribution of head pain. The cervical headache may radiate to the temporal and frontal areas and can be felt behind the eyes. Usually of mild to moderate severity, the headache is most often described as nagging. Associated factors are a history of pain on wakening, headache pain that endures several hours to days, and previous neck injury. Neck movements, particularly prolonged extension, aggravate the pain; neck stiffness and a grating sensation are common. Relief is obtained by heat, massage, and physiotherapy treatment.

Common Types of Headache

Three additional varieties of headache that not specifically related to sport are prevalent in the general population, and thus apply to the sporting community as well: migraine, tension, and cluster headaches.

Migraine Migraine is a common type of headache that is found in sports people and may not necessarily be related to exertion. A full discussion can be found in general medical texts.

- **Common Migraine** Common migraine is the most common variety. It has no aura and is usually a unilateral, pulsatile headache of moderate to severe intensity that can last all day. It is made worse by physical activity and is associated with photophobia, sonophobia, nausea, and perhaps vomiting.
- **Classic Migraine** Classical migraine typically commences with a visual or sensory disturbance that evolves to a headache of the common migraine type.

Treatment of attacks follows basic principles, and prophylaxis is emphasized to prevent acute episodes. The medications used for prophylaxis—beta-blockers, NSAIDs, antidepressants, and cal-cium channel blockers—may have detrimental effects on sporting performance; therefore, selection of these agents requires awareness of the demands of individual sports. Beta-blockers are banned by the International Olympic Committee under regulations regarding doping in sport.

Tension Headache Otherwise known as muscle contraction headache, tension headache can last from a few hours to weeks or months. It is often related to psychosocial stress, may often be of a mild, transient nature, and may be triggered by such factors as bright sunlight, squinting, and head trauma. Classically, a dull pressure like pain develops that is relatively constant and nonthrobbing. Commonly bifrontal and felt "behind the eyes," it could also be felt in other areas of the head and may be global. Exertion worsens symptoms and can lead to a migraine-type headache. Treatment most commonly involves use of simple analgesics and correction or avoidance of precipitating factors and underlying causes.

Cluster Headache Cluster headaches, which are thought to be vascular in origin, may follow head trauma but are relatively uncommon in that setting. The cluster is a series of headaches that generally occur over one or more weeks, with longer periods of remission. The headaches last 15 minutes to 2 to 3 hours, and may occur up to 10 times a day. They are unilateral, severe, and center around or behind the eye. Associated ipsilateral symptoms and findings include partial Horner's syndrome, facial sweating, conjunctival injection, lacrimation, and nasal congestion. Effective treatments for the acute attack include inhalation of 100% oxygen for up to 15 minutes and sumatriptan 6 mg subcutaneously. The most commonly used prophylactic drugs are prednisone, lithium, methysergide, ergotamine, and verapamil.

Posttraumatic Headache

Seven varieties of posttraumatic headache have been described:

1. **Chronic muscle contraction headache.** Identical to the tension headache previously discussed, chronic muscle contraction headaches can be a component of the postconcussion syndrome.

2. **Tension-vascular headache.** This headache shares features of both muscle contraction headache and migraine.
3. **Migraine.** "Footballer's migraine" is caused by heading the ball in soccer, and can also occur following blows to the head in boxing or other sports. Visual disturbances, motor and sensory symptoms, and severe headache are associated with nausea, and the headache is essentially the same as other migraines. A family history of migraine is commonly present, and prophylactic medication has very limited success. Similar cases have been described in boxers and wrestlers following head trauma.
4. **Dysautonomic cephalgia.** This condition is infrequently mentioned in the literature and is thought to be related to damage to cervical sympathetic nerve fibers in the anterior triangle of the neck at the time of head injury. The headache occurs up to months after the injury and is severe, unilateral, and frontotemporal in distribution. Accompanying features include ipsilateral pupillary dilatation, increased sweating on the face, blurred vision, photophobia, and nausea. A beta-blocker is the treatment of choice (IOC regulated).
5. **Headache associated with intracranial bleeding.** Headache often accompanies intracranial hemorrhage. The epidural, acute, and chronic subdural and intracerebral hematomas are discussed in the section on head injury and concussion.
6. **Second-impact catastrophic headache.** See the discussion of second-impact syndrome in the section on head injury and concussion.
7. **Head pain associated with local nerve entrapment.** These headaches are typically localized to a specific site of previous head trauma and are thought to arise from local nerve entrapment, consequent upon fibrosis and scarring as a component of the repair process.

NERVE ENTRAPMENTS OF THE LOWER LIMB

Nerve entrapments are common in the athletic population and easily recognized when symptoms are classic. However, they may stimulate variable and unusual symptoms that initially defy diagnosis. Nerve conduction studies and electromyography along with the response of symptoms to local anesthetic block at the potential site of compression help make the diagnosis. Management of many of these entrapments involves biomechanical correction, excision of space-occupying lesions, or excision of other structures impinging on neural tissue.

Interdigital Nerve

Compression of the interdigital nerves that supply sensation to the toes is relatively common. These nerves run over or against the deep transverse tarsal ligament that binds the metatarsal heads together, and compression is often associated with a Morton's neuroma, which classically occurs in the 3-4 interdigital space. The nerve angulates with the toes in hyperextension. The factors associated with compression include claw toe, high-heeled shoes, hallux valgus, abnormalities of foot posture, phalangeal fracture, a short gastrocnemius–soleus complex, and leg length inequality.

Interdigital nerve compression is a common condition in runners, and distal metatarsal pain with episodic lancinating pain into the toes occurs often in conjunction with dull throbbing pain when walking. Pain may radiate up the sciatic distribution. Palpation of the nerve as it passes across the deep transverse ligament with passive hyperextension of the toes reproduces the pain, and maximum tenderness is found between the metatarsal heads. Pain also occurs with compression of the transverse arch. There may be loss of sensation of the web space between the toes supplied by the nerve.

Treatment involves improvement of plantar flexion at the metatarsophalangeal joints, use of a metatarsal bar or pad, and correction of excessive pronation. If conservative measures fail, excision of the neuroma may be indicated.

Plantar Nerves

The plantar nerves are formed by the division of the posterior tibial nerve. In the tarsal tunnel the posterior tibial nerve splits into the medial and lateral plantar nerves and the calcaneal nerve. The plantar nerves pass through two openings in the medial superior origin of the abductor hallucis muscle at the calcaneus, and this is the common site of compression. If the heel is symptomatically involved, the site of compression is likely to be more proximal.

Hyperpronation and application of a heavy force to the dorsum of the foot are causative factors, and the usual presenting symptom is a burning pain in the plantar surface of the foot and toes. This is accompanied by loss of power of the intrinsic muscles of the foot, particularly in flexion, abduction, and adduction. These changes are most marked at the metatarsophalangeal joints. Sensory changes are found mainly on the sole of the foot. Marked tenderness is found at the site of compression, where continued pressure typically reproduces the symptoms.

First Branch of the Lateral Plantar Nerve

Compression of the first branch of the lateral plantar nerve, the nerve to the abductor digiti quinti, is a cause of chronic heel pain in athletes. It occurs most commonly in runners, but it can also occur in soccer, dance, tennis, and track and field athletes. Entrapment occurs between the deep fascia of the abductor halluces and the medial head of quadratus plantar.

On examination, the typical finding is tenderness over the nerve deep to the abductor hallucis muscle. Local muscle hypertrophy may be a factor in this condition; however, the most commonly associated biomechanical abnormality is hyperpronation. Rest and attention to biomechanical factors are often helpful. As with all nerve compression or entrapment problems, surgery may be useful in resistant cases.

Posterior Tibial Nerve (Tarsal Tunnel Syndrome)

The posterior tibial nerve runs behind and below the medial malleolus, accompanied by the tendons of tibialis posterior, flexor digitorum longus, and flexor hallucis longus. The lancinate ligament forms the roof of the tunnel and the posterior tibial nerve divides distal to this ligament (Fig 26-2).

Tarsal tunnel syndrome—compression of the posterior tibial nerve—can occur following local fracture or dislocation, or may be related to inflammatory edema consequent upon tendon pathology. Hyperpronation and local-space–occupying lesions such as lipomas, cysts, and varicose veins may be causative, but this condition is often idiopathic. It is not uncommon in runners, ballet dancers, and basketball players.

Diagnosis is made following complaints of burning pain in the toes, on the sole of the foot, and perhaps in the heel, often commencing at the medial malleolus. Retrograde referral may occur, and pain can be reproduced if pressure is applied at the tarsal tunnel or if a valgus stress is placed on the calcaneus. Treatment involves correction of underlying pathology, and perhaps decompression.

Deep Peroneal Nerve

The deep peroneal nerve supplies the skin of the cleft between the first and second toes; entrapment occurs on the dorsum of the foot or ankle as the nerve passes deep to the inferior extensor retinaculum. Potential etiologic factors are dorsal trauma over the tarsal bones, tight shoes, ankle sprains, and situps with the feet held under a bar. Runners, skiers, soccer players, and dancers are most commonly affected.

Pain is felt in the first toe accompanied by aching midfoot discomfort and dorsal foot pain. Careful examination reveals localized sensory loss. Weakness of toe extension, best demonstrated by extension with the ankle in full dorsiflexion, may be found.

Superficial Peroneal Nerve

The superficial peroneal nerve is a branch of the common peroneal nerve, and it arises at the neck of the fibula. It runs in association with peroneus longus and brevis, and its two branches innervate the distal, lateral part of the leg, dorsum of the foot, and dorsum of the first four toes (Fig 26-3). The opening where it pierces the deep fascia is the site of entrapment. There is no motor involvement, thus pain and altered sensation are the only symptoms.

Superficial peroneal nerve injury is most common in runners, but is also seen in soccer, hockey, and tennis players, body builders, and dancers.

Tibial Nerve

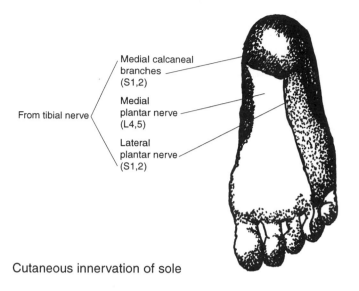

From tibial nerve

Medial calcaneal
branches
(S1,2)

Medial
plantar nerve
(L4,5)

Lateral
plantar nerve
(S1,2)

Cutaneous innervation of sole

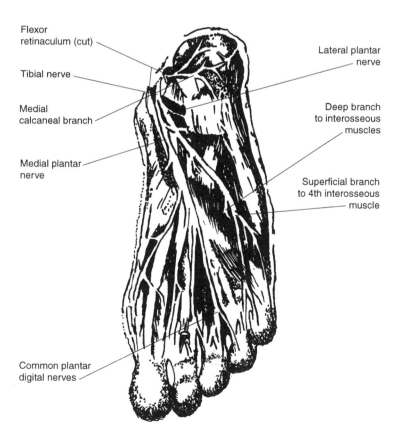

Flexor
retinaculum (cut)

Tibial nerve

Medial
calcaneal branch

Medial plantar
nerve

Lateral plantar
nerve

Deep branch
to interosseous
muscles

Superficial branch
to 4th interosseous
muscle

Common plantar
digital nerves

Branches of the Posterior Tibial Nerve

Figure 26-2. Anatomical location of the tibial nerves.

Common Peroneal Nerve and Branches

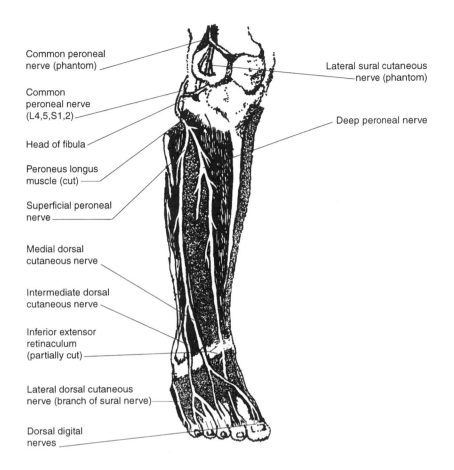

Common peroneal nerve (phantom)

Common peroneal nerve (L4,5,S1,2)

Head of fibula

Peroneus longus muscle (cut)

Superficial peroneal nerve

Medial dorsal cutaneous nerve

Intermediate dorsal cutaneous nerve

Inferior extensor retinaculum (partially cut)

Lateral dorsal cutaneous nerve (branch of sural nerve)

Dorsal digital nerves

Lateral sural cutaneous nerve (phantom)

Deep peroneal nerve

Cutaneous innervation

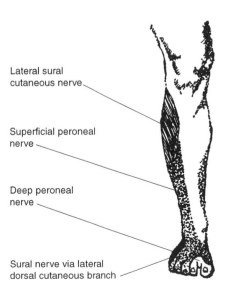

Lateral sural cutaneous nerve

Superficial peroneal nerve

Deep peroneal nerve

Sural nerve via lateral dorsal cutaneous branch

Figure 26-3. Anatomical location of the peroneal nerve.

The mechanism of injury involves forced plantar flexion, inversion, or a combination of these, direct trauma, or tight boots. The patient complains of burning, superficial pain associated with increased or decreased sensation in the above-mentioned distribution. The symptoms are exacerbated by local pressure or by activity.

Use of a lateral sole wedge to increase eversion, relaxing the fascia on the lateral aspect of the leg, may be helpful. If conservative measures fail, surgery is curative.

Common Peroneal Nerve

Entrapment of the common peroneal nerve occurs at the neck of the fibula at the sharp fibrous edge of the peroneus longus origin. Injury is characterized by pain in the lateral aspect of the leg and foot, induced by running. Sensory changes and motor weakness, particularly weakness of eversion of the foot and dorsiflexion of the ankle and toes, result.

Common causes of this injury include direct trauma from a tight plaster or a direct blow; it may also occur in association with a spiral fracture of the fibula, injury to the lateral collateral ligament of the knee, or inversion-plantar flexion forces at the ankle. Relief of external pressure, rest, and time often lead to resolution. Occasionally, surgery is required.

Obturator Nerve

The obturator nerve arises from the second, third, and fourth lumbar nerve roots, and it is vulnerable to compression at the obturator canal/obturator membrane. This nerve passes through the obturator canal, a hole in the obturator membrane close to the pubic bone, and it then innervates the skin of the medial thigh. Pain in the medial aspect of the thigh and weakness of adduction are the characteristic clinical features. Increased intra-abdominal pressure or hip motion increases pain, but the clinical examination at rest is often normal.

Compression may arise as a complication of surgery, local edema in osteitis pubis, and obturator hernia, and is occasionally seen as a consequence of athletic activity. The diagnosis is made on electromyogram (EMG) or nerve conduction findings and can be confirmed by fluoroscopically controlled injection of the nerve at the obturator fora-

men using local anesthetic. Conservative treatment options include massage, stretches, neuromeningeal stretches, and corticosteroid injection. Failure of these warrants surgical decompression at the level of the obturator foramen (14).

Ilio-Inguinal Nerve

The ilio-inguinal nerve arises from the first and second lumbar nerve roots, traverses the abdominal muscles to terminate in the spermatic cord or round ligament, and is most vulnerable to compression at the anterior superior iliac spine. The most frequent mechanism of injury involves sudden tension of abdominal muscles and pain in the groin. Radiation to the inner aspect of the thigh, aggravated by increasing tension in the abdominal wall is the usual symptom. Tenderness medial to the anterior superior iliac spine is often present (15). Nerve conduction studies and local anesthetic nerve-block may be useful diagnostic procedures, and treatment is initially conservative.

Lateral Femoral Cutaneous Nerve

Compression of the lateral femoral cutaneous nerve of the thigh, a condition also known as meralgia paresthetica, is most likely to occur at the anterior superior iliac spine (Fig 26-4). Arising from the second and third lumbar nerve roots, this nerve runs around and down the pelvis on the iliacus, then forward to the lateral end of the inguinal ligament and through the inguinal ligament at the anterior superior iliac spine. Compression may occur as a result of direct trauma, and is associated with tight clothing, obesity, hip adduction (as with a short limb), or crossing of the thighs. Burning pain and paresthesia develop over the anterior and lateral aspects of the thigh. Gymnasts are the most commonly affected athletes. Correction of the above-mentioned factors may effect a cure, but surgery may be required.

Piriformis Syndrome

In piriformis syndrome the sciatic nerve is compressed beneath or within a tight or damaged piriformis muscle (Fig 26-5). Numbness, paresthesia, and pain are felt in the posterior thigh and buttock, and occur in the absence of lower back pain. Active or resisted external rotation increases the symptoms, as does forced passive internal rota-

Lateral Femoral Cutaneous Nerve

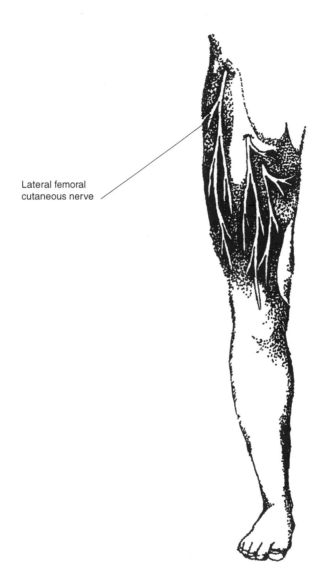

Lateral femoral
cutaneous nerve

Figure 26-4.   Distribution of the lateral femoral cutaneous nerve.

tion (Freiberg's sign), but there are usually no specific sensory or motor findings unless the compression has been severe and of long duration. Three clinical signs may be present:

1. Visible fasciculation in the hamstring muscle with direct compression of the sciatic nerve at the level of the piriformis.
2. Weakness of ankle eversion.

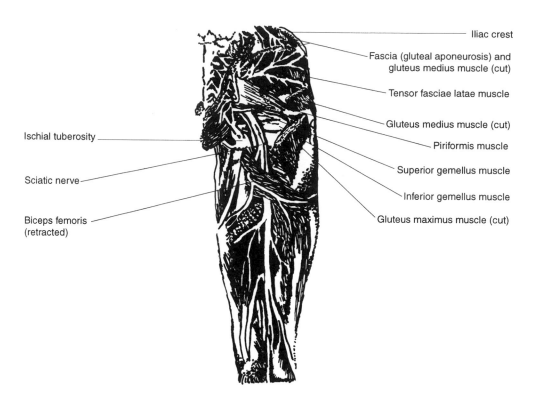

Figure 26-5.   Position and entrapment of sciatic nerve under the piriformis muscle.

3. Reproduction of symptoms with straight leg raising and passive internal rotation of the hip (16).

On biomechanical assessment, lumbosacral muscle tightness and restricted hip external rotation are commonly found. Treatment involves anti-inflammatory medication, alteration of activity, massage, piriformis stretches, and strengthening hip rotators. Injection with corticosteroid may be tried with variable results.

NERVE ENTRAPMENTS OF THE UPPER LIMB

Suprascapular Nerve

The suprascapular nerve is derived from the upper trunk of the brachial plexus, which is formed by the roots of cervical vertebrae C5 and C6. It passes under the trapezius to the suprascapular notch and supplies branches to the supraspinatus muscle and the glenohumeral and acromioclavicular joints. The nerve then passes though the spinoglenoid notch to innervate the infraspinatus muscle.

The notches are potential sites of compression. Extremes of shoulder motion, particularly horizontal adduction such as may occur in the follow-through phase of a throw, are important in the etiology. Deep, poorly localized pain is the most common feature, and weakness of abduction and external rotation accompanied by wasting of supraspinatus and infraspinatus is found. The EMG can be positive, and surgical decompression is often required.

Median Nerve

The median nerve originates from the brachial plexus formed by fibers from the sixth, seventh, and eighth cervical and first thoracic nerve roots. At the anterior aspect of the elbow, the median nerve travels under the lacertus fibrosis or bicipital aponeurosis, which expands to blend with the antebrachial fascia covering the superior anterior forearm muscle group. The nerve then passes through the two heads of the pronator teres and gives off a branch to flexor carpi radialis. At the distal margin of the pronator passage, 5 to 8 cm distal to the lateral epicondyle, the anterior interosseous nerve arises.

At the wrist, the median nerve passes through the osteofibrous carpal tunnel, which is bordered by the transverse carpal ligaments superiorly, the pisiform and hamate bones medially, and the scaphoid and trapezium bones laterally. The lunate, capitate, and trapezoid bones form the deep aspect of the tunnel.

Median Nerve Compression at the Elbow
There are four potential sites of compression at or near the elbow:

1. The most proximal and least common site of compression is the ligament of Struthers, a fibrous band running from a supracondylar process, 5 to 7 cm proximal to the medial epicondyle, to the medial epicondyle. The brachial artery travels under this ligament when present, and thus may also be compressed, leading to forearm claudication.
2. The lacertus fibrosis—the bicipital aponeurosis as it spans the flexor muscles of the forearm—may be a site of compression.
3. The most common site is at pronator teres where the median nerve passes between the deep and superficial heads of this muscle.
4. Compression may also occur at the proximal margin of flexor digitorum superficialis (Fig 26-6).

Clinical features include pain in the proximal volar aspect of the forearm usually of insidious onset. Activity exacerbates the pain (particularly repetitive forearm pronation and wrist flexion) and prompts fatigue of wrist flexion and of the thenar intrinsic muscles of the hand. Numbness and paresthesia occur in part or all of the median nerve distribution in the hand (radial 3.5 digits). It is most commonly seen in throwing or racket sports, weightlifting, and gymnastics.

Provocative tests may help in differentiation of the site of compression. If the following sites are involved, the resisted movements shown may lead to the onset of symptoms:

1. At pronator teres, resisted pronation of forearm/flexion of wrist.
2. At lacertus fibrosis, resisted supination of forearm/elbow flexion.
3. At flexor digitorum superficialis, resisted flexion of middle finger.

Investigation with EMG or nerve conduction studies is usually normal.

Treatment modalities include rest, muscle stretching, alteration of technique or occupational activities, splinting, NSAIDs, and, in resistant cases, decompression surgery.

Anterior Interosseous Syndrome The anterior interosseous nerve is susceptible to compression by fibrous bands from the deep head of the pronator teres or flexor digitorum superficialis, aberrant or anomalous vessels, anomalous muscles, or following aggressive forearm exercise. The clinical findings include proximal forearm pain that is increased by activity; weakness of flexor pollicis longus, pronator quadratus, and flexor digitorum profundus to the second and third digit; and an abnormal pinch attitude with inability to form typical "OK" sign due to flexion weakness of the distal thumb and finger joints. There is an absence of sensory symptoms or sensory loss. Treatment is essentially the same as that for median nerve compression.

Carpal Tunnel Syndrome Carpal tunnel syndrome is a compression neuropathy of the median nerve at the wrist. Associated conditions include overuse tenosynovitis and tenosynovitis associated with rheumatoid arthritis, intrinsic or extrinsic pressure, and the metabolic or vascular consequences of diabetes, pregnancy, and excessive weight. Carpal tunnel syndrome is common in wheelchair athletes but rare in other athletes. Occasional cases appear among cyclists, pitchers and throwers, and tennis players.

Symptoms and signs include wrist or hand pain; occasional proximal radiation to the forearm, elbow, shoulder, and neck; and sensory abnor-

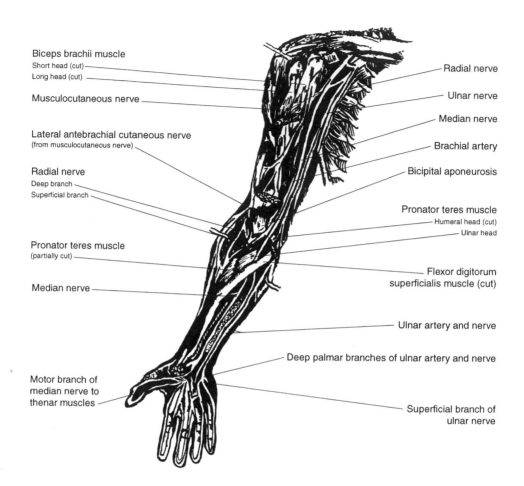

Figure 26-6. Nerves of the upper extremity.

malities, particularly numbness and paresthesia in the radial 3.5 digits, sparing the thenar eminence. Pain, numbness, and paresthesia are frequently worse at night. Tinel's and Phalen's signs are often positive, and motor deficits including weakness and clumsiness are variable. In relation to strength deficits, weakness of the abductor pollicis brevis is the most common finding. The sensitivity of nerve conduction studies is approximately 85% to 90%.

Treatment modalities include rest, immobilization, splints, anti-inflammatory modalities, NSAIDs, local injection of corticosteroid, physiotherapy, stretching techniques, and biomechanical modification where appropriate. Surgical intervention is occasionally warranted.

Ulnar Nerve

The ulnar nerve is derived from the eighth cervical and first thoracic nerve roots and is a terminal branch of the medial cord of the brachial plexus. At the elbow the ulnar nerve passes posterior to the medial epicondyle in the posterior condylar groove. The cubital tunnel begins just distal to the posterior condylar groove. The ulnar nerve later passes under the aponeurotic arch between the two heads of the flexor carpi ulnaris.

At the wrist, the ulnar nerve and artery enter an osteofibrous canal termed the canal of Guyon. This canal is a groove between the pisiform and the hook of the hamate. Distal to the canal, the deep branch, which is exclusively motor, innervates the three hypothenar muscles, the abductor digiti quinti, the flexor digiti quinti, and the opponens digiti quinti, all the palmar and dorsal interossei, the two medial lumbricals, the adductor pollicis, and the deep head of the flexor pollicis brevis.

Cubital Tunnel Syndrome Within the cubital tunnel compression can occur at several distinct sites. Commonly the ulnar nerve is compressed proximally under the arcuate ligament or flexor carpi ulnaris. The ulnar nerve is prone to tension overload at the elbow such as may occur in a thrower with laxity of the medial ligamentous structures of the elbow. A narrowed posterior condylar groove or poorly developed soft tissue constraints can lead to nerve subluxation anterior to the medial epicondyle. Extreme flexion and extension of the elbow, such as may occur during pitching a baseball or serving a tennis ball, may lead to hypermobility of the nerve, subluxation, or frank dislocation. Repetitive motions can lead to fibrosis or traction spurring, which either further narrows the groove or tethers the nerve in the groove making it prone to traction neuritis. Compression of the ulnar nerve has been described in association with hypertrophy of the medial head of the triceps and anconeus such as may occur in expert pitchers and weightlifters (17).

The usual clinical presentation of ulnar neuropathy of the elbow is aching pain in the medial elbow, sometimes radiating to the hand, and sensory disturbance including numbness, paresthesia, or dysesthesia over the hypothenar eminence, dorsoulnar hand, fifth digit, and ulnar half of the fourth digit. A positive Tinel's sign is frequently present over the ulnar nerve at the elbow. Weakness if present is usually mild or occurs late in the course, but clumsiness in the hand and fingers may be an early symptom. Provocative tests include ulnar nerve subluxation by rapid extension and flexion of the elbow, manual subluxation of the nerve, and a positive elbow flexion test holding the elbow fully flexed for up to 5 minutes.

Ulnar Tunnel Syndrome Most ulnar nerve injuries at the wrist are due to compressive force. Handlebar palsy is common in bicyclists and is caused by weight bearing on a dorsiflexed wrist with subsequent compression of the nerve in the canal of Guyon. Other etiologic factors include ulnar artery thrombosis by direct trauma, ganglions related to carpal joints, hamate fractures, or fibrotic arches in the palm. Ulnar nerve compression of the wrist may present with pure motor, pure sensory, or mixed findings; the classifications are listed as follows:

- Type I, a combined motor and sensory loss, is the most common variant. All the ulnar innervated hand muscles are weak. In addition, there is sensory loss over the ulnar area of the palm (hypothenar eminence) and the ring and little fingers.
- Type II is solely motor loss. This implies pressure injury of the deep motor branch only with sparing of the superficial sensory branch.
- Type III manifests only sensory changes. Hypesthesia is noted over the hypothenar eminence and volar ring and little fingers. There is no muscle weakness.

Compression may be progressive or acute. In the progressive presentation sensory changes occur first. The acute form may follow a very long bicycle ride, possibly over rough terrain, and both sensory and motor changes may be noted.

Preventative measures include a correct fit of the cycle, padding for the cyclist's gloves and handle bars, correct riding technique, and intermittent partial release of gripping pressure. Surgery is rarely required as most cases resolve following rest and correction of the above-mentioned factors.

The Lateral Ante-Brachial Cutaneous Nerve

The lateral ante-brachial cutaneous nerve is the terminal sensory branch of the musculocutaneous nerve and is derived from the fifth and sixth cervical nerve roots and the lateral cord of the brachial plexus.

Compression neuropathy of the antebrachial cutaneous nerve has been described in baseball pitchers, racket sport players, and in backstroke swimmers. The usual mechanism is forced pronation or sudden movement from supination to pronation with the elbow fully extended. The site of compression is at the lateral free margin of the bicipital aponeurosis that compresses the nerve between the biceps tendon and the brachial fascia. Symptoms include lateral elbow pain and sensory disturbance along the course of the nerve in the forearm.

Treatment involves relative rest, local anti-inflammatory measures, and perhaps splinting that limits the last 30° of extension. Surgery may also be required.

Radial Nerve

The radial nerve is derived from the C5–C8 nerve roots and arises from the posterior cord of brachial plexus. It runs in the spiral radial groove on the posterior aspect of humerus and across the radio-capitellar joint at the elbow, and then divides into posterior interosseous nerve (motor) and superficial cutaneous branch (sensory).

There are five potential sites of compression:

1. Fibrous bands tethering the posterior interosseous nerve to the radial head.
2. The edge of extensor carpi radialis brevis.
3. Recurrent radial artery and vein.
4. Arcade of Frohse.
5. Distal edge of supinator.

Clinical features include aching pain in the extensor aspect of the forearm with possible radiation to the dorsal aspect of the wrist. This is associated with repetitive movements of the forearm. Sensory symptoms and signs are rarely present as the posterior interosseous branch is more commonly involved. Tenderness occurs 3 to 4 cm distal to the lateral epicondyle. Supination at 30° elbow flexion (to exclude biceps function) is weak and painful.

Passive pronation with or without wrist flexion may increase the pain, and resisted middle finger extension with elbow extension is painful, but may also be painful in lateral epicondylitis. Ulnar deviation of the wrist may be weak. The location of symptoms leads to confusion with lateral epicondylitis, particularly when radial nerve compression affects branches innervating the periosteum of the lateral epicondyle.

Treatment of an acute radial tunnel syndrome involves rest, NSAIDs, assessment of sport tech-

nique, and perhaps immobilization for a short period. However, if the condition becomes chronic, surgical decompression is required.

Brachial Plexopathies

Brachial Plexus Injuries   Brachial plexus injury is not uncommon in sport, but American football poses a unique risk as up to 50% of players at some point experience a "stinger" or "burner" (18). The mechanism of injury usually involves lateral flexion of the neck away from the involved side in association with depression of the ipsilateral shoulder. Hyperextension injury of the neck or extension-compression can produce a similar clinical picture, and the presence of spinal stenosis increases the risk of injury. Brachial plexus lesions are more likely in younger players with less well-developed neck muscles; these lesions are essentially traction injuries in which the upper trunk of the plexus is most commonly affected (Fig 26-7).

The most important differential diagnosis is a root lesion in which compression of the nerve root or dorsal root ganglion occurs in the intervertebral foramen. In the older athlete this is associated with cervical disc disease or stenosis; and hyperextension or hyperextension-lateral flexion is the usual mechanism.

Brachial plexus injuries are graded as follows:

- Grade 1 injury is a *neurapraxia*. These injuries represent a transient loss of nerve function with a finite recovery time of less than 2 weeks. Physiologic function is impaired (conduction block or slowing), but no anatomic damage to the nerve is expected.
- Grade 2 injury is an *axonotmesis*. These are more severe injuries with physiologic function impaired and definite axonal damage (axon and myelin sheath disrupted but epineurium intact). Motor deficits last longer than 2 weeks (sensory changes are variable). The prognosis for recovery is good, but some deficits last up to a year.
- Grade 3 injury is a *neurotmesis*. These are severe injuries usually implying laceration or complete severance of the nerve with little chance of recovery of function.

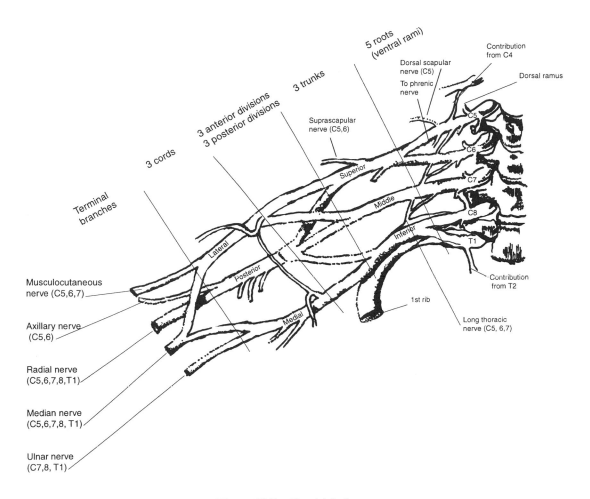

Figure 26-7. Brachial plexus.

Ninety percent of all brachial plexus injuries are mild, and the characteristic scenario is one of a football player running off the field shaking his arm after a tackle. The athlete may complain of stinging, burning, and of the arm "going to sleep"; or a player may feel a heaviness, numbness, and inability to move the arm. All symptoms resolve in 1 to 2 minutes and return to play is allowed once the examination is normal, serious injury to the neck has been excluded, and the player has been observed for 5 to 15 minutes. Reexamination should take place after the game and again in 48 to 72 hours to be sure no delayed findings occur.

Persistence of symptoms or neurologic signs indicates more serious injury and warrants repeated physical examinations, cervical spine radiographs, and perhaps CT or MRI scanning.

Return to play is allowed following resolution of both pain and paresthesia. The player should have a normal neurologic examination and demonstrate a full, pain-free range of cervical motion and normal strength of the affected limb. An abnormal EMG does not preclude participation.

Acute Brachial Neuritis Acute brachial neuritis is an uncommon condition seen in athletes that can be confused with a brachial plexus injury (19). This condition is characterized by rapid onset of significant shoulder pain in the absence of trauma. Weakness appears as the pain decreases, and it most commonly involves one or more of the deltoid, supraspinatus, serratus anterior, biceps, and

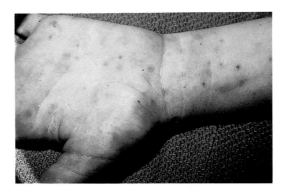

Plate 4. Rocky Mountain spotted fever rash on palm and wrist. (Photograph courtesy of Timothy W. Lane, MD.)

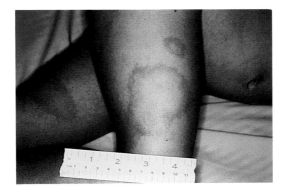

Plate 5. Erythema chronicum migrans with satellite lesions on the leg of a patient with Lyme disease. (Photograph courtesy of Centers for Disease Control.)

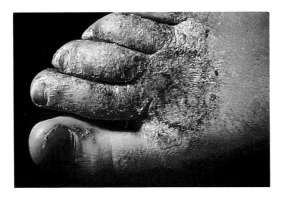

Plate 6. Classic tinea pedis (athlete's foot). (Photograph courtesy of the American Academy of Dermatology.)

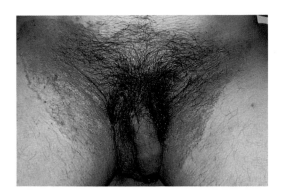

Plate 7. Classic tinea cruris (jock itch). (Photograph courtesy of the American Academy of Dermatology.)

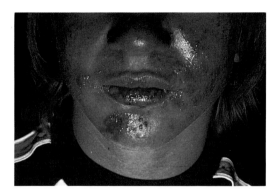

Plate 8. Herpes simplex exacerbated by sun exposure in a skier. (Photograph courtesy of the American Academy of Dermatology.)

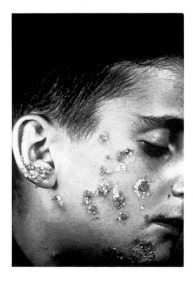

Plate 9. Impetigo. (Photograph courtesy of The Upjohn Company.)

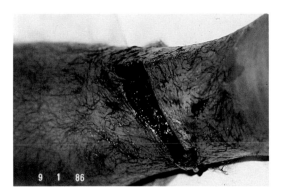

Plate 16. A laceration on the front of the lower leg caused by the barb of a stingray. Some venom from the barb integument may also be deposited into such a wound. (Reproduced by permission from Williamson J, Fenner P, Acott C. Medical aspects of marine envenomation and poisoning. In: Covacevich J, Davie P, Pearn J, eds. Toxic plants and animals: a guide for Australia. South Brisbane: Queensland Museum, 1987:215–240.)

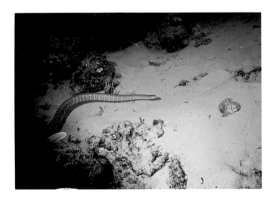

Plate 17. The "olive sea snake" *Aipysurus laevis* photographed in the northern Australian region. Note the paddle-shaped tail and the absence of gills, characteristics that distinguish it from an eel. (Photograph courtesy of Bob Halstead, Cairns, Queensland.)

Chapter 27
Nephrology in Sport

Mark E. Batt

RENAL PHYSIOLOGY DURING EXERCISE

At rest, the kidneys receive 17% to 25% of the cardiac output, 90% of which perfuses the renal cortex. Exercise causes renal blood flow to fall, and it may drop to 25% of the resting value with resultant changes in renal function, electrolyte, and protein excretion (1). The fall in renal blood flow is related to exercise intensity; through renal autoregulation, the glomerular filtration rate (GFR) remains relatively preserved (2). Alteration of renal blood flow during exercise is brought about by increased sympathetic activity and catecholamine release.

Antidiuretic hormone (ADH) level also increases with intense exercise, producing reduced urine output through control of renal tubular water reabsorption. Thus, a protection mechanism against excess body water loss during exercise exists, and this is related to hydration level, and exercise intensity and duration (3).

These effects, particularly GFR, are influenced by the state of hydration. Dehydration has a more pronounced effect, as hyperhydration does not appear to influence significantly postexercise urine output (4). The key element of body fluid homeostasis is total body sodium. Its excretion is largely unchanged by exercise—principally as a result of increased renal tubular uptake, rather than large changes in GFR, during exercise. Due to elevated sympathetic tone and plasma sodium level, aldosterone and thus renin are released during prolonged intense muscular activity. They combine to preserve both body sodium and water (5). Prolonged physical activity in itself has been shown to produce minimal net urinary electrolyte loss, thus warranting no specific replacement therapy (6).

RENAL ABNORMALITIES WITH EXERCISE

Proteinuria

Postexertion proteinuria occurs after both contact and noncontact sports and was first documented in exercising soldiers in 1878 (7). The etiology is complex and appears to be related to exercise intensity, not duration (8). At rest in the glomerulus, proteins smaller than albumin are filtered from plasma with subsequent extensive proximal tubular reabsorption. During exercise, a glomerular pattern of protein loss occurs with enhanced glomerular filtration of macromolecules (principally albumin) due to sluggish glomerular blood flow and increased glomerular basement membrane permeability. As exercise intensity increases, tubular reabsorption of small proteins declines, leading to higher urinary concentrations of low molecular weight proteins (B_2-microglobulin) and thus proteinuria of a mixed glomerular–tubular type (8).

Critical to the diagnosis of exercise-induced proteinuria is the rapid and predictable clearance of proteinuria after exercise. Protein loss is maximal within 30 minutes of stopping exercise and should cease within 24 to 48 hours. Peak levels register 2+ or 3+ on dipstick testing or with quantitative measurement 100 to 300 mg (9). The extent of proteinuria and speed of resolution differentiates exercise-induced proteinuria from more serious causes.

Normal urine collected under resting conditions contains up to 200 mg per day of protein. Dipstick tests for proteinuria are sensitive and may detect and indicate "trace proteinuria" at urinary protein levels of 100 mg/L physiologic proteinuria (8). When daily urine output exceeds 2 li-

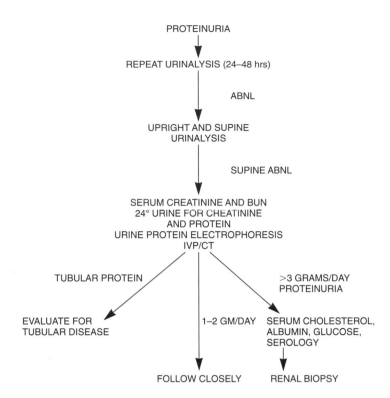

Figure 27-1. Evaluation of the athlete with proteinuria. NL = normal; ABNL = abnormal. (Reproduced by permission from Cianflocco AJ. Renal complications of exercise. Clin Sports Med 1992; 11:437–451.)

ters, negative testing with dipsticks occurs; more concentrated urine may register as positive, making this form of test a less reliable indicator of nonphysiologic proteinuria. Remembering that false-positive tests for proteinuria can occur is important when assessing concentrated postexercise or alkaline urine. A clinical yardstick is to combine the urinary specific gravity with protein dipstick estimates of trace or 1+ proteinuria: the last two digits of the specific gravity give an indicator of the upper limit of normal for that specimen of urine (e.g., 1.030 sp g = 30 mg/dL expected upper limit of normal for protein in that specimen) (10).

A training effect exists with reduced proteinuria for bouts of consistent exercise, but any increase in workload or intensity further elevates urinary protein levels (2). Follow-up urine samples of exercise-induced proteinuria may demonstrate

progressive resolution of proteinuria within 2 days. Such patients require repeat urinalysis at 48 hours after cessation of exercise. Prone and upright samples may be necessary to exclude benign orthostatic proteinuria. If high levels of proteinuria on dipstick testing persist, more detailed investigation is warranted (Fig 27-1).

Proteinuria is common during childhood and peaks in adolescence. The natural history is typically of a transient condition—less than 1:1000 have anything other than a benign cause (11). For this reason, the utility of urinalysis during adolescent preparticipation examinations has been questioned. In 1986, Peggs et al. (12) demonstrated proteinuria in 62% of the adult athletes screened. Half of the athletes presented for screening for 2 successive years, but only 28.5% demonstrated proteinuria on two successive occasions. Considering the transient nature of this phenomenon, routine screening is not recommended for this age group.

Dehydration and Renal Failure

The kidneys play a key role in the maintenance of fluid and electrolyte homeostasis during exercise. Mechanisms exist to protect the kidney while it maintains plasma volume. This balance may be upset, albeit rarely, by a metabolic milieu that results in renal compromise and, in some instances, acute renal failure. Specifically, the combined effects of exercise-to-exhaustion, dehydration, hyperpyrexia, hyperkalemia, and rhabdomyolysis are liable to produce renal damage. Trained and professional athletes have developed rhabdomyolysis through exhaustive exercise (13), but the most typical cases are untrained athletes such as military recruits, who develop renal damage early in their training courses as a result of renal ischemia and nephrotoxins (14).

Renal failure from exercise-induced rhabdomyolysis and resulting myoglobinuria is not inevitable, as was demonstrated by Sinert's retrospective cohort study of subjects with exercise-induced rhabdomyolysis, none of whom developed acute renal failure (15). This contrasts with the previous reports of rhabdomyolysis in nonexercising populations that described an incidence of renal failure of 17% to 40% (15).

An unidentified nephrotoxic cofactor has been suggested in other forms of rhabdomyolysis that is not thought to be present when rhabdomyolysis is exercise induced. Preventive measures to prevent exercise-induced rhabdomyolysis should include adequate fluid intake to enhance excretion of myoglobin; a carbohydrate-rich diet and rest to prevent glycogen depletion; and avoidance of repetitive exhaustive exercise (14). These measures minimize muscle damage, promote myoglobin elimination, and maintain extracellular volume, thus maintaining renal blood flow and preventing renal ischemia.

Hematuria in Sport

Macroscopic and microscopic hematuria can occur following exercise, regardless of sport. Gross hematuria following renal trauma clearly requires aggressive follow-up to exclude significant renal tract disruption. The more frequent and more puzzling phenomenon is urine discoloration in athletes who have no definite history of trauma.

The normal urine contains small numbers of red blood cells, which are dysmorphic and originate from glomeruli. This innocent microscopic hematuria in the general population is common, and its cause remains controversial. Spurious, asymptomatic "macroscopic hematuria," which may arise from urinary contaminants other than intact red blood cells, may discolor the urine red or brown. For example, vegetable dyes such as beetroot and medications such as nitrofurantoin and rifampicin may discolor the urine. Hemoglobinuria from the lysis of red blood cells may likewise discolor the urine and may occur due to repetitive foot strike in runners ("march hemoglobinuria" [16]). Additionally, myoglobinuria may occur in isolation or in combination with hemoglobinuria, discoloring the urine and producing a dipstick result positive for blood.

Dipstick tests react with hemo-groups that may present as intact red blood cells, or as myoglobin, or as free hemoglobin (hemoglobinuria). Due to this extreme sensitivity, the utility of urine dipstick testing for blood has been questioned (it detects as few as 1×10^6/L red blood cells in unspun urine); urine microscopy therefore remains the gold standard (17). Microscopy should be performed on a centrifuged and resuspended sample, and an intact red cell count of more than 100×10^6/L is regarded as abnormal. Any abnormal dipstick test should be repeated after 24 and 48 hours, then followed by repeat urine microscopy for red blood cells using morphology to attempt to distinguish glomerular from nonglomerular bleeding (17).

The implications of microscopic hematuria vary with the age of the patient. Patients over 40 years of age have greater likelihood of significant urologic abnormality than do those who are younger, but even young athletes with hematuria have been found with bladder malignancies. Important in both groups is the persistence of hematuria—sports hematuria is typically short lived, clearing after 48 hours (17,18).

There is no single cause of hematuria following exertion, and the variable pathogenesis relates in part to the nature of the physical activity. Runners frequently develop hematuria, and cystoscopy has revealed reciprocal lesions on the flexible posterior wall of the bladder and the thicker more rigid trigone. This suggests trauma, as the bladder wall strikes the interureteric ridge during running (19). The resultant superficial lesions may bleed briskly, producing a frank, short-lived terminal hematuria. Interestingly, this phenomenon may be intermittent for a given individual; it has been speculated that a lack of urine in the bladder facilitates apposition and trauma of the bladder walls.

Hematuria is common in long-distance runners. The incidence varies between 17% to 69%, with the highest incidence being reported in ultramarathon runners (16). Athletic psuedonephritis, the combination of hematuria with casts and proteinuria, may also occur in runners. Nephron ischemia and hypoxia leads to increased glomerular permeability with elevated filtration pressure and stasis, enhancing red blood cell and glomerular protein excretion (20,21). This mechanism probably also explains swimmer's hematuria, for which the magnitude also relates to the level of exertion. In both swimmers and runners the longer and more strenuous races produce a greater incidence and severity of hematuria (21,22). Hematuria may also arise from perineal trauma from bicycle seats and bumpy terrain among bicycle motocross and recreational cyclists (23,24). This may be alleviated by angling the nose of the saddle downward (25).

Finally, because hematuria may be a symptom of other medical conditions, such as sickle cell disease, schistosomiasis, and von Willebrand's disease, a thorough medical history is important. This history should include an accurate drug history, including anticoagulants and nonsteroidal antiinflammatory drugs (NSAIDs). NSAIDs, which are used widely in athletics, have less obvious side effects that should not be forgotten. NSAID usage of 54% was reported in a group of patients found to have idiopathic hematuria, thus suggesting it may be a potential cause (26). Furthermore, indomethacin has been shown to compromise renal function during sustained exercise and may itself potentiate the development of renal failure through changes in renal blood flow (27).

Incontinence

Incontinence is a common, underreported complaint of women. The prevalence rates are definition dependent. A prevalence of 8.5% was found in women aged 15 to 64 years of whom only 0.2% were recognized by care agencies (28). Higher prevalences of stress incontinence have been reported (40% to 52%), with the highest levels in parous women (29).

Sports that require running, jumping, high-impact landings, or maintenance of a Valsalva maneuver may lead to or exacerbate stress incontinence. In a study of elite nulliparous athletes with a mean age of 20 years, 28% reported urine loss during sports activity. The sports with greatest risk included gymnastics, basketball, tennis, and field hockey (30). Deficiency of the urethral closure mechanism may be helped by the use of pelvic floor exercises that provide a degree of symptomatic relief (31). The use of a vaginal tampon may be of help to some women with mild stress incontinence during exercise (32).

RENAL CONDITIONS AND EXERCISE

Renal Calculi

Renal calculi occur with approximately 12% of men and 5% of women experiencing an episode of renal colic during their lifetime (33). The majority of calculi contain calcium and are radiopaque: 60% are principally calcium oxalate, a further 20% contain principally calcium phosphate of apatite. Noncalcium stones are radiolucent and consist principally of uric acid (7%), cystine (3%), or struvite (7%). The latter is a magnesium-ammonium-phosphate stone created by a urinary tract infection of urea-splitting organisms such as *Proteus* or *Pseudomonas*. The pathogenesis of other stones is typically multifactorial but may have one core metabolic fault, such as cystinuria, hyperuricosuria, or hypercalcemia. Several solutes normally exist in the urine in high concentrations and are prevented from crystal-forming by other factors such as urinary pH. Alteration of urinary pH may change solute solubility and result in crystal deposition (33).

Nearly all renal calculi are preventable with adequately dilute urine. The supersaturation of solutes in the kidney promoted by dehydration is very pertinent to athletes. A urine volume of 2 liters daily is the ideal, and it should be specifically targeted because many individuals produce less than 1 liter of urine daily. Adequate postexercise hydration should be promoted; measuring pre- and postexercise weights can detect suspected fluid loss and provide a patient with guidance, especially in hot and humid environments. Adequate hydration is particularly important for wheelchair athletes, as renal calculi occur more frequently in athletes with a spinal cord injury. This is related to osteoporosis, hypercalcemia, and hypercalciuria (34).

Dietary advice for prevention and treatment of stones is frequently overlooked. During strength training, athletes are frequently encouraged to eat a high-protein diet, but the high urinary urate levels that arise from purine rich foods such as meat, compounded by high alcohol intake, can cause purine nucleotide degeneration. Serum urate concentration is not a reliable indicator of urine urate excretion as it does not correlate with renal urate excretion.

Following an accurate stone analysis, further dietary manipulation may be desirable, such as reducing dietary oxalate (chocolate, tea, spinach). Because any dietary change must lifelong, the regimen must be reasonable and sustainable. Also, the use of potassium citrate has been advocated to elevate pH and inhibit crystal formation (35).

End-Stage Renal Disease

Patients with chronic renal failure and end-stage renal disease (ESRD) have reduced exercise capacity (36). This reduced capacity may be further depressed by the coexistence of concurrent medical problems such as heart disease or diabetes mellitus. Reduced exercise capacity for these patients affects their ability to perform the activities of daily living and thus impacts their quality of life (37).

That patients who have received a renal transplant return to near normal aerobic capacity suggests that uremia is a cause of reduced aerobic activity. The diminution of aerobic capacity in uremia is mediated both peripherally and centrally, although the latter plays the most significant role through reduced maximal heart rate and cardiac output (36). The anemia of ESRD limits the delivery of oxygen, although peripheral oxygen extraction remains high.

Hemodialysis patients who exercise are capable of increasing their exercise capacity. These patients may exercise with a recumbent bicycle during dialysis. Consequently, further benefits of exercise may accrue, such as reduced blood pressure, improved lipid profile, and glucose tolerance (38). Erythropoietin may allow patients with ESRD to increase exercise loads and may alleviate symptoms of fatigue (36). Patients who undergo peritoneal dialysis may also exercise and are often most comfortable if this is performed when the peritoneal cavity is relatively empty of dialysate.

Exercise testing in patients with ESRD is controversial because the frequency of abnormal resting electrocardiograms coupled with low workloads achieved by ESRD patients leads to equivocal test results. If such testing is required, a radioisotope scan with dipyridamole is preferred (36).

Among patients who have had a renal transplant, maximal heart rate recovers and $\dot{V}o_2$max values approach those for sedentary controls (39). Exercise programs may improve the patient's endurance and quality of life, and may also counteract some of the adverse effects that immunosuppressants (particularly corticosteroids) have on muscle strength (36).

Renal Anomalies

Children's kidneys are less well protected than those of adults, because their kidney's size is proportionally larger and has less protection from perinephric fat, muscles, and thoracic cage. Children are therefore at greater risk of blunt trauma through contact and collision sports. In one study, sport accounted for 28% of conservatively treated blunt renal injuries in children (40). Among 240 children with blunt renal trauma, 11 had congenital anomalies, 4 of whom required surgery, yet of the remaining 229 only 5 required surgery. In situations where the injury appears to be greater than that expected from a magnitude of trauma, the presence of a renal anomaly should be considered (41).

Renal anomaly (solitary or horseshoe kidney) or previous trauma produces the clinical situation of a solitary organ, a scenario that has implications for sports participation—particularly for contact or collision sports. Although recommendations for participation in competitive sports do exist for this controversial area, no absolute rules exist to regulate this type of anomaly for the preparticipation examination (42). Generally, when these anomalies are recognized a child should be steered away from a sport where blunt renal trauma is more likely.

When a child does participate in sports, adequate and well-fitting protective equipment should be encouraged. All parties, including coaches, must be adequately informed of the potential risks and sequelae of this condition. The patient's notes should include this information; institutions may use a form of legal waiver regarding unpaired organs that can be signed jointly by the institution and the parties involved.

SUMMARY

Proteinuria and hematuria are common occurrences in exercising individuals. Fortunately, these conditions are typically benign; however, appropriate evaluation should exclude more serious pathology. Sports can predispose to serious renal problems, such as renal failure related to rhabdomyolysis, painful conditions such as kidney stones, and troublesome occurrences such as incontinence. A knowledge of renal physiology and the effects of exercise on renal function helps guide the sports medicine physician to the appropriate treatment of athletes. Exercise at some level is beneficial to almost all individuals: with appropriate precautions, exercise can be prescribed for chronic renal failure, congenital renal anomalies, and most nephrologic problems.

REFERENCES

1 Zambraski EJ. Renal regulation of fluid homeostasis during exercise. In: Gisolfi CV, Lamb DR, eds. Perspectives in exercise science and sports medicine, Vol. 3: Fluid homeostasis during exercise. Carmel, IN: Brown & Benchmark, 1988:247–276.

2 Poortmans JR. Exercise and renal function. Sports Med 1984;1:125–153.

3 Wade CE, Claybaugh JR. Plasma renin activity, vasopressin concentration, and urinary excretory responses to exercise in men. J Appl Physiol 1980;49:930–936.

4 Castenfors J. Renal function during exercise. With special reference to exercise proteinuria and the release of renin. Acta Physiol Scand 1967;70(suppl):1–44.

5 Galbo H. Endocrinology and metabolism in exercise. Int J Sports Med 1981;2:203–211.

6 Refsum HE, Strömme SB. Relationship between urine flow, glomerular filtration, and urine solute concentrations during prolonged heavy exercise. Scand J Clin Lab Invest 1975;35:775–780.

7 von Leube W. Uber ausscheidung von Eiwess in harn des gesunden Menschen. Wirkows Arch 1878;72:145–147.

8 Poortmans JR. Postexercise proteinuria in humans. JAMA 1985;253:236–240.

9 Goldszer RC, Siegel AJ. Renal abnormalities during exercise. In: Strauss RH, ed. Sports medicine. Philadelphia: WB Saunders, 1984:156–166.

10 Abuello JG, Kleeman CR, Norman ME. When proteinuria spells trouble. Patient Care 1990; 24:73–78,86,89–90,93–96.

11 Maxson WT. Benign proteinuria of childhood and adolescence: a survey. Clin Pediatr 1963; 2:662–668.

12 Peggs JF, Reinhardt RW, O'Brien JM. Proteinuria in adolescent sports physical examinations. J Fam Pract 1986;22:80–81.

13 Knochel JP. Rhabdomyolysis and myoglobinuria. Semin Nephrol 1981;1:75–86.

14 Olerud JE, Homer LD, Carroll HW. Incidence of acute exertional rhabdomyolysis. Serum myoglobin and enzyme levels as indicators of muscle injury. Arch Intern Med 1976;136:692–697.

15 Sinert R, Kohl L, Rainone T, Scalea T. Exercise-induced rhabdomyolysis. Ann Emerg Med 1994; 23:1301–1306.

16 Eichner ER. Haematuria—a diagnostic challenge. Physician Sports Med 1990;18:52–54,56–58,61–63.

17 Froom P, Ribak J, Benbassat J. Significance of microhaematuria in young adults. Br Med J 1984;288:20–22.

18 Bullock N. Asymptomatic microscopic haematuria [editorial]. Br Med J 1986;292:645.

19 Blacklock NJ. Bladder trauma in the long-distance runner: "10,000 metres haematuria." Br J Urol 1977;49:129–132.

20 Boileau M, Fuchs E, Barry JM, Hodges CV. Stress

hematuria: athletic pseudonephritis in marathoners. Urology 1980;15:471–474.

21 Abarbanel J, Benet AE, Lask D, Kimche D. Sports hematuria. J Urol 1990;143:887–890.

22 Alyea EP, Parish HH, Jr, Durham NC. Renal response to exercise: urinary findings. JAMA 1958;167:807–813.

23 Salcedo JR. Huffy-bike hematuria [letter]. N Engl J Med 1986;315:768.

24 O'Brien KP. Sports urology: the vicious cycle [letter]. N Engl J Med 1981;304:1367–1368.

25 Nichols TW Jr. Bicycle-seat hematuria [letter]. N Engl J Med 1984;311:1128.

26 Kraus SE, Siroky MB, Babayan RK, Krane RJ. Hematuria and the use of nonsteroidal anti-inflammatory drugs. J Urol 1984;132:288–290.

27 Walker RJ, Fawcett JP, Flannery EM, Gerrard DF. Indomethacin potentiates exercise-induced reduction in renal hemodynamics in athletes. Med Sci Sports Exerc 1994;26:1302–1306.

28 Thomas TM, Plymat KR, Blannin J, Meade TW. Prevalence of urinary incontinence. Br Med J 1980;281:1243–1245.

29 Crist T, Shingleton HM, Koch GG. Stress incontinence and the nulliparous patient. Obstet Gynecol 1972;40:13–17.

30 Nygaard IE, Thompson FL, Svengalis SL, Albright JP. Urinary incontinence in elite nulliparous athletes. Obstet Gynecol 1994;84:183–187.

31 Kegel AH. Physiologic therapy for urinary stress incontinence. JAMA 1951;146:915–917.

32 Feneley RCL. Urological aspects of incontinence. In: Mandelstam D, ed. Incontinence and its management. London: Croom Helm, 1980:35–54.

33 Emmerson BT. Urinary calculi. In: Whitworth JA, Lawrence JR, eds. Textbook of renal disease. London: Churchill Livingstone, 1994:291–300.

34 Fallon KE. The disabled athlete. In: Bloomfield J, Fricker PA, Fitch KD, eds. Science and medicine in sport. 2nd ed. Melbourne: Blackwell Scientific, 1995:550–575.

35 Coe FL. Prevention of kidney stones. Am J Med 1981;71:514–516.

36 Painter P. The importance of exercise training in rehabilitation of patients with end-stage renal disease. Am J Kidney Dis 1994;24(suppl):S2–S9, discussion S31–S32.

37 Evans RW, Manninen DL, Garrison LP Jr, et al. The quality of life of patients with end-stage renal disease. N Engl J Med 1985;312:553–559.

38 Goldberg AP, Geltman EM, Gavin JR III, et al. Exercise training reduces coronary risk and effectively rehabilitates hemodialysis patients. Nephron 1986;42:311–316.

39 Parmley WW. Recommendations of the American College of Cardiology on cardiovascular rehabilitation. Cardiology 1986;7:4–5.

40 Kuzmarov IW, Morehouse DD, Gibson S. Blunt renal trauma in the pediatric population: a retrospective study. J Urol 1981;126:648–649.

41 York JP. Sports and the male genitourinary system. Part 2: genital injuries and sexually transmitted diseases. Physician Sports Med 1990;18:92–96,98–100.

42 American Academy of Pediatrics Committee on Sports Medicine. Recommendations for participation in competitive sports. Pediatrics 1988; 81:737–739.

Chapter 28
Endocrinologic Conditions

Peter Brukner
Peter A. Fricker

This chapter reviews the more common and significant endocrine disorders that affect people of all ages, discussing the various complications and a wide range of exercise-related concerns. The discussion that follows is necessarily brief, given the large proportion of medical practice devoted to endocrine disorders. It deals primarily with information the practitioner needs to know, and its focus on athletes is unique.

DIABETES MELLITUS

There are two distinct types of diabetes: insulin-ependent (type I) and non-insulin-dependent (type II).

Type I Diabetes   Insulin-dependent diabetes mellitus (IDDM), or type I diabetes, was previously known as juvenile-onset diabetes and is thought to be an inherited autoimmune disease. Type I diabetes represents approximately 10% to 15% of diabetic cases in the Western world, but the incidence of type I varies throughout the world. Type I diabetes is characterized by an absence of endogenous insulin production. It occurs commonly in childhood and adolescence but can become symptomatic at any age. Insulin administration is essential to prevent ketosis, coma, and death.

Type II Diabetes   Type II diabetes mellitus, commonly called non-insulin-dependent diabetes mellitus (NIDDM), was previously known as maturity-onset or adult-onset diabetes. Approximately 90% of individuals with diabetes have type II, and this disease affects 3% to 7% of people in Western countries (1). The prevalence of NIDDM increases with age. The pathogenesis of NIDDM remains unknown (2,3), but is believed to be heterogeneous with a strong genetic factor (4). Approximately 80% of individuals with NIDDM are obese. NIDDM is characterized by diminished insulin secretion relative to serum glucose levels and peripheral insulin resistance, both of which result in chronic hyperglycemia.

Three major metabolic abnormalities characterize NIDDM:

1. Impairment in pancreatic β-cell insulin secretion in response to a glucose stimulus (5,6).
2. A reduced sensitivity to the action of insulin in major organ systems, such as muscle, liver, and adipose tissue (5,7,8).
3. Excessive hepatic glucose production in the basal state (9,10).

Both type I and type II diabetes cause serious complications such as accelerated atherosclerosis, which increases the risk of acute myocardial infarction two to threefold (11). As peripheral arterial disease incidence elevates dramatically, the risk of cerebral stroke doubles. The life expectancy of someone with diabetes is reduced to two-thirds that of a nondiabetic individual (12).

Type I diabetes is treated by administering exogenous insulin with the therapeutic aim of achieving and maintaining near-normal blood glucose levels. Diet is also closely monitored to achieve the same. For both type I and type II patients a low-fat, carbohydrate-controlled diet, with the emphasis on complex carbohydrate intake and reduction of simple carbohydrates, is recommended. In type II diabetes, exogenous insulin is occasionally required, but more frequently diet, weight loss, and exercise are the keys to treatment. Oral hypoglycemic agents are also widely used in the treatment of type II diabetes.

Exercise and Type I Diabetes

The relationship between diabetes mellitus and exercise has two important aspects: the adjustments the athlete with diabetes makes if he or she wishes to exercise, and the short-term and long-term risks and benefits of exercise to the patient with diabetes.

Prior to commencement or increase in intensity of an exercise program, a full examination should be performed with particular attention to the sites of diabetic complications—the cardiovascular system, the feet, and the eyes. A general fitness examination includes flexibility, muscular strength, and endurance, and assessment of cardiovascular fitness. An ECG is recommended for those over 35 years of age or those with diabetes of 15 years' duration. An exercise ECG should also be considered, as diabetics may have major coronary artery disease in the absence of ischemic symptoms. Long-term glucose control should be evaluated by measuring fructosamine or hemoglobin A_1 levels as well as by reviewing the patient's self-monitoring records. Blood glucose, cholesterol, and triglyceride levels should also be measured.

Control of Blood Glucose   Control of blood glucose is achieved by adjustment of carbohydrate intake, exercise levels, and insulin dosage. The meal plan and insulin dose vary according to the patient's response to exercise. Diabetics need to carefully monitor their blood glucose levels before and after every workout. Patients who track blood glucose before, during, and after exercise can learn their own response patterns. If no means exists to identify blood glucose levels before a workout, then the workout should be of short duration and low intensity with an oral glucose supply available.

Moderate exercise of less than 30 minutes rarely requires any insulin adjustment, although a small snack or glucose-containing drink just prior to exercise helps avoid hypoglycemia, especially if the blood glucose level is less than 5 mmol/L (90 mg/dL). Longer periods of exercise usually require snacks every 30 to 60 minutes, and some diabetics require snacks after exercise.

If short-acting insulin is used, it may be necessary to reduce the dose if exercise lasts more than 45 to 60 minutes. Prolonged exercise sessions usually require approximately a 20% reduction in the short-acting component (as determined by monitoring), although a decrease in total daily insulin may ultimately be required. Those involved in a long-term fitness program may notice the total daily insulin requirements decrease by as much as 30%.

Exercise and Type II Diabetes

Individuals with type II diabetes on diet therapy alone do not usually need to make any adjustments for exercise. Patients taking oral hypoglycemic drugs may need to halve their doses on days of prolonged exercise or withhold it altogether, depending on blood glucose levels. They are also advised to carry some glucose with them and be able to recognize the symptoms of hypoglycemia.

Diabetic athletes participating in team sports need to have a good knowledge of their normal glucose profiles in response to exercise. As competition may require interstate travel and altered eating patterns, the diabetic athlete should practice the "match day" routine at home and have snacks available as necessary. Good control of blood glucose levels may require regular access to carbohydrate-containing drinks. This not only serves to improve the glucose profile, but also aids rehydration during prolonged exercise. All patients with diabetes should carry an identification card or bracelet identifying them as diabetic. They should remain alert to the early signs of hypoglycemia for at least 6 to 12 hours after exercise and have their glucose tablets (or an alternative source of glucose) with them throughout this period. Dehydration during exercise should be prevented by adequate fluid consumption. One additional safety measure recommended to the diabetic athlete is to have an exercise partner in case of adverse reactions.

Dietary Management   The importance of a high-carbohydrate, low-fat diet for optimal diabetic control is well established. Fortunately, this conforms to the guidelines for maximizing athletic performance. Some older type II diabetic patients may have been educated to have low-carbohydrate diets. These individuals may have depleted glycogen stores, which impairs performance. Although carbohydrate requirements for exercise vary considerably among athletes, carbohydrate

Table 28-1   Adjustment of Food Intake with Exercise

Activity Level and Exercise Time	Blood Glucose Level (mmol/L)	Carbohydrate (CHO) Adjustment
Low level ½ hour	<5.5 (~ 100 mg/dL)	10 gram CHO (small serving of fruit, bread, cookie, yogurt, or milk)
	>5.5	No extra food
Moderate intensity 1 hour	<5.5	20–30 gram CHO (½–2 servings of fruit, bread, cookies, yogurt, and/or milk)
	5.5–10 (~ 100–180 mg/dL)	10 gram CHO (small serving of fruit, bread, cookie, yogurt, or milk)
	10–16.5	No extra food (in most cases)
	>16.5 (~ 300 mg/dL)	No extra food. Preferably do not exercise, as blood glucose level may go up.
Strenuous activity 1–2 hours	<5.5	45–60 gram CHO (1 sandwich and fruit and/or milk or yogurt)
	5.5–10	25–50 gram CHO (½ sandwich and fruit and/or milk or yogurt)
	10–16.5	15 gram CHO (1 serving of fruit, bread, cookies, yogurt, or milk)
	>16.5	Preferably do not exercise, as blood glucose level may go up.
Varying intensity Long duration	Variable glucose levels	Insulin may best be decreased.
	Must monitor	(Conservatively estimate the decrease in insulin peaking at time of activity by 10%. A 50% reduction is not common.)
½–1 day	Variable glucose levels	Increase carbohydrate before, during, and after activity by 10–50 gram.
	Must monitor	CHO per hours, such as diluted fruit juice

SOURCE: Adapted with permission from Brukner P, Khan K. Clinical sports medicine. Sidney: McGraw-Hill, 1993:605.

restriction is not recommended (see Table 28-1 for a general guide).

Athletes involved in endurance events who carbohydrate-load prior to competition may need to increase their insulin dosage transiently to cope with the increased carbohydrate intake. It is important that carbohydrate is ingested before, during, and after the event.

All insulin-dependent diabetic athletes should seek individual counseling from a sports dietitian and physician to arrange a specific dietary and training program. Generally, all diabetic athletes should be aware of the following:

- Athletes need to learn the effects of different types of exercise under different environmental conditions on their blood glucose levels.
- When exercising away from home, the athlete should carry carbohydrate foods such as fruit, fruit juice, barley sugar, or cookies.

- After vigorous exercise, blood glucose levels may continue to drop for a number of hours. Postexercise carbohydrate ingestion ensures replenishment of glycogen stores and prevents hypoglycemia.
- Dehydration may be confused with hypoglycemia. All athletes should consume plenty of fluid before, during, and after exercise.
- Alcohol should be discouraged following exercise as it lowers blood glucose levels and has a dehydrating effect.
- The best time for training is when blood glucose levels are above fasting level, but not high. About 1 to 2 hours after a meal is ideal.
- For intermittent exercise, the athlete should take some form of carbohydrate during breaks to control blood glucose levels and prevent hunger.
- During long-duration exercise, most diabetic athletes require regular carbohydrate intake in the form of food or liquids.

- Exercise speeds up the absorption of insulin from exercising limbs. This can be moderated by injecting into parts of the body away from the exercising muscle (e.g., the abdomen).

Complications of Exercise in the Diabetic Athlete

The diabetic athlete may suffer hypoglycemia, diabetic ketoacidosis, and other problems associated with the complications of diabetes.

Hypoglycemia   Hypoglycemia is the major fear among athletes with type I diabetes. Initial symptoms of hypoglycemia include sweating, nervousness, tremor, and hunger. The symptoms of impending hypoglycemia may be difficult to differentiate from symptoms experienced during vigorous exercise. If hypoglycemia is not corrected, confusion, abnormal behavior, loss of consciousness, and convulsions may occur.

Nocturnal hypoglycemia may follow late-afternoon or evening training or competition. Symptoms include night sweats, unpleasant dreams, and early morning headaches.

At the first indication of hypoglycemia, the athlete should ingest oral carbohydrate in solid or liquid form. Diabetic athletes should carry rapidly digestible forms of carbohydrate (e.g., glucose tablets, barley sugar) or have a glucose–electrolyte solution available. The semiconscious or unconscious diabetic patient urgently requires intravenous glucose administration (50 mL of 50% solution).

Prevention of hypoglycemia depends on adjustment of carbohydrate intake and insulin dosage to meet the individual athlete's needs. A continual source of glucose must be available during exercise, and, as a rule of thumb, athletes usually require between 15 and 30 gram of glucose per half hour of vigorous exercise.

Diabetic Ketoacidosis in the Athlete   Exercise commonly causes diabetic ketoacidosis when the athlete's diabetes is poorly controlled and circulating insulin levels are too low at the beginning of exercise. Individuals with blood glucose levels of 20 or 25 mmol/L and above are especially at risk of precipitating diabetic ketoacidosis if they exercise vigorously. This occurs because the counter-regulatory hormone response to exercise (glucagon, catecholamines, growth hormone, and glucocorticoids) pushes glucose levels higher at a time when there is insufficient insulin to prevent ketosis. An athlete must have satisfactory diabetic control before exercise and those with "brittle diabetes" must be very cautious in reducing insulin doses before exercise.

Risks and Benefits of Exercise   A thorough screening examination and an appropriate exercise program minimizes the risks of regular physical activity in patients with diabetes. The main risk is hypoglycemia, whereas the multiple benefits of exercise include improved insulin sensitivity, improved blood lipid profiles, decreased heart rate, and blood pressure at rest, decreased body weight, and possible decreased risk of coronary heart disease. In IDDM, exercise does not clearly improve glycemic control, although insulin requirements may be decreased slightly.

Exercise and the Complications of Diabetes

Exercise is often neglected when secondary complications of diabetes arise. Some unique concerns for the patient with diabetes that warrant close scrutiny include autonomic and peripheral neuropathy, retinopathy, and nephropathy, all of which are worsened by poor glucose control.

Autonomic Neuropathy   Abnormal autonomic function is common among those with diabetes of long duration. The risks for exercise in those with autonomic neuropathy include hypoglycemia, abnormal responses (e.g., postural drop) in blood pressure and heart rate, impaired function of the sympathetic and parasympathetic nervous systems, and abnormal thermoregulation. Patients with autonomic neuropathy have a higher risk of sudden death and myocardial infarction so that they should undergo submaximal exercise testing before exercise. High-intensity activity should be avoided, as should rapid changes in body position and extremes in temperature. Suitable exercises include water activities and stationary cycling.

Peripheral Neuropathy   Peripheral neuropathy (typically manifested as loss of light-touch sensation and two-point discrimination) usually begins symmetrically in the extremities and progresses proximally. Nonweightbearing activities such as swimming, cycling, and arm exercises are recommended in those with insensitive feet. Activities that improve balance are also appropriate choices. Regular close inspection of the feet and use of proper footwear are important, and the patient should avoid exercise that can cause trauma to the feet. Feet and toes should be kept dry and clean.

Diabetic Retinopathy The incidence of diabetic retinopathy is directly proportional to the severity and duration of the diabetes. Jarring of the head during exercise in contact sports may cause detachment of the retina. In individuals with proliferative retinopathy, only submaximal exercise tests should be conducted. Greenlee (13) recommends that heart rates not exceed the rate that elicits a systolic blood pressure of 170 mm Hg for individuals with proliferative retinopathy. Exercise resulting in a large increase in systolic pressure (such as weightlifting) can cause retinal hemorrhage and worsen the retinopathy. Exercise for these patients should involve stationary cycling, walking, and swimming. If possible, blood pressure should be monitored during the exercise program. Exercise is contraindicated if the individual has had recent photocoagulation treatment or surgery. Activities such as bungee jumping are ill-advised because of the potential for retinal damage.

Nephropathy Those diabetic patients with some degree of nephropathy may benefit from the reduction in risk factors with exercise; however, vigorous hemodynamic exercise should be avoided. This includes lifting heavy weights and high intensity aerobic activities. Activities that are weightbearing yet low impact are preferable, and it is important to wear well-cushioned shoes. Renal patients should be fully evaluated before commencing any exercise program. Fluid replacement is extremely important in these patients. Specific training programs for patients undergoing hemodialysis are advised (14). Because of the potential for hypoglycemia, diabetic patients are advised against activities such as scuba diving, parachuting, and rock climbing.

Conclusion

The athlete with diabetes needs a good understanding of the effects of exercise on blood glucose levels. With regular monitoring and appropriate adjustments to insulin dosage and carbohydrate intake, the athlete with diabetes can participate fully in most sporting activities.

MENSTRUAL IRREGULARITIES ASSOCIATED WITH EXERCISE

Exercise is associated with disorders of the menstrual cycle such as delayed menarche, luteal dysfunction, and amenorrhea.

Delayed Menarche

The average age of menarche is between 12 and 13 years. Menarche (the onset of menstrual bleeding) usually occurs 1 to 2 years after the commencement of the pubertal growth spurt. The exact mechanisms determining the timing of menarche are not known, although genetic factors play an important role.

Evidence suggests that the age of menarche correlates with athletic performance, so high-performance athletes tend to have a later age of menarche than the normal population (15). These high-performance athletes fall into two groups: those who commence intense physical training prior to menarche, and those who commence training after menarche. The presence of delayed-onset menarche in both groups indicates that there may be a combination of factors causing this condition.

intense training in premenarcheal years, as occurs commonly in ballet dancers and gymnasts, is associated with delayed-onset menarche (15). This association does not necessarily imply cause and effect. Thinness, which may occur as a result of intense training, may be the most important factor preventing the onset of menses. The combination of intensive exercise and low body weight may affect the hypothalamic secretion of hormones, thus delaying the onset of menarche. Also of note is that breast development and menarche may be delayed, but the development of pubic hair is not.

The observation that high-performance female athletes have a history of delayed-onset menarche, even without a history of intense training prior to menarche, suggests that delayed menarche may confer some athletic advantage. Athletes may inherit a tendency for a slower rate of maturation, and this may lead to prolonged bony growth (due to delayed closure of the bony epiphyses). Late maturity is associated with longer legs, narrower hips, less weight per unit height, and less relative body fat than the early maturer, and these factors can be advantageous to athletic performance. There may also be a sociologic component to this process.

Luteal Phase Defects

Abnormal luteal function is common among athletes (16). The luteal phase extends from the time of ovulation to the onset of menstruation; it is normally associated with high levels of estrogen and progesterone, and its normal length is 14 days. A shortened luteal phase of less than 10 days is commonly found in exercising women and is usually associated with lower than normal levels of progesterone. This abnormality of the luteal phase is often not recognized because the women still menstruate regularly. There may be an associated slightly prolonged follicular phase resulting in normal or near-normal lengths of the menstrual cycle (28 days). This condition may only be recognized by plotting basal body temperature, which fails to show the expected rise seen in a normal luteal phase. Low progesterone levels in the luteal phase of the cycle may also be an indicator of luteal phase defect.

There appears to be a direct relationship between the amount of exercise and the development of luteal phase defects. It is uncertain whether this luteal insufficiency is a stage in a continuum of menstrual cycle irregularity proceeding to oligomenorrhea or amenorrhea, or whether it is a separate entity. The main effects of luteal phase defects are infertility or subfertility. Another concern is the possibility of an increased risk of endometrial carcinoma due to the effect of unopposed estrogen activity with reduced progesterone levels.

Oligomenorrhea and Amenorrhea

The incidence of oligomenorrhea (irregular menstruation) and amenorrhea (absent menstruation) is increased in the sporting population. Studies have shown the incidence of these conditions in athletes to be between 10% and 20% (17,18), compared with the incidence in the general population of 5%. The incidence in runners and ballet dancers has been found to be particularly high compared with swimmers and cyclists (19). It is

thought that as many as 50% of competitive distance runners have reduced or absent periods (19). These conditions are associated with reduction of the pulse frequency of luteinizing hormone (LH) and low levels of the hormones estrogen and progesterone.

Causes of Exercise-Associated Menstrual Irregularities

The mechanism producing menstrual cycle irregularity in the athlete is centered on the hypothalamus. A variety of interacting factors probably cause hypothalamic dysfunction and subsequent reduction in the release of gonadotrophin-releasing hormone (GnRH), which controls the release from the pituitary gland of the reproductive hormones follicle-stimulating hormone (FSH) and luteinizing hormone (LH). These hormones directly control the events of the menstrual cycle, including the production of estrogen and progesterone. Athletic amenorrhea is therefore one form of hypothalamic amenorrhea. Other forms of hypothalamic amenorrhea include psychogenic amenorrhea, anorexia nervosa, and amenorrhea associated with malnutrition or drugs (e.g., phenothiazines).

As the hypothalamic and pituitary changes in response to exercise are found not only in women with menstrual irregularities but also in those with normal, regular menstrual cycles, there must be another important factor in the etiology of these conditions. Certain women may show a particular susceptibility to such exercise-induced hypothalamic and pituitary changes. This group may be classed as those with "immature" reproductive systems.

A summary of the causes of menstrual cycle irregularity is shown in Figure 28-1. The factors that may contribute to hypothalamic dysfunction include low body fat, psychological stress, level of exercise, and an immature reproductive system.

Low Body Fat

There is a clear association between reduced body fat and the incidence of menstrual cycle irregularity (17,18). This is not to say that there is a critical level of body fat below which menstrual cycle irregularities develop as was once thought. There is considerable individual variation, and there may

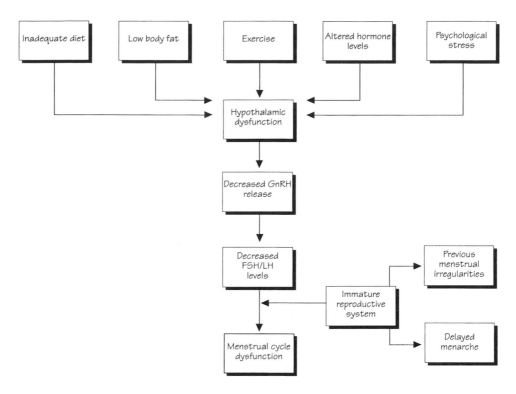

Figure 28-1. Causes of menstrual cycle irregularities. (Reproduced by permission from Brukner P, Khan K. Clinical sports medicine. Sidney: McGraw-Hill, 1993:547.)

be a critical level for each individual. There have been numerous examples reported where amenorrheic athletes have increased their percentages of body fat for some reason (e.g., reduction in activity or injury), and normal menstruation has resumed.

Inadequate Diet
Inadequate dietary intake may be a factor in the production of menstrual cycle irregularities (17,20–22). The most likely dietary causes are inadequate caloric intake or inadequate levels of dietary components such as protein, carbohydrate, or calcium. Whether this dietary inadequacy has its effect on menstrual cycle irregularity directly or by a reduction in body fat is uncertain.

Psychological Stress
Studies establish that psychological stress affects hypothalamic function, and many athletes experience high levels of psychological stress either re-

lated to their sporting activity or to outside factors such as work, family, or relationships. Psychological stress may be a contributing factor in the development of menstrual irregularities in athletes, but as yet no convincing evidence has emerged (17).

Level of Exercise
There appears to be a relationship between menstrual irregularities and the level of exercise performed, as determined by either the total amount of exercise or the intensity of the activity. As mentioned previously, normal menstruation often resumes with cessation of athletic activity from injury or retirement, or even with reduction of exercise during a precompetition taper or during the off-season. Frequently menstruation then ceases on resumption of the previous level of exercise.

Exercise, as a form of stress, may have a direct effect on the hypothalamus; alternatively, it may have its effect through the actions of one or more of the hormones whose levels are elevated by exercise. Two hormones that are elevated during exercise and may affect the hypothalamus are cortisol and the opioid peptides. Cortisol levels have been shown to increase with exercise. This may be associated with increased corticotropin and corticotropin releasing hormone (CRH). It is possible that CRH may inhibit secretion of LH from the pituitary. Opioid peptides such as beta endorphins are elevated with exercise and may have a negative feedback effect on the hypothalamus.

The "Immature" Reproductive System   The factors above may all interact to affect hypothalamic and pituitary function in athletes. Why then do only certain athletes develop menstrual cycle irregularities? One theory suggests that certain women are susceptible to these irregularities, possibly because of immaturity of the reproductive system (23). This may explain why the incidence of menstrual cycle irregularities is more common in younger women, women who have not been pregnant, women with a family history or past history of menstrual irregularity, and those with a history of delayed menarche.

Complications of Exercise-Associated Menstrual Cycle Irregularities

There are two major problems associated with menstrual cycle irregularities. These are reduced fertility and reduced bone mass.

Reduced Fertility   Intensely exercising females have reduced fertility compared with their sedentary counterparts. Anovulatory cycles are common in athletes and may be associated with amenorrhea, oligomenorrhea, and luteal phase defects, or may occur in otherwise normally menstruating athletes. A good indication that ovulation has occurred in a particular cycle is the presence of either premenstrual symptoms at the end of the cycle or ovulation pain in midcycle. Ovulation may be confirmed with the use of the basal body temperature, which rises between 0.2 °C and 0.6 °C at the time of ovulation and remains elevated during the luteal phase.

The athlete should not automatically assume that amenorrhea necessarily means infertility. There have been many examples of athletes with long histories of amenorrhea becoming pregnant. If pregnancy is desired, ovulation and a normal menstrual cycle can usually be induced by reducing the level of exercise or increasing the level of body fat. If this does not induce ovulation, the athlete should be referred for gynecologic assessment; if necessary ovulation can be induced by pharmacologic means.

Reduced Bone Mass   Since 1984 it has become clear that there is an association between exercise-associated amenorrhea and reduced bone density (24). This reduction in bone density relates to the low estrogen levels associated with amenorrhea. This condition is similar to that which occurs after menopause and appears to affect mainly trabecular bone rather than cortical bone. Lack of estrogen has been shown to have a negative effect on bone density, but exercise, especially weightbearing exercise, has been shown to have a positive effect at specific weightbearing sites. In females with exercise-associated amenorrhea, the negative effect of lack of estrogen may have a marked effect at nonweightbearing sites, but minimal effect at weightbearing sites.

Hypoestrogenic athletes have been found to lose bone mass in a similar way to postmenopausal women. Bone is lost rapidly in the first 2 or 3 years following loss of estrogen at a rate of approximately 4% per year. After the first few years, the rate of loss continues at a slower rate. This is an important consideration in the treatment of amenorrheic athletes because the reduction of bone mass in athletes can have two detrimental effects: a possibly increased susceptibility of developing fractures and postmenopausal osteoporosis.

Stress Fractures   Stress fractures occur in both males and normally menstruating females; however, it seems that the incidence of stress fractures in amenorrheic females is higher than among normally menstruating females (25,26). This higher incidence may not be related to a decrease in bone mass. The reduction in bone mass appears to occur primarily in trabecular bone, with little or no effect on cortical bone, but stress fractures occur mainly in the cortical bones of the lower limb, such as the tibia. Also, a reduction in bone density in athletes with stress fractures has not been demonstrated (27). Bone density does not necessarily relate to bone strength, but it is the only parameter that can be easily measured. Unfortunately, bone density has not, until recently, been measured in fractured bones; thus far, the indications are that there is no relationship between decreased bone density and the incidence of stress fractures.

Postmenopausal Osteoporosis   The reduction in bone mass among amenorrhea suffers may increase the susceptibility of these athletes to the development of postmenopausal osteoporosis. Postmenopausal osteoporosis is a major health problem in Western societies, characterized by the high incidence of osteoporosis-related traumatic fractures, especially of the spine, hip, and wrist. These fractures are associated with a high morbidity and mortality. The most important means of prevention of postmenopausal osteoporosis is the attainment of a high peak bone mass. Peak bone mass, which is now thought to be attained as early as 16 to 20 years of age, is dependent on a number of interrelated factors including genetics, nutrition (especially calcium intake), exercise, and hormonal status. Of these factors, probably the most important is hormonal status. The presence of estrogen is necessary for the attainment of adequate peak bone mass. Lengthy periods of hypoestrogenism associated with delayed menarche or hypoestrogenic athletic amenorrhea during the vital bone-forming years of ages 10 to 20 result in lowered peak bone mass, thus increasing the likelihood of postmenopausal osteoporosis.

Treatment of Exercise-Associated Menstrual Irregularities

Delayed Menarche   If menstruation has not occurred by the age of 16 years, medical evaluation should be considered. It is important to exclude any other possible cause of delayed menarche. For example, genetic abnormalities and ovarian failure are rare causes of delayed menarche, and the possibility of an eating disorder such as anorexia nervosa should also be considered.

In compiling the patient history, the physician should ask about the development of secondary sexual characteristics, weight changes, virilizing changes, possibility of pregnancy, drug use, emotional problems, or increased psychological stress. A family history of any delay in menarche or chromosomal disorders should also be determined.

A thorough examination should look for evidence of neurologic disorders or endocrine disorders (e.g., thyroid, adrenal, and pituitary disorders),

and should include assessment of visual fields and visual acuity. Ideally, a pelvic examination should also be performed, but in the sexually inactive patient it may be more appropriate to perform a transabdominal pelvic ultrasound examination to exclude any gynecologic abnormality. A blood test should be performed to assess prolactin, FSH and LH levels, and thyroid function tests (TFT). The presence of adequate levels of estrogen may be assessed by measuring the serum estradiol.

The combination of an ultrasound scan that demonstrates the presence of a uterus and adequate serum estradiol levels excludes most gynecologic causes of primary amenorrhea. Performing a progesterone challenge is an alternative method of assessment. This involves the patient taking a 5-day course of the progesterone derivative medroxyprogesterone acetate (Provera). If a withdrawal bleed occurs after completion of the course, the endometrium (lining of the uterus) has been stimulated by estrogen. If no bleed occurs, the patient should be regarded as hypoestrogenic.

Delayed menarche secondary to intense training is characterized by low FSH and LH levels typical of prepubertal levels. The bone age may also be delayed. Bone age may be assessed by plain x-ray. If genetic abnormalities are suspected, blood tests show a raised FSH level, or if the patient is 18 years or older, a blood karyotype should be performed and the athlete referred for specialized assessment.

Management of the young athlete with delayed menarche involves reassurance to the girl and her parents that there is no structural or endocrine abnormality and that the delay in menarche is related to her level of exercise. She should be informed that a reduction in the level of exercise and a slight increase in the level of body fat will probably result in the commencement of menstruation. However, should the girl wish to maintain or increase her level of exercise, then estrogen replacement should be commenced if there is evidence of hypoestrogenism—evidence shows that the maximum amount of bone loss in the hypoestrogenic athlete occurs in the first 2 or 3 years. The girl should be given the option of commencing estrogen therapy either in the form of the oral contraceptive pill or as the combination of estrogen and progesterone therapy used by post-menopausal women.

Luteal Phase Defects   Luteal phase defects do not require treatment unless fertility is required. If fertility is desired, treatment should be along the lines mentioned in the section discussing fertility.

Oligomenorrhea and Amenorrhea   As in the case of athletes with delayed menarche, one must not automatically assume that amenorrhea in an athlete is caused by exercise. Other possible causes of amenorrhea must be excluded, notably pregnancy. Psychological stress, anorexia nervosa, polycystic ovaries, thyroid disease, prolactinoma, oral contraceptive pills, drugs, and constitutional disorders should also be considered in the differential diagnosis.

A thorough history and examination should be performed to detect all possible causes of amenorrhea. Blood tests should be performed to assess levels of prolactin, FSH, LH, TFT, and serum estradiol. Typical findings in exercise-associated amenorrhea are low levels of FSH, LH, and estradiol. A bone density examination should be considered if the period of amenorrhea exceeds 1 year, or if a stress fracture is present.

The main object of treatment of athletes with hypoestrogenic amenorrhea is to ensure adequate estrogen levels. This objective may be achieved by the athlete reducing the level of exercise or increasing the percentage of body fat, either of which usually results in the spontaneous resumption of normal menstruation. Restoration of bone mass lost as a result of exercise-induced amenorrhea may occur with natural resumption of menses, particularly when the period of amenorrhea has been less than 4 years (28,29).

If the athlete is unwilling to reduce the level of exercise, estrogen replacement should be commenced as early as possible after the onset of amenorrhea because bone loss is maximal in the first 2 to 3 years after onset. Estrogen replacement may restore bone mass lost from hypoestrogenic amenorrhea of up to 3 years' duration. When the period of amenorrhea is longer than 3 years, estrogen replacement should still be given in order to prevent further bone loss.

Estrogen may be given in the form of the oral contraceptive pill or as combined estrogen–progesterone therapy. The oral contraceptive pill, which has the advantage of providing contraception for the sexually active amenorrheic woman who wishes to avoid pregnancy, should be provided as one of the monophasic pills. Alternatively, cyclical estrogen and progesterone can be given as conjugated equine estrogens, 0.625 mg daily on days 1 to 25 of the calendar month, and medroxyprogesterone acetate, 5 mg on days 14 to 25 of the month. Following cessation of the tablets, a withdrawal bleed usually occurs.

Contraindications to estrogen therapy include hypertension, abnormal liver function, any history of deep venous thrombosis, breast or endometrial carcinoma, and undiagnosed abnormal vaginal bleeding.

Calcium is an important factor in maximizing bone mass. The recommended daily intake of calcium in hypoestrogenic women is 1500 mg per day. Adolescents and young adults are advised to take 1200 mg per day.

Unfortunately, the first presentation of the amenorrheic athlete may be a stress fracture. Bone density examination should be performed on all amenorrheic athletes with a stress fracture, and this should be repeated at 12-month intervals. The probable relationship between the stress fracture and the athlete's amenorrhea should be discussed with the athlete. Advice should be given regarding calcium and estrogen therapy as well as specific activity. Regardless of estrogen status, the physician should also assess the presence of any other predisposing factors (such as biomechanical faults) to the development of stress fractures; if other factors are present, these must be corrected before the athlete resumes activity.

THE MALE REPRODUCTIVE SYSTEM

Physical activity can have a range of effects on male reproductive function, depending on the intensity and duration of the activity and the fitness of the individual. In particular, endurance training may be associated with reduction in circulating testosterone levels.

Testosterone
Testosterone has an important anabolic role, so alteration in reproductive hormone profiles may

have detrimental skeletal consequences similar to those seen in females with menstrual disturbances (30).

The main functions of the testes, steroid biosynthesis and spermatogenesis, are controlled by higher structures of the hypothalamic–pituitary–gonadal (HPG) axis operating under a negative feedback system. Testosterone is the major gonadal regulatory hormone (31). GnRH, secreted in pulses by the hypothalamus, stimulates the pituitary gland to secrete two gonadotrophic hormones: LH and FSH. LH stimulates the testis to secrete testosterone, and FSH facilitates sperm production.

Approximately 95% of circulating serum testosterone comes from production in the testis, and the remainder is produced in the adrenal glands. Testosterone is found in plasma primarily bound to proteins, albumen, and sex hormone–binding globulin (SHBG); a small proportion (3%) circulates unbound and is referred to as free testosterone (30). The biologically active forms of testosterone are those that are bound to albumen and the small unbound or free portion (32).

As well as being responsible for the development and maintenance of secondary sex characteristics and for spermatogenesis, testosterone is a powerful anabolic hormone that stimulates tissue growth and development. Testosterone has important effects on bone mass, as demonstrated by findings that hypogonadism in males is a risk factor for osteoporosis (33–35). Testosterone may have direct effects on bone formation, given that androgen receptors have been identified on osteoblasts (36). It may also act indirectly by augmenting the nocturnal secretion of growth hormone and subsequently insulin-like growth factor 1 (IGF-1), particularly during puberty, and by increasing muscular activity and stresses on the skeleton (promoting bone mass at local sites).

Effect of Exercise on Testosterone Levels

Relatively short-duration exercise bouts at maximal or near-maximal intensity appear to increase serum testosterone levels, with measurable changes evident within minutes (37–42). However, prolonged acute submaximal exercise bouts of approximately 2 hours or longer suppress circulating testosterone, and levels may remain low for several days (38–43). Controversy exists regarding the effects of chronic intense exercise on basal testosterone levels. Apparently some male athletes who train intensely may experience reductions in testosterone levels.

Long-term exercise-associated suppression of serum testosterone levels may result from decreased production levels, decreased protein binding, or increased clearance (44). Of these, the most likely mechanism is decreased testosterone production arising from either intrinsic failure of the testis to maintain adequate steroid biosynthesis, perhaps due to testicular microtrauma and temperature elevation (45), or from central dysfunction in the HPG axis.

Osteopenia   Limited studies have failed to establish a relationship between lowered circulating testosterone and osteopenia in male athletes (46–49). However, there are a number of methodologic problems with these studies. Bone density in male athletes can be lower without a concurrent decrease in testosterone, suggesting that bone density and testosterone levels are not closely related. Further research is necessary to monitor concurrent changes in bone density and testosterone over a period of time in exercising males. In any case, the effect of exercise on the male reproductive system does not appear as extreme as it is on the female system, and any impact on bone density is not nearly as evident.

The study results imply that factors apart from testosterone levels must be responsible for the observed osteopenia in some male athletes. Many factors have the potential to adversely affect bone density independently of alterations in reproductive functions, including low calcium intake, energy deficit, weight loss, psychological stress, and low body fat. All of these factors may be associated with intense endurance training (50).

Puberty   Although a delayed onset of menarche can be assessed in females, there is no physiologic index comparable to assess age of menarche and pubertal development in males. Longitudinal data indicate that sporting participation has little effect on attained stature, the timing of peak height velocity, rate of statural growth, or sexual maturation in males (51). Whether these results necessarily apply to intense endurance exercise is unclear as most studies do not focus on such extreme forms of exercise. Although males with delayed puberty have been found to exhibit significant osteopenia, the pubertal delay in these reports is not attributed to sporting pursuits but to some disease process or congenital disorder.

THYROID GLAND

Approximately 5% of the human population is affected by either hypo- or hyperthyroidism, with women being overrepresented (52). As changes in thyroid state affect both cardiovascular and skeletal muscle tissues, altered thyroid function may affect the ability to perform exercise.

Hypothyroidism

Hypothyroidism is associated with decreased exercise tolerance (53). Inadequate blood flow to skeletal muscle contributes significantly to exercise intolerance through insufficient oxygen delivery and suboptimal delivery of blood-borne substrates such as glucose and free fatty acids (54–56). Exercise intolerance may also be related to mucopolysaccharide abnormalities interfering with muscle metabolism. Reduced skeletal muscle oxidative capacity is a feature of hypothyroidism (57–59), and impaired lipid oxidation (56) results in a greater reliance on intramuscular carbohydrate (60,61).

Treatment of hypothyroidism follows established principles, with replacement therapy using synthetic hormones L-thyroxine and L-triiodothyronine in the majority of cases. Return to a normal metabolic state over a period is recommended for most patients, as sudden physiologic change can affect cardiac function adversely. The maintenance dose of thyroxine, approximately 1.7 μg per kilogram body weight per day, provides serum levels of thyroxine at the upper normal range. Once stabilized, the patient should be permitted to exercise as he or she wishes with the proviso that medical review be undertaken every few months.

Hyperthyroidism

Hyperthyroid individuals have reduced exercise tolerance, although the mechanism for this association is unclear (53). Hyperthyroidism increases cardiac output and reduces total peripheral resistance (52,62,63), changes that result in increased blood flow to skeletal muscle during exercise. As this hyperperfusion ought to improve exercise capacity, other factors must explain the exercise intolerance noted in hyperthyroidism. Resting glycogen levels are reduced in hyperthyroid humans (64,65), and studies show that glycogen is depleted at a faster rate during submaximal exercise (66). These findings probably account for the higher blood lactate and muscle lactate levels reported during submaximal exercise in the hyperthyroid state. It appears that these effects on glycogen metabolism account in large part for the reduced endurance characteristics of hyperthyroid individuals. Another factor that may contribute to reduced endurance is a relative hyperthermia in the hyperthyroid state. Internal body temperatures are higher during submaximal exercise in hyperthyroidism, possibly due to greater heat production and/or impaired heat dissipation (67).

Treatment of hyperthyroidism depends on careful assessment of thyroid status, as this can vary unpredictably and even result in a hypothyroid state (after chronic thyroiditis, for example). In general, long-term antithyroid therapy with propylthiouracil (100 mg three or four times a day) or methimazole (10 mg three or four times a day) is used for children, young adults, or pregnant women, and sometimes L-thyroxine is added to guard against accidental hypothyroidism. Good control is manifest by normal thyroid function tests and clinical signs. The practitioner must monitor for side effects, including the recognized complication of leukopenia from drug therapy.

Iodide has its place in more severe thyrotoxicosis and the reader is referred to appropriate texts for comprehensive discussion of this therapy.

Beta-blockers such as propranolol (40 to 120 mg/day) counter the adrenergic effects of thyrotoxicosis, such as sweating, tremor, and tachycardia. These agents are banned in competition under Olympic regulations, and patients who wish to compete in this context should apply to the appropriate sport governing body to obtain dispensation for reasons of health.

Radioactive therapy and surgery for hyperthyroid conditions are potential therapeutic options discussed in appropriate texts.

With appropriate treatment and careful supervision, patients can exercise. High-intensity activities or prolonged exercise are not recommended for physiologic reasons, especially in cases that manifest cardiac involvement. Walking, golf, gentle swimming, or cycling should all be possible for the well-managed patient.

Growth Hormone Excess: Acromegaly and Gigantism

An excess of growth hormone (GH), whether from a pituitary adenoma or from self-administration, results in acromegaly, a condition characterized by bony and soft tissue hypertrophy. When GH excess develops prior to closure of epiphyses, gigantism results, and this is typified by accelerated linear growth. The enlargement of tissues produces the recognizable signs of large hands and feet, prognathism, enlarged tongue, spaced teeth, coarse facial features, skin tags, acanthosis nigricans, and oily skin.

Presentation   Although acromegaly is rare, it can be found in sport because of the height advantage given by the disease—currently at least three athletes with known acromegaly are playing at the national and international level. The disease produces muscle weakness (despite muscle size) and fatigue. The basal metabolic rate increases and causes increased sweat and sebaceous gland activity. Many patients complain of headaches, nerve entrapments (such as carpal tunnel syndrome or ulnar neuropathy), and/or arthralgia of large joints. Hypertension commonly develops and leads to increased left ventricular wall thickness and congestive cardiac failure. Amenorrhea may occur (with or without hyperprolactinemia), and hirsutism is common. Thyroid goiter is common, and 3% to 7% of patients are hyperthyroid (68). Some studies report inguinal hernias and abdominal pain each in approximately one-third of patients, and intracranial aneurysms coexist in up to 10% of patients (67).

Acromegaly patients have shortened life expectancies; death results from cerebrovascular, cardiovascular, or respiratory disease, or from associated diabetes mellitus (a product of growth hormone's anti-insulin effect). Associated endocrinopathies include hyperparathyroidism (with hypercalciuria and renal stones), hyperprolactinemia (with galactorrhea, amenorrhea, and loss of libido), pancreatic islet cell tumors, pheochromocytoma, and hyperaldosteronism. Pituitary adenomas are found in most patients with acromegaly and giantism. Tumors are more aggressive in younger patients (hence, contributing large adolescents to sports such as basketball) and GH levels in blood correlate with tumor size.

Diagnosis   Basal or random GH levels may be elevated in normal persons, with diabetes mellitus, renal failure, or stress, thus diagnosis relies on measurements of glucose-suppressed GH concentration (<2 μg/L 60 to 120 min after 100 gram oral glucose is recommended [58]) and estimation of insulin-like growth factor 1/somatomedin-C (IGF-1/SM-C) concentrations in serum. Measurements of serum IGF-1/SM-C concentrations correlate with disease activity.

Imaging of the sella turcica with computed tomography or magnetic resonance imaging is recommended, as the yield is 90% for finding the pituitary tumor in the acromegalic patient. Skeletal x-rays may show tufting of the distal phalanges of the hands or feet, enlarged vertebral bodies with anterior lipping, bowing of the long bones of the lower limb, and thickening of the ribs and clavicles. Soft-tissue radiographs show thickening of the heel pad (>18 mm in females, >21 mm in males).

Testing of pituitary insufficiency is recommended, together with screening for hyperprolactinemia. Large adenomas can impair visual fields and produce oculomotor and/or abducens neuropathy.

Treatment   Patients should be treated as a matter of urgency. The aims of therapy are to return levels of GH and IGF-1/SM-C to normal, prevent tumor enlargement, and preserve pituitary function. The range of modalities used in treatment include trans-sphenoidal surgery, pituitary irradiation, and chemotherapy with bromocriptine and/or octreotide (which inhibits GH secretion). Management requires long-term follow-up and attention to associated disorders such as diabetes mellitus, together with regular screening for colonic cancer.

Acromegaly and Gigantism in Athletes   In distinct contrast to the wealth of research published on aspects of growth hormone use and abuse in sport, there has been scant discussion of acromegaly (or gigantism) in the literature. For the clinician managing an athlete with acromegaly or gigantism, the best advice is to work closely in consultation with specialist management to gain control of the disease as quickly as possible.

Those who have cared for athletes with acromegaly know that playing a sport such as basketball at an elite level is entirely possible, despite active disease. Such athletes typically pass off complaints of fatigue or arthralgia of knees and ankles as the usual aches and pains associated with competitive sport. Treatment, however, can have dramatic effects. One of the authors (PF) diagnosed acromegaly in a 23-year-old female basketball player at the international level during a medical examination at the start of her contract with a new team. Surgery to the pituitary for a large active adenoma resulted in rapid diminution of fatigue, headaches, and (some) weight, accompanied by markedly improved on-court performance in running, jumping, and cutting. Her personality changed from pleasant and cheerful to positively buoyant, and her contribution to the team's efforts grew accordingly. The time lost to her sport was of the order of 3 to 4 months, and her postoperative recovery (12 months) was uneventful.

Conclusion

Clinicians must be aware of the possibility of pathogenic mechanisms for tall or large athletes. Conditions such as acromegaly and gigantism certainly do not prevent participation at elite levels of sport, but are nevertheless insidious diseases with the potential to shorten life.

ADRENAL GLAND DISORDERS

The adrenal cortex is stimulated by the polypeptide adrenocorticotrophic hormone (ACTH) to synthesize the steroids glucocorticoids (cortisol), mineralocorticoids (aldosterone), and adrenal androgens (dehydroepiandrosterone). Distinct zones of the adrenal cortex produce specific hormones. This is a result of each zone having its particular enzymes to carry out the processes of hydroxylation and molecular transformations. The outer zone (zona glomerulosa) produces mainly aldosterone, and the inner zone (zona fasciculata reticularis) is the site of androgen and cortisol synthesis.

Cushing's Syndrome

Cushing's syndrome is a hyperfunction of the adrenal cortex. Cushing originally described the syndrome as truncal obesity, hypertension, fatigability and weakness, amenorrhea, hirsutism, purple abdominal striae, edema, glucosuria, osteoporosis, and a basophilic tumor of the pituitary gland (69). Most cases are due to bilateral adrenal hyperplasia, which may result from excess pituitary ACTH secretion or from neuroendocrine tumors (e.g., bronchogenic carcinoma, pancreatic carcinoma). Pituitary-dependent adrenal hyperplasia is three times more common in women than in men and typically presents in the third and fourth decades. Cushing's syndrome is rare in children and adolescents, usually results from pituitary tumor, and is characterized by weight gain and growth retardation (70).

Many of the symptoms and signs of Cushing's syndrome can be deduced from the action of cortisol. The features of muscle weakness and fatigue, osteoporosis, and the evidence of connective tissue breakdown (such as striae and the tendency to bruise easily) are all direct effects of glucocorticoid excess. The complication of diabetes mellitus (seen in 20% of patients), hypertension, and the tendency to deposit adipose tissue (resulting in truncal obesity, "moon" facies, and the "buffalo hump") are also results of this abnormal physiologic state. Increased androgen production results in hirsutism, acne, and oligo- or amenorrhea. Mood state is often disturbed, ranging from emotional lability to overt psychosis (69).

The diagnosis of Cushing's syndrome depends on demonstrating increased cortisol production and the failure to suppress this with dexamethasone administration. Further investigation is necessary to determine the source of the stimulus to excess adrenal activity; particular attention is paid to possible pituitary or other (neuroendocrine) tumors. (The appropriate texts on the syndrome contain more detailed discussion.)

Therapy for this condition depends on diagnosis. Tumor excision or ablation (at adrenal, pituitary, or other sites), chemotherapy, and adrenalectomy are potential options. Appropriate replacement therapy follows definitive treatment and requires constant surveillance to maintain satisfactory management.

Adrenal Hypercortisolism and Exercise
There is a dearth of literature on the subject of Cushing's syndrome and exercise, but it would appear that patients who are appropriately managed and in remission on maintenance therapy (as appropriate) should be permitted to exercise as they wish. This clinical condition should be compatible with low-intensity exercise such as walking, swimming, and golf. Exercise may help promote well-being and perhaps counter osteoporosis. Given the problems of skin susceptibility to bruising, infection, and laceration (with poor healing), and underlying conditions such as hypertension and diabetes mellitus, advising patients against intense exercise or any activity with the potential for contact or physical injury is sensible.

Hypofunction of the Adrenal Cortex: Addison's Disease

Addison's original description of "general languor and debility, remarkable feebleness of the heart's action, irritability of the stomach, and a peculiar change of color of the skin" summarizes the dominant clinical features of primary adrenocortical deficiency, or Addison's disease (71). Addison's disease is quite rare, can occur at any age, and affects both sexes equally. As a result of the therapeutic use of steroids, secondary adrenal insufficiency is becoming more common (71).

Addison's disease is an autoimmune disorder that produces its effects after 90% of the adrenal cortex has been destroyed. In a recent series of 91 patients with this disorder, autoimmune adrenalitis was considered the cause of 91% and tuberculosis the cause of another 7%. The patients with autoimmune disease displayed conditions as follows (72):

20%	associated primary hypothyroidism
10%	vitiligo
8%	nontoxic thyroid goiter
7%	(of women) premature menopause
6%	Graves' disease
5%	pernicious anemia
2%	Sjögren's disease
1%	hypoparathyroidism
1%	diabetes mellitus
1%	coeliac disease

Autoantibodies to the adrenal were detected in 83% of these patients, with antibodies against microsomal antigens, thyroglobulin, parietal cells, pancreatic islet cells, and the ovary also detected (in decreasing order of frequency from 58% to 4%) (72).

The other significant causes of adrenal insufficiency are primarily infectious. They include AIDS, cytomegalovirus, *Mycobacterium avium intracellulare*, cryptococcus, histoplasmosis, and coccidioidomycosis.

Symptoms The cardinal symptom of Addison's disease is asthenia—typically of gradual onset, but often dramatic in its intensity. Pigmentation of the skin results in a diffuse tanned appearance of areas of the body both exposed and unexposed to the sun. The mucous membranes may bear blue-black patches, and patchy vitiligo may develop.

Postural hypotension and arterial hypotension per se are typical findings, together with gastrointestinal signs, and symptoms of anorexia, weight loss, vomiting, and diarrhea, and vague abdominal pain. Mood change is common, and the loss of pubic and axillary hair in females may result from androgen loss.

The diagnosis depends on demonstrating depleted adrenal reserve by administration of ACTH, together with low urinary cortisol and other steroid production and various electrolyte disturbances (such as hyponatremia, hyperkalemia, hypercalcemia, and acidosis).

Treatment All patients with Addison's disease should receive specific hormone replacement. Most patients are managed on 25–37.5 mg cortisone daily in divided doses (or prednisone 7.5 mg/day in divided doses), with two-thirds given in the morning with food and one-third in the evening with food. In addition, 0.05–0.1 mg fludrocortisone is given daily to maintain adequate mineralocorticoid levels, and 3–4 gram per day of sodium is recommended to help maintain intravascular volume.

During periods of illness, doses of cortisone should be increased to 75–150 mg per day (in divided doses), and similar provisions must be made for patients undergoing surgery. The appropriate texts contain more detailed discussions of these concerns.

Adrenal crisis results from a physiologic demand for increased cortisol—such as during bouts of infection, trauma (or surgery), gastrointestinal upsets, or significant stress (including exercise). Crisis, which is manifested by profound circulatory collapse and a worsening of any or all preexisting symptoms and signs, requires urgent hospital-based resuscitation.

Addison's Disease and Exercise   For Addison's disease patients who wish to exercise at any intensity—and certainly whenever sweating for any period of time is anticipated—doses of cortisone should be increased as previously discussed for illness or stress; also, fludrocortisone should be increased to double the usual dose, supplemented by added salt intake. Regular exercise with regular levels of steroid therapy are obviously easier to manage than intermittent bouts and dose adjustments. Any adjustments of dosage and exercise levels must be closely monitored and followed up over ensuing days.

The question of bone mineral density in patients with Addison's disease has been examined. In a group (n = 30) of men and women patients on cortisone replacement therapy, two analyses over 12 months showed no significant lumbar (trabecular) bone loss in premenopausal women and men compared with controls, and slight loss only in postmenopausal patients (73). The effect of exercise was not studied. By contrast, another study on Addison's disease patients that involved 9 females and 5 males, aged around the mid-50s, reported that the women had a greater than expected reduction in bone mineral density (74). This latter study examined the lumbar spine and femoral neck, but did not evaluate exercise.

The available reports provide mixed messages, but it is clear that bone mineral density is a concern for patients on glucocorticoid therapy, and that weightbearing exercise may be therapeutic. Certainly younger patients would do well to undertake regular low-intensity workouts (such as walking, cycling, and perhaps swimming) to promote bone health through gentle impact and muscle exercise. Similarly, older patients may at least attempt to minimize any demineralization associated with their therapy. Beyond this, regular, gentle aerobic exercise is believed to promote a sense of well-being and a positive outlook, which may themselves be beneficial.

REFERENCES

1   World Health Organisation Study Group. Technical report series No 727. Geneva, Switzerland, 1985.
2   Leahy JL, Boyd AE III. Diabetes genes in non-insulin-dependent diabetes mellitus. N Engl J Med 1993;328:56–57.
3   Pfeiffer EF, Dolderer M. Etiopathogenesis of type II diabetes. Medicographia 1987;9:22–26.
4   Fajans SS, Cloutier MC, Crowther RL. The Banting Memorial Lecture, 1978: clinical and etiologic heterogeneity of idiopathic diabetes mellitus. Diabetes 1978;27:1112–1125.
5   DeFronzo R, Ferrannini E, Koivisto V. New concepts in the pathogenesis and treatment of non insulin dependent diabetes mellitus. Am J Med 1983;74(suppl. 1A):52–81.
6   Halter JB, Graf RJ, Porte D Jr. Potentiation of insulin secretory responses by plasma glucose tolerance and plasma glucose levels in U.S. population aged 30–74 years. Diabetes 1979;36:523–534.
7   DeFronzo R, Deibert D, Hendler R, et al. Insulin sensitivity and insulin binding to monocytes in maturity onset diabetes. J Clin Invest 1979; 63:939–946.
8   Olefsky JM, Kolterman OG, Scarlett JA. Insulin action and resistance in obesity and non-insulin-dependent type II diabetes mellitus. Am J Physiol 1982;243:E15–E30.
9   Gerich JE. Assessment of insulin resistance and its role in non insulin dependent diabetes mellitus. J Lab Clin Med 1984;103(4):497–505.
10   Revers RR, Fink R, Griffin J, et al. Influence of hyperglycemia on insulin's in vivo effects in Type II diabetes. J Clin Invest 1984;73:664–672.
11   Garcia MJ, McNamara PM, Gordon T, Kannel WB. Morbidity and mortality in diabetes in the Fra-

mingham population. A sixteen year follow up study. Diabetes 1974;23:105–111.

12 Campaigne BN, Lampman RN. Exercise in the clinical management of diabetes. Champaign, IL: Human Kinetics, 1994.

13 Greenlee G. Exercise options for patients with retinopathy and peripheral vascular disease. Prac Diabet 1987;6:9–11.

14 Painter P. Exercise in end stage renal disease. Exerc Sport Sci Rev 1988;16:305–340.

15 Malina RM, Spirduso WW, Tate C, Baylor AM. Age at menarche and selected menstrual characteristics in athletes at different competitive levels and in different sports. Med Sci Sports Exerc 1978;10:218–222.

16 Prior JC, Cameron K, Ho Uen B, et al. Menstrual cycle changes with marathon training: Anovulation and short luteal phase. Can J Appl Sports Sci 1982;7:173.

17 Schwartz B, Cumming DC, Riordan E, et al. Exercise-associated amenorrhea: a distinct entity? Am J Obstet Gynecol 1981;141:662.

18 Shangold MM, Levine HS. The effect of marathon training upon menstrual function. Am J Obstet Gynecol 1982;143:862.

19 Sanborn MM, Martin BJ, Wagner WW. Is athletic amenorrhea specific to runners? Am J Obstet Gynecol 1982;143:85–89.

20 Calabrese LH, Kirkendall DT, Floyd M, et al. Menstrual abnormalities, nutritional patterns, and body composition in female classical ballet dancers. Physician Sports Med 1983;11:86.

21 Frisch RE, Botz-Welbergen AV, McArthur JW, et al. Delayed menarche and amenorrhea of college athletes in relation to age of onset of training. JAMA 1981;246:1559.

22 Deuster PA, Kyle SB, Moser PB, et al. Nutritional intakes and status of highly trained amenorrheic and eumenorrheic women runners. Fertil Steril 1986;46:636.

23 Brukner P, Khan K. Clinical sports medicine. Sydney: McGraw-Hill, 1993:547.

24 Cann CE, Martin MC, Genant HK, Jafle RB. Decreased spinal mineral content in amenorrheic women. JAMA 1984;251:626.

25 Marcus R, Cann C, Madvig P, et al. Menstrual function and bone mass in elite women distance runners. Ann Int Med 1985;102:158.

26 Warren MP. The effects of exercise on pubertal progression and reproductive function in girls. J Clin Endocrinol Metab 1980; 51:1150–1157.

27 Carbon R, Sambrook PN, Deakin V, et al. Bone density of elite female athletes with stress fractures. Med J Aust 1990;153:373–376.

28 Lindberg JS, Powell MR, Hunt MM, et al. Increased vertebral bone mineral density in response to reduced exercise in amenorrheic runners. West J Med 1987;146:39–42.

29 Drinkwater BL, Bruemer B, Chesnut CH III. Bone mineral density after resumption of menses in amenorrheic athletes. JAMA 1986;256:380–382.

30 Arce JC, De Souza M. Exercise and male factor infertility. Sports Med 1993;15:146–169.

31 Hackney AC. Endurance training and testosterone levels. Sports Med 1989;8:117–127.

32 Pardridge WM. Serum bioavailability of sex steroid hormones. Clin Endocrinol Metab 1986; 15:259–278.

33 Seeman E, Melton LJ, O'Fallon WM, Riggs BL. Risk factors for spinal osteoporosis in men. Am J Med 1983;75:977–983.

34 Krabbe S, Christiansen C, Rodbro P, Transbol I. Effect of puberty on rates of bone growth and mineralization with observations in male delayed puberty. Arch Dis Child 1979;54:950–953.

35 Finkelstein JS, Neer RM, Biller BMK, et al. Osteopenia in men with a history of delayed puberty. New Engl J Med 1992;326:600–604.

36 Colvard DS, Eriksen EF, Keeting PE, et al. Identification of androgen receptors in normal human osteoblast-like cells. Proc Natl Acad Sci USA 1989;86:854–857.

37 McColl EM, Wheeler GD, Gomes P, et al. The effects of acute exercise on pulsatile LH release in high-mileage male runners. Clin Endocrinol 1989;31:617–621.

38 Guglielmini C, Paolini AR, Conconi F. Variations of serum testosterone concentrations after physical exercise of different duration. Int J Sports Med 1984;5:246–249.

39 Kraemer RR, Kilgore JL, Kraemer GR, Castracane VD. Growth hormone, IGF-1, and testosterone responses to resistive exercises. Med Sci Sports Exerc 1992;24:1346–1352.

40 Gray AB, Telford RD, Weidemann MJ. Endocrine response to intense interval exercise. Eur J App Physiol 1993;66:366–371.

41 Hakkinen K, Pakarinen A, Alen M, et al. Neuromuscular and hormonal adaptations in athletes to strength training in two years. J App Physiol 1988;65:2406–2412.

42 Cadoux-Hudson TA, Few JD, Imms FJ. The effect of exercise on the production and clearance of testosterone in well trained young men. Eur J App Physiol 1985;54:321–325.

43 Tanaka H, Cleroux J, de Champlain J, et al. Persistent effects of a marathon run on the pituitary–testicular axis. J Endocrinol Invest 1986;9:97–101.

44 Cumming DC, Wheeler GD, McColl EM. The effects of exercise on reproductive function in men. Sports Med 1989;7:1–17.

45 Kandeel FR, Swerdloff RS. Role of temperature in regulation of spermatogenesis and use of heating as a method of contraception. Fertil Steril 1988;49:1–23.

46 MacDougall JD, Webber CE, Martin J, et al. Rela-

tionship among running mileage, bone density, and serum testosterone in male runners. J App Physiol 1992;73:1165–1170.

47 Hetland ML, Haarbo J, Christiansen C. Low bone mass and high bone turnover in male long distance runners. J Clin Endocrinol Metab 1993;77:770–775.

48 Bilanin JE, Blanchard MS, Russek-Cohen E. Lower vertebral bone density in male long distance runners. Med Sci Sports Exerc 1989;21:66–70.

49 Smith R, Rutherford OM. Spine and total body bone mineral density and serum testosterone levels in male athletes. Eur J App Physiol 1993;67:330–334.

50 Bennell KL, Brukner PD, Malcolm SA. Effect of altered reproductive function and lowered testosterone levels on bone density in male endurance athletes. Br J Sports Med 1996;30:205–208.

51 Malina RM. Physical activity and training: effects on stature and the adolescent growth spurt. Med Sci Sports Exerc 1994;26:759–766.

52 Klein I. Thyroid hormone and the cardiovascular system. Am J Med 1990;88:631–637.

53 McAllister RM, Sansone JC, Laughlin MH. Effects of hyperthyroidism on muscle blood flow during exercise in the rat. Am J Physiol 1995;268:H330–H335.

54 Wieshammer S, Keck FS, Waitzinger J, et al. Left ventricular function at rest and during exercise in acute hypothyroidism. Br Heart J 1988;60:204–211.

55 Burack R, Edwards RHT, Green M, et al. The response to exercise before and after treatment of myxedema with thyroxine. J Pharmacol Exp Ther 1971;176:212–219.

56 Graettinger JS, Muenster JJ, Checchia CS, et al. A correlation of clinical and hemodynamic studies in patients with hypothyroidism. J Clin Invest 1988;37:502–510.

57 Baldwin KM, Hooker AM, Herrick RE, et al. Respiratory capacity and glycogen depletion in thyroid-deficient muscle. J Appl Physiol 1980;49:102–106.

58 McAllister RM, Ogilvie RW, Terjung RL. Functional and metabolic consequences of skeletal muscle remodeling in hypothyroidism. Am J Physiol 1991;260:E272–E279.

59 Dudley GA, Tullson PC, Terjung RL. Influence of mitochondrial content on the sensitivity of respiratory control. J Biol Chem 1987;262:9109–9114.

60 Kaciuba-Uscilko H, Brzezinska Z, Kobryn A. Metabolic and temperature responses to physical exercise in thyroidectomized dogs. Eur J Appl Physiol 1979;40:219–226.

61 Kaciuba-Uscilko H, Brzezinska Z, Kruk B, et al. Thyroid hormone deficiency and muscle metabolism during light and heavy exercise in dogs. Pflugers Arch 1988;412:336–337.

62 Freedberg AS, Hamolsky MW. Effects of thyroid hormones on certain nonendocrine systems. In: Greer MA, Solomon DH, eds. Handbook of physiology. Vol 3. Bethesda: American Physiological Society, 1974:435–468.

63 Morkin E, Flink IL, Goldman S. Biochemical and physiologic effects of thyroid hormone on cardiac performance. Prog Cardiovasc Dis 1983;25:435–464.

64 Wiles CM, Young A, Jones DA, Edwards RH. Muscle relaxation rate, fibre-type composition and energy turnover in hyper- and hypothyroid patients. Clin Sci 1979;57:375–384.

65 Celsing F, Blomstrand E, Melichna J, et al. Effect of hyperthyroidism on fibre-type composition, fibre area, glycogen content and enzyme activity in human skeletal muscle. Clin Physiol 1986;6:171–181.

66 Sestoft L, Saltin B. Working capacity and mitochondrial enzyme activities in muscle of hyperthyroid patients before and after 3 months of treatment. Biochem Soc Trans 1985;13:733–734.

67 Nazar K, Chwalbinska-Moneta J, Machalla J, et al. Metabolic and body temperature change during exercise in hyperthyroid patients. Clin Sci Mol Med 1978;54:323–327.

68 Daniels GH, Martin JB. Neuroendocrine regulation and diseases of the anterior pituitary and hypothalamus. In: Isselbacher KJ, Braunwald E, Wilson JD, et al., eds. Harrison's principles of internal medicine. 13th ed. New York: McGraw-Hill, 1994:1899–1902.

69 Williams GH, Dluhy RG. Cushing's syndrome. In: Isselbacher KJ, Braunwald E, Wilson JD, et al., eds. Harrison's principles of internal medicine. 13th ed. New York: McGraw-Hill, 1994:1960–1965.

70 Magiakou MA, Mastorakos G, Oldfield EH, et al. Cushing's syndrome in children and adolescents. N Engl J Med 1994;331:629–636.

71 Williams GH, Dluhy RD. Hypofunction of adrenal cortex. In: Isselbacher KJ, Braunwald E, Wilson JD, et al., eds. Harrison's principles of internal medicine. 13th ed. New York: McGraw-Hill, 1994:1970–1973.

72 Zelissen PM, Bast EJ, Croughs RJ. Associated autoimmunity in Addison's disease. J Autoimmun 1995;8:121–130.

73 Valero MA, Leon M, Ruiz-Valdepenas MP, et al. Bone density and turnover in Addison's disease: effect of glucocorticoid treatment. Bone-mineralization 1994;26:9–17.

74 Florkowski CM, Holmes SJ, Elliott JR, et al. Bone mineral density is reduced in female but not male subjects with Addison's disease. N Z Med J 1994;107:52–53.

Chapter 29
Dermatologic Problems in Athletes

Wade A. Lillegard
Janus D. Butcher
Karl B. Fields

Skin lesions, which often are readily apparent to the affected athlete, team members, and coaches, are the primary reason for approximately 21% of college training room visits (1). Sports physicians are expected to diagnose, treat, and provide advice regarding the contagiousness of the dermatitis and to determine when a return to competition is safe. Athletes are usually affected by the same disorders found in the general population, although sports activities can increase the risk of specific dermatologic conditions. This chapter describes the characteristics, treatment, and sports-related restrictions of the more common skin disorders.

CLASSIFICATION OF SKIN DISORDERS IN SPORT

Skin problems in sports typically fall into five general categories based on the etiology. Skin infections cause particular concern due to the potential for contagious spread; they are caused by fungal, bacterial, and viral agents and can be manifestations of systemic infections. Traumatic skin injuries—such as blisters, calluses, corns, contusions, and abrasions—limit participation only through the pain they cause. Sports also expose athletes to environmental extremes that damage skin. Excessive sun exposure may arise from snow reflection, water magnification, or lengthy periods in bright, sunny conditions. Types of skin problems precipitated by the sun include sunburn, photodermatitis, solar elastosis, and skin cancers. Extreme heat may contribute to intertrigo, miliaria, and can sometimes trigger urticaria. Extreme cold can also induce urticaria as well as conditions like chilblain, Raynaud's phenomenon, and frostbite.

Sports also have the potential to exacerbate preexisting skin conditions. Three of the most commonly affected chronic skin problems are eczema, acne, and psoriasis. In addition, a variety of miscellaneous skin conditions occur in athletes, such as contact dermatitis, insect bites, and insect stings. Finally, poorly understood conditions that cause skin manifestations include exercise-induced urticaria, angioedema, and anaphylaxis.

INFECTIOUS SKIN CONDITIONS IN ATHLETES

Tinea Pedis

Tinea pedis occurs so often in conjunction with sports that the popular name is "athlete's foot." This infection generally causes an erythematous and often scaling eruption on the plantar surface of the foot. The skin between the toes is often macerated with painful fissures (Plate 6). Skin breakdown and concomitant fungal infection can lead to a special presentation called "podopompholyx," which is characterized by single or multiloculated vesicular lesions that may spread to the tissue below the surface of the skin. The most common etiologic agent is *Trichophyton rubrum,* followed by other dermatophytes such as *T. mentagrophytes* and *Epidermophyton floccosum. Candida* is a less common cause of tinea pedis.

Diagnosis Clinical appearance typically leads to the diagnosis. The differential diagnosis includes eczema, contact dermatitis, and pustular psoriasis; in questionable cases, skin scrapings will demonstrate fungal elements on a KOH preparation. Fungal cultures can also be used for confirmation.

Prevention   Tinea pedis is contracted from direct contact with the fungus through shared surfaces such as locker or shower room floors. Warm, moist conditions facilitate growth of fungus, so tinea pedis rarely occurs in populations who do not wear shoes. The infection may be prevented by keeping the feet clean and dry, using absorbent cotton athletic socks, and avoiding direct skin to surface contact in high-risk environments.

Treatment   Topical antifungal medications effectively treat most cases of tinea pedis. Nystatin, miconazole, and clotrimazole are each effective when applied two to three times per day over the affected area for 2 to 4 weeks. Moist infections between the toes resolve more quickly with the addition of drying agents such as powders. In resistant cases, a trial of the newer azole antifungals such as ketoconazole, econazole nitrate, or oxiconazole may be tried. Some of these preparations require only once a day application.

Resistant cases of fungal scaling of the sole may respond better to a topical allylamine (Naftifine, terbinafine) than an imidazole. One study demonstrated a mycologic cure rate of 97% at 6 weeks using a 1-week course of terbinafine, compared to an 84% cure rate with a 4-week course of clotrimazole (2).

Oral medication is rarely needed, but in cases resistant to topical therapy ultramicronized griseofulvin, 500 mg two times per day, is generally effective. Alternative oral regimens include ketoconazole, fluconazole, and itraconazole, but safety data for these need to be established before assessing the risk-benefit ratio.

Treatment failures tend to come from using products that rely on tolnaftate; noncompliance with treatment regimens; misdiagnosis, or secondary bacterial infections.

Tinea Cruris

Tinea cruris is a similar process to tinea pedis and is caused by the same organisms. Common association with sport has led to the popular name "jock itch." All of the same measures that benefit tinea pedis work for tinea cruris, but rarely do these infections become severe enough to require oral medications. Hygiene may be a factor. Drying is very helpful, and in mild cases simple cornstarch is effective and appears to work as well as commercial drying agents.

Diagnosis   The rash appears as reddened, scaly patches, usually with sharp margins covering the moist folds of the groin and inner thighs but sparing the scrotum and penis (Plate 7). Symptoms include pain and pruritus and occasionally a weeping discharge. The differential diagnosis includes contact dermatitis, mechanical intertrigo, candida intertrigo, and erythrasma.

Treatment   Standard treatments include the same topical antifungal agents used in tinea pedis. Topical low-potency steroid compounds may be used in combination with antifungals to lessen pruritus. Other approaches to drying (such as bathing the lesions in a 1:10 vinegar/water soak followed by drying with a blow dryer before application of topical medication) may facilitate response for the first 3 to 4 days of treatment. In addition, use of powdered antifungals and talcum powder may be alternative approaches to weeping lesions.

Tinea Corporis

Tinea corporis (tinea gladiatorum, ring worm) refers to a superficial tinea infection of nonhairy portions of the skin (i.e., the face, trunk, and limbs). Clinical characteristics include an erythematous scaling ring with slightly raised borders or smaller lesions that may appear as erythematous irregular-shaped patches. These are often pruritic and widespread. This infection is quite contagious, and epidemics among wrestlers occur.

Diagnosis   Diagnosis is based on clinical appearance and the characteristic hyphae seen on KOH prepared skin scrapings.

Treatment   Treatment with topical antifungal agents as outlined under tinea pedis may be effective in superficial, isolated lesions. More extensive involvement or resistant cases should be treated with oral antifungal medications such as ultramicronized Griseofulvin, 500 mg twice a day (3). Infection control measures direct that all lesions be treated with antifungal agents and covered with a gas-permeable membrane (such as ProWrap) and stretch tape before a wrestler can compete (4). If the athlete has lesions that cannot be covered in this fashion, he or she must be disqualified from competition.

Onychomycosis

Onychomycosis is a fungal infection of the toenail that manifests as irregular thickening and pigmentation (white, yellow, orange) of the nail plate. In some cases onycholysis may be seen. The most common causative agents are dermatophytes (primarily *Trichophyton rubrum*), and rarely other organisms like *Candida*, which may spread to the nail from a coexistent tinea pedis infection.

Treatment   Topical antifungals are ineffective against onychomycosis. Fungal infection penetrates deeply into the nail and this, along with the very slow rate of growth in the nail bed, causes difficulty in getting effective antifungal treatment to eradicate the infection. Recurrence rates, even with extended regimens like oral griseofulvin, 500 mg twice a day for 6 to 8 months, remain unacceptably high (5). New antifungal medications, including itraconazole and terbinafine, show more promise. Terbinafine, at a dose of 250 mg once daily for 12 weeks, results in high cure rates (82% mycologic cure) with low recurrence (6). The oral form of terbinafine is not yet available in the United States but is widely used in Europe. Itraconazole, given in a pulse regimen of 200 mg twice a day for the first 7 days of 3 consecutive months, has shown a similar cure rate (84%) with recurrence rates of less than 15% (7).

Tinea Versicolor

Tinea versicolor is a common superficial skin infection caused by the yeast *Pityrosporum orbiculare*. Skin changes result in hypopigmented or hyperpigmented macules, primarily on the trunk, neck, and upper extremities.

Diagnosis   In patients with darker skin pigmentation, hypopigmented lesions are the rule. The diagnosis is confirmed by KOH staining of a skin scraping showing a "spaghetti and meatballs" appearance that represents the active fungal form (*Malassezia furfur*) of the yeast. In cases where the scraping is not confirmatory, a differential diagnosis should consider vitiligo, pityriasis alba, sebhorrheic dermatitis, and possibly secondary syphilis and pityriasis rosea.

Treatment   Treatment options for tinea versicolor vary with the extent of the rash. For mild or moderate skin involvement, topical treatment with selenium sulfide lotion 2.5%, applied once weekly overnight for 3 to 4 weeks or 10 minutes daily for 7 days, may suffice. Alternatively, topical antifungals and sodium thiosulfate (Tinver) may be used twice daily for 3 to 4 weeks, but these are very expensive considering the quantity needed.

Oral regimens are easy and are preferred by patients. A typical regimen would be oral ketoconazole, 400 mg once weekly for 2 to 4 weeks. The athlete is encouraged to exercise, sweat, and not to shower until the next day to make the regimen more effective. Concentration of the drug in sweat makes this an effective way to apply the antifungal preparation over all the skin. An alternative regimen uses oral keotoconazole, 200 mg per day for 3 days, before exercise. The concern with any oral regimen of this class of medication is the potential for hepatotoxicity, as ketoconazole has caused documented hepatic necrosis. The athlete should be informed that the pigment changes may take 6 to 8 weeks to resolve.

Pitted Keratolysis

Pitted keratolysis presents with a number of superficial pits ranging from 1 to 3 mm in diameter. The distribution of lesions is primarily over the heel, but sometimes extends to the entire sole of the foot (Fig 29-1). The appearance may also mimic flat plantar warts. The number of names that have been coined for this condition (including "stinky foot" or "tennis shoe foot") basically reflect the tendency of this condition to be malodorous. The etiologic agent causing pitted keratolysis is *Corynebacterium*, which thrives on dead scaly skin, in a warm moist environment.

Treatment   The infection appears to have an association with excess sweating, so drying agents (e.g., 20% aluminum chloride or 5% benzoyl peroxide) and frequent changes of shoes, socks, or insoles are all helpful in eradication. Generally, topical erythromycin antibiotics are adequate to control outbreaks when applied four times daily, although more extensive involvement may warrant a course of oral erythromycin.

Cutaneous Herpes Simplex

Cutaneous herpes simplex virus/herpes gladiatorium (HSV-1) is allowed entry through traumatic breaks in the skin, thus athletes who have frequent skin abrasions are at special risk. Contagious

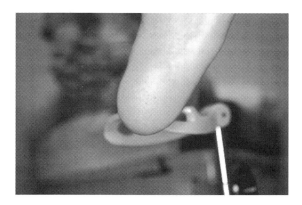

Figure 29-1. Pitted keratolysis involving plantar surface of the heel. (Courtesy of the American Academy of Dermatology.)

spread has been best documented among wrestlers, in whom outbreaks have been traced to infected individuals and to infected fomites (e.g., mats, towels, or clothing). Occurrences are known in rugby (herpes rugbiformus or scrum pox), football, and many other sports. In athletes participating in contact sports, lesions most often occur on the head and may involve the eyes, leading to a conjunctivitis or blepharitis. However, the vesicles do occur anywhere on the body where skin breakdown develops (8). For example, an HSV-1 outbreak in kayakers developed on the skin over the lumbosacral area. The infection among these boaters was probably related to abrasions caused by pressure on the backrest and inoculation via an infected spray skirt.

Presentation Herpes simplex infection leads to multiple vesicles on a confluent erythematous base. Prodromal symptoms such as pain, itching, and burning often precede lesions and may be accompanied by fever, sore throat, headache, and painful adenopathy. The most common sites of nonsexually transmitted herpes in athletes are the mouth (orolabial), finger (herpetic whitlow), and sites of skin trauma (herpes gladiatorum).

In orolabial herpes, active lesions tend to cluster around the mucocutaneous junction of the lips and may be accompanied by neuralgia and swollen lymph nodes (Plate 8). Trigger factors include both emotional and physical (infection, trauma, sun, cold, wind) stresses. Most individuals do not recall their initial infection, but approximately 90% of the infected population experiences orolabial herpes in early childhood. Following the initial infection, the virus enters a dormant phase by residing in neural ganglion and later activating to cause the individual recurrent attacks (9). Twenty to forty percent of the population in developed nations have recurrences of orolabial herpes.

Diagnosis Clinical diagnosis usually suffices for most cases of HSV-1 infection. However, several confirmatory tests are available including a Tzanck smear, viral titers, immunologic tests, monoclonal antibody tests, and cultures. The differential diagnoses for these infections include herpes zoster, coxsackievirus, staphylococcal furuncles, and impetigo.

Treatment If acyclovir is used to treat outbreaks, treatment of HSV-1 should begin immediately with the onset of any prodromal symptoms. Unfortunately, much of the data for treatment efficacy rely on trials of HSV-2 treatment, and whether the same results can be expected is not known. Acyclovir oral, 400 mg three to five times a day for 5 to 7 days, is generally considered the treatment of choice, although a number of alternatives exist. For example, some prefer a lower dosage of 200 mg five times daily extended to 10 days. Famciclovir (Famvir) is a new antiviral drug that is effective against herpes simplex viruses and may prove efficacious in this condition. The recommended dosage is 250–750 mg three times daily. In athletes with active lesions, the advantages of treatment with oral acyclovir include shortening the duration of active disease and reduction of viral shedding by approximately 50%.

Adjunctive treatment with capsaicin cream or viscous lidocaine is helpful for symptomatic relief. Nonsteroidal anti-inflammatory medications may also be useful for the neuralgia associated with an acute outbreak. Some clinicians use acyclovir ointment to hasten the resolution of lesions, but this adds expense and the data supporting this are minimal at present. The acute treatment chosen probably does not affect recurrences. In patients with frequent recurrences, prophylaxis with acyclovir, 200 mg five times a day or 400 mg twice daily throughout the year or during times of increased stress may be beneficial (10). Prophylactic treatment may also be useful for an entire team when two or more athletes have developed active lesions.

Prevention   High attack rates ranging from 25% to 67% after close contacts of HSV-1 patients have led to the efforts to remove athletes with active infection from participation. Through these efforts, sports officials hope to prevent future epidemics (11). Most sports associations prohibit athletes with active, cutaneous HSV-1 infections from direct contact sports such as football, wrestling, and rugby. In the United States, for example, the National Collegiate Athletic Association (NCAA) Wrestling Committee recommends that an athlete not participate in a tournament unless he or she is free of new lesions for 3 days and has no active lesions, the lesions are crusted, and the athlete is on acyclovir at the time of the tournament (4). In addition, all lesions must be covered during competition.

Routine skin examinations by trainers, coaches, and officials should help detect those athletes reluctant to report skin infections. Additionally, infection control efforts should include routine cleansing of mats for wrestling (1:10 solution of bleach), clean clothes and towels in all sports, and education for the athletes.

Herpetic Whitlow

Herpetic whitlow is a painful, reddened inflammation at the base and corners of a single fingernail, often resembling bacterial or candidal paronychia. The infection results from HSV-1 or HSV-2 contracted by spread from direct contact or autoinoculation from genital herpes or herpetic stomatitis (12).

Diagnosis   Pruritus and pain often precede an outbreak of clear vesicles on an erythematous base. Generally, only one finger is involved at the nail margins, and there is a progression to ulceration at the margins of the lesion. If the vesicles coalesce, the fluid usually appears cloudy, and this along with erythematous streaking in the forearms can mimic a bacterial infection. Key differentiating features from a bacterial paronychia are a history of oral or genital herpes and the presence of superficial vesicles. A positive Tzanck smear and/ or viral cultures can help confirm the diagnosis. Candidal paronychia and coxsackievirus infection (which can often involve fingers, feet, and the mouth) are other differential diagnoses.

Treatment   The infection is self-limited, with primary infections lasting 2 to 6 weeks (13), but oral acyclovir, 200–400 mg five times per day for 5 days at the outset of symptoms, can speed resolution. Incision and drainage, the standard treatment for bacterial paronychia, should be avoided, as drainage only leads to viral seeding. Athletes with this condition are highly contagious, and their lesion should be completely covered with an occlusive dressing prior to practice.

Acute Bacterial Paronychia

Acute baterial paronychia is a painful suppurative inflammation of the nailfold surrounding the nail plate. This often occurs as the nail edge is pushed into the fold. The infection may be due to bacteria or fungi, but the most common agents are staphylococci and streptococci.

Treatment   When identified early (before abscess formation), acute bacterial paronychia can be treated with frequent warm soaks, elevation, and 10 days of any oral antistaphylococcal agent (such as dicloxacillin, cephalexin, or erythromycin). Abscesses usually are superficial and subcuticular. Drainage is needed and can be accomplished by elevating the eponychium by sliding the flat edge of a No. 11 blade into the nail sulcus. After extruding any pus, the area is gently probed to open all pockets, and gauze is then placed under the eponychium fold to facilitate drainage. Deeper abscesses or ones that extend under the base of the nail may need a more extensive incision (12) or even removal of a long section of nail to allow drainage. Postsurgical treatment consists of warm soaks and antibiotic treatment as described above.

Chronic Paronychia

Chronic paronychia probably relates to frequent exposure to water with the accompanying presumed stretching and relaxation of the nailfold (14); thus, individuals who participate in water sports are at greater risk. A mixture of organisms including *Candida, Streptococcus,* and *Pseudomonas* colonizes the area; both yeast and bacterial cultures are needed to identify the offending organisms.

Treatment   Bacterial infections require antibiotic treatment covering staphylococcus. Yeast infections are treated with an imidazole-containing topical antifungal cream. Oral ketoconazole is indicated for yeast infections resistant to topical therapy, although griseofulvin does not work against *Candida*, and surgical excision of 2 to 3 mm of the nailfold may be necessary to decrease the dead space. The area affected needs to be kept as dry as possible until the condition resolves, and the involved finger should be covered prior to practice or competition (14).

Impetigo

Impetigo commonly occurs secondary to a skin infection caused by staphylococcus and group A β-hemolytic streptococcus species. The characteristic skin eruption begins as erythema, but may develop rapidly into blisters or honey-colored crusted lesions (Plate 9). Impetigo spreads quickly to multiple areas of the body and, on rare occasions, can lead to deeper invasive infections. Contagious spread of impetigo has been reported in both soccer and football.

Treatment These organisms are highly susceptible to erythromycin, dicloxacillin, amoxicillin-clavulanate, or a first-generation cephalosporin. Oral penicillin is still very effective in streptococcal infections, but does not work against staphylococcus. Intramuscular (IM) benzathine penicillin can still be used to treat noncompliant patients.

Topical treatment works best when coupled with an effort to remove crusts with warm soaks applied for 10 to 15 minutes. Topical application of mupirocin, four times a day for 10 days after skin cleansing, is effective in 90% of cases, although cost and frequent application are drawbacks.

Most sports organizations have regulations to prevent spread of impetigo. For example, one set of guidelines for wrestlers requires completion of at least 3 days of antibiotic therapy and/or no new lesions in the 48 hours prior to competition. All lesions must be covered prior to competition (4).

Folliculitis

Folliculitis is an infection of the hair follicles, typically caused by *Staphylococcus aureus* (15) or by common skin bacteria seen in acne. Inflammatory changes typically occur at the base of hair follicles and include a spectrum of erythematous macules, papules, pustules, and possibly some crusted lesions. A predilection for outbreak of the rash is in skin areas traumatized by maceration (e.g., under shoulder pads, under sweaty garments, and on the legs, arms, and trunk of wrestlers). Erythema and tiny pustules remain near the skin surface in superficial folliculitis, whereas deep folliculitis produces abscesses (furuncles or boils). Sometimes infected furuncles communicate to produce a carbuncle with multiple points through the epidermis.

Treatment Keeping the area clean and dry is the initial treatment in each of these conditions. Mild cases of folliculitis respond to a variety of measures including antibacterial soaps, 10% benzoyl peroxide, topical bacitracin or mupirocin twice a day plus oral tetracycline or erythromycin 250–500 mg four times a day for 10 days. More severe cases require a medication more effective against staphylococcus, such as dicloxacillin, 125–250 mg four times a day for 10 days.

Furuncles and carbuncles are treated with the application of local heat and incision, and drainage is needed for those that become fluctuant. For contact sports, athletes may require a letter from the team physician verifying the diagnosis, appropriate antibiotic treatment, and dates of treatment (4). A typical guideline for wrestlers to compete or practice requires them to be without new lesions for 48 hours, have completed 3 to 5 days of antibiotic treatment, and/or have no moist, exudative or draining lesions.

Hot Tub Folliculitis "Hot tub" folliculitis differs from typical folliculitis in that the infection stems from *Pseudomonas aeruginosa*, commonly found in hot tubs and whirlpools. The papulovesicular/pustular lesions generally involve the axilla, breast, and pubic areas but occasionally extend over the trunk. This infection is generally self-limited in 7 to 10 days and requires no specific treatment (16).

Molluscum Contagiosum

Molluscum contagiosum is a pox viral infection of skin commonly affecting schoolchildren. Transmission occurs through auto-inoculation and close physical contact (17). Sports-related spread has been well documented. Infections in the hands,

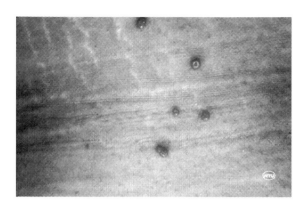

Figure 29-2. Molluscum contagiosum demonstrating umbilication. (Courtesy of the American Academy of Dermatology.)

face, and upper body locations are common in wrestlers and boxers, probably secondary to skin trauma. Outbreaks also have occurred among teammates in sports like cross-country running, in which the mode of spread is less logical.

Diagnosis Classically, the lesions appear as single or small groups of 1.5-mm smooth, dome shaped, pearly, or flesh-colored papules; larger ones show central umbilication (dimpling) and sometimes erythema around the base (17) (Fig 29-2). The lesions represent a viral inclusion body and do not become invasive. Common locations include the axilla and adjacent arm, chest wall, perineum, and upper thigh (18). The differential diagnoses include basal cell epithelioma, trichoepithelioma, ectopic sebaceous glands, or chalazion (of an eyelid) (19).

Treatment Overtreatment should be avoided as this is a benign process and may spontaneously regress after a few months. Treatment is gentle destruction using chemicals, cryotherapy, or curettage. Unroofing the papule with a needle or scalpel hastens resolution. Effective chemical treatments with retinoic acid, phenol, salicylic acid, lactic acid, or cantharidin may be tried, but cryotherapy is considered the treatment of choice. Each lesion is frozen using liquid nitrogen on a cotton-tipped swab, applied for 6 to 10 seconds. Treatment is repeated at 3-week intervals as needed (17).

Untreated infections generally last between 6 to 9 months but can persist for years (18). Wrestlers and athletes in close-contact sports need treatment to prevent spread and should have the lesions either curetted or covered with a gas-permeable membrane (e.g., Op-site) followed by wrapping and tape prior to participation.

Verruca Vulgaris (Common Warts)

Warts are caused by infections with the human papilloma virus and commonly affect all population groups. They typically appear as rough, hyperkeratotic papules and usually remain skin-colored. Variations in appearance include papules on a stalk, thickened cutaneous horns, and almost flat, macular-appearing lesions, some of which show slight erosion (plantar warts). Two diagnostic features are that warts interrupt normal skin lines and shaving of the top will reveal black dots representative of thrombosed capillaries.

Athletes experience the most trouble from warts when they occur on the plantar surface of the foot or on the hands. In either of these locations they are prone to trauma, and sports activity may cause significant irritation. When the irritation limits performance, aggressive modes of therapy may be indicated.

Treatment For the typical wart, patience remains a virtue as daily, topical application of salicylic acid, lactic acid, or a combination of the two results in resolution after 12 weeks of therapy in 70% to 80% of cases. During the course of treatment, appropriate coverage of the warts for contact sports helps lessen the low risk of transmission (20).

Other treatment approaches include cryotherapy with liquid nitrogen. To be effective, this requires a freeze deep enough to produce a blister. Often this type therapy can interrupt participation, so many athletes reserve this for off-season times.

Surgical removal or electrical desiccation, while effective, poses the risk of delaying participation. One negative aspect of a surgical approach is that scarring may be deeper than anticipated, as warts may extend well below the surface of the skin. Recurrence of a wart in an area of scar tissue can present a difficult treatment challenge. Desiccation with a CO_2 laser, while more expensive, minimizes tissue damage and may be a preferable alternative for difficult locations such as periungual warts.

The numerous therapies attest to the fact that an ideal antiviral therapy for warts has yet to emerge. In difficult cases, a dermatologist may assist with other treatments such as trichloroacetic acid, injectable bleomycin, 5-fluorouracil gel, and types of immunotherapy. Genital warts, a special class of warts with specific risks, are discussed in the chapter on sexually transmitted diseases.

Erythrasma

Erythrasma is a bacterial infection that often mimics a topical fungal infection but is caused by the bacterium *Corynebacterium minutissimum.* The typical rash develops as a reddish-brown patch with desquamation in the axilla and groin.

Diagnosis   Diagnosis hinges on the absence of fungal elements on KOH preparation, and the presence of coral-red fluorescence on examination with a Wood's light (16).

Treatment   Several treatments work for milder cases, such as topical erythromycin ointment applied four times a day or antibacterial soaps. However, more severe cases require oral erythromycin or tetracycline, 250 mg four times a day for 10 to 14 days.

Differential Diagnoses   The differential diagnosis for groin and axillary rashes can be confusing, but certain characteristics help identify each rash. *Candida* intertrigo appears basically like tinea cruris except that the rash extends to involve the scrotum and penis in men and vulva in women. Satellite lesions are also seen proximal to the main rash. (Extensive candida infections always raise the question of diabetes mellitus.) Tinea cruris usually has an elevated border. Erythrasma often itches less and has a more thickened appearance of the central rash than either of these conditions. Mechanical intertrigo may contribute to infection and sometimes appears similar to an infectious rash, but usually it is more shiny because it is caused by abrasion of the skin surface—causes include moist skin, cold conditions, rough garment material, and obesity with irritation of contiguous areas of skin. Contact or irritant dermatitis is caused by fabrics, soaps, or dye in undergarments or uniforms, and may appear blistery.

TRAUMATIC INJURIES TO SKIN FROM SPORT

Black Heel

Black heel (talon noir) is a blue or black heel discoloration over the heel from multiple calcaneal petechiae. It can be caused by the shearing forces associated with sudden stops. Certain sports predispose an athlete to this bruising of the posterior plantar surface of the heel, including volleyball, racket sports, running, lacrosse, and basketball. The condition is painless, does not require treatment, and may be prevented with properly fitted footwear with adequate padding. In recurrent cases, additional insoles, thick padded socks, or felt padding should be considered.

Subungual Hematoma

Subungual hematoma (runner's toe, tennis toe) is a splinter hemorrhage in the nail bed, usually involving the first or second toe. It may result from shearing forces of the distal nail pushing on the toebox of the shoe. Subungual hematomas are most common in cutting sports that require frequent stops and abrupt turns (tennis, racquetball, football), but distance runners also develop them.

Treatment   Drainage can lessen pain if the collection of blood beneath the nail hurts. Methods include "drilling" using an 18-gauge needle, puncturing with the tip of a heated paper clip, or penetrating the nail with a laser or an electric cautery device. As with any surgery on the foot, care must be taken to warn the athlete of signs of infection.

Prevention of subungual hematomas may be assisted by trimming the nails back beyond the distal edge of the toe, changing wet shoes, and wearing properly fitted footwear that provide adequate room in the toebox.

Ingrown Toenails

Ingrown toenails cause an erythematous, swollen area in the nailfold adjacent to the nail bed. With bacterial secondary infection, a purulent discharge and evidence of cellulitis develops.

Treatment   Mild cases respond to elevation of the nail edge by placing a petroleum-jelly–impregnated pledget of cotton or dental floss under the distal edge of the nail. This is changed weekly to allow the nail to separate from the nailfold. Oral antibiotics effective against staphylococcus, warm soaks, and shoes with a wide toe box will resolve most early infections.

Severe cases require minor surgery: partial removal of one-fourth to one-third of the involved side of the nail after local anesthesia with a digital block using 1% lidocaine. Chemical ablation of the nail matrix with phenol or similar compounds after removal of part of the nail may lessen recurrences.

Prevention of future problems hinges on better nail care including instructing patients to grow the nail edge beyond the lateral and medial skin folds of the nail bed and using shoes with a wide toebox.

Callouses

Callouses (tylomata) develop because of prolonged friction or pressure. They appear as hyperkeratotic lesions with diffuse thickening and no central core (as seen with planters warts). Callouses are typical stigmata of specific sports activity (e.g., hand callouses among weightlifters) and usually form over a bunion or bony prominence (e.g., the first metatarsal head).

Treatment   Treatment is unnecessary unless the callous causes symptoms of pain. Treatment begins with paring the thickened skin, followed by application of 40% salicylic acid plasters. Moisturizers or specific softening regimens, such as using a solution of two parts propylene glycol and one part water applied in an occlusive dressing, may lessen problems.

Prevention hinges on reducing friction and using padding to relieve pressure. Specific athletic gloves or other equipment may be effective.

Corns

Corns (helomata) are elevated, thickened, circumscribed skin nodules with a broad base, located between the toes and on the plantar surface of the foot. The apex of the nodule points toward the dermis. Repetitive friction and mechanical trauma, usually over an underlying bony exostosis, prompts the formation of corns. The most common location of corns on the plantar surface of the foot is the metatarsal arch, but they are also seen as soft corns between the toes of the fourth interdigital web space.

Diagnosis   Paring of these lesions helps make the diagnosis, as a disruption of the normal papillary skin at the border of the lesion is evident. This differs from plantar warts which have typical dermal papillae, and from callouses that do not have a disruption in papillary pattern.

Treatment   The first phase of treatment is reducing the thickness of the corn by paring it with a surgical blade or by applying 40% salicylic acid plasters. Friction can be reduced by felt pads or donuts. Surgical excision of an underlying bony exostosis provides definitive treatment, and prevention of recurrence may necessitate orthotics to correct poor foot biomechanics.

Blisters

Blisters are fluid-filled bullae that form at the site of friction. Any change in training activity (distance or intensity), equipment (new shoes), or environmental stress (running in wet shoes) may be the precipitating cause. They are probably the most common skin problem in sports, and they certainly limit performance. Blisters on the hand may severely affect grip in sports that require a racket or other hand-held equipment. Similarly, painful blisters on the feet may limit an athlete's performance in jumping or running sports.

Treatment   Treatment of blisters generally does not include unroofing them unless evidence of infection exists, as the overlying skin acts as a protective dressing. When blisters are likely to rupture or must be unroofed, they should be dressed with antibiotic ointment (Bacitracin, Neosporin, Bactroban) and covered with a soft protective dressing.

Large blisters may need to be drained when they interfere with activity. This is best accomplished by lancing with a large-gauge needle under sterile conditions. Symptoms can be reduced after draining by instilling 1% lidocaine into the blister and "tacking" the roof down with benzoin.

Prevention   The best approach for dealing with blisters is prevention. Toughening of the feet can be accomplished with tannic acid soaks: steep 2 tea bags in 1 cup of boiling water; dilute with cool water, and soak the feet for 5 to 10 minutes daily. The athlete should be advised that this will stain the feet. Another approach to toughening is to paint the feet daily with chemical agents like Benzoin, which will lead the skin to dry and thicken.

The opposite method is to reduce friction as much as possible by daily softening with petroleum jelly or lanolin-based products and frequent sock or glove changes.

Athletic trainers often try to speed an athlete's return to the sport by injecting blisters with zinc-oxide–based compounds that dry and toughen the skin under the surface of the skin. This may be effective, but it requires careful observation and sterile technique to lessen risk of introducing infection.

Abrasions

Abrasions (strawberries, mat burn, road rash) are scrapes of the epidermal layers that are often caused by falls or abrupt contact with a playing surface. Poorly fitted equipment also may cause scraping of epidermal layers.

Treatment   The first stage of treatment is careful cleansing by copious irrigation with sterile saline followed by removal of necrotic material and debris. Chlorhexidine-based antiseptic cleanser is preferred over hypochlorite or iodine as it does not damage normal tissue (21).

Once bleeding is controlled, the wound should be covered with a hydrogel (Geliperm, Vigilon, Scherisors) or hydrocolloid (Duoderm, Granuflex) dressing for about 3 days. These dressings promote healing more effectively than gauze and antibiotic ointment because 1) wounds heal better in a moist environment, 2) they decrease the pH of the wound (inhibiting bacterial growth), 3) they are nonirritant, and 4) they tend to reduce localized pain (21).

Prophylactic antibiotics and tetanus toxoid are reserved for particularly dirty or high-risk wounds (punctures, or hand injuries); otherwise, wounds should be observed for infection and treated with oral or topical antibiotics only when signs of infection appear.

ENVIRONMENTAL SKIN DAMAGE

Environmental skin damage in athletes is often caused by participation in or exposure to extreme conditions. Sun exposure is the most common environmental factor that leads athletes to seek medical care.

Sunburn

Triathalons, running, biking, water sports, baseball, tennis, and any activity done outside for a prolonged period can predispose an athlete to sunburn. Typically, sunburns occur early in the season when athletes have not "tanned" sufficiently or when a team from a colder region travels to a sunnier climate to participate. However, even well-acclimatized athletes may sunburn with the intense exposure that occurs during mountaineering, water sports, and skiing.

Prevention   Prevention of sunburn is desirable and can be accomplished with reduced sun exposure and a gradual schedule of increasing time in the sun. Other helpful measures include protective clothing and application of sunscreens or sunblock. *Sunscreens* contain PABA, which can extend one's time in the sun before burning. Rating systems give the multiple of time (the SPF or sun protective factor) that one can spend in the sun before burning. Sunscreens with an SPF 15 are most effective. *Sunblocks* rely on zinc oxide to try to completely shield the skin from UV light penetration.

Treatment   Treatment of mild to moderate sunburn (first or second degree) includes analgesics and cool compresses. A topical corticosteroid may help relieve the inflammation of mild burns but should be used with extreme caution on the face. Moderate burns sometimes necessitate an oral corticosteroid for symptom relief.

Severe sunburns mimic burns from any other source and require IV fluids, generous application of antibiotic creams, dressings, and strong analgesics. When individuals are aware that they cannot avoid excessive sun exposure, pretreatment with aspirin, nonsteroidal anti-inflammatory drugs, or an oral corticosteroid may reduce the severity of the subsequent burn.

Photodermatitis

Photodermatitis refers to a variety of conditions related to sun exposure. Often the sun exposure requires a cofactor to trigger the skin rash or reaction that occurs.

Medications commonly precipitate photosensitivity. Among the drugs known to increase sensitivity to sun are tetracycline, sulfonamide, griseofulvin, diuretics, phenothiazides, first-generation sulfonylurea oral diabetic agents, and Benadryl. In addition, a number of chemical substances found in perfumes or other cosmetics may help trigger reactions. These reactions are variable in nature and range from nodular ("sun poisoning"), to solar purpura, to solar-induced urticaria.

Treatment   Protection from excess sun exposure as well as removing any offending agent are keys to successful treatment.

Skin Cancer

Prolonged skin exposure ages and damages the skin. *Solar elastosis* refers to the thickening and wrinkling of the skin that often occurs over the back of the neck and face after years of damage. In addition, excess sun exposure may precipitate skin cancers:

- **Basal Cell Skin Cancer.** The presence of telangiectasias and actinic keratoses may herald the development of basal cell skin cancers. True basal cells are characterized by pearly borders, telangiectasias, and often a central nonhealing ulcer.
- **Melanoma.** Melanomas, the most serious skin cancers, are usually darkly pigmented lesions, but may present with a variety of colorations, shapes, nodularity, and sizes. Their increased occurrence in geographical regions with more intense sun is well known. In addition, their occurrence in certain anatomical locations such as the lower extremity has been linked to cer-

tain sports activities, hence the name "cyclist's melanoma."

Heat

Excessive heat may contribute to a number of conditions in athletes, including intertrigo or most of the conditions that affect the groin or axillae. Heat that causes excessive sweating may also worsen folliculitis or acne. Miliaria (heat bumps) are benign tiny papules that develop with excessive temperatures. In addition, heat can trigger a type of cholinergic urticaria.

Cold

Cold causes a number of specific skin problems. Cold air typically has low humidity, so dry skin is a common problem that can worsen eczema and other chronic skin conditions. Sweating from intense exercise may further deplete skin oils and worsen the chapping, cracking, or itching brought on by dryness.

Pernio (chilblains) is a reaction to cold and damp that is characterized by blue to reddish papules and nodules over the extremities. These lesions may itch or burn and take up to 3 weeks to completely resolve. Raynaud's phenomenon occurs in association with cold conditions. More extreme cold exposures can lead to frostnip or true frostbite.

EXACERBATION OF CHRONIC SKIN CONDITIONS BY SPORT

Acne Vulgaris

Acne vulgaris occurs in adults, but it is well-known as the most common skin condition among adolescents, with 70% to 80% developing some degree of acne. The typical rash consists of papules, pustules, comedones, nodules, and cysts located primarily on the face, back, shoulders, and chest.

Diagnosis   To confirm the clinical diagnosis, the presence of comedones (blackheads or whiteheads) is necessary. The severity of the acne is judged by the number of lesions, and is classified as either grade I mild, grade II moderate, grade III severe, or grade IV very severe (22). In addition to grading, acne vulgaris should be described by the predominant type of lesion—comedonal, papular, pustular, nodular, or cystic—as this may affect treatment.

The differential diagnoses include Gram-negative folliculitis, rosacea, steroid acne, and contact acne (caused by cosmetics, industrial agents, or chlorinated hydrocarbons). *Acne mechanica* arises in areas where sweat and occlusion from athletic garments or equipment aggravate the skin. This most commonly occurs under helmets, chin straps, shoulder pads, bra straps, jock straps, or other areas of friction.

Treatment   Topical therapy remains the mainstay for treatment of noninflammatory comedones and mild to moderate inflammatory acne. Tretinoin (Retin-A) is the most effective initial treatment as it normalizes follicular desquamation, promotes drainage, and potentiates penetration of topical antibiotics (23). Tretinoin can excessively dry skin; to minimize irritation, a mild cream formulation (0.025%) should be used initially and applied nightly. After a few weeks the 0.05% and 0.1% formulations can be used if stronger therapy seems needed. A gel formulation of 0.01% or 0.025% may be useful in athletes with oily skin or in humid climates. Good clinical improvement is generally seen by 6 weeks.

For mild acne, benzoyl peroxide, 2.5% to 10%, can be used as an alternative or in combination with Tretinoin. Higher strengths increase the dryness but not the bacteriocidal properties. For combination therapy, Tretinoin should be applied at night and benzoylperoxide in the morning.

Topical antibiotics such as erythromycin (2%) or clindamycin (1%) applied with benzoylperoxide typically are required for moderate acne. Oral antibiotics may often initiate a quicker response; tetracycline or erythromycin, 250 mg four times a day, can be used for moderate acne that is resistant to topical therapy and for severe acne. Some patients with resistant or severe acne vulgaris may need specialized treatments and should be referred to a dermatologist.

Eczema

Eczema classically worsens with either drying or irritation. Because sports lead to excessive sweating and often to friction and abrasions, eczema often worsens in athletes. Factors that may contribute to flares include uniforms, braces, wraps, dyes in clothing, ill-fitting equipment or clothes, and the detergents used to clean uniforms. Winter sports occur in conditions with low humidity and harsh temperatures that lead to chapping, and such environmental extremes may significantly flare eczema, even in athletes in whom control was satisfactory. Athletes known to have asthma or allergies often develop eczema. For this reason when an athlete develops a rash, eczema should be suspected unless an obvious cause is found.

Complications

- *Dyshidrosis eczema* refers to a subset of the atopic dermatitis group that leads to vesicles and bullae over the hands and feet. Hyperhidrosis often contributes to flares over the feet. The vesicles can also mimic tinea pedis. When these vesicles become large or develop a secondary bacterial infection, they can cause enough pain to limit effective participation.
- *Eczema herpeticum* is a serious complication of eczema. This generalized herpesvirus infection occurs after a patient with extensive eczema is exposed to herpesvirus.

Treatment   Treatment of all forms of eczema relies on mild soaps, generous use of moisturizing agents, and topical corticosteroids. Infected, more severe cases may also require oral antibiotics, wet compress dressings, careful cleansing, and nocturnal use of occlusive wraps with high-potency topical corticosteroid preparations underneath. Only in rare situations should oral corticosteroids be used in eczema.

Psoriasis

Psoriasis is one of the more common papulosquamous disorders seen in medicine. Several types of psoriasis exist, each having a different appearance. The most common findings include thick, well-demarcated plaques, with adherent silvery scale on extensor surfaces and over areas of bony prominences. Pitting of the fingernails and a thickened, scaly rash of the scalp that mimics severe sebhorrheic dermatitis are also suggestive of psoriasis. Psoriatic plaques tend to proliferate in areas of skin trauma. For this reason, contact sports, sports equipment, braces, and even tight clothing can all trigger the development of psoriatic plaques.

Treatment   Athletes may find that they need to dramatically increase their use of petroleum jelly or other emollients to prevent their psoriasis from worsening during competitive seasons. Topical steroid preparations, tar shampoos, calcipotriol (a vitamin D analogue), and increased sun exposure all may play a significant role in controlling this skin disorder.

MISCELLANEOUS SKIN CONDITIONS IN ATHLETES

Contact Dermatitis

Contact dermatitis develops when an external irritant or allergic agent causes a localized skin reaction. The reaction first manifests as erythema, edema, and occasional vesicles (24). Subsequently, papules and crusting form at the site of contact (Plate 10).

There are differences between irritant and allergic contact dermatitis. *Irritant dermatitis* typically is associated more with burning and pain, and erupts within 24 hours of contact. *Allergic dermatitis* reactions cause intense pruritus and become symptomatic 24 to 96 hours after contact in previously sensitized individuals (24). Common sensitizing agents seen in athletes include poison oak, sumac, and ivy; nickel (jewelry); chromate (chrome-tanned leather in helmet bands and some shoes); mercaptobenzothiazole (natural and synthetic rubber athletic shoes and equipment); and cosmetics. In addition to the point of first contact, allergic-contact dermatitis may spread locally or to distant sites.

Eczema is one of the most difficult conditions to distinguish from contact dermatitis. The differential diagnoses also include psoriasis, herpes simplex, herpes zoster, and scabies.

Treatment   Irritant, oozing skin eruptions respond to twice-a-day applications of medium to high potency steroid solutions, sprays, or creams. Steroid ointments or creams work best when the lesions begin to dry. No treatment offers long-term success without avoidance of the contact allergen or irritant. Lesions should be covered prior to practice, not to protect other athletes but rather to avoid further irritation.

Scabies

Scabies is an infestation with the mite *Sarcoptes scabiei,* which burrows into the skin and leaves sensitizing feces and eggs. This is one of the most pruritic lesions of any skin condition, and will even awaken patients from sleep. Lesions are papular or vesicular with surrounding erythema in the finger web spaces, axillae, genitalia, and around the nipples in females (Plate 11). Linear excoriations and scabbing of individual lesions commonly occurs. Transmission may occur in close contact sports such as wrestling, rugby, and football. Diagnosis can be made by microscopic examination of skin scrapings for the mites, eggs, or feces.

Treatment   Scabicides serve as the primary treatment. For example, lindane shampoo can be applied in a single dose and rinsed off after 3 minutes. Alternatively, Elimite cream (permethrin 5%), applied from the neck downward overnight (8 to 14 hours) and showered off in the morning is another effective regimen.

To control symptoms, adjunctive treatment with topical steroids (Triamcinolone 0.1%) and an oral antipruritic such as hydroxyzine (Atarax), 25–50 mg every 4 to 6 hours, is helpful but oral agents may be too sedating for many athletes.

Athletes should be advised that itching may persist for several weeks after treatment with a scabicide and does not indicate a persistent infection. To prevent reinfection, all linen and clothing should be washed to remove remaining parasites. Most sports guidelines require athletes in contact sports to have verification of treatment and a negative skin scraping prior to participation (4).

Pediculosis

Pediculosis or crab louse (*Pthirus pubis*) infestation is a readily transmissible, highly pruritic infection that affects the pubic area, abdomen, or axilla.

Treatment   Treatment with 5% permethrin cream applied at night (8 to 14 hours), effectively kills the parasite. Intimate contacts should be treated as well, and all clothing and bedding should be carefully cleansed. Athletes need verification of treatment and no evidence of active infection before they can participate in a contact sport.

SUMMARY

Athletes are at risk for any of the common dermatologic problems seen in the general population. Usually these skin problems fall into five broad categories: infections, traumatic skin injuries, environmentally mediated skin problems, common skin conditions worsened by sports participation, and miscellaneous problems. Sports physicians need good diagnostic and management skills for these frequently encountered conditions. In addition, recognition of how sports may affect the occurrence and control of these problems will enable the physician to prescribe treatment and give advice that allows maximal participation and minimal risk to other competitors.

REFERENCES

1 McGrew CA, Lillegard WA, McKeag D, Hough DO. Profile of patient care in a primary care sports medicine fellowship. Clin J Sports Med 1992;2:126–131.

2 Evans EG, Dodman B, Williamson DM, et al. Comparison of terbinafine and clotrimazole in treating tinea pedis. Br Med J 1993;307:645–647.

3 Scheinberg RS. Stopping skin assailants: Fungi, yeasts, and viruses. Physician Sports Med 1994;22:33–36,38–39.

4 Committee NW. NCAA wrestling championship handbook. NCAA Publications, 1993.

5 Roberts DT. Oral therapeutic agents in fungal nail disease. J Am Acad Dermatol 1994;31:S78–S81.

6 Goodfield M. Clinical results with terbinafine in onychomycosis. J Dermatol Treat 1990;1(suppl 2):55–57.

7 Roseeuw D, De Doncker P. New approaches to the tratment of onychomycosis. J Am Acad Derm 1993;29:45–50.

8 Higgins CR, Schofield JK, Tatnall FM, Leigh IM. Natural history, management and complications of herpes labialis. J Med Virol 1993;1(suppl):22–26.

9 Becker TM. Herpes gladiatorum: a growing problem in sports medicine. Cutis 1992;50:150–152.

10 Spruance SL. Prophylactic chemotherapy with acyclovir for recurrent herpes simplex labialis. J Med Virol 1993;1(suppl):27–32.

11 Belongia E, Goodman J, Holland E, et al. An outbreak of herpes gladiatorum at a high-school wrestling camp. N Engl J Med 1991;325:906–910.

12 Moran GJ, Talan DA. Hand infections. Emerg Med Clin North Am 1993;11:601–619.

13 Fitzpatrick TB, Eisen AZ, Wolf K, et al. Dermatology in general medicine. 4th ed. New York: McGraw-Hill, 1993.

14 Kvedar JC. Disorders of the nails. In: Olbricht SM, Bigby ME, Arndt KA, eds. Manual of clinical problems in dermatology. Boston: Little, Brown, 1992:118–123.

15 Schwartz RA, Fox MD. Office dermatology. Am Fam Physician Monogr 1992;Spring:1–24.

16 Sevier TL. Infectious disease in athletes. Med Clin North Am 1994;78:389–412.

17 Janniger CK, Schwartz RA. Molluscum contagiosum in children. Cutis 1993;52:194–196.

18 Highet AS. Molluscum contagiosum. Arch Dis Child 1992;67:1248–1249.

19 Degreef HJ, DeDoncker PR. Current therapy of dermatophytosis. J Am Acad Dermatol 1994;31:S25–S30.

20 Maytin EV. Warts. In: Olbricht SM, Bigby ME, Arndt KA, eds. Manual of clinical problems in dermatology. Boston: Little, Brown, 1992.

21 Ryan TJ. Wound dressing. Dermatol Clin 1993;11:207–213.

22 Durme DJV, Brozena SJ. Common dermatoses. In: Taylor RB, ed. Family medicine; principles and practice. 4th ed. New York: Springer-Verlag, 1994:920–928.

23 Leyden JJ, Shalita A. Rational therapy for acne vulgaris: an update on topical treatment. J Am Acad Dermatol 1986;15:907–915.

24 Krasteva M. Contact dermatitis. Int J Dermatol 1993;32:547–560.

Chapter 30
Rheumatology and the Athlete

Peter A. Fricker

This chapter outlines the rheumatic disorders most often seen in medical practice, and discusses the implications of exercise on the various disease states. Many individuals with osteoarthritis, rheumatoid arthritis, and ankylosing spondylitis enthusiastically pursue fitness and physical activity. They need to know just how their particular diagnoses might limit their ambitions, or indeed how their exercise might assist them in recovery and maintenance of health.

OSTEOARTHRITIS

Osteoarthritis is an ubiquitous condition. Although two terms used interchangeably with osteoarthritis are "osteoarthrosis" and "degenerative joint disease," the term osteoarthrosis should perhaps be reserved for a systemic illness with involvement of joints undergoing degenerative change (as in primary generalized osteoarthrosis).

The incidence of osteoarthritis (OA) increases with age as evidenced by radiographic studies, but only 30% of persons with radiographic evidence of OA complain of pain in the affected joints. The condition is believed to be multifactorial in origin, involving heredity, obesity, trauma, and overuse. OA can be classified into primary (generalized osteoarthrosis) and secondary forms, with the latter specifically related to a given antecedent.

Clinical Features

OA is the most common arthritis of both the central and peripheral skeleton. Hallmarks of the disease process include progressive deterioration and loss of articular cartilage, and reactive bony changes at the margins of the joints and in the sub-chondral layer. In a teleological sense, the osteophytes and other bony changes of this disease are seen as a healing response to injury, quite distinct from the erosive changes seen in conditions such as rheumatoid arthritis.

Clinically, OA manifests as gradual development of joint pain, joint stiffness, and joint enlargement, associated with gradual loss of range of motion. Joint pain worsens at the end of the day with activity. Synovitis is common; inflammation appears as a joint stiffness that requires the individual to devote a period of time to warming up prior to activity.

Primary Generalized Osteoarthritis Primary generalized OA is characterized by Bouchard's nodes at the proximal interphalangeal joints and Heberden's nodes at the distal interphalangeal joints of the fingers. Other features include involvement of large weightbearing joints such as the hips and knees. This condition is believed to be transmitted by a single autosomal gene that is dominant in females; the incidence in females is 10 times that in males.

Secondary Osteoarthritis Secondary OA typically follows trauma to a joint, particularly a weightbearing joint which is then subjected to repetitive stresses, and this is compounded by obesity. Other causes of degenerative joint disease include congenital dislocation of the hips, slipped capital femoral epiphysis, Legg-Calvé-Perthes disease, rheumatoid arthritis, gout, septic arthritis, hemophilia, acromegaly, hemochromatosis, and Paget's disease.

Pathology The pathology of OA consists of fissuring and pitting of the articular cartilage followed by erosive changes. These erosions become confluent and then leave the subchondral bone

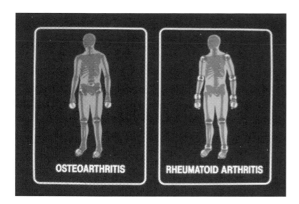

Figure 30-1. Comparison of joint involvement between rheumatoid arthritis and osteoarthritis. (Courtesy of Pfizer Inc.)

exposed. With continued joint movement, the denuded bone becomes polished (eburnation), and this is accompanied by subchondral bone thickening and sclerosis as evident on x-ray.

Osteophytes arise from bony proliferation at the joint margins. Subchondral cysts are thought to result from synovial joint fluid being pushed into the bone under high compressive forces, and/or from tissue breakdown related to focal areas of microfracture in the ischemic subchondral bone.

Synovitis results from the release of inflammatory mediators from articular cartilage breakdown and possibly from immune mediators that are "exposed" by the degenerative process.

Diagnosis

The clinical features of OA relate to the combination of mechanical and inflammatory factors that interplay in this disease. Pain after activity reflects the mechanical nature of bone wearing on bone; synovitis as such contributes symptoms of stiffness to joints that "warm up" and improve with exercise. Night pain occurs late in the disease, as well as pain on passive motion and crepitus. Synovitis, synovial effusion, and osteophyte formation produce enlargement of joints.

Joints involved in primary and secondary forms of OA are diverse (Fig 30-1). The acromioclavicular joint, the first metatarsophalangeal joint, and the patellofemoral joint are some of those that may

be affected, together with the more common hip, knee, and spine lesions. Spinal involvement encompasses the intervertebral discs, vertebral bodies, and zygapophyseal joints to produce secondary involvement of vertebral arteries, nerve roots, and the cauda equina.

Radiographs confirm the diagnosis by demonstrating the typical findings of loss of joint space, osteophyte formation, marginal sclerosis, and subchondral cysts (Fig 30-2). Blood tests and synovial fluid examination are rarely helpful, but synovial fluid may reveal a slight increase in white cell count as well as calcium pyrophosphate dihydrate and/or apatite crystals.

In general, OA is not a crippling disease, but its natural history is to progress. In weightbearing joints, pain can lead to immobility and secondary muscle wasting, which can contribute to a vicious cycle of pain and weakness from disuse atrophy. Occasionally OA may mimic rheumatoid or other systemic forms of arthritis; the primary concern in the differential diagnosis is the seronegative arthropathies; ankylosis is uncommon, except in the erosive inflammatory form of OA.

Management

Once joints have been damaged, overuse and repetitive impact forces pose special risks. Painful joints respond to analgesics in most cases; nonsteroidal anti-inflammatory drugs (NSAIDs) can be reserved for inflammatory symptoms and signs (stiffness, a requirement for warmup, synovial ef-

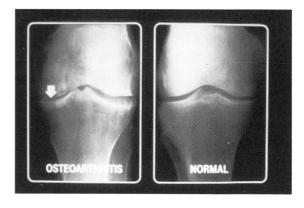

Figure 30-2. A joint with osteoarthritis compared with a normal joint. (Courtesy of Pfizer Inc.)

fusion) rather than long-term control. Walking sticks or canes can be used on an as-needed basis.

Obesity worsens OA, and nothing works for painful knees or hips as well as weight loss in the overweight patient. A weight-loss program should incorporate diet and exercise. Keeping the joint warm with an appropriate thermal sleeve or heat retainer is useful, but tight-fitting appliances over the muscles above the knee in particular can contribute to muscle wasting. Attention to biomechanical abnormalities (e.g., the use of orthoses and splints) is reasonable, but therapeutic effects in this area are still largely conjectural. Intra-articular injection of corticosteroids can be used for acute exacerbations of synovitis, but caution is advised with respect to repeated injections as these may produce crystals, which then produce their own arthropathy. There is also the risk of direct damage to articular cartilage by corticosteroids.

Surgery   Prosthetic hips have proven very successful, and there are many athletes (and ex-athletes) who manage to exercise gently but regularly (e.g., walking and golf) and maintain fitness on their new hips. Knee and ankle prostheses are a little more fragile, and activity on such joints really should be limited to nonweightbearing activities such as swimming and cycling.

Exercise and Osteoarthritis

Rehabilitation   Exercise is of prime importance in the rehabilitation of a joint affected by OA. Nonimpact exercise, swimming, cycling, and light weights are recommended for those who suffer from OA of the knees, hips, ankles, and back (in most cases). Obviously, particular exercises must be looked at for each case—a cervical spine with limited range of movement and nerve root involvement may not do well for swimming, for example.

Resistance training with machine weights, free weights, or equipment such as rubber bands also promotes muscle strength for those joints that need support. Quadriceps and hamstring exercises, for example, need only 10 minutes a day to maintain muscle strength and encourage range of movement of an affected knee. In all cases, physi-

cal therapists and/or specialists in physical medicine should encourage discussion with patients of appropriate exercise programs for particular joints.

Does Exercise Cause Arthritis?   The answer to this is "probably not." Several studies have examined the role of sport and exercise in producing OA in later years, and large studies have provided the reassuring finding that recreational sporting activities such as jogging probably do not produce higher rates of OA of knees and hips in exercisers compared with controls (1).

Studies of competitive or elite athletes such as marathoners generally provide reassuring findings, but some researchers caution that running in excess of 100 km (65 miles) per week may predispose an athlete to the development of OA (2). Activities such as throwing and hitting have also been blamed for the development of degenerative joint disease in elbows; baseball pitchers, especially at the elite or professional level, are particularly at risk for this. Limiting the number of innings pitched per week has been tried to good effect in younger pitchers, but the demands of professional sport can unfortunately overwhelm the need to allow appropriate recovery.

Contact sports that produce traumatic lesions of joints are a different proposition. The author believes that joint damage brought on by contact sport may be exacerbated by athletic activity and may produce OA in later years. Certainly knees partially or wholly removed of menisci (arthroscopically or by arthrotomy) run a high risk of degenerative changes over a few years (3,4). With this in mind, once OA is established, therapeutic exercise should be provided to maintain strength, flexibility, and function of joints, but the type of activity should not pose a risk of accelerated joint degeneration.

RHEUMATOID ARTHRITIS

Rheumatoid arthritis (RA) is a chronic, systemic, inflammatory condition that typically progresses to destroy joints and incapacitate the patient. The disease is characterized by immune or serologic markers and the manifestations of vasculitis. These include rheumatoid nodules, arteritis (of small blood vessels especially), lymphadenopathy, spleno-megaly, pericarditis, neuropathy, and scleritis. Women are affected two to three times more often than men, and the disease usually presents in the fourth decade or later. There is a juvenile form that is discussed later in this chapter.

Clinical Features

The onset of disease in RA varies from a mild pau-ciarticular illness of variable severity to an aggres-sive painful condition of quite rapid onset and re-lentless progress. Although the degree of joint involvement does not necessarily correlate with systemic symptoms or extra-articular manifesta-tions, erosive joint disease and extra-articular fea-tures are more often seen in those patients with high titers of rheumatoid factors.

Joint involvement causes pain, stiffness, and limitation of motion, associated with a duration of morning stiffness; these symptoms directly parallel the inflammatory activity of the synovial joints in-volved. The joints most often affected include the small joints of the hands, the wrists, knees, and feet. Generally joint involvement is bilateral, sym-metrical, and polyarticular, but any diarthrodial joint can be affected. It is vital that all joints be as-sessed as therapy necessarily depends on each and every joint's status.

Extra-articular manifestations of RA involve ten-dons, bursae, nerves, and the skin, and therapy for the affected patient requires consideration of all soft tissue structures as well as joints. Cardiac lesions occur, though they rarely cause clinical limitations; as valvular disease, myocarditis, and coronary arte-ritis have all been described in RA, a subclinical full assessment of cardiac status is encouraged. Pericar-ditis (which can be fatal) is not uncommon and may occur together with a pleural effusion.

Diagnostic tests are outlined in appropriate medical texts, but depend upon finding rheuma-toid factors in high titer, an elevated ESR, and asso-ciated blood findings such as leukocytosis and ane-mia of chronic illness. Radiographs of the hands and feet can be useful in assessing the severity of disease; these may show juxta-articular osteopenia

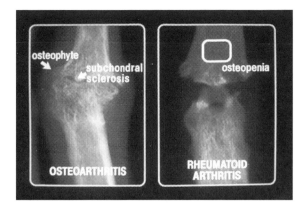

Figure 30-3. A comparison of radiographs in osteo-arthritis and rheumatoid arthritis. (Courtesy of Pfizer Inc.)

and the characteristic subarticular erosions of the metacarpophalangeal and metatarsophalangeal joints in particular (Fig 30-3).

Treatment

RA is a disease of remissions and exacerbations—it progresses over time, destroying and deforming joints. In some cases, the disease does appear to burn out, but this is unusual. The main objectives of treatment are 1) relief of pain, 2) reduction or suppression of inflammation, and 3) preservation of joint function and muscle strength through range of motion. Attention to these objectives should help maintain the patient's quality of life.

Pain Relief   Aspirin is still the drug of choice for initial drug therapy. An adequate dosage must be provided to maintain a serum salicylate level of 23–30 mg/dL, and overdosage must be avoided. If the patient cannot tolerate aspirin, other NSAIDs can be tried, although no evidence exists that they have superior efficacy. Every medical practitioner should be familiar with at least two or three alter-nate drugs. Among the alternative agents used for RA, the antimalarials (especially chloroquine) have a side effect of retinal lesions, requiring that the patient undergo regular ophthalmic reviews.

Inflammation Suppression   Currently, there is a trend toward instituting disease-modification therapies at an earlier stage of the disease. Sup-pressive therapies for erosive RA include D-penicillamine (which is not much used today), gold salts, and methotrexate. Because these agents have well-described toxic effects on blood parameters and the kidney in particular, extreme caution must be observed with respect to their use—practitioners should refer to specialists before initiating any pharmacologic therapy beyond NSAIDs. Corticosteroid injections should be used with caution for palliation only, as frequent injections pose a risk of soft tissue disruption (particularly tendons).

Physical Therapy   While joints are stiff, swollen, and painful, any activity worsens the condition and appropriate rest is advised. Splints (especially at night) to rest joints and prevent contractures are very useful, and canes or walking sticks can be used to provide relief for weightbearing joints in particular. Once inflammation and pain have been brought under control, activity for affected joints is recommended. Swimming in heated pools is a wonderful way of exercising as it provides warmth, weight support, and exercise to promote muscle strength and joint range of motion. Cycling can also be used when it is comfortable, and patients should be encouraged to walk while activity of the disease allows.

Does Exercise Affect Disease Severity?

Studies of the effects of physical training on moderately active RA patients do show beneficial results. Some research has shown decreased activity of the disease in "dynamically" trained patients, compared with nontrained patients who did not derive such benefits when treated with rest or bed rest. These studies have indicated that bed rest should be prescribed only for patients with very active disease. Exercise duration is also important to achieve the appropriate benefits. For example, one study indicated that exercise sessions of 15 or 25 minutes three times weekly led to improvements in mood, less fatigue, and better functional status of patients with moderate RA. Nonexercise controls and patients exercising 35 minutes a day three times weekly failed to show these results (5).

RA patients may need activity to regain physical health and well-being after immobilization, just as do healthy people. Lyngberg and co-workers (6) in

Denmark believe that a poor functional status is predictive of higher mortality in RA patients and that corticosteroid therapy in such patients is associated with a higher incidence of arteriosclerosis and osteoporosis. They believe that physical training, especially of RA patients taking corticosteroids, may produce beneficial effects, similar to those found in other RA patients and in healthy persons. Their study of physical training of a group of elderly RA patients on low-dose corticosteroid treatment demonstrated that 3 months of bicycle exercises, heel lifts, and step-climbing produced a doubling of work capacity and no increase in disease activity.

JUVENILE RHEUMATOID ARTHRITIS

Juvenile rheumatoid arthritis (JRA) is the principal form of chronic arthritic disease in children. JRA is classified into three subtypes (related to onset): systemic, polyarticular, and pauciarticular.

- *Systemic JRA* is typified by persistent intermittent fever with arthritis.
- *Pauciarticular JRA* is defined as JRA affecting four or fewer joints in the first 6 months of disease.
- *Polyarticular JRA* involves five or more joints in the first 6 months (and is exclusive of the systemic form).

JRA excludes other rheumatic diseases. Systemic lupus erythematosus, the vasculitic syndromes, ankylosing spondylitis, and rheumatic fever can all be diagnosed on their particular natural history and serology.

JRA produces symptoms of joint pain with activity (rather than pain at rest) and joint stiffness after immobility (morning stiffness). It can retard growth and reduce skeletal height, and physeal changes can affect the neighboring joints. There are no diagnostic tests for JRA although rheumatoid factors, antinuclear antibodies, and HLA-B27 markers can be used to produce subclassifications of the disease. HLA-B27 positivity, for example, is associated with the JRA that affects males rather than females, older children, often those with a family history of spondyloarthropathy, and those with negative tests for rheumatoid factors and antinuclear antibodies. JRA can also produce erythematous rashes, polyserositis, lymphadenopathy, hepatosplenomegaly, leukocytosis, and anemia (particularly in the systemic onset form); in the pauciarticular type, an iridocyclitis can affect up to 50% of patients.

Treatment

The outlook for most children with JRA is good, as at least 75% of patients undergo long remissions with minimal disability. Management relies on providing 1) symptomatic relief with aspirin (except during influenza attacks when Reye's syndrome may result), or in older children, with NSAIDs; 2) physical therapy and exercise to maintain joint position, function, and muscle strength.

Exercise Exercise is encouraged for JRA sufferers when activity of the disease permits it. Early mobilization can and should be encouraged, as it is now accepted that no harm is done and movement helps prevent contractures. This particularly applies to patients with more severe disease who are on corticosteroid therapy. Patients should lead normal lives, and swimming, cycling, rowing, sailing, and light weight training are all permitted. Contact sports, however, should be avoided. Because attention should be paid to eye disease in particular as it can be aggressive and destructive, an ophthalmologist should undertake regular review and help supervise management.

SYSTEMIC LUPUS ERYTHEMATOSUS (SLE)

Systemic lupus erythematosus (SLE), which affects young and old, is a multisystem disease associated with antibody formation to nuclear antigens. Children commonly present with fever, arthralgia, arthritis, and rashes of all forms (maculopapular, erythematous, urticarial, bullous, etc.). The classic butterfly rash occurs in about 30% of children at diagnosis. SLE is known for its widespread effects on kidneys, the pleura, pericardium, the brain and nerves, blood platelets (thrombocytopenia), ab-

dominal organs, lymph nodes—essentially all organ systems. It causes miscarriages early in pregnancy. The female to male ratio of sufferers is about 5:1, and a genetic or familial component is suspected.

Diagnosis

The diagnosis, which is described in greater detail in appropriate texts, rests on the demonstration of antinuclear antibodies, particularly those against DNA; these can be used to monitor the activity of the disease. IgM rheumatoid factor is often found, and low levels of C3 and C4 (of the complement pathway) denote either exacerbations of extrarenal involvement or advancing renal disease. Anemia occurs in many patients, but unless it is a hemolytic form, it is typically a mild, normochromic and normocytic variety. A low white cell count is often seen, as well as mild thrombocytopenia.

Management

Management of children and adults with SLE depends on the activity of the disease. Gentle exercise is certainly not contraindicated and should be encouraged when symptoms and clinical indicators permit. The activity of the disease can vary markedly, and the patient should be left to decide when and how much exercise is feasible. Pharmacologic management relies on anti-inflammatory medication. Aspirin in therapeutic doses remains the drug of choice, unless side effects require the use of other NSAIDs.

Patients with skin involvement or significant joint disease may respond to antimalarials such as chloroquine, but due care must be paid to the potential for retinopathy with this medication. Short, tapering courses of prednisolone may be used for relief of severe symptoms and signs, but a rheumatologist should be consulted before instituting any frequent use. Cytotoxic drugs such as cyclophosphamide may also be used in significant disease, but the serious side effects require that the patient receive careful blood and urine monitoring.

SLE is a complex problem and the clinician must be ever alert to the wide range of complications associated with this disease. The appropriate rheumatology texts contain detailed discussion of this disease and its management.

ANKYLOSING SPONDYLITIS (AS)

Ankylosing spondylitis (AS) is the prototype of the seronegative spondyloarthropathies, which include psoriatic arthropathy, Reiter's syndrome, the reactive arthropathies, and juvenile chronic polyarthropathy. All these disorders are associated with HLA-B27, absence of rheumatoid factor in the serum (hence seronegative), and lack of rheumatoid nodules. A feature of this group of diseases is the development of sacroiliitis and of enthesopathies such as plantar fasciitis and Achilles tendinitis where the tendon inserts into bone. AS has a reported prevalence of 0.1% to 0.4% of the population, with a male to female ratio of 2:1 (7).

Diagnosis

AS is suggested in a patient younger than 40 years by a history of progressive (lower) back stiffness and pain of gradual onset, with morning stiffness that eases with movement. Associated features such as anterior uveitis, nonsymmetrical arthritis of peripheral joints, enthesitis, and a family history of the condition (particularly affecting males) further support the diagnosis. On examination, typical features that confirm the clinical diagnosis include

- active and apparently painful fixation of the vertebral column
- abdominal breathing
- restricted flexion of the lumbar spine and diminished costovertebral joint movement
- tenderness and irritability of the sacroiliac joint(s)
- systemic hallmarks of skin lesions (psoriasis), nail changes (pitting), and uveitis

Laboratory tests are generally unhelpful; at best, a modestly elevated ESR may be the only abnormality. HLA typing is not mandatory as a diagnostic test, as HLA-B27 may be absent in 10% of AS sufferers (6).

Typical x-ray findings include evidence of bilateral sacroiliitis (sclerosis and irregularity), anterior spondylitis with squaring of the vertebral bodies, and syndesmophyte formation. Technetium 99m bone scanning may show sacroiliitis.

Prognosis

If an early diagnosis is made and appropriate management instituted, patients should do well, with the majority leading near-normal lives. The remainder are affected in the later stages of the disease by flexion deformities of the hips and knees, a straightened lumbar spine, and thoracic kyphosis. Women generally run a milder course than men but tend to have more peripheral joint involvement (7).

Management

The main risk to a patient with AS is ankylosis promoted by excessive rest (7). Treatment incorporates drug therapy with NSAIDs (in appropriate doses to promote mobility and comfort) and a regular exercise program of swimming, walking, and light resistance exercise, attention to ergonomics at home and work, and regular supportive review by the clinician. For the athlete, exercise is, of course, to be encouraged, but contact sports, repetitive impact, and extremes of weightbearing are inadvisable.

GOUT

Gout, the most common form of inflammatory joint disease in males, is characterized by recurrent attacks of joint inflammation caused by the release of monosodium urate monohydrate crystals into the joint cavity. Tophi (sodium urate deposits) form in and around the joints, in the kidneys, and in various subcutaneous sites (such as the ears and elbows). Some patients form renal stones of uric acid.

Hyperuricemia is associated with gout, as the causative agent, uric acid, is the end result of purine metabolism. Hyperuricemia is multifactorial, involving heredity, diet (purine foods), body weight, and some disease states. Hyperuricemia may result from an excessive rate of uric acid production (as in myeloproliferative disorders), a decrease in renal excretion, or a combination of both. (The appropriate texts contain more detailed discussions of purine and uric acid metabolism.)

Gout patients are almost always male, and they are typically 40 to 50 years old at disease onset. In the majority of patients, the disease presents with severe, acute, intermittent joint pains, usually affecting the first metatarsophalangeal joint. Joint involvement can extend to tarsal joints, ankles and knees, and, less often, to other joints. Olecranon bursitis is not uncommon.

Diagnosis

Hyperuricemia does not make the diagnosis. Definitive diagnosis depends on finding monosodium urate monohydrate crystals in the synovial fluid of an inflamed or asymptomatic joint and/or demonstrating these crystals in aspirates or tissue sections of tophaceous deposits.

The needle-shaped crystals range from 2 to 10 microns in length (but may be longer) and may be seen free in synovial fluid or as intracellular bodies in synovial leukocytes during an attack. They are strongly birefringent under polarized light with a first-order red compensator (8).

Plain radiography of affected joints in the early stages of disease shows soft tissue swelling only, but "punched out" lesions in the juxta-articular bone caused by tophaceous deposits are typical of chronic disease. There is no sclerotic reaction, and joint space is preserved until late stages of the disease.

Management

The prognosis for gout is good, provided treatment is instituted early and is tolerated by the patient. With appropriate uricosuric or allopurinol therapy, tophi and renal impairment can improve.

Acute attacks can be managed with NSAIDs such as indomethacin (300 mg on the first day, then 150 mg daily until the attack is settled) or diclofenac (300 mg on the first day, reduced by 50–100 mg daily until control is established). Colchicine is also extremely effective (0.6 mg hourly until diarrhea develops or the pain is controlled, to a maximum of 7.2 mg in any 24-hour period).

Long-term management for patients with tophi, elevated serum uric acid, or recurrent attacks centers on allopurinol (50 mg twice daily, up to 600 mg daily) or probenecid (2–3 grams per day in divided doses) to keep serum uric acid levels below 0.4 mmol/L (6 mg/dL). Colchicine in low doses is recommended to prevent acute attacks of gout while the serum uric acid levels alter with therapy.

Allopurinol is recommended for patients with extensive tophaceous gout or with renal impairment, or for patients undergoing antimitotic therapy or after failed uricosuric therapy. The side effects of allopurinol include hypersensitivity syndrome, skin rashes, nonspecific symptoms, and bone marrow depression, so patients require cautious monitoring. Estimates suggest that 5% of patients stop allopurinol therapy because of the side effects; in hospitalized individuals, 1 in 260 placed on treatment will develop a life-threatening reaction (9). Probenecid also causes side effects in 8% to 10% of patients, including gastric irritation, skin rashes, nephrotic syndrome, status epilepticus, and hepatic necrosis (10).

Gout and the Athlete

There is no reason to exclude a patient with gout from undertaking exercise. As rapid changes in hydration may precipitate acute attacks of gout, patients should frequently stop for drinks during prolonged exercise. Anticipating a change in fluid status with prophylactic medication is recommended. If necessary, colchicine can be used in the doses previously recommended. There is no need to adjust doses of allopurinol or probenecid.

If joint disease is established, appropriate attention must be paid to protecting each involved joint. For example, orthoses can be very useful in supporting an affected great toe.

CALCIUM PYROPHOSPHATE DEPOSITION DISEASE (PSEUDOGOUT)

Calcium pyrophosphate deposition disease, or pseudogout, describes the acute inflammatory gout-like attacks that occur in patients with intra-articular calcium pyrophosphate dihydrate (CPPD) deposits. Surveys have revealed that about 6% of individuals over 80 years old have such deposits. As with classic gout, men are affected more often than women (1.4:1), but the incidence of disease is about half that of gout.

Acute pseudogout is characterized by an inflammation in one or more joints that lasts several days. Attacks may be abrupt and are self-limited; they can be provoked by trauma to the joint, surgery, or severe illness. The knee is most often affected, but any synovial joint can be involved. The joints most often affected include the knees, wrists, metacarpophalangeal joints, hips, shoulders, elbows, and ankles. Although this condition is primarily an inflammatory process (often resembling rheumatoid arthritis), degeneration of joints may be seen later in the disease.

Diagnosis

The diagnosis of psuedogout is made by identifying CPPD crystals in the synovial fluid. These are strongly negative in birefringence under polarized light. Crystals may be found in asymptomatic joints. Radiography may reveal evidence of CPPD deposits within articular cartilage, fibrocartilage (as in the pubic symphysis), and in tendons, ligaments, and joint capsules. (The term "chondrocalcinosis" is used in association with such x-ray findings, but similar calcification can result from deposits of calcium oxalate, hydroxyapatite, or dicalcium phosphate dihydrate.)

There are hereditary forms of CPPD disease, but metabolic diseases can also produce CPPD arthropathy. These diseases include hyperparathyroidism, hemochromatosis, hypothyroidism, gout, hypomagnesemia, and hypophosphatasia. Therefore, appropriate screening is mandatory in assessment.

Management

There is no means available for removing CPPD crystals from joints. Treatment of any underlying disorder such as hyperparathyroidism or hemochromatosis does not result in resorption of crystals—in fact, thyroid hormone replacement is reported to lead to the presentation of symptoms (11).

Acute attacks can be managed with NSAID therapy, together with judicious joint aspiration with or without intra-articular corticosteroid injection. Oral colchicine does not appear to be as predictably reliable in pseudogout as it is for the the treatment of gout.

Pseudogout and the Athlete

Athletes should be advised that mechanical trauma may liberate CPPD crystals from articular cartilage and precipitate an acute attack of arthritis. Trial and error seems to be the only method of establishing whether a particular athlete is at risk of exercise-induced (and thus trauma-associated) arthritis.

Although there is no evidence to suggest that changes in the state of hydration (e.g., during exercise) precipitate acute attacks, common sense dictates that adequate hydration should be maintained by the athletic patient. All the principles of care should be applied to the care of affected joints, as CPPD disease is a destructive, irreversible process.

OTHER RHEUMATOLOGICAL DISEASES

Many rheumatologic conditions affect athletes at all ages. Among these are the connective disorders: progressive systemic sclerosis and mixed connective disease; the polymyositis/dermatomyositis conditions; and the various forms of arteritis (or vasculitis). All of these require careful diagnosis and specific management, but all allow for some capacity to exercise. Patients must strike a balance between physical activity and appropriate rest during inflammation.

Although the juvenile conditions Osgood-Schlatter disease and Sinding-Larsen-Johannson syndrome are very common, this chapter does not discuss them because of their apophyseal etiology, rather than being true joint diseases. These conditions are well described in other texts (see [12] for a comprehensive discussion of these conditions in the young athlete).

CONCLUSION

The practice of rheumatology promotes health and well-being through a combination of pharmacotherapy, mechanical support, protection for joints, and therapeutic exercise. An athlete with an arthropathic disease should be encouraged to control the attacks of inflammation as quickly as possible, to use appropriate orthoses and splints, and exercise judiciously (moving from nonweightbearing to weightbearing) as the condition permits.

REFERENCES

1 Murphy L, Fallon K, Fricker P, McDonald W. Does long distance running cause osteoarthritis? Sport Health 1995;13:15–26.

2 Marti B, Knobloch M, Tschopp A, et al. Is excessive running predictive of degenerative hip disease? Controlled study of former elite athletes. Br Med J 1989;299:91–93.

3 Jackson J. Degenerative changes in the knee after meniscectomy. Br Med J 1968;II:525–527.

4 Rangger C, Klestil T, Gloetzer W, et al. Osteoarthritis after arthroscopic partial meniscectomy. Am J Sports Med 1995;23:240–244.

5 Clark SR, et al. The use of exercise to treat rheumatic disease. In: Golberg L, Elliot DL, eds. Exercise for prevention and treatment of illness. Philadelphia: FA Davis, 1994:83–106.

6 Lyngberg K, Harreby M, Bentzen H, et al. Elderly rheumatoid arthritis patients on steroid treatment tolerate physical training without an increase in disease activity. Arch Phys Med Rehabil 1994;75:1189–1195.

7 Rijswijk M. Management of ankylosing spondylitis. In: Folia rheumatologica. Basel: Documenta Geigy, 1994:8–23.

8 Gatter RA. The compensated polarized light microscope in clinical rheumatology. Arthritis Rheum 1974;17:253–255.

9 Wallace SL, Singer JZ. Treatment of gout. In: Schumacher HR Jr, ed. Primer on the rheumatic diseases. 9th ed. Atlanta: Arthritis Foundation, 1988:202–206.

10 Gout. In: Hall H, ed. The new medicine, vol. I: Rheumatology. Lancaster, UK: MTP Press, 1983: 75–78.

11 Dorwart BB, Schumacher HR. Joint effusions, chondrocalcinosis and other rheumatic manifestations in hypothyroidsim: a clinicopathologic study. Am J Med 1975;59:780–790.

12 Bloomfield J, Fricker PA, Fitch KD, eds. Science and medicine in sport. 2nd ed. Melbourne: Blackwell Science, 1995.

Chapter 31
The Athlete with Anemia

Karl B. Fields

Anemia, one of the most common medical conditions, occurs in all age groups and populations. Typically, anemia is defined as a decreased number of red blood cells (RBCs) or hemoglobin concentration (HGB). Anemia carries a less serious progonosis for athletes, who are generally an active and healthy population. However, all the pathologic conditions that cause anemia can occur in sports participants, thus the specific diagnosis must be clearly established.

CAUSES OF ANEMIA

Red Blood Cell Production

Complex cellular and biochemical processes are required to produce the red blood cell. Development of RBCs begins with a pluripotent stem cell in the bone marrow. This cell differentiates into specific colony-forming units that produce the entire red blood cell line. Erythropoietin, a hormone formed in the kidneys, stimulates production of RBCs. In order to carry oxygen, RBCs must incorporate hemoglobin. A complex of iron plus porphyrin forms heme, which has a strong affinity for oxygen. Heme binds with the carrier protein ferroglobin to form hemoglobin. Any breakdown in this process results in fewer RBCs being formed (1).

A reduction in RBCs occurs as a result of inadequate development, excessive destruction, or blood loss.

Inadequate Development

Other important substances in RBC formation include pyridoxine (vitamin B_6), folic acid, and vitamin B_{12}. Pyridoxine serves as a catalyst for one of the essential steps in hemoglobin formation. Folic acid and vitamin B_{12} promote the formation of DNA and RNA for the nucleus of the precursor cells in the red blood cell line. Low levels of any of these substances or any problems in this process leads to reduced production and abnormal formation of RBCs.

Excessive Destruction

Excessive destruction of RBCs typically results from disorders that alter the red blood cell membrane. Congenital conditions such as spherocytosis or elliptocytosis that affect the shape and stability of red cells are examples of this mechanism. In addition, acquired changes in the RBC can alter the membrane and lead to excess destruction. Specific external agents such as bacteria, viruses, drugs, and chemicals have been implicated in RBC damage. Autoimmune diseases have a myriad of effects on the body including hemolytic anemia in which antibodies are directed at the RBC (2).

Blood Loss

In most individuals, blood loss occurs from heavy menses or gastrointestinal (GI) or genitourinary (GU) sources. Athletes in endurance sports frequently develop low-grade GI bleeding. GU bleeding has been recognized in association with physical activity for years, as evidenced by the classic reports of "march hemoglobinuria" in soldiers (3,4). GU bleeding can occasionally occur from trauma in contact and collision sports. In endurance athletes, menses generally tend to lessen in quantity. While blood loss does occur in athletes, the association of significant blood loss from athletic activity remains rare.

In the athlete that does demonstrates significant blood loss, the diagnostic search should focus on the common pathologic conditions known to precipitate bleeding from the GI or GU systems. For example, although hematuria is a well-known phenomenon in runners, case reports of bladder cancer in young athletes suggest that even common findings need thorough evaluation (5).

CLASSIFICATION OF ANEMIA

Classification of anemia relies on the size of the RBC. RBC indices, particularly the mean corpuscular volume (MCV), generally place anemia into one of three categories: microcytic, normocytic, and macrocytic. All of the categories tend to develop in specific conditions (Table 31-1).

- *Microcytic* anemia is considered to be a MCV less than 75 fL.
- *Normocytic* anemia is a MCV of 75 to 95 fL.
- *Macrocytic* anemia is a MCV greater than 95 fL.

This classification works well for major anemia. Thus, the first screening tests typically focus on microcytic anemia to establish a diagnosis of iron deficiency, the most common problem in this category. Macrocytic anemias are less frequently encountered, but an initial evaluation with laboratory screening for serum B_{12}, serum folic acid, and thyroid function tests generally diagnoses a significant number of cases (6).

The classification shown in Table 31-1 often fails when complex factors contribute to the anemia. For example, a mix of iron deficiency in an individual taking a folic acid antagonist medication makes the blood morphology difficult to predict. Similarly, RBC morphology may be normocytic early in a hematopoietic malignancy, but in a later phase of the same illness it may become macrocytic. Numerous hemoglobin variants exist throughout the world, and increasing travel and intermarriage of different races lead to combinations of hemoglobin about which little medical information exists (7–11).

Table 31-1   Categories of Anemia

Microcytic
  Iron deficiency
  Thalassemia minor
  Lead poisoning
  Sideroblastic anemia
Macrocytic
  Folate deficiency
  B_{12} deficiency
  Hypothyroidism
  Drugs
  Liver disease
  Malignancy
Normocytic
  Chronic disease
  Hemolysis
  Rapid bleeding
  Aplastic anemia
  Malignancy
Variable
  Aplastic anemia
  Chronic blood loss
  Mixed nutritional causes
  Hemoglobinopathy

CONDITIONS COMMON IN ATHLETES

Sports Anemia (Dilutional Pseudoanemia)

The finding that many endurance athletes have somewhat low hemoglobin led Yoshimura to coin the term *sports anemia* in 1970 (3). Runners and swimmers typically have hemoglobin levels of 0.5 to 1 gram lower than expected, a finding that seems particularly true of the more elite competitors. Why these healthy, competitive individuals have lower hemoglobin levels than sedentary counterparts has prompted further investigation. Numerous physiologic studies have demonstrated that these athletes have actually increased total numbers of RBCs and a high RBC mass along with normal indices. The difference in HGB level was explained not by decline in RBC parameters but by an increase in plasma volume. Thus the concept of a dilutional "pseudoanemia."

Additional studies have looked at blood volume after training, and all show an increase in plasma volume with minimal change in RBC mass. During the active phase of exercise, plasma volume decreases because of a number of actions. Fluid is pushed into soft tissue by muscle contraction and then diffuses into tissue because of osmotic pressure changes from the production of metabolites such as lactic acid. Additional fluid loss occurs through sweating. The net effect of the loss in plasma volume is that HGB levels normalize during the exercise (12).

Why the body undergoes these changes remains speculative, but several teleologic explanations have been suggested. One thought is that the increased plasma volume lowers viscosity, which decreases the likelihood of hypercoaguable problems during exercise. In addition, a larger blood volume increases cardiac output and may increase oxygen delivery, both advantageous adaptations for exercise. Finally, sweating is a key mechanism for heat dissipation and increased sweating associated with high plasma volume may reduce the risk of hyperthermia with exercise.

Dilutional pseudoanemia does not appear to be pathologic but rather an adaptation to endurance training (13). Therefore, this condition should not be classified as a true anemia, but rather as a training change or physiologic adaptation expected in endurance athletes. Several studies of elite distance runners with low HGB levels show that other blood parameters are normal even when there is an increase in RBC mass. This indicates that iron supplementation or other treatment is not necessary.

Iron Deficiency Anemia

Iron deficiency is the most common true anemia found in athletes (14). Iron must be incorporated into the formation of hemoglobin; several problems, including inadequate intake, inadequate absorption, and excessive loss, can limit the available iron for this process. Special groups with a greater risk of iron deficiency anemia are women with heavy menstruation, any athlete who diets, and adolescent athletes. In adolescent athletes the key concern is that rapid growth, particularly in the Tanner 3 stage, requires greater quantities of iron, something often difficult to obtain due to the typical adolescent's less-than-ideal dietary intake. Also, there continues to be a risk of iron deficiency anemia associated with certain parasitic infections such as hookworm, and athletes from tropical countries where such parasites are more common may require diagnostic testing to exclude an infectious cause of their anemia.

Controversy exists over the true prevalence of iron deficiency anemia. Nevertheless, it is the most common nutritional deficiency in the United States and many other countries. Statistics point to the magnitude of the problem with studies showing that as many as 20% of menstruating women have low ferritin (3). In addition, at some point during their menstrual years approximately 20% of women develop an iron deficiency anemia. Low ferritin indicates decreased storage of iron, but the number of patients with low ferritin who develop anemia is unclear.

Diagnosis   Underdetection of iron deficiency anemia is the norm as most athletes are asymptomatic. When symptoms occur they include weakness, lassitude, palpitations, and shortness of breath. Occasionally, an unexplained symptom called "pica"—the craving for starch, ice, or clay—may be the first manifestation of iron deficiency anemia. Fatigue and underperformance are two principal reasons for athletes to seek medical care. The first step in this evaluation is screening for anemia, as low hemoglobin levels definitely worsen performance.

Physical findings typically occur in more advanced anemia and signs include paleness, glossitis, angular cheilitis, and koilonychia (spoon-shaped nails) (6). In the case of a suggestive history or pathognomonic physical findings, additional testing for anemia is warranted. The specific laboratory findings used to confirm iron deficiency anemia include the following:

- Low HGB level in adults: <12 g/dL female or <14 g/dL males
- MCV <75 fL
- Peripheral smear: hypochromic, microcytic red cells
- Serum iron low with high total iron-binding capacity
- Serum ferritin <12 ng/mL
- Bone marrow: decreased iron staining indicative of depleted iron stores (1)

In difficult cases all of these tests may be needed, but in practice most physicians rely on a complete blood count, peripheral smear, and serum ferritin to confirm the diagnosis.

Differential Diagnoses In general, the differential diagnosis of a microcytic anemia falls between iron deficiency and a hemoglobinopathy, particularly thalassemia minor. Sideroblastic anemia and lead poisoning remain rare. MCV levels below 60 fL occur much more commonly in thalassemia minor and make the diagnosis of iron deficiency less likely. Nevertheless, atypical microcytic presentations of anemia, of chronic disease or of conditions like aplastic anemia, while rare, should prompt the clinician to confirm the diagnosis of iron deficiency, particularly when the anemia persists. Most athletes use nonsteroidal antiinflammatory drugs (NSAIDs), which are among the most common medications associated with aplastic anemia.

Risk Factors At one time, endurance athletes and runners in particular were considered at high risk for iron deficiency. This seemed logical based on the demonstration of GI and GU blood loss in athletes as well as foot-strike hemolysis and loss of iron in sweat. Studies of distance runners reported extremely high levels of suspected iron deficiency (range: 40% to 82% of females, 17% to 29% of males), but these reports were based on serum ferritins of <25 ng/mL (13). In reality, these levels are borderline and are probably artificially lowered by the dilutional effects of increased plasma volume (3). Similar data arose from studies that showed declining ferritin levels with the progression of a cross-country season, but these were not controlled for increasing plasma volume.

More recent studies no longer suggest that athletes are at greater risk of iron deficiency anemia (13). One study of athletes in three sports found no difference in male and female distance runners, male triathletes, and female ballet dancers versus matched controls in the incidence of individuals with true anemia (range: 1.7% to 3.3% in the three groups) (15).

Of the various factors causing blood loss, GI problems and menstruation are the two that normally cause enough blood loss to lead athletes to develop iron deficiency anemia. Blood loss accounts for a small minority of athletes with iron deficiency anemia. The number one cause of iron deficiency in women is caused by inadequate iron in

their diet. Vegetarian and other special diets may not contain enough iron to prevent anemia. In sports that emphasize "thinness," a finding of iron deficiency anemia should raise serious concern: is the anemia associated with amenorrhea? The amenorrheic athlete whose sport has an emphasis on thinness may have the markers for much larger problems including eating disorders, bone loss, anemia, and menstrual irregularity. Dietary insufficiency in athletes who have adequate access to food suggests a careful review of nutritional history to differentiate poor nutritional habits from abnormal eating behaviors.

Treatment Treatment of iron deficiency anemia requires the administration of a palatable form of elemental iron, such as 50 mg given three times daily as ferrous gluconate, sulfate, or lactate. Absorption is best between meals and may be improved with intake of orange juice or ascorbic acid. Dietary changes can make a major difference in iron intake by increasing iron-rich foods like red meat, poultry, and fish. Foods that may block iron absorption are those high in tannin, phytate, or phosphate. GI intolerance is the fundamental problem causing inadequate iron supplementation, and in these cases parenteral iron may be needed.

In an athlete with borderline amenia an empiric treatment trial of iron is warranted for approximately 2 months to determine whether there is a 1 gram increase in HGB.

Anemic patients treated with iron improve their exercise capacity, but treatment of iron deficiency in the absence of anemia has not been shown to improve performance (13). Most physicians suggest dietary changes or iron supplements (50 mg daily as opposed to therapeutic doses) in athletes with low ferritin but no evidence of anemia. Similarly, women with a history of recurrent, documented iron deficiency should be given either daily or every-other-day doses of iron prophylactically. No documentation of the efficacy of this approach exists, but the risk/benefit ratio weighs strongly toward treatment.

Foot-Strike Hemolysis

A number of well-designed experiments show the occurrence of foot-strike hemolysis. The magnitude of red cell destruction appears low and probably represents breakdown of older, more fragile cells. Overt hemoglobinuria rarely occurs, but descriptions of this phenomenon were first described by Fleischer in 1881, who coined the term *march hemoglobinuria* after soldiers on vigorous marches developed this condition (3,4). Marathon runners are the athletes most prone to foot-strike hemolysis. Recent reports regarding role of foot-strike hemolysis in hematologic changes of runners suggest that the contribution is not strong enough to regard this is a true cause of anemia (13).

Interestingly, foot strike is not the only etiologic factor, as the same hemolysis occurs in swimmers and rowers who do not have the same impact problems. Other postulated causes include increased body temperature and altered flow dynamics in vigorous sport. Clinically significant hemolysis in athletes should trigger a search for problems that traditionally cause hemolytic anemia, and foot-strike hemolysis from athletic participation should remain a diagnosis of exclusion.

Treatment requires different shoes, orthotic foot supports, changes in running surface, and/or modification of the training program (14).

Macrocytic Anemia

B_{12} deficiency and true pernicious anemia rarely occur in athletes. Folic acid deficiency is also unusual in normally nourished individuals. However, athletes traveling from certain African nations and individuals following extreme diets or who have eating disorders may have an increased risk of folate deficiency. Otherwise, two of the most common causes for macrocytic anemia in athletes include drugs and hypothyroidism.

Drugs should always be suspected when a megaloblastic anemia is noted. Agents associated with megaloblastic changes include triamterene, sulfasalazine, sulfamethoxazole-trimethoprim, oral contraceptives, and anticonvulsants including phenytoin, primidone, and phenobarbital. Hypothyroidism causes a macrocytic anemia in which fatigue is a prominent feature. As both hypothyroidism and anemia have been found in athletes who are underperforming, thyroid function should be checked any time a macrocytic anemia is identified (16).

Hemolytic Anemia

Hemolytic anemias are uncommon but can be triggered by a number of common illnesses and medications. Causes include antigen–antibody reactions that lead to red cell membrane breakdown, abnormal red cells that have fragile membranes, and defects of the red cell itself.

Drugs   Drug-induced hemolytic anemia occurs following ingestion of one of a number of medicines including

- penicillin and cephalosporin
- quinidine and quinine
- sulfonamide
- isoniazid
- phenacetin

Acute Illnesses   Acute illnesses known to trigger hemolytic anemia include

- mycoplasma pneumonia
- infectious mononucleosis
- malarial infections
- sepsis from a variety of bacteria
- certain idiopathic types of hemolytic anemia (suspected to be viral mediated) (10)

Of these acute illnesses both mycoplasma pneumonia and infectious mononucleosis (glandular fever) frequently occur in athletes. The diagnosis of either of these suggests follow-up of the complete blood count before the athlete returns to competition. Presence of an anemia should lead to a search for hemolysis including Coomb's test and a check for cold and warm antibodies.

Chronic Illnesses   Chronic illnesses and congenital conditions also trigger hemolysis in some individuals. Although most collagen vascular diseases cause some degree of anemia, lupus erythematosus remains the most common disorder identified in athletes. Another condition that occurs throughout the world is G6PD (glucose-6-phosphate deydrogenase) deficiency. Individuals with this disorder develop hemolysis following bacterial or viral infection.

A variety of substances including sulfa drugs, antimalarials, and other specific agents such nitrofurantoin, nalidixic acid, or even the ingestion of fava beans can trigger hemolysis in affected individuals.

Heredity   American and African black males are at highest risk, although a different variety affects Mediterranean and Asian populations. Rarer causes of hemolytic anemia include congenital red cell anomalies such as hereditary spherocytosis and hereditary elliptocytosis, most of which are diagnosed before the age of sports participation (17). Hemoglobinopathies are discussed in this chapter.

HEMOGLOBINOPATHIES

Thalassemia

Thalassemia occurs from a defect in synthesis of one or more HGB subunits. Variants include α and β thalassemia. The latter, β thalassemia, is caused by complex variations in β-globulin synthesis that lead to a range of clinical presentations. The most common is thalassemia minor, which rarely causes severe illness. Thalassemia major does cause severe problems, but fortunately it is rare. Laboratory testing differentiates the two conditions: α thalassemia shows a decrease in HGB A_2, whereas β thalassemia shows an increase in HGB A_2 and an increase in HGB F.

Anemia occurs with both variants, although it is less common with α thalassemia. Hemolytic anemia with Heinz bodies can occur. β Thalassemia minor causes more changes including a mild anemia characterized by slight icterus, modest splenomegaly, and basophilic stippling on peripheral smear. Thalassemia minor frequently mimics iron deficiency because of the marked microcytosis and the mild anemia. Differentiating features include normal iron studies, an extremely low MCV, and a peripheral smear with basophilic stippling. MCVs may be 60 fL or less in many cases of thalassemia minor, which would be an unusual finding in iron deficiency.

Distribution of thalassemia is worldwide. Mediterranean, African, and Middle Eastern patients commonly have α thalassemia. About 2% of the U.S. African-American population has α thalassemia without symptoms. β Thalassemia occurs in 1% of Southern Italians, and is common in Central Africa, the Middle East, Southeast Asia, and the South Pacific. Thalassemia should, thus, be a part of the differential diagnosis for anemia in athletes wherever they compete.

More study is needed to understand the impact on performance, but currently no treatment is recommended for mild anemia associated with thalassemia (9).

Sickle Cell Anemia

Sickle Cell Disease   Sickle cell disease is a severe hemoglobinopathy characterized by a chronic hemolytic anemia that leads to extremely low HGB levels, usually in the range of 6 to 7 grams per deciliter. A myriad of complications leads to significant morbidity and a shortened life expectancy.

Sickle cell patients have a substitution of valine for glutamic acid at the sixth position of the β-hemoglobin chain, a mutation that provides protection against malaria. However, RBCs containing the sickle hemoglobin (HGB S) change into elongated cells with a sickle-like appearance and other bizarre forms that can occlude distal capillaries. The result of this is significant end-organ damage to the lungs, heart, spleen, bone, brain, and other tissue. A higher risk of some infections leads to more frequent sepsis, pneumonia, and ostcomyclitis.

No deaths from exercise in sickle cell disease have been reported, perhaps because the severity of the anemia may limit exercise tolerance. Limited sports performance is possible in a minority of patients who have persistently high levels of fetal hemoglobin, which lead them to a milder form of the disease.

Sickle Cell Trait   Athletes with homozygous HGB SS disease are rare, but many athletes with heterozygous HGB AS compete. This condition, *sickle cell trait*, varies in severity by each individual, with most having about 40% HGB S. Performance limitations with sickle cell trait, are rare and welltrained HGB AS individuals perform similarly to HGB AA (normal) athletes in both anaerobic and aerobic training. Sickle cell trait does not cause anemia and often goes undetected. Typically, no limitations have been placed on HGB AS athletes and most data support this. For example, no complications were noted for athletes with HGB AS in competition at the Mexico City Olympics where the altitude was 2135 meters (18).

Epidemiologic and physiologic studies have begun to question whether sickle trait is truly benign. For individuals with HGB AS, the effects of exercise—including dehydration, increased body temperature, hypoxia, and acidosis—all increase the likelihood of sickling. This is confirmed by tests showing that exercise to exhaustion usually produces small numbers of reversibly sickled cells in HGB AS athletes. In addition, rare reports suggest that severe hypoxia at high altitudes (10,000 feet) has led to splenic infarction in HGB AS individuals, and that infarction of the renal medulla can also occur.

Clinical syndromes common to sickle cell disease have not been the primary problems in HGB AS athletes. Unexpected death is the worst potential outcome of HGB AS disease and is most often associated with severe exertional rhabdomyolysis. U.S. military data are alarming, as black soldiers with HGB AS have 20 to 30 times the risk of exertional death compared to black soldiers without HGB S (19). Reports from a U.S. Army base at Fort Bliss show that all exercise-related deaths between 1965 and 1981 were associated with HGB S (5 with HGB AS and 1 with HGB SC) (19). The same risk pattern apparently exists in high school and college athletes, as recent sudden death statistics have found sickle cell trait as the cause in 7 of 136 cases (20). Currently, the only recommendation for athletes with HGB AS is to advise caution when exercising at high altitude or following a recent illness. The statistical relationship with sudden cardiac death suggests that further research is needed.

Additional Hemoglobin Variants

Over 500 strains of HGB have been identified worldwide. HGB C occurs in about 2% of black Americans, but rarely causes complications when coupled as HGB AC. HGB CC or HGB SC, however, can result in hemolytic anemia and other clinical syndromes.

HGB E occurs as one of the most common variants in Southeast Asia. HGB AE causes few problems, but HGB EE and HGB E β thalassemia both can cause severe anemia. With the substantial migration of Southeast Asians into all corners of the globe, new HGB combinations are more common. The implications of these for disease and for sports performance remain undetermined. For example, will HGB SE athletes have similar risks to HGB AS individuals?

As the world becomes more of a global village, further study of hemodynamic implications of HGB variants is needed to clarify sports-specific risks.

SPECIAL CONSIDERATIONS OF ANEMIA IN ATHLETES

Some situations should alert the clinician that more serious problems exist than the degree of anemia suggests. For example, iron deficiency anemia in a nonmenstruating female athlete, a male wrestler, or any athlete in a sport requiring weight control sport may be associated with an eating disorder. Similarly, a true normochromic and normocytic anemia in any athlete suggests a systemic disease. Anemia in athletes using regular medications warrants a careful review of the hematologic effects of those products. Aplastic anemia, bone marrow suppressive agents, and hematologic malignancies all lower granulocyte counts as well as produce anemia. For this reason, the combination of low granulocyte counts plus anemia should raise serious concern. Changes on peripheral smears that include target cells, basophilic stippling, or unusual RBC forms should prompt hemoglobin electrophoresis as a part of the anemia workup.

Evaluation of the Athlete with Anemia

A rational approach to the athlete with anemia is to consider a medical condition as the primary cause unless "sports anemia" seems the only logical conclusion. Recent-onset anemia in athletes on NSAIDs are worrisome as most NSAIDs have been reported to cause aplastic anemia and varying degrees of bone-marrow suppression. Careful medical evaluation, nutritional assessment, and sometimes psychological referral may be needed to delineate particularly difficult diagnostic cases with anemia.

Sports activity does not cause significant hemolysis or enough iron loss to explain the occurrence of anemia. A systematic review of the athlete's history, physical findings, and standard laboratory testing helps classify most anemia into categories that have a limited differential diagnosis. Treatment of the anemia and the underlying cause should return all but the rare athlete to full sports activity.

REFERENCES

1 American Board of Pediatrics. Program for renewal of certification in pediatrics: guides for record review—anemia. Pediatr Rev 1994 (suppl).
2 Bunn HF. Pathophysiology of the anemias. In: Isselbacher KJ, Braunwald E, Wilson JD, et al., eds. Harrison's principles of internal medicine. New York: McGraw-Hill, 1994:1717–1721.
3 Balaban EP. Sports anemia. Clin Sports Med 1992;11:313–325.
4 Fleischer R. Uber eine neue Form von Hamoglobinurie beim Menschen. Klin Wochenschr (Berlin) 1881;18:691.
5 Elliot DL, Goldberg L, Eichner ER. Hematuria in a young recreational runner. Med Sci Sports Exerc 1991;23:892–894.
6 Bridges KR, Bunn HF. Anemias with disturbed iron metabolism. In: Isselbacher KJ, Braunwald E, Wilson JD, et al., eds. Harrison's principles of internal medicine. New York: McGraw-Hill, 1994:1721–1726.
7 Babior BM, Bunn HF. Megaloblastic anemias. In: Isselbacher KJ, Braunwald E, Wilson JD, et al., eds. Harrison's principles of internal medicine. New York: McGraw-Hill, 1994:1726–1732.
8 Bunn HF. Anemia associated with chronic disorders. In: Isselbacher KJ, Braunwald E, Wilson JD, et al., eds. Harrison's principles of internal medicine. New York: McGraw-Hill, 1994:1732–1734.
9 Bunn HF. Disorders of hemoglobin. In: Isselbacher KJ, Braunwald E, Wilson JD, et al., eds. Harrison's principles of internal medicine. New York: McGraw-Hill, 1994:1734–1743.
10 Rosse W, Bunn HF. Hemolytic anemias. In: Isselbacher KJ, Braunwald E, Wilson JD, et al., eds. Harrison's principles of internal medicine. New York: McGraw-Hill, 1994:1743–1754.
11 Rappeport JM, Bunn HF. Bone marrow failure: aplastic anemia and other primary bone marrow disorders. In: Isselbacher KJ, Braunwald E, Wilson JD, et al., eds. Harrison's principles of internal medicine. New York: McGraw-Hill, 1994:1754–1757.
12 Selby GB, Eichner ER. Hematocrit and performance: the effect of endurance training on blood volume. Semin Hematol 1994;31:122–127.
13 Eichner ER. Sports anemia, iron supplements, and blood doping. Med Sci Sports Exerc 1992;24:S315–318.
14 Eichner ER. Hematologic problems. In: Grana WA, Kalenak A, eds. Clinical sports medicine. Philadelphia: WB Saunders 1991:209–216.
15 Weight LM, Klein M, Noakes TD, Jacobs P. Sports anemia—a real or apparent phenomenon in endurance-trained athletes? Int J Sports Med 1992;13:344–347.
16 Colon-Otero G, Menke D, Hook CC. A practical approach to the differential diagnosis and evaluation of the adult patient with macrocytic anemia. Med Clin North Am 1992;76:581–597.
17 Tabbara IA. Hemolytic anemias. Med Clin North Am 1992;76:649–668.
18 Gozal D, Thieiet P, Mbala E, et al. Effect of different modalities of exercise and recovery on exercise performance in subjects with sickle cell trait. Med Sci Sports Exerc 1992;24:1325–1331.
19 Kark JA, Ward FT. Exercise and hemoglobin S. Semin Hematol 1994;31:181–225.
20 Van Camp SP, Bloor CM, Mueller FO, et al. Nontraumatic sports death in high school and college athletes. Med Sci Sports Exerc 1995;27:641–647.

Chapter 32
Immune Function and Exercise

David B. Pyne

This chapter discusses the influence of exercise and training on immune function, which may ultimately alter resistance to infectious agents. The interaction between exercise and immune function has important clinical implications in the fields of preventive and rehabilitative sports medicine. The primary focus in the context of sports medicine is whether strenuous exercise and training suppress immune function and increase the risk of common upper respiratory tract and gastrointestinal tract infections. Most of the infections sustained by athletes are normally mild and self-limiting, but the physician may, on occasions, have to deal with a more debilitating defect in host defense. The complexity and diversity of the immune system, coupled with the influence of many biological and environmental variables including exercise and training, can provide a significant challenge to the sports medicine practitioner.

ORGANIZATION OF THE IMMUNE SYSTEM

The immune system is a complex network of interacting cellular and humoral (soluble) components that protect host tissues from invading microorganisms, trauma, and foreign substances. Within this network some elements form the specific (acquired) division of host defense involving antigen–antibody interaction, whereas others form the nonspecific (innate) division involving direct lysis or phagocytosis of pathogenic agents (1). These elements generally act in concert to detect and degrade molecules targeted for destruction. Apart from host defense, the immune system also plays an important role in allergic and inflammatory reactions, and in the processes of wound repair and tissue remodeling. Activity of the immune system is regulated by a balance between the wide range of immunopotentiating and immunosuppressive mediators (2). It is likely that immune dysfunction in otherwise healthy athletes is caused primarily by transient exercise-induced changes in immunoregulatory mechanisms rather than by any inherent or congenital defect.

The immune system is sensitive to a wide range of biological and environmental variables. In addition to the effects of exercise and training, various physical stresses including direct tissue injury, surgery, burns, and hemorrhagic shock influence immune function. The clinician also needs to consider the age and gender of the patient, sleep patterns, underlying psychological stress, and the presence of conditions such as hypoxia and hyperthermia when evaluating immune function. Given the potential interaction of these behavioral and environmental influences, it is obvious that the immune system must be flexible and adaptable to cope with isolated and cumulative stress.

THE EFFECT OF EXERCISE ON THE IMMUNE SYSTEM

Exercise can affect both the distribution (circulating concentration) and/or the functional activity of the cellular and humoral parameters. Research shows that intense exercise suppresses most immunologic functions for up to several hours after exercise, but it is not clear whether these changes have any significant or lasting clinical effects (3,4). It is likely that the functional activity of immune cells and soluble factors may have to fall below a critical threshold before susceptibility to infection increases (2). For moderate exercise, results have been conflicting, but in general this type of activity elicits an improvement in both immune function and resistance to infection.

Much research has been directed toward study of the apparent paradox between exercise intensity and immune function. Experimental evidence generally supports the long-held beliefs and anecdotal reports by elite athletes and fitness enthusiasts that physical activity influences immunity. The suppression of discrete aspects of immune function after intense exercise may provide an opportunity for infectious agents to take advantage of a temporarily suppressed host defense (5).

Although a suppressed immune system may have direct clinical effects in terms of the resistance to illness and infection, other physiologic modifications may explain the experimental evidence and clinical findings. The exercise- or training-induced immunosuppression observed in elite athletes may be an adaptive response that limits inflammation and reduces the risk of autoimmune reactions damaging host tissues (6).

Changes in the Distribution of Immune Cells

In general, acute exercise causes an increase in the circulating number of immune cells (leukocytes), yet indices of functional activity are often decreased. Some alterations may be due to changes in total leukocyte number rather than functional changes at the single cell level. Most studies show transient immunosuppression after intense exercise (>80% of maximal oxygen uptake), but there is conflicting evidence regarding the effects of moderate exercise (<60% maximal oxygen uptake) on functional measures and changes in the concentration of soluble components such as complement, cytokines, and immunoglobulins (7). The conflicting results may be attributable to biological variability in immune parameters or to the methodologic differences in the experimental procedures employed.

The leukocytosis of exercise is a well-described but short-term phenomenon that generally has limited clinical implications. The increase in the number of circulating leukocytes is the result of intensity-dependent elevations in cardiac output and in the concentration of immunomodulatory hormones such as adrenaline and cortisol (8). Leukocyte (total white cell count), granulocyte (predominantly neutrophils), and lymphocyte count all increase during exercise. After increasing during and immediately after exercise, the lymphocyte count may decline (even below resting levels) in the first few hours of recovery as these cells leave the circulation in large numbers. Even mild exercise can elicit an elevation in the circulating number of leukocytes, and for this reason, athletes should refrain from exercise for at least 12 hours prior to hematologic evaluation. An acute and/or a prolonged elevation in the white cell count may be evidence that an infection has become established.

Enumeration of lymphocyte subsets has also been used to show that exercise exerts a transient effect on the distribution of the lymphocyte population. Intensive exercise causes a transient decrease in the $CD4^+/CD8^+$ (T-helper/T-suppressor cell) ratio, while prolonged training may lead to a decrease in the circulating concentration of natural killer (NK) cells. A prolonged decrease in the T-helper/T-suppressor ratio may be evidence of underlying pathology or impaired immunocompetence. A decrease in the circulating number of NK-cells, a key mononuclear leukocyte that exerts antitumor and antiviral activity, may signify a reduction in the ability to counter the viral infections commonly observed in athletes.

Changes in Functional Measures

Exercise and training may cause significant changes in measures of immune cell function such as lymphocyte proliferation, NK-cell activity, and aspects of phagocytosis including chemotaxis, adherence, ingestion, degranulation, and activation of the respiratory (oxidative) burst. Although the number of lymphocytes in the circulation increases with intense exercise, their ability to proliferate in vitro following stimulation decreases. NK-cell activity generally increases during exercise, yet conversely it is often suppressed during the first few hours of recovery (9). Most of these in vitro techniques show that exercise causes short-term (up to several hours) perturbations in distribution and functional activities, but baseline levels are normally restored within a few hours.

Changes in Soluble Immune Components

Exercise may also cause changes in the peripheral concentration of key soluble immune components. This is especially evident in mucosal immunity, which forms a first line of defense against infectious agents. The mucosal tissues and soluble factors form a physical and chemical barrier against colonization by pathogenic microorganisms. The concentration of serum and salivary immunoglobulins (particularly IgA and IgG) is known to decrease after intense exercise and during a prolonged season of athletic training (10). IgA is the major immunoglobulin found in seromucous secretions, where it defends external body surfaces. The concentration of salivary IgA correlates more closely with resistance to certain viruses than do serum antibodies. IgG is the most abundant immunoglobulin in internal body fluids and is very effective in neutralizing toxins and bacterial pathogens in the extravascular environment.

Investigation and Assessment of Immune Function

Clinical investigation of an athlete suspected of suffering an infection normally involves a thorough history and examination. The following clinical findings may be evidence of host defense failure: infection, recurrent infection, allergy, lymphadenopathy, diarrhea, or manifestations of autoimmune disease.

Management of an infected athlete is guided by clinical assessment and follows traditional lines for viral and/or bacterial infections (1). In cases of inflammation, traditional clinical measures such as erythrocyte sedimentation rate, or key acute phase proteins such as C-reactive protein should be considered. Nutritional assessment may identify deficiencies in key nutrients (e.g., vitamins, minerals, glucose, or amino acids, which are all essential for immunocyte growth and replication) as possible factors contributing to immunosuppression and recurrent infection.

Quantitative assessment of immune status, where no clinical defect in host defense is suspected, normally involves a simple full blood examination (FBE), which provides the numbers and percentages of leukocytes (granulocytes, lymphocytes, and monocytes) in peripheral blood as a basic immune profile. Less often, where a moderate failure in host defense is suspected, a full biochemical profile should be conducted. In rare cases of major breakdown in host defense, a full battery of hematologic and immunologic testing is indicated. The nature and extent of laboratory investigation depends on the clinical evaluation, type of infection (if any), and whether any abnormalities are detected with initial screening (11).

In cases of severe or recurrent infection, a failure of host defense may be the first evidence of hematologic or immunologic disease. The history and type of infection may indicate the nature of the defect in the immune system. More specialized assessment of host defense may include immunophenotyping of lymphocyte subsets (T-cells, B-cells, and NK-cells), enumeration of serum and/or salivary immunoglobulin concentration, or measurement of functional activities such as lymphocyte proliferation, NK-cell function, or aspects of phagocytic function (Table 32-1). Future research may establish the functional significance of various phenotypic markers expressed by activated leukocytes. For many of these functional measures, normal reference ranges have not yet been established. Congenital or acquired immunodeficiency is usually diagnosed by the virtual absence of functional activity rather than by minor fluctuations within homeostatic limits (2). Until sports-specific guidelines are established, practitioners will need to rely on the interpretation provided by each clinical laboratory.

SUMMARY

The immune system is a complex and diverse network of cellular and soluble components influenced by a wide range of biological and environmental variables. Changes in immune function with exercise and training may represent some form of adaptive (protective) response in addition to the clinical manifestations of altered resistance to infection. Monitoring training stress, nutritional status, and inflammation may be useful in the clinical and practical management of immune

Table 32-1   Specific Clinical and Laboratory Tests of Immune Function

General
  Full blood examination (FBE) including white cell differential
  Immunophenotyping of lymphocyte subsets (e.g., CD3, CD4, CD8)
  Erythrocyte sedimentation rate (ESR)
  Delayed hypersensitivity skin test (cellular-mediated immunity)
  Activation status of leukocyte subpopulations
Nonspecific
  Phagocytic function
  Attachment
  Chemotaxis
  Phagocytosis
  Degranulation
  Respiratory burst
  Serum complement assays
  Acute phase response (plasma concentrations of proteins)
Specific
  T-cells
    Proliferation
    Activation status
  B-cells
    Proliferation
    Antibody production
      Immunoglobulins (plasma and salivary concentration) such as IgA, IgG, IgM, IgD, IgE
      Titers of induced or acquired antibodies
  NK-cell
    Cytotoxicity

function in athletes. Guidelines for the prescription of exercise necessary to optimize immunologic responses, and/or counter the adverse effects of strenuous and/or prolonged training, are yet to be fully described.

REFERENCES

1 Pyne DB, Gray A, McDonald WM. Exercise, training and immunity. In: Bloomfield J, Fricker P, Fitch K, eds. Textbook of science and medicine in sport. 2nd ed. Melbourne: Blackwell Science, 1995:602–615.
2 Smith JA. Guidelines, standards and perspectives in exercise immunology. Med Sci Sports Exerc 1995;27:497–506.
3 Cannon JG. Exercise and resistance to infection. J Appl Physiol 1993;74:973–981.
4 Pyne DB. Exercise, training and the immune system. Sports Med Training Rehabil 1994;5:47–64.
5 Nieman DC. Exercise, upper respiratory tract infection, and the immune system. Med Sci Sports Exerc 1994;27:128–139.
6 Pyne DB, Baker MS, Fricker PA, et al. Effects of an intensive 12-wk training program by elite swimmers on neutrophil oxidative activity. Med Sci Sports Exerc 1995;27:536–542.
7 Rhind SG, Shek PN, Shephard RJ. The impact of exercise on cytokines and receptor expression. Exerc Immunol Rev 1995;1:97–148.
8 McCarthy DA, Dale MM. The leucocytosis of exercise: a review and model. Sports Med 1988;6:333–363.
9 Gannon GA, Shek PN, Shephard RJ. Natural killer cells: modulation by intensity and duration of exercise. Exerc Immunol Rev 1995;1:26–48.
10 Gleeson M, McDonald WA, Cripps AW, et al. The effect on immunity of long term intensive training in elite swimmers. Clin Exp Immunol 1995;102:210–215.
11 Isbister JP, Pittiglio DH. Clinical hematology: a problem-oriented approach. Baltimore: William & Wilkins, 1988:151–160.

Chapter 33
The Effects of Training at High Altitude

David F. Gerrard

[D]ire predictions preceded the Games. No previous Summer Games had been held at an elevation of higher than 658 feet above sea level. . . . It was thought that competition for long distance swimmers and runners would not be possible in the oxygen-thin atmosphere. Alarmists thought that deaths might occur from the exertion. Some physicians and ex-athletes thought that the Games were dangerous and unfair and should be boycotted (1).

One could argue that the 1968 Mexico City Olympics did for sport science what World War II did to accelerate the advancement of aircraft design. In the rarified air of Mexico City (2300 meters), Olympic athletes from sea level were predicted to be at physiologic disadvantage; some even predicted that competitors could die. As a result, the international sport science community focused on the issue of physical exertion at altitude. There was vigorous collaboration between scientists and clinicians to determine how the altitude might affect individual performances.

Mindful of the physiologic changes stimulated by a decrease in barometric pressure and oxygen partial pressure, the conclusions were that events exceeding 2-minutes' duration (e.g., 1500 meter track, 400 meter swim) would be slower, and performance in events that involved effort against a decreased air resistance (e.g., long jump, triple jump, and sprints) would be enhanced. These predictions in fact proved true, as perhaps best illustrated by Bob Beamon's remarkable long jump record of 8.90 meters (29 feet 2.5 inches). At the same time, track athletes habituated to high altitude were clearly dominant in the middle and longer distances. The record book confirms that during the 1968 Olympics, world or Olympic records were established on the track in the men's 100 meter, 200 meter, 400 meter, 800 meter, and 1500 meter plus the long jump and the pole vault. In contrast, the 3000 meter steeplechase, the 10,000 meter, and the marathon were 4%, 7%, and 8.5% slower than the existing world records or best times (2).

THE ATMOSPHERE AND PHYSICAL GAS LAWS

The atmosphere has a universal and consistent composition. It comprises 78.08% nitrogen, 20.95% oxygen, and a small trace of other gases including argon, neon, carbon dioxide, hydrogen, and helium. The weight exerted by the atmosphere at any given point is termed the barometric or atmospheric pressure; this reduces, together with the partial pressure of oxygen (PO_2), in relationship to increasing altitude.

At sea level, at a temperature of 15 °C, the barometric pressure is 760 mm Hg and the PO_2 is 159.2 mm Hg. At the altitude of Mexico City (2300 meters) the barometric pressure is 586 mm Hg, and PO_2 is 122 mm Hg. To understand the effects these changes have on the body, it is necessary to acknowledge three important physical gas laws (3,4).

1 **Dalton's Law of Partial Pressure** deals with the pressure exerted by gases at differing altitudes: the total pressure of a gas mixture is the sum of the individual or partial pressures of all the gases in the mixture (Fig 33-1).
2 **Boyle's Law** relates to the expansion of gases: when the temperature remains constant, the volume of a given mass of gas varies inversely to its pressure (Fig 33-2).
3 **Henry's Law** explains the solubility of gases within a liquid: the quantity of gas dissolved in

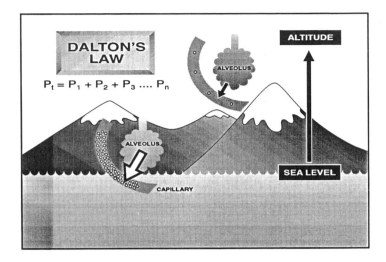

Figure 33-1.   Dalton's law. (Modified with permission from Blumen IJ, Dunne MJ. Flight physiology. Emergency 1992;24:37–43.)

1 mL of a liquid is proportional to the partial pressure of the gas in contact with the liquid (Fig 33-3).

Collectively, these physical laws help explain the behavior of gases, particularly oxygen, at various altitudes. If one considers the physical laws of gases and how readily oxygen is released from hemoglobin (oxygen dissociation curve), it is possible to anticipate the theoretical limitations to physical activity at altitude.

SIGNIFICANT PHYSIOLOGIC RESPONSES TO ALTITUDE

The past two decades have seen an explosion of interest in the effects of training at altitude, but the ultimate goal of improved sea-level performance has proven elusive. Study results are ambiguous or inconclusive, in part due to the variable study designs, the locations of studies in differing altitudes, the wide variety of physical activities compared,

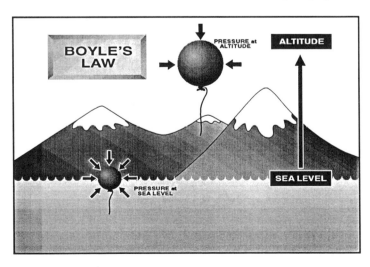

Figure 33-2.   Boyle's law. (Modified with permission from Blumen IJ, Dunne MJ. Flight physiology. Emergency 1992;24:37–43.)

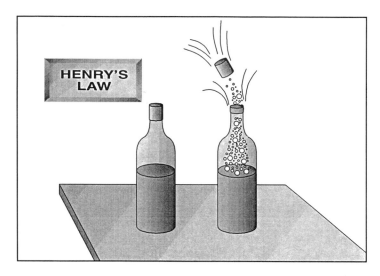

Figure 33-3. Henry's law. (Modified with permission from Blumen IJ, Dunne MJ. Flight physiology. Emergency 1992;24:37–43.)

and the absence of any identified control groups. Thus, the postulated benefit of altitude training for sea-level athletic performance remains one of the most contentious issues in contemporary sport science, and no unequivocal scientific evidence has conclusively confirmed or repudiated the proposed benefits of altitude adaptation. Agreement exists, however, that the physiologic rate-limiting factors associated with altitude limit the intensity of training in such environments.

After the Mexico City Olympics, the outstanding performances of residents from high altitudes stimulated researchers to consider whether being "temporarily" exposed to high altitude would confer some significant performance benefits on those who lived habitually at sea level. Although it

Table 33-1   Physiologic Changes in Response to Altitude: A Time Frame for Reference

Physiologic Change	Time at Altitude for Change	Time for Maximal Change
Hyperventilation	Immediate	Weeks
Increased heart rate	Immediate	Weeks
Increased hemoglobin	Days to weeks	Weeks
Increased capillary density	Weeks	Months/years
Increased aerobic enzyme activity in muscle	Weeks	Months?
Increased mitochondrial density in muscle	Weeks	Months
Stimulated erythropoiesis	Days	Weeks

SOURCE: Adapted from Sutton JR. Exercise at high altitude: does it improve endurance performance at sea level? Sports Sci Exchange 1993;6:289–303.

is well recognized that altitude training improves athletic performance at high altitude, how this translates to performance at sea level remains a hotly debated issue (5). An overriding premise is that our ability to transport and utilize oxygen improves at altitude in response to lower barometric pressure and oxygen partial pressure. There are numerous, documented physiologic responses, and these are summarized as follows:

- Hyperventilation
- Increased heart rate
- Increased hemoglobin concentration
- Increased capillary density
- Increased aerobic enzyme activity in muscle
- Increased mitochondrial density in skeletal muscle
- Stimulated rate of erythropoiesis

Pulmonary Adaptation

An immediate effect of exposure to altitude is a respiratory compensation that results in an increased tidal volume and an increase in the frequency of breathing. This hyperventilatory response gives rise to a respiratory alkalosis as the result of the increased elimination of CO_2. By way of compensation, the renal excretion of bicarbonate is stimulated, and this reduces the buffering capacity of the blood. As a result, lactic acid production from the anaerobic or oxygen independent metabolic pathway is less readily tolerated. The so-called lactate paradox demonstrates a reduction in blood lactic acid at altitude for a given exercise intensity; this is thought to be linked to phosphofructokinase availability as the rate-limiting step. At high altitudes (hypoxic conditions) lactic acidosis can impair ATP production and excitation-contraction coupling, thus necessitating the reduction of training intensity. However, an increase in dietary carbohydrate is considered by many to be a factor in reestablishing acid-base balance.

Another important consideration linked to the hyperventilatory response is the increased loss of fluid through the respiratory tract. This is accentuated not only by hyperventilation, but also by the reduced relative humidity at altitude which demands that athletes be more aware of adequate hydration than they are at sea level.

Cardiac Adaptation

A further, well-recognized early response to exercise at altitude is the rapid increase of heart rate and cardiac output during rest and submaximal activity. However, as adaptation occurs linked to a catecholamine response, many observers have noted that resting heart rate approximates to normal (5).

Hematologic Adaptation

A number of significant hematologic adaptations to altitude have been reported (6). These include an increase in both hemoglobin concentration and hematocrit. They follow a rapid decrease in plasma volume and a subsequent stimulus to erythropoiesis. Governed by the fact that hypoxia is a fundamental stimulus to erythropoietin (EPO) production, research has shown that as brief a period as 6 hours at an altitude of 2000 meters will increase EPO production by approximately 40%. The same researchers described a secondary decrease in EPO after 1 week, reaching a steady-state level by 1 to 2 months. Despite this phenomenon, the increase in hemoglobin concentration at altitude is considered to be a result of the reduction in plasma volume rather than a true increase in erythropoiesis (5).

Nutritional considerations at altitude include the availability of adequate iron stores, essential for the maintenance of erythropoiesis and the synthesis of hemoglobin. Clearly then, the adequacy of iron stores is a well-recognized prerequisite for adaptation of training at altitude.

Red blood cells contain 2,3-diphosphoglycerate ($2,3\text{-}P_2Gri$), which is linked closely to the ability to give up oxygen at tissue level. The younger the cell population, the higher the $2,3\text{-}P_2Gri$ concentration. Given the stimulation to erythropoiesis at altitude, there is a larger population of immature erythrocytes and a corresponding enhancement of oxygen release, particularly during submaximal exercise (7). However, $2,3\text{-}P_2Gri$ concentration is reported to fall rapidly after descent to sea level (7).

Muscle Adapation

Another well-recognized response to prolonged altitude exposure is an increase in both the density of mitochondria and capillaries in skeletal muscle. This would tend to suggest the conferment of enhanced aerobic capacity in skeletal muscle, but there is clear evidence that this is secondary to a reduction in muscle mass, and may be linked to an altered testosterone/cortisol ratio reflecting a relative catabolic response (2,5).

Altitude Training: Advantages and Disadvantages

The interest in the subject of altitude training has been longstanding, and has embraced a history of autotransfusion techniques (blood-doping or blood-boosting), specified altitude training camps, and the contemporary use of synthetic EPO. The common hypothesis still remains that stimulated erythropoiesis equates directly to an increased capacity for tissue oxygenation and consequent improved athletic performance. Of a less quantifiable nature is the important "training camp effect": simply bringing athletes together for a period of concentrated training, testing, and observation is known to enhance performance.

Sports physicians and exercise scientists who guide high-performance athletes and offer advice on the relative merits of altitude training would do well to revisit a number of important physiologic principles. The contemporary interest in high-altitude training seems driven primarily by the view that the hypoxic stimulus induces an adaptive polycythemia. It is assumed that the legacy of an increased population of red blood cells translates directly into a potential for enhanced athletic performance.

Disadvantages of High-Altitude Training An inability to maintain training intensity at altitude, the resulting reduction of maximum work capacity ($\dot{V}o_2$max), the earlier onset of fatigue at altitude, and a reduction in plasma volume are considered disadvantages. So too, in extreme cases, is the possibility of developing high-altitude pulmonary and cerebral edema.

Acute "mountain sickness" associated with rapid ascent and vigorous exercise at altitude (2,8) is accompanied by the attendant symptoms of headache, nausea, vomiting, irritability, malaise, and insomnia. These well-documented symptoms in alpine climbers are considered secondary to the presence of cerebral edema (2). Such sequelae are clearly unlikely at the modest altitudes selected by coaches to undertake altitude training (usually between 1500 and 2000 meters), but if any competition is planned at an altitude similar to that of the Mexico City Olympics (2300 meters), then wisdom suggests that a period of adaptation is prudent. In fact, many authorities suggest that for levels above 1500 meters lower work intensity and adequate recovery periods are essential to gain the maximum benefits of physiologic adaptation (9). The debate still wages as to the duration of the optimal adaptive period, but there seems to be some consensus that for altitudes up to 2000 meters at least 14 days' adaptation is required.

Live High, Train Low Studies

Recent studies by sports scientists from Finland and the United States have focused on the concept of living habitually at altitude but training at sea level (the so-called "live high, train low" theory). Theoretically, this scenario allows athletes to maintain training intensity while at the same time receiving the benefits of altitude habituation. To test this theory where it is geographically impossible to effect a local change, athletes are living in specially designed "nitrogen houses," so constructed that the introduction of nitrogen gas simply displaces oxygen and thereby creates a physiologic environment that simulates hypoxia. Athletes are then free to continue their training at sea level at an intensity that is not subjected to the same hypoxic, rate-limiting influences of altitude; in the evenings, they return to eat and sleep in relative hypoxia. These studies are in their experimental infancy, but their exciting potential is demanding international attention.

CONCLUSION

Training at high altitude has been shown to improve performance at high altitude; however, the translation of this effect to subsequent sea level performances has not been conclusively demonstrated. The theory seems physiologically sound, but the studies have remained ambiguous and inconclusive.

The hypoxia of high altitude induces a number of hematologic changes including a secondary polycythemia, an alteration in acid-base balance, and an increase in hemoglobin concentration and hematocrit (due to decreased plasma volume). The well-recognized stimulus to erythropoiesis decreases after 2 or 3 days, reaching steady-state levels by about 3 weeks.

Major nutritional concerns at altitude are the availability of adequate iron stores and increased carbohydrates, and the need for increased fluid to meet the requirements of stimulated erythropoiesis and fluid loss from decreased humidity and hyperventilation.

The answers to adequate altitude acclimatization, and the maximization of the benefits thought to be induced by the physiologic stimulus of hypoxia, might well come from contemporary studies that are exploring the concept of living at altitude and training at sea level (the "live high, train low" theory).

REFERENCES

1 Henry B, Yeomans PH. An approved history of the Olympic games. Los Angeles: Alfred Publishing, 1984:331.
2 Milledge JS. High altitude. In: Harries M, Williams C, Stanish WD, Micheli LJ, eds. Oxford textbook of sports medicine. Oxford: Oxford Medical, 1991: 217–230.
3 Blumen IJ, Dunne MJ. Flight physiology. Emergency 1992;24:37–43.
4 Blumen IJ, Abonethy MK, Dunne MJ. Flight physiology. Clinical considerations. Clin Care Clin 1992;8: 597–618.
5 Sutton JR. Exercise at high altitude: does it improve endurance performance at sea level? Sports Sci Exchange 1993;6:289–303.
6 Bergland B. High-altitude training. Aspects of hematological adaptation. Sports Med 1992;14:289–303.
7 Hahn AG. The physiological rationale for altitude training—state of the art review. Aust Sports Comm 1992;31:2–12.
8 Coote JH. Medicine and mechanisms in altitude sickness. Sports Med 1995;20:148–159.
9 Pyke FS, Sutton JR. Environmental stress. In: Bloomfield J, Fricker PA, Fitch KD, eds. Textbook of science and medicine in sport. Melbourne: Blackwell Scientific, 1992:114–133.

PART III
SPECIAL MEDICAL PROBLEMS IN THE ATHLETE

Chapter 34
Hyperthermia and Heat-Related Illnesses

Robert C. Gambrell

Hyperthermia and heat-related illnesses are common occurrences each summer. Although the actual incidence of heat-related illnesses is unknown and many cases go unreported, heat stroke causes nearly 4000 deaths each year in the United States (1,2). Elderly or debilitated individuals face increased risk, but athletes exercising in the heat are also vulnerable. Heat stroke is the third most common cause of death among American athletes (3): from 1955 to 1990, reports listed 84 deaths from heat stroke in American football (1). The most disturbing aspect of these deaths is that heat illness among athletes is predictable and preventable when appropriately anticipated. Coaches, trainers, and physicians must understand the causes, prevention, and treatment of heat-related illnesses to allow athletes to participate safely in heat.

Heat-related illnesses include heat cramps, heat edema, heat syncope, heat exhaustion, and heat stroke. Heat cramps, heat edema, and heat syncope are minor illnesses that usually respond to rest and hydration. Heat exhaustion and heat stroke span a continuum from serious to life-threatening; heat stroke is distinguished from heat exhaustion by the presence of central nervous system (CNS) dysfunction (4).

PATHOPHYSIOLOGY

Heat illness results when heat production exceeds heat loss. Heat production comes from both endogenous and exogenous sources. *Endogenous* heat arises from muscle activity and metabolism. *Exogenous* heat transfers to the body when environmental temperature exceeds body temperature. Heat loss occurs by conduction, convection, radiation, or evaporation. At rest, when environmental temperature is below body temperature, thermoregulation is maintained principally by convection of heat to the skin surface and radiation of heat to the environment (5). Evaporation of moisture from the lungs during respiration also accounts for small amounts of heat loss.

As an individual begins to exercise and heat production increases, sweating provides compensatory heat loss through evaporation. When environmental temperature equals or exceeds body temperature, sweating is the predominant mechanism of heat loss (3); athletes exercising in these conditions rely almost exclusively on evaporative heat loss to regulate body temperature (1,5).

Acclimatization is the essential component of an athlete's adaptation to exercise in the heat. Acclimatization through repeated exposure to a hot environment promotes several physiologic changes that improve heat dissipation. Heat exposure lasting 60 to 90 minutes per day for 1 to 2 weeks is required for adequate adaptation of the cardiovascular, endocrine, and exocrine systems (1,3,6). Physiologic changes include increased cardiac output, extracellular fluid volume expansion, diminished sweat sodium concentration, and increased sweat volume (3). Once acclimatized, an individual experiences a smaller rise in rectal temperature at any given workload in the heat (3).

A number of environmental, individual, and medical factors interact to increase the risk for heat illness. The risk for heat stroke increases with temperature and humidity. How hot one feels and the actual environmental heat stress experienced vary with temperature, relative humidity, wind, and degree of cloud cover. Environmental heat stress is measured using the wet bulb globe temperature (WBGT) index, which is a temperature/humidity/radiation index. To lose heat, the athlete produces sweat and the sweat must evaporate. Increased humidity, heat-retaining clothing, lack of wind, and inadequate acclimatization inhibit this process. Predisposing individual and medical factors that interfere with heat exchange include age extremes, obesity, dehydration, cardiovascular disease, sweat gland dysfunction, drugs, alcohol, past history of heat stroke, sunburn, and mid-day overeating (1,6). A variety of medications increase an athlete's risk for heat illness. Thyroid hormones and amphetamines increase heat production. Antihistamines, anticholinergics, phenothiazines, and benztropine mesylate decrease sweat production. Sedatives and haloperidol decrease thirst recognition (2,4,7).

MINOR HEAT-RELATED ILLNESSES

Minor heat-related illnesses include heat cramps, heat edema, and heat syncope. Minor heat-related illnesses generally respond well to removal from heat, rest, and hydration. All mild heat illnesses require rehydration.

Heat Cramps   Heat cramps usually affect the large muscles of the legs but occasionally involve abdominal or other muscles. Heat cramps probably result from excessive salt and electrolyte loss from sweating, and occur even in highly acclimatized individuals who drink large volumes of water to replenish fluids lost by sweating (3,6). Heat cramps are easily treated by rest, massage, and 1% oral salt solutions (3,6).

Heat Edema   Heat edema is swelling that often occurs in unacclimatized individuals exposed to heat stress. The swelling results from peripheral vasodilation, decreased intravascular volume, and increased hydrostatic pressure in response to aldosterone-mediated sodium retention (3,6). Heat edema responds to elevation of the extremities, ambulation, and acclimatization (3,6), but should not be treated with diuretics (3).

Heat Syncope   Heat syncope arises from the same mechanisms as heat edema, but the changes are severe enough to cause orthostatic hypotension and loss of consciousness. Heat syncope may be avoided by sitting or lying down whenever the

symptoms of light-headedness or weakness are experienced.

HYPERTHERMIA

Heat exhaustion from excessive sweating in a hot and humid environment leads to extreme enough volume contraction to interfere with heat dissipation. Core body temperature rises but remains less than 40 °C (104 °F), and the athlete typically cannot continue activity in the heat. Common symptoms of heat exhaustion include generalized malaise, weakness, headache, anorexia, nausea, vomiting, tachycardia, and hypotension. Major neurologic impairment is absent. Because heat exhaustion and heat stroke appear similar clinically, heat exhaustion is a diagnosis of exclusion that can only be made when history, physical, and laboratory examination do not indicate heat stroke.

Diagnosis

Heat stroke is an emergency that requires immediate treatment because core body temperatures in excess of 40 °C (104 °F) may rapidly cause irreversible central nervous system damage. Heat stroke falls into two categories: classic and exertional. In both cases the body's ability to dissipate heat is overwhelmed.

- **Classic heat stroke** generally occurs in elderly or debilitated individuals who are overwhelmed by exceedingly high environmental temperatures. Classic heat stroke includes the triad of hyperthermia (40 °C or higher), anhidrosis, and CNS changes.
- **Exertional heat stroke** develops in young, healthy athletes and individuals exercising or working in hot humid environments. Exertional heat stroke may be accompanied by profuse sweating.

Core body temperature greater than 40 °C (104 °F) is usually present, but is not an absolute criterion for diagnosis (3,6) because some cooling may have lowered the core body temperature even though cellular and organ damage has already occurred. Accurate core body temperature measured rectally is essential (3). Esophageal or bladder temperatures have also been used but oral, aural, or axillary temperatures do not reflect core body temperatures and may be misleading (2).

Extreme or prolonged periods of elevated core body temperature exceeding 40 °C (104 °F) cause widespread cellular injury and even multisystem organ failure (6). Signs of central nervous system injury include headache, confusion, seizures, stupor, and coma. Evidence of serious CNS dysfunction or other organ-system damage identifies individuals with heat stroke even with lower core body temperatures (3,6). In addition to an elevated core body temperature, the presenting symptoms of heat stroke may include hypotension, vomiting, diarrhea, and mental status changes.

Early mortality reflects injury to the central nervous system, but other organ systems are also vulnerable to heat injury (4). Complications of heat stroke include permanent CNS injury, rhabdomyolysis, acute renal failure, liver injury, pulmonary edema, and disseminated intravascular coagulation (DIC). Athletes with heat stroke should be monitored for several days following the injury because organ system damage, especially to the hepatic system, may not be apparent initially (6). Poor prognostic indicators are core body temperature greater than 42.2 °C (107.6 °F), aspartate aminotransferase greater than 1000 during the first 24 hours, and coma of greater than 2 hours' duration (4). Mortality correlates with the duration and intensity of hyperthermia.

The differential diagnoses of a hyperthermic patient with CNS changes include infections such as meningitis, encephalitis, malaria, or typhoid; drugs that may cause hyperthermia or precipitate neuroleptic malignant syndrome; delirium tremens; thyrotoxicosis; pheochromocytoma; or rarely hypothalamic dysfunction due to midbrain hemorrhage (6). The clinical setting and history aid in differentiating these from heat stroke. Whenever heat stroke is suspected, treatment should not be delayed and must be accomplished rapidly to prevent injury. Cooling will not harm patients who are hyperthermic for other reasons.

Treatment

The first step in treatment for heat stroke is to lower the core body temperature to below 39 °C (102 °F) (3,6). The athlete should be moved to a cooler lo-cation and be disrobed, and active cooling measures should be instituted. Active cooling measures include ice water immersion, ice packs, ice water cooling blanket, warm water mist with fanning, or a combination of these measures.

Internal cooling such as cold water irrigation of the stomach or rectum, peritoneal lavage, and cardiopulmonary bypass are effective, but no more efficacious than properly performed external cooling measures (2). Invasive cooling measures should be reserved for individuals who have failed external cooling measures.

Ice water immersion has been the most widely used method for many years and clearly lowers core body temperature. However, one concern is that ice water immersion may stimulate cutaneous vasoconstriction and reflexive shivering that interfere with heat loss. The use of warm water mist with cooling fans is at least as effective as ice water immersion and avoids these complications (2,6).

While beginning active cooling measures, intravenous hydration should be started at a controlled rate in the hyperthermic patient who is at increased risk of cerebral or pulmonary edema (2,4,6). Blood and urine tests monitor organ damage. Core body temperature monitoring helps avoid overcooling or rebound hyperthermia.

Medications have limited use in the treatment of heat stroke. Chlorpromazine can control reflex shivering that results from cooling (2,4,6). Mannitol is useful in the treatment of cerebral edema and renal failure secondary to rhabdomyolysis (2,4). Steroids, antipyretics, and dantrolene have no role in the treatment of exertional heat stroke (2,4,6).

Heat stroke can lead to permanent CNS, hepatic, and renal dysfunction. Athletes suffering heat stroke may have heat intolerance for up to a year (4). No variables predict recovery from heat intolerance, so all athletes with a history of heat stroke should undergo an exercise trial in the heat to determine their heat tolerance status (4).

SPECIAL CONSIDERATIONS IN ATHLETES

Exercising in the heat presents several unique challenges to athletes and to the individuals caring for their health. Successful athletes tolerate tremendous levels of physical pain and fatigue during competition and may ignore symptoms of heat illness until it is too late. Individuals responsible for the health of athletes exercising in hot, humid environments should be familiar with unique risks of heat illnesses in sport and should closely observe athletes in extreme conditions.

Exertional heat stroke in athletes relates to demand on the cardiovascular system. Cardiac output must maintain blood pressure, increased blood flow to the skin for heat transfer, and raise circulation to skeletal muscle by 20-fold. Thus, adequate hydration is necessary to meet these demands (5,8). In the athlete with no underlying cardiovascular disease, exercise performance is often maintained even as the risk of heat injury increases (7).

Heat exhaustion is primarily a function of hypohydration, and, conversely, well-hydrated individuals tolerate a higher core body temperature during exercise (4,5,7,8). Rectal temperatures during athletic events of 40 °C to 42 °C (104 °F to 107.6 °F) exceed established survival limits (35 °C to 40 °C), and efficient thermoregulation allows this to occur in apparently asymptomatic individuals (7). CNS symptoms may develop rapidly in the athlete suffering exertional heat stroke as he/she may continue performing well up to the point of severe heat injury.

Organizing Events in Hot, Humid Conditions

Organizers responsible for athletic events scheduled in hot, humid environments must take adequate precautions based on environmental conditions. The American College of Sports Medicine recommends that when the WBGT is above 28 °C (82 °F) consideration should be given to rescheduling or delaying events until safer conditions prevail (Table 34-1) (9). Additionally, summer events should be scheduled for early morning and an adequate supply of water should be available before and during events. Medical directors of tournaments or sports festivals held in the summer should monitor the WBGT index and be prepared to modify rules to allow unlimited substitutions or change games scheduled for the heat of the day to earlier or later times (3).

Table 34-1 Guidelines for Team Activities Based on Wet Bulb Globe Temperature (WBGT) Index

WBGT		
Fahrenheit	**Celsius**	**Activity**
<65	18	Follow regular schedules; allow full access to fluids
65–72	18–22	Add quarterly fluid breaks; allow free access to fluids
73–82	23–28	Shorten games or allow unlimited substitutions; add quarterly fluid breaks; allow full access to water
82–85	28–30	Establish an alternate schedule in advance to move mid-day games to earlier and later hours; allow unrestricted substitution at all age levels; shorten game times; add quarterly fluid breaks; allow fluid breaks during play
>85	>30	Cancel all exertion and avoid sun exposure at rest

SOURCE: American College of Medicine. Position of Thermal Injuries During Distance Running. Position Statement, 1985.

Heat Preparation for Endurance Events

The treatment of heat injuries in athletes participating in mass endurance events such as marathons or triathlons poses unique challenges. Triaging a number of runners with possible heat injuries requires proper planning and preparation. Races scheduled during hot, humid conditions frequently have multiple participants who need care. In the 1977, 1978, and 1979 Peachtree Road Race (held in July in Atlanta, Georgia) there were 56, 31, and 29 runners who had severe heat injuries (10).

In addition to the usual medical preparations, medical race directors responsible for competitions in the heat must ensure that adequate water is available along the course. Coordination with local emergency departments can ensure the rapid transport of affected individuals. Review of prior race experiences, education and training of the medical staff in the management of heat illness, and establishment of treatment protocols facilitate the effectiveness of the team. Preparing the medical treatment area to provide active cooling measures requires an adequate supply of water and ice, large circulating fans, and a well-ventilated, shaded, and/or air-conditioned treatment area. Cooling measures must be planned to accommodate the expected number of participants.

The established protocols for the treatment of runners collapsing or suspected of heat illness guides triage and management of symptomatic individuals. Athletes suspected of heat illness should quickly be moved to a cooler location, the active cooling measures instituted, and their vital signs monitored frequently. If the runner can take oral fluids, this should be encouraged; those unable to tolerate fluids or who are vomiting need an intravenous infusion.

In races where medical treatment is set up on site, a rectal temperature should gauge the level of hyperthermia and guide treatment. Athletes with signs and symptoms of heat exhaustion can frequently be treated on site with cooling and hydration. Anyone suspected of heat stroke, especially those with marked elevations in core body temperature over 40° C (104 °F) or with marked CNS dysfunction, should be transported immediately to the emergency department while cooling measures, intravenous fluids, and monitoring are continued.

Heat Preparation for American Football

Another sport with special risks is American football, particularly in practice sessions conducted in the heat of summer. Temperatures over 90 °F, relative humidity over 70%, unacclimatized athletes, and equipment (particularly helmets) that interferes with heat loss are instigators of heat stroke. Coaches and trainers need to be educated in the prevention, warning signs, symptoms, and initial treatment of heat illness.

Coaches should allow unrestricted access to water, have frequent water breaks, and modify the practice schedule as guided by the WBGT index. Athletes should be monitored closely for dehydration, with prepractice weigh-ins to check for excessive weight loss. Athletes losing more than 5% of body weight during training should be held out of

physical activity, be advised to rest, and be reevaluated in 24 hours. Athletes losing more than 7% of total body weight should be evaluated by a physician (1). Obese or overweight athletes, those known to be in poor physical condition, and those with a previous heat illness should be monitored even more closely during exercise in the heat (1). By gradually increasing the length and intensity of workouts, the coaching staff can limit the amount of heat stress experienced by their athletes during the period of acclimatization. For early season practices, athletes should wear shorts and tee-shirts before going straight into full equipment.

SUMMARY

Prevention of heat-related illness and hyperthermia in athletes exercising in the heat should be our goal. Ensuring adequate hydration, allowing for proper acclimatization of athletes, and modifying activities based on environmental heat stress are essential. A reduction in the number of heat-related illnesses and heat strokes can be accomplished with proper preparation and management of athletic events held in hot, humid environments.

REFERENCES

1 Allman FL. The effects of heat on the athlete. J Med Assoc Georgia 1992;81:307–310.
2 Lee-Chiong TL, Stitt JT. Heatstroke and other heat-related illnesses. Postgrad Med 1995;98:26–36.
3 Bracker MD. Environmental and thermal injury. Clin Sports Med 1992;11:419–436.
4 Tom PA, Garmel GM, Auerbach PS. Environment-dependent sports emergencies. Med Clin North Am 1994;78:305–325.
5 Nadel ER. Temperature regulation and hyperthermia during exercise. Clin Chest Med 1984;5:13–20.
6 Tek D, Olshaker JS. Heat illness. Emerg Med Clin North Am 1992;10:299–310.
7 Hubbard RW. An introduction: the role of exercise in the etiology of exertional heatstroke. Med Sci Sports Exerc 1990;22:2–5.
8 Sutton J, Coleman MJ, Millar AP, et al. The medical problems of mass participation in athletic competition, the "city-to-surf" race. Med J Aust 1972;2:127–133.

9 American College of Sports Medicine. Prevention of thermal injuries during distance running. Position Statement. 1985.

10 England AC, Fraser DW, Hightower AW, et al. Preventing severe heat injury in runners: suggestions from the 1979 Peachtree Road Race experience. Ann Intern Med 1982;97:196–201.

Chapter 35
Hypothermia

Janus D. Butcher
Robert C. Gambrell

It is far from easy to determine whether Nature has proved to man a kind parent or a merciless stepmother
—Pliny the Elder, 1st century

Throughout time, humans have battled for survival against hostile elements. Humans are ill designed to live in all but a few idyllic regions, but through the manipulation of technology have flourished in nearly every environment on the planet. For most of the developed world today, the environmental challenges faced by our ancestors are little more than inconveniences. However, in spite of our technological advances, environmental injuries remain commonplace, and physicians must supplement preventative measures with a sound understanding of the diagnoses and treatment of environmental injuries.

ACCIDENTAL HYPOTHERMIA

The formidable risk of hypothermia is not confined to cold climates or traditional winter sports, but rather applies to a wide variety of sports. The risks of some sports are intuitive, but others are much less obvious. For example, in addition to winter sports, hypothermia occurs commonly in water sports (boating, swimming, scuba, whitewater rafting) and mountaineering. Endurance events also pose a risk, as an exhausted participant is unable to maintain the heat production necessary to overcome environmental losses (1–3). Major risk factors can be classified in two categories: 1) those that result in greater heat losses (through impaired thermoregulation), and 2) those that lead to reduced thermogenesis. The latter risk factors include age (the very old and young), underlying diseases (cardiovascular, endocrinopathies), exhaustive exercise, alcohol intoxication, and trauma (Table 35-1).

Pathophysiology

Two factors are required for hypothermia to develop:

1. The ambient temperature must be below core body temperature (CBT).
2. The body's ability to generate heat must be less than ongoing heat losses (4).

Humans function optimally in a relatively narrow temperature range. At ambient air temperatures above 28 °C (82.4 °F) heat produced by basal metabolism is adequate to maintain CBT at 37 °C (5). In conditions below this temperature, the body must produce additional heat to remain thermoneutral. *Thermogenesis* is accomplished through increased physical activity and autonomically mediated shivering, a normal physical response of healthy individuals in a moderate environment. In other groups, such as the elderly, ill, or traumatized patient, or even the fatigued endurance athlete, the heat-generating potential can be severely impaired while at the same time heat losses are increased. Certain environmental conditions can also overwhelm the thermogenic potential, as is seen in cold water immersion or extreme windchill.

Heat loss occurs through four transfer processes: conduction, convection, evaporation, and radiation.

- **Conductive heat loss** describes the transfer of heat by direct contact between objects. The rate

Table 35-1   Risk Factors for Accidental
Hypothermia

Impaired Thermogenesis (Decreased Production)
- Endocrine diseases
    Hypothyroidism
    Diabetes mellitus
    Adrenopituitary dysfunction
- Cardiovascular disease
- Exhaustive exercise
- Malnutrition
    Chronic alcoholism
    Anorexia
- Neoplasia
- Infection/Sepsis

Impaired Thermoregulation (Increased Losses)
- Age (very old and young)
- Trauma
- Severe burns
- Chronic disease
    Diabetes mellitus
- Neurologic disease or injury
    CVA
    Spinal cord injury
    Multiple sclerosis
    Intercranial hemorrhage
    Hypothalamic dysfunction
- Toxins
    Drug overdose
    Ethanol
- Neoplasia

Increased Environmental Losses
- Cold water immersion
- Windchill
- Inadequate clothing and/or equipment

of loss is determined by both the intrinsic conductive properties of the objects and the temperature difference between the two.
- **Evaporation** results in heat loss through the conversion of liquid (sweat or through the respiratory mucosa) to a vapor. This is the most important process for eliminating excess heat in warm conditions.
- **Convection** refers to the transfer of energy to a flowing media such as air or water.
- **Radiant heat transfer** occurs through electromagnetic radiation into the surrounding environment.

Each of these processes may contribute to hypothermia; however, conduction and convection play the major role in the setting of immersion injuries. Because of the high conductivity of water (32 times greater than air) and the potential for significant convective losses in moving water, CBT can fall rapidly when the body is immersed. Even in relatively warm ambient conditions, immersion in cold water can lead to rapid, fatal heat losses.

Cold affects the function of multiple body systems including the cardiovascular, pulmonary, renal, hemocoagulation, and central nervous systems. A full review of the physiology of cold injury is beyond the scope of this chapter, but the important physiologic effects and associated symptoms are summarized in Table 35-2.

CLINICAL PRESENTATION OF HYPOTHERMIA

Hypothermia, defined as a CBT below 35 °C, can be further divided into stages:

- Mild (CBT 32 to 35 °C)
- Moderate (CBT 28 to 32 °C)
- Severe (CBT <28 °C)

These three categories are not definitive; however, as the clinical findings generally parallel the drop in CBT, these stages provide useful landmarks for defining the optimal therapeutic options.

Mild Hypothermia

The findings in mild hypothermia are consistent with the body's attempt to increase heat production and reduce thermal losses. Thus, the manifestations are tachycardia, uncontrolled shivering, and peripheral vasoconstriction. Cold diuresis, common in the early stages of hypothermia, occurs in response to the increasing central blood pool caused by peripheral vasoconstriction. If the temperature continues to fall, the initial polyuria ends and oliguria, due to renal hypoperfusion, develop (6). The intravascular volume losses from cold diuresis are often excessive and result in hypovolemic shock as external rewarming procedures open constricted peripheral vascular beds.

Aggressive monitoring and fluid replacement are required during rewarming to avoid serious hy-

Table 35-2   Physiologic Changes of Hypothermia and Associated Symptoms

System	Physiologic Changes	Symptoms/Signs	
Cardiovascular	Conduction disturbances • Bradycardia • Arrhythmias Cardiac output	Bradycardia J wave on ECG	
Renal	GFR early GFR late	Cold diuresis Oliguria	
Hemocoagulation	Thrombocytopenia Impaired coagulation cascade	Increased bleeding time	
Central Nervous System	Decreased cerebral blood flow	Amnesia Confusion Stupor	Poor judgment Obtundation Coma
Neuromusculoskeletal	Peripheral vasoconstriction	Extreme ataxia	Muscle rigidity

povolemic complications. Many other findings are described in mild hypothermia, including dysarthria, extremity ataxia, skin pallor, perioral cyanosis, and muscle rigidity. Other reported signs and symptoms are listed in Table 35-2.

Moderate Hypothermia

When core body temperature falls below 32 °C, the body's ability to respond becomes significantly impaired. The shivering reflex is lost, and heat production falls sharply. Worsening cognitive functions prevent the victim from recognizing his or her danger and seeking warmth—in extreme cases, the victim may exhibit paradoxical behavior by undressing, which results in further heat losses. At these temperatures, hypotension and bradycardia are common and are associated with reductions in cardiac output, cerebral blood flow, and renal perfusion.

Central nervous system function continues to deteriorate as the temperature drops, leading to obtundation, stupor, and coma. Pupillary dilation, muscular rigidity, loss of reflexes, and unresponsiveness may lead to the mistaken conclusion that the victim is dead (7).

Cardiac arrhythmias occur infrequently above 32 °C, but as the temperature drops below this level a variety of conduction disturbances are seen. Atrial fibrillation frequently occurs in the moderate hypothermic range and is probably due to atrial distention (8). Supraventricular tachycardia is also common, particularly during rewarming.

Severe Hypothermia

As the core body temperature falls below 28 °C, ventricular irritability leads to more severe arrhythmias, including ventricular tachycardia and fibrillation. The pathophysiology of ventricular arrhythmias lies in slowed conduction through the His–Purkinje system. Disproportionate slowing of conduction velocity and lengthening of the absolute refractory period lead to a reentry phenomenon (6). Because of the irritability of the cold myocardium, minimal manipulation of the hypothermic patient may precipitate fatal ventricular arrhythmias. Spontaneous asystole or fine ventricular fibrillation occurs at temperatures below 20 to 25 °C.

The characteristic ECG change associated with hypothermia is the Osborne wave (J wave). The Osborne wave forms at the junction of the QRS complex and T wave giving the ST segment a characteristic "J" shape. It is typically seen at temperatures below 32 °C in leads II and V_6, but as temperature falls it becomes prominent in leads V_3 and V_4 (6). The Osborne wave is not pathopneumonic for hypothermia, but is reported in up to 80% of patients with a CBT below 30 °C.

TREATMENT

Early recognition and prompt rewarming are critical in the hypothermic athlete. Treatment must be individualized based on the presenting

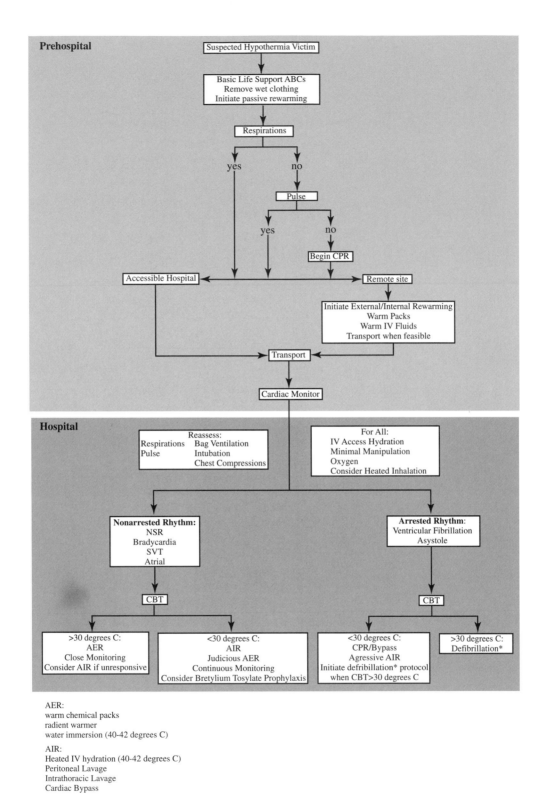

Figure 35-1. Treatment algorithm for hypothermia as outlined in the textbook of *Advanced Cardiac Life Support,* 1994 (Copyright American Heart Association).

circumstances, degree of hypothermia, and the underlying health of the victim. The following discussion provides an outline for management of these casualties, but algorithms do not supplant clinical judgment. Also, rescuers should keep in mind that full recovery even from extremely low temperatures may be possible; therefore, full resuscitative efforts should usually be undertaken even for severely hypothermic patients (9,10).

Rewarming Strategies

There are two modalities for rewarming the hypothermic patient:

- **Passive** rewarming insulates the victim from heat loss and promotes rewarming through internal thermogenesis.
- **Active** rewarming applies extrinsic heat sources to a victim to increase CBT.

Active rewarming strategies are further divided as *external* or *internal,* based on the modality used (Fig 35-1).

One potentially fatal complication during rewarming is CBT afterdrop. *Afterdrop* refers to the continued core cooling during early rewarming. Two factors may contribute to this phenomenon (11):

1. Conductive loss: equilibration of blood temperature as the cold blood from the extremities is mobilized and mixes with the central pool
2. Convective loss: the cooling of warm blood from the central pool as it perfuses the cold peripheral tissues

Another possible contributor to afterdrop is the conductive loss of heat from the warm solid tissues of the core directly to the solid tissues of the extremities. The temperature drop due to the afterdrop phenomenon can be significant and may lead to a worsening condition in the face of aggressive rewarming.

Passive Rewarming   Prehospital measures involve stemming heat loss by removing wet clothing, drying the victim, and initiating passive rewarming by covering with an insulated material. The patient should be transferred to an appropriate treatment

facility as quickly as possible. Active rewarming in the field must be done with great caution due to the risks associated with hypovolemia and CBT afterdrop. If the treatment facility is near and the patient stable, then basic life support (BLS) measures, monitoring, and passive rewarming during transport are appropriate. The treatment decisions become more complicated if a treatment facility is not readily accessible, as may be the case in wilderness activities. If the benefits of initiating active rewarming outweigh the risks associated with hypotension and afterdrop, then active rewarming strategies should be initiated in the field.

Active Rewarming: External   Active external rewarming (AER) techniques are usually adequate to warm the mildly hypothermic patient. These measures include chemical hot packs (applied to the groin, axilla, neck, and thorax), warming blankets or pads, and radiant heat lamps. Warm water baths (40 to 42 °C) are also very effective but complicate the monitoring of the patient. Aggressive external rewarming measures result in a warming rate of approximately 0.5 to 1.0 °C per hour (6). Although AER techniques serve as the main rewarming modalities in mild hypothermia, they may also serve as adjuncts to active internal rewarming in severely hypothermic patients.

Active Rewarming: Internal   Active internal rewarming (AIR) refers to the introduction of heat directly to the victim's core. Techniques range from augmenting the mildly hypothermic victim's external rewarming with warm oral or IV fluids to the use of extracorporeal blood rewarming for the severely hypothermic patient. The modality chosen for rewarming will be based on several factors, including the degree of hypothermia, the victim's cardiac status, available equipment, and the level of training of the treatment personnel.

Several highly effective techniques for AIR can be performed in most emergency departments. Rewarming should be initiated quickly and in a controlled fashion. The patient should be handled very gently with continuous cardiac and blood pressure monitoring. The accurate assessment of the CBT is also crucial. A rectal or esophageal thermometer, placed 15 to 20 cm into the lumen of the viscera, provides an efficient means for continuous

CBT monitoring. Alternatively, tympanic thermometers provide an accurate intermittent measure of CBT.

Heated Inhalation Therapy (HIT)   Although recent reviews have brought into question its efficacy (12), HIT has been used for decades for central rewarming. The technique involves the use of heated humidified air or oxygen (42 to 46 °C) delivered through an endotracheal tube or mask. Theoretically, this method provides heat through the condensation of warm fluid in the airway mucosa. This technique is safe, noninvasive, and readily available in most advanced rescue vehicles for early care of the hypothermic victim. At low temperatures (32 °C) the heat provided by inhalation therapy equals endogenous production (6).

Heated Intravenous Fluid Therapy   Hydration with heated IV fluid has a dual indication in the hypothermic patient: it is both a rewarming technique and a means to provide intravascular volume replacement. An initial bolus of 500 cc of isotonic crystalloid solution (normal saline) with 5% glucose, warmed to 40 to 42 °C, should be used. Lactate buffered fluids should be avoided because the hypothermic liver has a decreased ability metabolize lactate. Subsequent fluid replacement depends on the patient's clinical response, although those with long-term exposure may have large fluid requirements.

Peritoneal Lavage   The decision to employ the more aggressive rewarming strategies is based on temperature (less than 32 °C), cardiac arrhythmias or arrest, failure to respond to less aggressive measures, or the presence of underlying illness/ trauma requiring more rapid rewarming. Hollow viscous lavage has been described, but it offers limited benefit in situations of severe hypothermia. A much more effective method for AIR is the use of peritoneal lavage. Several techniques have been described including the "mini-laparotomy" and transperitoneal large-bore needle placement. A very simple and relatively safe technique involves the introduction of a plastic catheter over a guide wire. Following the percutaneous placement of a an 8 Fr catheter into the pelvic gutter, warmed isotonic dialysate (40 to 45 °C) is introduced in allocates of 1 to 2 liters. This fluid is aspirated after 20 to 30 minutes. A 6-liter-per-hour exchange rate

(10–20 mL/kg) results in rewarming at 1 to 3 °C per hour (6). This technique is further simplified by the availability of preassembled kits, which are commercially available and are stocked in most emergency departments.

Closed thoracic lavage is also effective, but requires greater technical expertise. Two 36 Fr thoracostomy tubes are placed: the anterior (afferent) tube in the third intercostal space along the midclavicular line, and the posterior (efferent) tube at the fifth or sixth intercostal space along the midaxillary line (6). Single-pass continuous infusion using degree-normal saline (40 to 42 °C) at approximately 180 cc/minute results in a rewarming rate of 1.5 to 2.0 °C per hour (13). Alternatively, a single thoracostomy tube can be used with intermittent infusion of 300 cc boluses of normal saline (40 to 42 °C). This is then aspirated after 10 to 15 minutes and repeated.

Extracorporeal Rewarming (ECR)   Extracorporeal rewarming is a highly effective method for rewarming the severely hypothermic patient. Advantages with ECR include the ability to control the rate of rewarming and continue tissue perfusion and oxygenation in the setting of cardiac arrest (14). Unfortunately, this modality requires specialized equipment and personnel and is generally limited to larger hospitals and medical centers that offer cardiothoracic surgery services.

An alternative technique for direct core rewarming is continuous arteriovenous rewarming (CAVR). An 8.5 Fr catheter is placed in the femoral artery and attached to the inflow port of a Rapid Fluid Warmer (Level I Technologies, Marshfield, MA). A second line from the warmer outflow port is placed in the subclavian vein. The heat exchange is accomplished using continuous water (40 °C) flow in the exchange chamber. This method is technically less difficult, yet allows rewarming of 3 to 4 °C per hour (15). Because CAVR requires spontaneous cardiac activity to drive the circulatory fistula, it is not effective in the setting of cardiac arrest.

Other Resuscitation Considerations

Cardiopulmonary Resuscitation (CPR)   As in all emergency treatment situations, the principles of basic life support (BLS) should be followed. Difficulty in checking pulse and respiration may occur due to the presence of peripheral vasoconstriction, bradycardia, and muscular rigidity. In the hypothermia victim with cardiac arrest, CPR should be initiated in the field. Although chest compressions are less efficient in the hypothermic patient, viability can be maintained because of reduced metabolic requirements of the cold body. This is supported by the findings of a large multicenter report that recommended the use of CPR except in the following circumstances: 1) preexisting and verified "do not resuscitate" orders, 2) obvious lethal injuries, 3) situations where CPR is technically impossible, 4) when signs of life are present, or 5) when performing CPR would endanger the life of the rescuer (16).

Arrhythmias The peculiarities of arrhythmia management in the hypothermic patient prompted the American Heart Association to develop a specific hypothermia management protocol (17). The main difficulty is that the arrhythmias tend to be resistant to treatment as long as the patient remains cold. As a result, every effort must be made to increase the CBT while maintaining cardiopulmonary perfusion. In the ideal setting, cardiopulmonary bypass can be used to accomplish both; but this modality is not widely available, so collateral resuscitation efforts are usually required to maintain perfusion and aggressively rewarm the patient.

The predominant atrial arrhythmia in hypothermia is fibrillation with a slow ventricular response. Atrial fibrillation usually resolves with rewarming and seldom requires specific therapy. Supraventricular tachyarrythmias are also common, particularly during rewarming, and they tend to resolve as CBT rises.

Spontaneous ventricular fibrillation and asystole develop at temperatures below 28 °C and resist all forms of cardioversion including electrical, chemical, and pacing. In these patients, aggressive rewarming must elevate the CBT above 28 to 30 °C before cardioversion is successful (18).

Medications used in the setting of hypothermia are less effective and caution must be taken to avoid excessive dosing, which can lead to toxic levels as the patient becomes euthermic. Bretylium tosylate may be a useful antiarrhythmic in hypothermic patients and appears to lower the defibrillation threshold in this setting.

Discontinuing Resuscitation The decision to discontinue resuscitative efforts is complex. The unofficial guideline that "patients aren't dead until they are *warm* and dead" has shown merit many times in the past with heroic saves of profoundly hypothermic victims (9,10). More objective prognostic criteria are lacking, although there are several potential poor outcome indicators, including hyperkalemia (19), severe trauma (20), underlying medical illnesses, and need for prehospital CPR (18). A hypothermia-outcome score based on several criteria (including BUN, CPR, intubation, systolic blood pressure, and nasogastric tube placement) has been developed, but it is not a tool for determining prognosis (21).

The decision to stop resuscitation should be based on the complete clinical picture, not on selected criteria. If there is no clear insult that is incompatible with life (i.e., major trauma), cardiopulmonary support should continue until a CBT greater than 35 °C has been achieved, at which point the utility of resuscitative efforts can be better judged.

PREVENTION AND PREPARATION FOR ENDURANCE EVENTS

Planning for mass-participation endurance events should include preparation for the treatment of hypothermic patients. This is true even when the event will be held in moderate conditions (T < 28 °C or 82.4 °F), and it is particularly important when precipitation seems likely. Equipment, supplies, and personnel requirements vary based on the type of event, anticipated weather conditions, and event duration, but several factors merit universal consideration:

- Warm fluids for oral and IV hydration should be available at all aid stations. IV bag warmers or microwave ovens should be present to ensure that fluids can be warmed for late completions. The best fluid for IV hydration of the hypothermic endurance athlete is normal saline with 5% dextrose. Lactated fluids should be avoided.

- Low temperature thermometers, preferably tympanic, should be available to treatment personnel.
- A warm, dry changing area should be established at the finish area to allow the athletes to recover from the event and escape further environmental heat losses.
- Readily accessible, appropriate transportation to a treatment facility capable of supporting AIR (peritoneal lavage, thoracic lavage, cardiopulmonary bypass) should be on standby. The transportation vehicles must be outfitted for PER, along with the capability to monitor the patient's cardiac status and provide heated IV hydration and inhalation therapy.

REFERENCES

1 Jones BH, Rock PB, Smith LS, et al. Medical complaints after a marathon run in cool weather. Physician Sports Med 1985;13:103–108.
2 Adner MM, Scarlet JJ, Casey J, et al. The Boston marathon medical team: ten years of experience. Physician Sports Med 1988;16:99–106.
3 Robertson J. Sports medicine manual for long distance running. Athletic Congress/USA, 1986.
4 Tom PA, Garmel GM, Auerbach PS. Environment-dependent sports emergencies. Med Clin North Am 1994;78:305–325.
5 Gentilello LM. Advances in the management of hypothermia. Surg Clin North Am 1995;75:243–256.
6 Danzl DF, Pozos RS, Hamlet MP. Accidental hypothermia. In: Auerbach PS, ed. Wilderness medicine: management of wilderness and environmental emergences. 3rd ed. St. Louis: Mosby, 1995:51–103.
7 Weinberg AD. Hypothermia. Ann Emerg Med 1993;22:370–379.
8 Varon J, Sadovnikoff N, Sternbach GL. Hypothermia: saving patients from the big chill. Postgrad Med 1992;92:47–59.
9 Bolte RG, Black PG, Bowere RS, et al. The use of extracorporeal rewarming in a child submerged for 66 minutes. JAMA 1988;260:377–379.
10 Southwick FS, Dalglish PH. Recovery after prolonged asystolic cardiac arrest in profound hypothermia. JAMA 1980;243:1250–1253.
11 Romet TT. Mechanism of afterdrop after cold water immersion. J Appl Physiol 1988;62:1535–1538.
12 Sterba J. Efficacy and safety of prehospital rewarming techniques to treat accidental hypothermia. Ann Emerg Med 1991;20:896–901.
13 Iverson RJ, Atkin SH, Jaker MA, et al. Successful CPR in a severely hypothermic patient using continuous thoracostomy lavage. Ann Emerg Med 1990;19:1335–1337.
14 Vretenar DF, Urschel JD, Parrott JCW, Unruh HW. Cardiopulmonary bypass resuscitation for accidental hypothermia. Ann Thorac Surg 1994;58:895–898.
15 Gentilello LM, Rifley WJ. Continuous arteriovenous rewarming: report of a new technique for treating hypothermia. J Trauma 1991;31:1151–1153.
16 Danzl DF, Hedges JR, Pozos RS. Hypothermia outcome score: development and implications. Crit Care Med 1989;17:227–231.
17 American Heart Association. Advanced cardiac life support, 1992.
18 Zell SC, Kurtz KJ. Severe exposure hypothermia: a resuscitation protocol. Ann Emerg Med 1985;14:339–344.
19 Schaller M, Fischer AP, Perret CH. Hyperkalemia: a prognostic factor during acute severe hypothermia. JAMA 1990;264:1842–1857.
20 Jurkovich GJ, Greiser WB, Luterman A, Curreri W. Hypothermia in trauma victims: an ominous predictor of survival. J Trauma 1987;27:1019–1024.
21 Danzel DF, Pozos RS, Auerbach PS, et al. Multicenter hypothermia survey. Ann Emerg Med 1987;16:1042–1055.

Chapter 36
Altitude Illness

Janus D. Butcher

The relationship between high altitude and illness has been recognized for centuries—the first written descriptions were recorded by Chinese traders traveling through mountainous areas en route to Eastern Europe in 30 B.C. (1). Although we have no direct evidence of altitude illness in prehistoric man, the recent discovery of the "Ice Man" in the Austrian-Italian Alps at an elevation of 10,530 feet has prompted speculation that he may have been an early victim of altitude illness (2). Today, the mobility of our society makes travel to high and remote destinations possible for large segments of our population. As a result, many health care providers, even those who live at low altitudes, are seeing increasing numbers of patients with altitude illness due to the popularity of sports such as skiing, snow boarding, mountaineering, and trekking. Sports medicine practitioners require a general knowledge of the pathophysiology, treatment, and prevention of altitude illness to adequately counsel patients prior to travel.

Our current understanding of the physiology of altitude exposure comes from research done over the past 50 years by investigators such as John Sutton. Through a combination of innovative research design and physical stamina, he and others have probed the intricacies of altitude illness. A comprehensive understanding is still evolving, but the work of these researchers serves as a model for future study.

THE PHYSIOLOGY OF ASCENT

The primary physiologic insult in ascent to high altitude is hypoxia. At sea level, the partial pressure of oxygen is approximately 155 mm Hg; at 8848 meters (Mount Everest's summit), the partial pressure of oxygen falls below 60 mm Hg. The arterial blood oxygen saturation declines from 99% at sea level to less than 60% at 8848 meters (3). Many physiologic changes occur in response to hypoxia as the body attempts to allow individuals to function at high altitudes. *Acclimatization* describes the adaptive processes that increase the availability of oxygen to tissues in a low-oxygen environment. These adaptations affect every step in oxygen delivery, including respiratory rate, circulation, blood carrying capacity, and peripheral oxygen extraction.

Several cardiovascular changes occur with increasing elevation. Maximal heart rate decreases, while resting heart rate increases. At extreme altitudes, maximal and resting heart rate are nearly equal. Stroke volume is reduced due to decreased cardiac contractility, shortened filing time, and reduced preload (3). Cardiac output increases slightly with ascent but maintains a constant relationship with work intensity (i.e., the same cardiac output remains for a given work intensity at sea level versus high altitude) (4). In addition, there is a marked reduction in maximal oxygen uptake (3–5).

Respiratory rate increases dramatically as the partial pressure of oxygen decreases. This hypoxic ventilatory response (HVR) is a major determinate of an individual's ability to acclimatize. The HVR appears to be genetically determined; significant variation is seen between individuals, such that those with greater HVR generally experience fewer symptoms of altitude illness (6). The increased ventilation results in respiratory alkalosis and hypocapnia, which have a negative feedback on respiratory rate. In the low-oxygen environ-

Acute Mountain Sickness

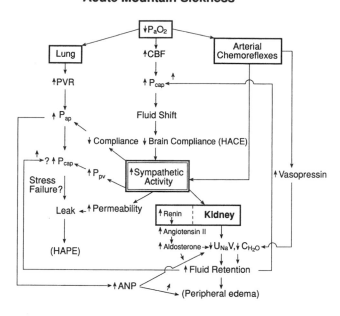

Figure 36-1. Central role of elevated sympathetic activity in the edemas of altitude. Hypoxemia (PaO$_2$) elevates cerebral blood flow (CBF), which, in turn, raises cerebral capillary hydrostatic pressure (Pcap) such that a transcapillary fluid shift occurs. The resulting high-altitude cerebral edema (HACE) reduces brain compliance. Elevated intracranial pressure and distortion of central neural structures provokes elevations of peripheral sympathetic activity above levels normally produced by stimulation of peripheral chemoreflexes. Hypoxia raises pulmonary vascular resistance, which raises pulmonary artery pressure (Pap). Elevated sympathetic activity to the lungs decreases compliance of pulmonary arteries and provokes pulmonary venous constriction and increased capillary permeability. The precise influence of hypoxic pulmonary vascular responses combined with increased pulmonary sympathetic activity on pulmonary capillary hydrostatic pressure is unclear. The relative importance of pulmonary capillary stress failure is uncertain. Only small elevations of Pcap are required to cause large fluid fluxes if permeability is increased such that HAPE occurs. Increased sympathetic activity is associated with a neurogenic antinatriuresis such that fluid retention and peripheral edemas occur. Increased aldosterone from sympathetic stimulation of renin or from ACTH and increased vasopressin from stimulation of chemoreflexes add to the tubular alpha-adrenergic antinatriuresis and opposes natriuretic effects from atrial natriuretic peptide (ANP) released by elevated central blood volume. However, ANP could contribute to peripheral edema, HAPE, or HACE. Renal fluid retention contributes to elevated Pcap in lung, brain, and peripheral tissues. (Reproduced by permission from Krasney JA. A neurogenic basis for acute altitude illness. Med Sci Sports Exerc 1994; 26:195–208.)

ment of high altitudes, the hypoxic ventilatory drive dominates.

Oxygen carrying capacity rises through an increase in hemoglobin concentration. This is initially due to hemoconcentration from diuresis, and later from erythropoiesis (7). The magnitude of increase in hemoglobin varies, but it can be as much as 33% during a gradual climb to extreme altitude (8). In addition, 2,3-diphosphoglycerate (2,3-DPG) facilitates oxygen delivery to tissue by causing a left shift in the oxyhemoglobin dissociation curve. This is offset somewhat by an alkalosis-driven right shift in the oxyhemoglobin dissociation curve. Other adaptive responses include an increase in skeletal muscle capillary density and intracellular mitochondrial hyperplasia (7). These appear to be less important in the acute adaptation, and occur after weeks of high-altitude exposure.

The pathophysiology of altitude illness can be summarized as the rate of ascent exceeding the individual's ability to acclimatize. Recent research suggests a primary role for the central nervous system in altitude illness, triggered by hypoxic cerebral vasodilation. This hypothesis postulates that cerebral vasodilation causes increased intracranial pressure, which leads to cerebral edema, decreased brain compliance, and a systemic sympathetic discharge (Fig 36-1) (9). The observed increases in intracranial pressure are dramatic, ranging from 60 to 300 mm Hg above baseline in victims of acute mountain sickness (AMS) (9–10). The subsequent sympathetic discharge further increases intracranial pressure and initiates the vascular changes observed in the pulmonary and renal systems.

In most people, the response to hypoxic respiratory alkalosis is increased urine output as the kidneys eliminate excess bicarbonate (HCO_3-). The development of AMS and more severe altitude illness may, in part, relate to inappropriate fluid retention, which occurs through a combination of sympathetic mediated sodium retention and the hormonal effects of increased aldosterone and atrial natriuretic factor (9). Fluid retention accentuates the direct hypoxic and sympathetic effects on both the pulmonary and cerebral vasculature.

HIGH ALTITUDE SYNDROMES

Altitude illness develops at elevations above 2000 to 2400 meters, the elevation of most ski resorts. Millions of recreational athletes visit these areas each year. Of "lowland" residents visiting these altitudes, approximately 25% will develop AMS (11,12). A much greater percentage develop individual symptoms of altitude illness, mainly headache. Risk increases at high elevations: as many as 54% of people who travel abruptly to altitudes above 4000 meters develop AMS (13). Most severe altitude illnesses (high-altitude pulmonary or cerebral edema) occur between 3049 meters (10,000 feet) and 5488 meters (18,000 feet). The reported incidence ranges from 0.01% to 15.5% of those ascending to high altitude (14).

The risk of developing altitude illness relates to several factors including individual physiology, rate of ascent, altitude attained, and length of time spent at that altitude. The typical victim lives at low altitude and flies or drives to a high elevation (>2400 meters). Altitude illness spans a spectrum of disease, with AMS representing the most common and fortunately the least serious form. The other major entities are high-altitude cerebral edema (HACE), which is the most ominous of these illnesses, and high-altitude pulmonary edema (HAPE), which is less dramatic than HACE in presentation but is responsible for the highest number of deaths from acute altitude illness (15).

Acute Mountain Sickness

AMS can be triggered by rapid ascent from low altitude to an altitude above 2400 meters. Other factors that contribute to the development of AMS include alcohol consumption, sedative use, extreme exertion, and tobacco smoke.

Presentation The symptoms of AMS are vague and can mimic other processes such as ethanol hangover and viral illness. Common symptoms include throbbing headache, malaise, lethargy, anorexia, sleep disturbances, nausea, vomiting, and mild peripheral edema. Occasionally, victims exhibit a dry cough or mild dyspnea. These symptoms typically develop within 8 to 24 hours of ascent, and in most individuals they resolve without specific treatment over 24 to 72 hours. A small proportion of victims with AMS progress to more severe altitude illness, warranting close observation to identify a worsening status. The physical findings in AMS are nonspecific, thus respiratory rales, cyanosis, or truncal ataxia are indicators of progression to a more severe altitude illness.

Treatment   Treatment of AMS is aimed at facilitating acclimatization. If climbing or hiking when symptoms develop, the individual should stop ascent and wait for acclimatization (usually 24 to 48 hours). Occasionally, a brief descent of 500 to 1000 meters is necessary to allow symptoms to resolve before continuing. Individuals flying or driving to elevations above 2400 meters should avoid alcohol and tobacco smoke and limit exercise to moderate levels for the first 24 hours.

Several medications aid in the treatment of AMS. Acetazolamide, a carbonic anhydrase inhibitor, has been used in the treatment and prevention of AMS and functions by stimulating ventilation which improves arterial oxygenation (16). Acetazolamide also decreases sleep disturbances by minimizing periodic breathing (17). The recommended dosage of acetazolamide is 125 to 250 mg one to two times a day. Dexamethasone (4 mg every 6 hours for 6 doses) also effectively relieves AMS acutely and prophylactically at altitudes above 2700 meters but appears of little use at lower altitudes (18). Ibuprofen is effective in relieving the headache associated with AMS (19).

Prevention   The prevention of AMS focuses on the facilitation of acclimatization. A gradual ascent should limit elevation gain to 600 meters per day at altitudes above 2500 meters. The athlete should follow a high-carbohydrate diet (70%) beginning 24 hours before ascent, avoid alcohol, and begin with consistent but moderate exertion (15). Extreme exercise should await acclimatization.

High-Altitude Pulmonary Edema

HAPE is a life-threatening form of AMS. The mortality in HAPE is as high as 44%, making it the most common cause of death related to high-altitude illness (21). HAPE typically develops in climbers above 3000 meters, usually within 2 to 4 days of ascent (15). The risk factors include elevation attained, speed of ascent, and a history of previous HAPE. Strenuous exercise performed immediately upon arrival to the high altitude may also contribute (22).

Characteristically, the victim has pulmonary arterial hypertension with normal cardiac function, and requires immediate action to improve oxygenation. As with all forms of AMS, the pathophysiology is probably multifactorial, involving increased sympathetic vascular tone and hormonally mediated fluid retention. These factors lead to stress capillary failure and pulmonary edema (20).

Presentation   HAPE is usually preceded by AMS symptoms. While severe the headaches and lethargy continue, the victim develops pulmonary complaints including severe dyspnea and a productive cough. Physical findings include pulmonary rales, tachycardia, and cyanosis. Chest radiography demonstrates patchy infiltrates separated by areas of normal aeration (Fig 36-2). Objective criteria developed to diagnose HAPE are shown in Table 36-1 (23). A high index of suspicion for HAPE must be maintained in the setting of AMS, particularly when a cough or peripheral edema are present.

Treatment   The most effective treatment in HAPE is descent. The use of portable oxygen, either by mask or in a hyperbaric chamber, will provide relief during descent. The most effective medication in the treatment and prevention of HAPE is nifedipine (Aldalat, Procardia) (24). Acutely nifedipine is given sublingually (20 mg), followed by 20 mg slow release every 6 to 8 hours. This treatment has also been shown to prevent recurrence of HAPE in susceptible individuals (25).

Prevention   As with the other forms of altitude illness, prevention is aimed at facilitating acclimatization. For individuals residing below 2400 meters, climbing to moderate or extreme altitudes should involve stages of ascent (as described for AMS). The axiom "climb high, sleep low" should be followed, and sleeping altitude should not increase by more than 600 meters per day. An additional day for acclimatization should be allowed for each elevation gain of 600 meters (15).

High-Altitude Cerebral Edema

Presentation   The development of central nervous system symptoms in the setting of AMS is an ominous sign. Typical symptoms of HACE include

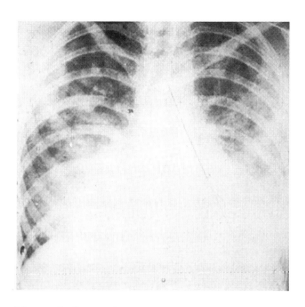

Figure 36-2. In high-altitude pulmonary edema (HAPE), chest radiography demonstrates patchy infiltrates separated by areas of normal aeration. (Reprinted from Bloomfield J, Fricker PA, Fitch KD. Science and medicine in sport. 2nd ed. Oxford: Blackwell Science, 1995:145.)

unrelenting headache associated with vomiting, truncal ataxia, impaired mental status (confusion, poor judgment, delirium), and severe lassitude. Hemiparesis, hemiplegia, seizures, and coma are less common, but suggest the progression of this syndrome. HACE can develop within 24 hours of

Table 36-1   Diagnostic Criteria for High-Altitude Pulmonary Edema (HAPE)

1. Two or more of the following symptoms:
   Dyspnea at rest
   Cough
   Weakness
   Impaired exercise performance

AND

2. Two or more of the following signs:
   Rales/wheezes in one or both lung fields
   Central cyanosis
   Tachycardia
   Tachypnea

AMS, but typically will be delayed 1 to 3 days (15). The mean altitude for occurrence is 15,500 feet, although it has been reported as low as 8200 feet (22).

Treatment   Descent should be initiated immediately upon recognition of neurologic symptoms in the setting of AMS. Supplemental oxygen should be delivered during descent either by oxygen mask or portable hyperbaric oxygen chamber. Dexamethasone (4–8 mg IM or IV, followed by 4 mg every 6 hours) is the medication of choice in the field. In severe cases, intubation with hyperventilation or intravenous mannitol may be helpful to decrease intracranial pressure but may not be possible in the field. Diuretics should be used only when intravascular volume status can be adequately monitored, and thus are generally not used outside the hospital (15).

High-Altitude Retinal Hemorrhage

High-altitude retinal hemorrhages (HARHs) are a common finding at elevations above 14,000 feet, with an incidence as high as 40% (26). They are usually asymptomatic but can lead to complaints of visual changes, floaters, or scotomata. Funduscopic exam reveals arterial and venous engorgement and retinal hemorrhages (Fig 36-3). HARH is commonly seen in victims of HAPE and HACE. HARHs usually resolve without specific treatment in 7 to 14 days, and rarely have any sequelae (15).

SUMMARY

Altitude illnesses have become more common with the increased mobility of modern society. Acute mountain sickness, high-altitude pulmonary edema, high-altitude cerebral edema, and high-altitude retinal hemorrhage are the medical problems commonly associated with high-altitude activity. In each condition, new treatments have improved clinical outcomes, but prevention always should be the primary strategy.

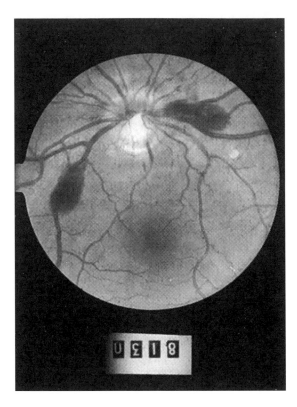

Figure 36-3. In high-altitude retinal hemorrhage (HARH), a funduscopic exam reveals arterial and venous engorgement. (Reprinted from Bloomfield J, Fricker PA, Fitch KD. Science and medicine in sport. 2nd ed. Oxford: Blackwell Science, 1995:146.)

REFERENCES

1 Gilbert DL. The first documented report of mountain sickness: the China headache mountain story. Respir Physiol 1983;52:315.

2 Roberts D. The iceman. Natl Geographic 1993; 183:37–67.

3 Reeves JT, Graves BM, Sutton JR, et al. Operation Everest II: preservation of cardiac function at extreme altitude. J Appl Physiol 1987;63:531–539.

4 Pugh LGCE. Cardiac output in muscular exercise at 5800 meters. J Appl Physiol 1964;19:441–447.

5 West JB, Boyer SJ, Graber DJ, et al. Maximal exercise at extreme altitudes on Mount Everest. J Appl Physiol 1983;55:688–698.

6 Milledge JS. The ventilatory response to hypoxia: how much is good for a mountaineer? Postgrad Med J 1986;63:169–172.

7 Sutton J. Mountain sickness. Neurol Clin 1992; 10:1015–1030.

8 Sutton JR, Reeves JT, Groves BM, et al. Oxygen transport and cardiovascular function at extreme altitude: lessons from operation Everest II. Int J Sports Med 1992;13:S13–S18.

9 Krasney JA. A neurogenic basis for acute altitude illness. Med Sci Sports Exerc 1994;26:195–208.

10 Singh I, Khanna PK, Srivastana MC, et al. Acute mountain sickness. N Engl J Med 1969;280:175–184.

11 Montgomery AB, Mills J, Luce JM. Incidence of acute mountain sickness at intermediate altitude. JAMA 1989;261:732–734.

12 Honigman B, Theis MK, Koziol-McLain J, et al. Acute mountain sickness in a general tourist population at moderate altitudes. Ann Int Med 1993;118:587–592.

13 Houston CS. Altitude sickness. In: Strauss RH, ed. Sports medicine. 2nd ed. Philadelphia: WB Saunders, 1991:389–408.

14 Rabold M. High altitude pulmonary edema: a collective review. Am J Emerg Med 1989;7:426–433.

15 Hackett PH, Roach RC. High-altitude medicine. In: Auerbach PS, ed. Wilderness medicine: management of wilderness and environmental emergencies. 3rd ed. St. Louis: Mosby, 1995:1–37.

16 Grissom CK, Roach RC, Sarnqist FH, Hackett PH. Acetazolamide in the treatment of acute mountain sickness: clinical efficacy and effect on gas exchange. Ann Int Med 1992;116:461–465.

17 Sutton JR, Houston CS, Mansell AL, et al. Effect of acetazolamide on hypoxemia during sleep at high altitudes. N Engl J Med 1979;301:1329–1331.

18 Montgomery AB, Luce JM, Micheal P, Mills J. Effects of dexamethasone on the incidence of acute mountain sickness at two intermediate altitudes. JAMA 1989;261:734–736.

19 Burtscher M, Likar R, Nachbauer W. Ibuprofen versus sumatriptan for high altitude headache. Lancet 1995;346:254–355.

20 West JB, Tsukimoto K, Mathieu-Costello O, Prediletto R. Stress failure in pulmonary capillaries. J Appl Physiol 1991;70:1731–1742.

21 Lobenhoffer HP, Zink RA, Brendel W. High altitude pulmonary edema: analysis of 166 cases. In: Brendel W, Zink RA, eds. High altitude physiology and medicine. New York: Springer, 1982:219–231.

22 Tom P, Garmel GM, Auerbach PS. Environment-dependent sports emergencies. Med Clin North Am 1994;78:305–325.

23 Sutton JR, Houston CS, Coates G, eds. Hypoxia and molecular medicine: proceedings of the 8th international hypoxia symposium held at Lake

Louise, Canada, February 9–13, 1993. Burlington, VT: Queen City, 1992:327.

24 Oelz O, Maggiorini M, Ritter M, et al. Prevention and treatment of high altitude pulmonary edema by a calcium channel blocker. Int J Sports Med 1992;13:S65–S68.

25 Bartsch P, Maggiorini M, Ritter M, et al. Prevention of high-altitude pulmonary edema by nifedipine. N Engl J Med 1991;325:1284–1389.

26 McFadden DM, Houston CS, Sutton JR, et al. High altitude retinopathy. JAMA 1981;245:381–386.

Chapter 37
Diving Medicine

Kevin Boundy

Any diver using underwater breathing apparatus is at risk of dysbaric illness. Although dysbaric illness often requires treatment in a recompression chamber, appropriate first aid minimizes the insult to a sick diver and maximizes chances of a full recovery.

BAROTRAUMA

In sea water, the pressure exerted on a submerged body increases by 1 atmosphere every 10 meters in depth. This means that if the pressure exerted at the surface is 1 atmosphere absolute (1 ATA) then it will be 2 ATA at 10 meters, 3 ATA at 20 meters, and so on.

Boyle's law states that at a constant temperature the volume of a given mass of gas is inversely proportional to the absolute pressure. Put simply, as the pressure on a gas increases, the volume occupied by that gas decreases. Gas enclosed within the body obeys this law, and this is the basis for barotrauma.

Gas-filled spaces undergo their greatest volume changes near the surface. Diving to a depth of only 10 meters results in a volume change of 50%. In contrast, going from a depth of 20 meters to 30 meters results in a volume change of 24%. Since the greater changes in volume occur near the surface, any pressure-related contraindication to diving must be considered absolute: shallow dives are just as dangerous as deep dives.

Middle Ear Barotrauma
The most common form of barotrauma affects the middle ear. As a diver descends, the increase in ambient pressure causes the tympanic membrane (TM) to bow inward, producing local pain. Pressure in the middle ear can be equalized with the external environment by performing a Valsalva maneuver. Divers who cannot clear their ears before entering the water should not dive. If the diver is unable to equalize the pressure, the relatively negative pressure within the middle ear causes the mucous membranes lining this cavity, including those around the entrance to the Eustachian tube, to become edematous.

On surfacing, the diver may complain of the ear feeling full, blocked, or painful. On examination the TM may appear normal or show an increase in vascularity, frank hemorrhage, or even rupture, depending on the severity of the condition. The changes in the appearance of the TM mirror the degree of engorgement of the mucous membrane lining the middle ear.

Treatment Treatment is symptomatic: decongestants and cessation of all diving until clinical resolution, which usually occurs within 7 days if the TM is not ruptured. If the TM is ruptured, topical antibiotics should be considered (1), and an opinion from an ear, nose, and throat specialist may be advisable. A ruptured eardrum is an absolute contraindication to diving (2). All cases of middle ear barotrauma should have an audiogram at the time of presentation to ensure there is no coexisting inner ear barotrauma.

Inner Ear Barotrauma
Any barotrauma of the middle ear can affect the inner ear and cause vertigo. Vertigo while diving can be fatal. Persisting vertigo or tinnitus are indicative of damage to the inner ear, usually a rupture of the wide window (known as a perilymph fistula). There may also be ataxia, disorientation, and some degree of hearing loss.

Treatment If inner ear barotrauma is suspected, an ENT review should be sought urgently. The patient should rest sitting up in bed. Activities that raise intracranial pressure, such as coughing or straining to defecate, should be discouraged by the use of sedatives and laxatives (1). Serial audiograms will help assess clinical progression.

Sinus Barotrauma

Sinus barotrauma, although less common than middle ear barotrauma, still occurs relatively frequently in divers. Most often the frontal and maxillary sinuses are involved, presenting pain over the affected sinus. If airflow into the sinus is blocked during descent, the relative negative pressure within the sinus causes the mucous membranes to become engorged and eventually hemorrhage. The gas trapped within the sinus expands again on ascent, forcing the blood out into the nasopharynx. Often the blood appears in the face mask.

Treatment Symptoms usually settle over a few days with use of a nasal decongestant.

Pulmonary Barotrauma and Cerebral Arterial Gas Embolism (CAGE)

The most serious barotrauma affects the pulmonary system and is second only to drowning as a cause of death in divers (2,3). Pulmonary barotrauma arises most often after rapid or uncontrolled ascent. If a diver fails to exhale during ascent, the overexpansion of gas within the alveoli can lead to alveolar rupture (2,4). This phenomenon is most common in people who hold their breath during ascent, but it is also seen in those who are predisposed to air trapping because of asthma or some other inflammatory disorder of the lung. Because of this risk, asthma is considered an absolute contraindication to diving. Alveolar rupture can present as local pulmonary tissue damage, surgical emphysema, pneumothorax, or an arterial gas embolus.

The most serious complication of pulmonary barotrauma is an arterial gas embolism, caused by gas escaping from ruptured alveoli into the pulmonary circulation. The gas travels to the left side of the heart where bubbles are distributed to all parts of the systemic circulation. The most profound pathology is caused by bubbles that migrate to the brain and produce a cerebral arterial gas embolism (CAGE).

Signs of a CAGE include *any* neurologic symptom, ranging from confusion to unconsciousness that develops just before or soon after surfacing. Almost all CAGEs present within 5 minutes of reaching the surface (4–6). The clinical picture can fluctuate as the cerebral bubbles redistribute, occasionally giving the picture of a spontaneous recovery. Clinicians should be aware that a CAGE can present without any clinical evidence of pulmonary barotrauma.

Treatment for CAGE Urgent recompression is the major priority (6), even in cases of spontaneous recovery, because redistribution of bubbles can lead to a further deterioration in the clinical condition (7). The first-aid treatment for CAGE consists of the following (Table 37-1):

1 Keep the diver horizontal to minimize the risk of further bubbles floating up into the carotid system.
2 Provide 100% oxygen, either by a tight-fitting mask or an endotracheal tube, to help raise the partial pressure of oxygen in tissues that may have been rendered ischemic by the embolus (5).
3 Give appropriate intravenous therapy to correct dehydration and maintain blood pressure prior to recompression. Hypertonic solutions should not be used unless required acutely because of the risk of a rebound increase in intracranial pressure (3,8).

Note that the head-down position is *not* recommended, because it is believed that the increased intracranial pressure generated by such a maneuver is likely to complicate cerebral injury (9). An

Table 37-1 First-Aid Treatment of a Cerebral Arterial Gas Embolism (CAGE)

1 Lay the patient down flat.
2 Give 100% oxygen, either by a well-fitting mask or an endotracheal tube.
3 Establish intravenous access and give only enough fluid to maintain urinary output and adequate blood pressure.

indwelling urinary catheter should be inserted if bladder control is affected.

Other than oxygen, few drugs are of help in the first-aid situation. If a patient is seizing, diazepam or midazolam reduces cerebral activity. This not only controls the fit, but also reduces the demand for oxygen by the ischemic brain.

If a recompression facility is not readily available, prevention of secondary complications such as arrhythmias and renal failure should be based on conventional medical principles. Arrhythmias are not uncommon, and the patient should be monitored throughout the period prior to recompression. If associated pulmonary barotrauma has produced a pneumothorax, surgical emphysema, or other pulmonary tissue damage, these should be treated according to standard protocols.

Miscellaneous Barotrauma

Dental barotrauma (pain in or around the teeth when changing depth) and mask squeeze (facial pain secondary to the development of a relatively negative pressure within the face mask) are less serious forms of barotrauma that may present after a dive. They should be treated in the same fashion as other forms of trauma to these areas.

DECOMPRESSION SICKNESS (DCS)

Henry's law states that at a constant temperature the amount of a gas that dissolves in a liquid is proportional to the pressure of the gas over the liquid. Thus, as the diver descends and the ambient pressure rises, the partial pressure of the gas being breathed increases. This results in more gas dissolving in the bloodstream, and thence being delivered to the tissues.

Decompression sickness (DCS) is a direct result of the nitrogen gas that was previously dissolved in body fluids while the diver was under pressure coming out of solution when the pressure is reduced during ascent. Longer, deeper dives result in more nitrogen being absorbed by the body, so decompression stops should be allowed during ascent to give the diver time to expel this extra gas from the tissues before bubble formation becomes a problem.

Almost any organ system can be affected by bubble formation either directly or indirectly, and symptoms may develop gradually in the hours after a dive. Classic symptoms in over 90% of cases of DCS are persisting lethargy, fatigue, and general malaise. Serious DCS, however, can develop within minutes of a dive.

Vascular DCS

Most vascular bubbles form in the venous circulation. The bubbles in the bloodstream increase the permeability of the vascular endothelium, encouraging platelet aggregation and activation of clotting systems. This results in diminished plasma volume, increased blood viscosity, and decreased blood flow. To lessen complications from these changes, all patients with DCS should have intravenous fluids administered at the onset of treatment.

Pulmonary DCS

Venous bubbles are usually filtered at the lungs, which prevents them from passing into the arterial system and becoming arterial gas emboli. If more than 10% of the pulmonary vascular bed is obstructed, a clinical syndrome known as "the chokes" develops. Clinical features of the chokes include pleuritic chest pain and tachypnea associated with a cough. Impairment of the pulmonary circulation can result in decreased pulse rate and blood pressure, with eventual circulatory collapse.

Neurologic DCS

Nitrogen is readily taken up from the blood into fatty tissues including the myelin sheaths of nerves. The clinical picture of neurologic involvement in DCS can vary from a silent lesion within the cerebrum (10) to paraplegia, depending on the site of the lesion. When a peripheral nerve is affected the neurologic picture may appear bizarre. The patient may present with glove or stocking anesthesia or an area of paresthesia not consistent with any particular nervous distribution.

Musculoskeletal DCS

Musculoskeletal DCS, commonly known as "the bends," is DCS of the muscles, tendons, and other soft tissues. It typically produces a vague diffuse pain.

Table 37-2 First-Aid Treatment of Decompression Sickness (DCS)

1 Have the patient rest, preferably lying down.
2 Give 100% oxygen, either by a well-fitting mask or an endotracheal tube.
3 Establish intravenous access and ensure the patient is well hydrated.

Cutaneous DCS

DCS of the skin often presents as a rash, sometimes with cyanotic mottling and marbling of the skin. This is indicative of bubbles present in both the skin and its blood vessels, and is asociated with DCS elsewhere.

Treatment of DCS

Because of the risk of a "silent" neurologic lesion coexisting with other forms of DCS, all suspected clinical cases should have early initiation of recompression treatment. The quicker this therapy begins, the greater the chance of a full recovery from even serious lesions (10). Much can be done, however, for a patient with DCS while awaiting recompression (Table 37-2).

As with a CAGE, the patient should be laid flat and given 100% oxygen, either by a tight-fitting mask or an endotracheal tube. Oxygen is useful because the bubbles that cause DCS are almost 100% nitrogen. Saturating the tissues with oxygen increases the concentration gradient for the nitrogen and helps reduce the bubbles' size (6). Because prolonged exposure to oxygen has toxic effects on both the lungs and the central nervous system, patients who require prolonged oxygen therapy should be given "air breaks." If patients require more than 18 hours of oxygen therapy prior to recompression, the oxygen should be supplied on a 1-hour-on, 1-hour-off basis (4).

As previously noted, hydration and IV access are initial treatments in DCS, but alert patients should be encouraged to drink. Well-hydrated patients have a better outcome, particularly if the hematocrit can be maintained at less than 50%. Blood pressure and fluid balance require monitoring throughout treatment.

Although corticosteroids have been used in an attempt to reduce spinal or cerebral edema, no proven benefits have been associated with their use (11). They have, however, been shown to increase the patient's susceptibility to oxygen toxicity (3).

Benzodiazepines help control the vertigo, nausea, and vomiting associated with labyrinthine DCS. They are also useful in patients suffering from toxic or confusional states, as these patients can be difficult to transport to or to control in a recompression chamber. Because benzodiazepines can mask any clinical improvement seen with recompression, they should not be administered without the approval of the medical officer at the recompression chamber. Once given, they will also mask the further development of DCS, so patients requiring such treatment should be recompressed as a matter of course. Whenever possible, benzodiazepines should only be administered with the approval of the medical officer at the recompression chamber.

SUMMARY

All divers face some risk of dysbaric illness, but the risks can be minimized by appropriate diving precautions. Two major types of clinical syndromes occur, related to either barotrauma or to decompression sickness. The mainstay of treatment is the recompression chamber, but physicians who care for underwater athletes should be aware of the clinical conditions and the appropriate therapy that can be instituted while preparing the athlete for recompression.

REFERENCES

1 Stiernberg CM, Strunk CL. Ear injuries in sport. Texas Med 1986;82:32–36.
2 Arthur LCDR DC. A synopsis of diving medicine for emergency physicians: Part 1. US Navy Med 1985;2:19–28.
3 Edmonds CW, Lowry CJ, Pennefather JW. Diving and subaquatic medicine. Mosman, Australia: Diving Medical Centre, 1983.
4 Gorman DF. Decompression sickness and arterial gas embolism in sports scuba divers. Sports Med 1989;8:32–42.
5 Kizer KW. Dysbaric air embolism in Hawaii. Ann Emerg Med 1987;16:535–541.

6 Neuman TS. Diving medicine. Clin Sports Med 1987;6:647–661.

7 Orton J. Medical problems of recreational diving. Aust Fam Physician 1989;18:674–685.

8 Dutka AJ. A review of the pathophysiology and potential application of experimental therapies for cerebral ischemia to the treatment of cerebral arterial gas embolism. Undersea Biomed Res 1985;12:403–421.

9 Dutka AJ. Recommendations made for diving accident management. Pressure 1990;19. [As quoted in editorial.]

10 Arthur LCDR DC. A synopsis of diving medicine for emergency physicians: Part 2. US Navy Med 1985;3:21–27.

11 Francis TJR, Dutka AJ. Methyl prednisolone in the treatment of acute spinal cord decompression sickness. Undersea Biomed Res 1989;16:165–174.

Chapter 38
Marine Envenomation

John A. Williamson

Envenomation implies the entry of a toxin into the human body by penetration of the skin or mucous membrane. Thus, some marine envenomations are accompanied by simultaneous trauma (e.g., a puncture wound from a stingray barb). *Poisoning* implies entry into the body by oral ingestion and absorption from the gastrointestinal tract. The term *toxin* covers both venoms and poisons. This chapter will consider some aspects of only one form of marine poisoning: tetrodotoxin poisoning. This type of poison is the most common, and it serves as an archetype of toxins as it can also act as a venom.

PREVALENCE OF ENVENOMATION INJURIES

The people most affected by marine envenomations and poisonings are those living in tropical maritime communities. However, water sports participants such as scuba divers, windsurfers, and recreational boaters are increasingly being affected. There are around 2 million recreational scuba (self-contained underwater breathing apparatus) and hookah (surface-supply breathing apparatus) dives made annually in Australia alone.

Table 38-1 lists, in approximate descending order, the comparative prevalence of mortality and morbidity resulting from marine envenomation worldwide. Recent international scrutiny of the statistical data on morbidity and mortality resulting from marine envenomation has revealed that previous data had been skewed in favor of mortality. Morbidity is common and may be serious.

Pathophysiology of the Toxins
Most marine venoms are complex mixtures of proteins, polypeptides, and enzymes. The toxic effects are usually dose-dependent and cause immediate, severe localized pain and tissue inflammation at the site of entry. They are also antigenic, and may induce allergic reactions in susceptible individuals, such as people with asthma, allergic eczema, or rhinitis. Anaphylaxis has also been documented, but is rare. Venoms may exhibit systemic effects including myocardial depression, vasoconstriction and systemic hypertension, central respiratory disturbance, acute pulmonary edema, shock, and syncope. Local effects include again vasoconstriction and vesiculation of skin with underlying tissue necrosis, and severe pain may occur as part of an intense inflammatory response. Secondary infection, scarring, or keloid may result. In vitro hemolysis has been repeatedly documented experimentally, but its clinical significance is unclear.

Marine poisons vary widely in their chemical composition. For example, the highly potent ciguatoxin is a large, complex set of molecules. Conversely, tetrodotoxin—the principal venom component in the bite of the blue-ringed octopus (*Hapalochlaena* species; Plate 12) and also the poison found in puffer fish flesh (ingested as *fugu* in Japan)—is a simple, small molecule. Tetrodoxin has a molecular weight of 419, is relatively nonantigenic, and produces no local tissue effects. It specifically blocks sodium (Na^+) channels in excitable membranes, producing neurogenic respiratory paralysis without initial loss of consciousness.

CORAL CUTS/ABRASIONS/STINGS

Common Symptoms
Coral cuts, abrasions, and stings are injuries that may occur over coral reefs. Coral abrasions and lac-

Table 38-1   Comparison of the Relative Frequencies of Mortality and Morbidity in Human Victims from Marine Animals, in Descending Order of Respective Prevalence

Mortality	Morbidity
Pufferfish poisoning*	Coral cuts, abrasions, stings (including wound infections)
Paralytic shellfish poisoning	Jellyfish stings (especially *Physalia* spp.)
Chirodropid jellyfish stings	Ciguatera poisoning
Ciguatera poisoning	Spiny fish stings (including stingray)
Turtle flesh poisoning	Other marine animal poisoning from ingestion
Sea snakes	
Spiny fish injuries	
Physalia (Portuguese man-of-war) stings	

NOTE: The relative morbidities are informed estimates only.
*Although pufferfish are poisonous and not venomous, they can be unpredictably aggressive. Some species grow to considerable size (e.g., 50 cm long) and have been known to attack people in the water and inflict serious bite injuries. (Reproduced by permission from Williamson JA, Fenner PJ, Burnett JW. The injuries, their incidence and the toxins that produce them. In: Williamson JA, Fenner PJ, Burnett JW, Rifkin JF, eds. Venomous and poisonous marine animals: a medical and biological handbook. Sydney: University of New South Wales Press, 1996:77.)

erations are more common than stings, and they can produce serious morbidity if neglected. In the usual scenario, an initial abrasion often passes unnoticed, and coral debris is introduced into the wound. When the debris is not removed, inflammation and indolent infection with pain, itching, and discharge may result. The symptoms may persist for days. Allergies to the embedded protein coral polyp material have also been documented.

Physical Findings and Diagnostic Features

Stings   Injuries inflicted by stinging corals are accompanied by immediate stinging pain, then itching and wheal formation wherever contact has been made. Divers or snorkelers who touch stung skin then rub their face or eyes will transfer the nematocysts and produce additional stings in those areas. (See the section on cnidarians for more information on nematocysts.)

Cuts and Abrasions   Neglected coral cuts and abrasions quickly become inflamed, itchy, and swollen, with a circumferential, spreading erythema, regional lymphadenopathy, and discharge. Secondary infections with terrestrial or marine

pathogenic microorganisms (e.g., *Vibrio* species) may result in months of difficult-to-treat morbidity.

Treatment

1 Remove the injured person from the water and gently remove any superficial debris from the wound.
2 Within no longer than 4 hours of the injury, cleanse the wound with fresh water, a weak detergent/antiseptic (chlorhexidine), and a soft bristle brush. Although severe pain usually does not accompany the cleansing process, individuals with special anesthetic needs, such as children, may require formal medical referral.
3 Bandage the wound with a soft dressing, elevate the affected part, and seek medical advice.

Medical follow-up includes possible x-ray of the wound, further cleansing or removal of deeply embedded foreign bodies under appropriate anesthesia, tetanus prophylaxis, and microbiologic consultation.

Pharmacologic Treatment   If toxic or allergic symptoms persist, medical advice should be sought before attempting oral antihistamine or steroid therapy. Topical antihistamines have proven disappointing for marine stings. As systemic antihistamines are associated with the side effect of drowsiness, their use is generally incompatible with continued athletic participation on that day.

CNIDARIAN (JELLYFISH) STINGS

Common Symptoms

Cnidarians, or jellyfish, are characterized by the possession of *nematocysts,* intrinsic stinging micro-apparatus (Fig 38-1). Injuries from nematocyst stings are common worldwide, and are characterized by extensive morbidity and some mortality. Because of their smaller body size and lack of hairy skin, women and children are particularly susceptible to serious effects after skin contact with cnidarians.

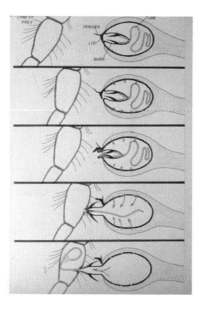

Figure 38-1. A sequential diagrammatic representation of a firing cnidarian nematocyst penetrating the cuticle of a prawn's leg. The combination harpoon/injection syringe deposits a microdose of venom through the skin into the dermis. Tentacles may contain millions of such nematocysts. (Drawing conceived by Dr. Robert F Hartwick, PhD, James Cook University. Reproduced by permission from Williamson JA. Classification. In: Exton D, ed. The marine stinger book. 3rd ed. Brisbane, Queensland. Surf Life Saving Queensland, 1985:xvii–xxi.)

The typical sting results in immediate, sometimes severe, pain and edema, and avulsed tentacle material may remain attached to the victim's skin. Untreated pain can persist for many hours. The powerfully antigenic venom mixtures may induce local itching and swelling, and delayed local and distal eruptions may occur up to 6 weeks later. Dyspnea, disturbance of consciousness, and even circulatory arrest have been recorded following the sting of certain box jellyfish (chirodropids) (Plate 13) and at least one species of *Stomolophus* found in the China seas.

Physical Findings and Diagnostic Features

As the victims seldom see the offending animal in the water, even when it is large, taking a thorough history can be difficult with some cnidarian stings. Thus, much ignorance persists concerning the role of cnidarian stings in marine envenomation.

Chirodropid (Multitentacled Box Jellyfish) Stings   On contact with the box jellyfish, the victim will experience an immediate, severe pain that may render him or her difficult to control and, in worst cases, incoherent. The simultaneous discharge of the venom contents of millions of tentacular nematocysts results in a massive, rapid envenomation process through the epidermis, and the tentacles can remain adhered to the victim's skin. Stung skin immediately exhibits an intense, acute inflammatory reaction. Whealed, blanched skin where actual tentacle contact has occurred may darken with threatened necrosis (Plate 14). Nausea and vomiting follow, and progressive impairment of consciousness may develop quickly in worst cases. With life-threatening envenomation, shock, a rapid weak pulse, and respiratory and/or cardiac arrest may occur quickly.

Irukandji Syndrome   A tiny carybdeid box jellyfish, such as the four-tentacled *Carukia barnesi* (Plate 15), can induce a moderate sting with very little skin marking. The symptoms of envenomation, which follow in 30 to 40 minutes, are a prostrating syndrome of generalized muscle pain, vomiting, headache, and systemic hypertension. Less commonly, myocardial failure and pulmonary edema can subsequently occur.

Physalia* Species   *Pacific Bluebottle   The source of the world's commonest jellyfish sting, the Pacific bluebottle jellyfish appears as a blue, gas-filled float with a grouping of short, dark-blue tentacles and one long, stinging tentacle hanging underneath. This jellyfish's sting results in instant, moderately severe local skin pain, which is usually short lived. The longitudinal wheal on the victim's skin is typically composed of a series of elliptical white wheals, surrounded with an angry red flare. Systemic effects are unusual.

Atlantic Portuguese Man-of-War The Portuguese man-of-war, a large crested jellyfish with multiple long tentacles, also belongs to the genus *Physalia*. The Atlantic variety is quite dangerous, and several human deaths have been recorded on the South Carolina and Florida coasts. Sting effects are similar to those of a bluebottle sting (above), but additionally muscle and back pain, prostration, vomiting, and, in worst cases, cardiovascular collapse may occur.

Treatment

Box Jellyfish Stings *Nonserious Stings* For a recognized box jellyfish sting, immediately douse the entire sting with 2 to 3 liters of household vinegar (4% to 6% acetic acid in water) to render the unfired nematocysts harmless. (Do *not* apply vinegar to any other type of jellyfish sting.) Following the vinegar application, simply apply ice or cold packs to the stung skin for pain relief. Seek medical aid if pain is unrelieved.

Serious Stings For serious box jellyfish stings, resuscitation (DRABC) should always take absolute priority. Do not waste time picking off tentacle bites—a vinegar treatment can render them harmless. After vinegar has been applied, apply compression immobilization bandages over stings on limbs without interfering with resuscitation efforts. Make arrangements for urgent ambulance attendance and specific antivenom administration.

Other Jellyfish or Cnidarian Stings

1 Pick off, or use fresh seawater to wash off any adherent tentacle material. Do *not* apply fresh water, vinegar, or methylated spirits.
2 Apply cold packs or wrapped ice to the stung area for pain relief. Seek medical advice for unrelieved pain.

SPINY FISH INJURIES AND ENVENOMATION

The world's seas contain a bewildering array of fishes equipped with venomous spines for capturing prey or self-defense. They do not attack human beings—many of the reported injuries have been among aquarium keepers rather than individuals on the open sea. Fish spines may be located on fins (dorsal, pectoral, caudal, ventral) or near the mouth (labial), are often erectile, and are usually connected to or coated with glands producing a powerful venom mixture. The stingray, for example, possesses a long, powerful tail barb that can inflict a serious laceration (Plate 16) or stab wound and deposit a powerful tissue-necrosing venom along the wound track. The crown-of-thorns sea star (*Acanthaster planci*), which is not actually a fish, also can inflict injuries with its spines.

Common Symptoms
The typical spiny fish injury produces immediate and often devastating local pain and swelling. Spines or barbs (such as the stingray's) may break off and be visible in the wound. The pain will immobilize the injured part (usually the hand or foot), and the suffering will leave the victim distraught. In serious cases, the pain in an untreated injury does not abate appreciably. In the absence of a major blood vessel injury, local circulatory embarrassment or excessive bleeding is uncommon.

Physical Findings and Diagnostic Features
Immediate and severe pain is the rule with all fish-spine injuries. The sting of the stonefish (*Synanceia* species) is a classic—and most painful—example. Because stonefish have superb camouflage and prefer stationary, bottom-dwelling positions, the victim's puncture wounds typically occur on the sole of the foot or less commonly on the hand; often, the victim may have stood on the unseen fish, or may have mistaken it for a "funny looking rock" and attempted to pick it up.

The puncture wound has a surrounding purplish discoloration, and rapid and impressive local edema. Systemic effects are rare, but the intense pain can generate incoherence, nausea, vomiting, and sweating. Fragments of the spine may be retained in the wound depths, requiring radiography for detection. Among the many thousands of recorded stonefish stings, only three human deaths have been (somewhat unconvincingly) documented.

Secondary infection (including tetanus) is a possibility in any neglected marine-spine wound. Following stingray spine wounds, inexorable tissue necrosis will occur along the barb path; thus, stingray injuries to any part of the trunk (the chest, back, or abdomen) are medical emergencies.

Treatment

All spiny fish injuries will ultimately require medical consultation, but the preliminary care should follow the following guidelines:

1 Do not attempt to remove any deeply embedded spine material, and do not apply compression bandages to spiny fish wounds.
2 Immerse the envenomated part (usually a limb) in comfortably hot (*not* boiling) water for pain relief. The rescuer should test the water temperature before immersing the victim's limb. Maintain immersion of the limb and the comfortable water temperature en route to medical aid.

Medical attention for spiny fish wounds includes

- local anesthetic block for pain relief
- radiologic examination of the wound for spine fragments
- possible removal of retained spine fragments, and or surgical excision of tissue, according to surgical consultation
- appropriate antivenom administration (for stonefish wounds)
- tetanus prophylaxis
- selected antibiotic prophylaxis and follow-up assessment

SEA SNAKES AND OCTOPUSES

Sea Snakes

Sea snakes are distributed worldwide, but are more prevalent in warmer seas. Sea snakes are distinguished from eels by the absence of gills (sea snakes are lung breathers), their paddle-shaped tails, and the flap over each of their paired nostrils (Plate 17). They are agile swimmers and are known to exhibit curiousity; contrary to popular belief, sea snakes seldom attack human beings, but they will defend themselves or their territories if they perceive a threat. One of the most widely distributed venomous animal is the beaked sea snake (*Enhydrina schistosa*).

Common Symptoms Sea snakes have an effective biting mechanism and very toxic venoms. Deaths and near-fatalities from sea snake bites are well documented. The bite is sometimes painless, with little local reaction. The venom produces myotoxicity with muscle pains and red urine (myoglobinuria). In significantly envenomed victims, nausea, vomiting, dizziness, and dry throat may precede postsynaptic neuromuscular paresis or paralysis and respiratory failure. Coagulation disturbances or hemolysis typically do not occur.

Blue-Ringed Octopuses

These small, attractive animals (one can fit in the palm of an unwary hand) are agile swimmers and are known to inhabit tropical and temperate seas throughout the Indo-Pacific region.

Common Symptoms The bite from the small, parrot-like beak of this mollusk is usually painless—a drop of blood on the skin is often the only initial clue to envenomation. Bites never occur when both the human and the animal are fully immersed in the sea (a single record exists of a scuba diver accidentally kneeling on a blue-ringed octopus while taking underwater photographs). The primary danger is to beachcombers or waders—especially children—who unknowingly may handle these animals.

Most bites do not seriously envenomate. In those that do, the first symptoms are usually circumoral paresthesia and numbness, followed by blurred vision, dysphagia, and difficult breathing.

Physical Findings and Diagnostic Features

Sea snake and blue-ringed octopus bites almost invariably result from unwarranted or unintentional interference with the animal. Often, a victim will have hauled aboard a net-captured sea snake or handled a "pretty little octopus."

Sea Snake Bites With sea snake envenomation, vomiting, shallow breathing and rapid pulse may precede respiratory failure from neurotoxicity. The muscle pains from sea snake venom myotoxicity may produce a reluctance in the victim to move, and trismus may develop—such signs may be mistaken for those of neurotoxicity.

Blue-Ringed Octopus Bites   The paralyzed victim of blue-ringed octopus (tetrodotoxin) envenomation may remain fully aware prior to succumbing to the effects of acute hypoxia. Thus, rescuers should be cautious regarding any remarks within the victim's hearing during resuscitation efforts.

Treatment of Sea Snake and Blue-Ringed Octopus Bites

For initiating treatment of sea snake or blue-ringed octopus bite, an oral account of the patient's encounter is sufficient: do not attempt to capture the sea snake, or handle the octopus. Species identification of the snake or the octopus for adequate treatment is not required, and a single octopus can deliver more than one serious bite.

First aid for the bites should proceed as follows:

1 Further activity by the victim is absolutely contraindicated: immobilize the victim and the bitten limb immediately.
2 Do not wait for symptoms to occur: immediately apply a compression immobilization bandage to the bitten site and limb, then splint the limb as for a fracture. Note the time of application of the bandages, and, if possible, the time of the bite. Do *not* remove the bandages and do *not* apply an arterial tourniquet, nor cut or incise the wound.
3 In paresis victims, airway protection and resuscitation take absolute priority. Full recovery can be anticipated provided hypoxic damage is prevented by adequate ventilation (initially as expired air resuscitation).
4 Obtain medical advice and aid to permit appropriate antivenom administration. Management of any possible renal and/or electrolyte complications should follow in medical hands as soon as possible.

SPECIAL CONSIDERATIONS IN ATHLETES

Likelihood of Marine Envenomation

Scuba Divers   There is now clear evidence that scuba divers are at increased risk of sustaining ma-

rine envenomation. Death and serious morbidity in scuba divers and snorkelers (breath-hold divers)* have been documented from jellyfish envenomation, stingray injury/envenomation, coral abrasion complications (e.g., *Vibrio vulnificus* infection), and rarely sea anemone stings.

Surf Lifesavers and Ironman Competitors   Copious records now exist concerning the risk of cnidarian stings on surf lifesavers performing patrol and rescue duties in the sea. Competitors in ironman competitions have also sustained impressive stings. Additionally, surf carnivals have been canceled due to swarms of stinging jellyfish such as bluebottles and mauve stingers (*Pelagia noctiluca*).

Transocean and Channel Endurance Swimmers   Despite their protective layer of insulating grease, endurance swimmers remain at risk for cnidarian stings, both from intact smaller animals and from fragments of detached tentacle material. Media publicity tends to focus on the safety of shark cages, but jellyfish (and sea snakes) can be dangerous, and they easily penetrate such enclosures.

Surfers and Windsurfers   Interestingly, windsurfers and surfboard riders do not often suffer serious marine envenomation, probably due in part to their custom of wearing of protective wet suits or stinger suits (Fig 38-2).

Risks and Presentation in Athletes

Given that athletes are healthy and generally have larger muscle mass, a venom dose might be expected to have less systemic effect; however, the high metabolic rate and physical exertion (muscle pump effect) in the envenomated athlete during an event can greatly enhance venom absorption, leading to more rapid onset and more serious systemic effects. Children and female athletes are at especial risk for cnidarian envenomation effects, but the severity of irukanji envenomation in large ironman competitors has been equally severe.

An additional clinical consideration in athletes is that the athlete's intense concentration, motiva-

---

*Fatalities among scuba divers and snorkelers have also occurred from shark attack (Australia) and from needlefish stab wounds (Okinawa, Japan). Trauma that does not involve envenomation is beyond the scope of this chapter.

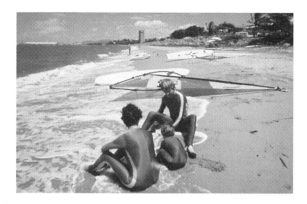

Figure 38-2. A water sports family in northern Australia all wearing nylon-spandex stinger suits. Women and children without stinger suit protection are particularly vulnerable to the effects of box jellyfish envenomation. The suits also provide significant protection from sunburn.

tion, and physical effort may mask any sightings (as during spear fishing competitions) or early symptoms. Athletes ignoring or hiding pain during competition is well known, and the more advanced effects of any serious envenomation may develop before either the athlete or his or her attendants become aware of the problem.

Management of Marine Envenomation in the Athlete

The first aid and medical measures recommended for marine envenomation either will not interfere with an athlete's performance or are employed in situations where it is imperative that the athlete withdraw immediately from competition on that day. Consequently, most of the treatment options described above for nonathletes apply equally to athletes.

Return to Training and Competition   The coordination of ongoing treatment for envenomation with the athlete's return to training and competition must be individualized to each patient and episode:

- The vast majority of marine envenomations do not produce serious or life-threatening effects,

and the return to training can be measured in hours or days.
- Serious skin damage requires consultation with a medical specialist, and generally precludes training and competition until healing is complete.
- Athletes who have had antivenom administered require several days of rest from full training, and follow-up for any delayed side effects. The persistence of any systemic envenomation symptoms or any evidence of local infection contraindicates return to training and/or competition.
- Athletes who have sustained the full-blown irukandji syndrome can expect to be unfit up to one month, because of muscle soreness, lassitude, and poor concentration.

Prevention of Marine Envenomation

Prevention of marine envenomation among athletes is important—even minor injuries can be distracting influences on the motivation to train, compete, and win. Athletes who observe the following precautions can avoid unnecessary injury.

- On tropical beaches in summer, swim in a stinger enclosure or in the vicinity of surf lifesaver patrols. When enclosures or supervision are not available, always wear a stinger suit.
- Never dive or snorkel without a wet suit or stinger suit (see Figure 38-2), especially in tropical waters.
- Do not run or duck-dive into the water in the tropics.
- Wear gloves when fishing.
- Never approach an unidentified marine animal.
- Never pull a live stingray or sea snake into a boat.
- Never handle even dead spiny fish, as they can still sting.
- Never handle blue-ringed octopuses, cone shells, or sea snakes.
- Never reach into hidden crevices underwater or handle marine life, even if you are wearing protective gloves.

Chapter 39
Envenomation: Insects, Spiders, and Snakes

Struan Sutherland

Although athletes are no more prone to suffer an envenomation than the general population, such an event may dramatically, if temporarily, curtail their performance. A bee sting would hardly improve the tennis player's serve, especially if he or she were allergic to the creature's venom. If a tiny insect enters a hurdler's or pole-vaulter's eye at a critical moment, the outcome might be replayed many times on television. Spider and snake bites add to the usual dangers faced by orienteers and mountain climbers, nor should the possibility of infectious diseases spread by mosquitoes and ticks be forgotten. For every human on earth there are a few thousand mosquitoes and midges, plus many spiders, wasps, bees, and a snake or two. Illnesses caused by these creatures are unpredictable, and this brief review highlights ways to lessen such accidents.

INSECTS

Insects can affect athletic performance in several ways. Tiny insects can become extremely irritating foreign bodies in the eye. Important stinging insects are the common honeybee, wasps of various types, hornets, and ants. The harm they may cause humans is either due to direct effects of venom or as a result of development of an allergy to venom components. Normal reactions to a sting consist of local pain and swelling with resolution over several hours. If the sting occurs at the back of throat, there is a risk that breathing may be obstructed; therefore, it is dangerous to drink directly from cans of soft drinks outdoors because an unobserved bee or wasp may have entered the container.

Treatment

Ocular Obstructions   Recommended first aid is to bathe the eye and instill local anesthetic to aid removal of the creature. If symptoms persist for more than 1 hour refer to an ophthalmologist.

Stings   Allergy to insects' venoms is a major problem. Fortunately, the investigation and treatment of most of these allergies are now on sound scientific footing. Bee venom allergy is particularly well understood, and the following generalizations can be made:

- One in ten persons stung by a bee may have an abnormal local reaction with marked swelling and itchiness persisting over several days.
- Others may have a systemic reaction ranging from a mild generalized rash to full blown anaphylaxis with urticaria, bronchospasm, and hypotension. Perhaps 1 in 120 persons suffers a life-threatening reaction to bee sting.

Generally persons that suffer any type of allergic reaction have had prior stings, but this is not always the case. Furthermore, the degree of reaction is usually more severe with subsequent stings.

Local reactions may be relieved by ice-water packs and, to a variable extent, by antihistamine or cortisone creams. Bee stings should be scraped off.

In anaphylaxis, the drug of choice is adrenaline (dosage: 0.3 mg intramuscularly, less for a child). It should be given by any route as a matter of urgency (1). Corticosteroids and antihistamines are drugs of secondary choice (recommended doses are hydrocortisone, 2 to 6 mg/kg IV, and promethazine, 0.5 to 1.0 mg/kg). Maintenance of airway, oxygen therapy, and infusion of colloid solutions to counter hypotension may all be required.

All patients who suffer significant allergic reactions to insect venoms should be referred to an allergist for investigation and possible therapy. Pure venom is now used for skin testing and laboratory investigations as well as immunotherapy. The response to therapy with bee venom may be successful in over 95% of cases. The patient's allergic state may sometimes alter with the passage of time, so yearly reviews of skin tests and serology should be considered.

Prevention

Care should be taken to reduce the population of stinging insects near sports grounds. Clover should be sprayed to discourage bees. Allergic persons should avoid wearing perfumes or bright clothing (which attracts insects) when outdoors. People who have had a life-threatening allergic reaction to an insect sting should always carry a form of injectable adrenaline. Preloaded syringes suitable for self-injection are commercially available.

SPIDERS

There are many species of spiders in the world and almost all are venomous. Fortunately, only a few are capable of causing human fatalities. Apart from the Sydney funnel-web spider (native to eastern Australia), which has killed children in less than 2 hours, illnesses caused by spiders develop relatively slowly (2). The most important group of spiders belongs to the genus *Latrodectus*, which includes the black widow spider of America and the Australian redback spider.

The development of necrotizing arachnidism is a poorly understood problem. Tissue damage of the type seen following bites by the brown recluse (fiddleback) spider has been reported in countries where these species are not found. Thus, although accurate figures are not available, it is possible many accidents and accidental injuries are a result of overreaction to bites or near bites from relatively harmless spiders.

Treatment

No specific first aid is required for most spider bites. Certainly the bite site should not be incised or interfered with, nor should arterial tourniquets be applied. If the bite is particularly painful, ice-water packs may give some relief.

Antivenins are available for the most dangerous spiders. In the case of the Sydney funnel-web spider, the immediate application of pressure and immobilization (Fig 39-1) has proven life-saving, particularly in young children. If significant system envenomation develops, the appropriate antivenin should be given in adequate quantity—preferably in a hospital, but any delay should be avoided. Should necrotizing arachnidism develop, hyperbaric oxygen therapy may be beneficial.

Prevention

As most bites occur when a passive spider is brought into direct contact with the human skin, close inspection of bedding or clothing that has been unused for a while is advisable. Two sport-related redback spider bite cases from Australia are good examples. In once instance, a cyclist was bitten on the ear by a redback spider that had taken up residence over the previous few weeks in her bicycle helmet. In the second instance, a scuba diver was bitten on the thigh while putting on a wet suit that had hung all winter in his garage. Both of these patients required antivenin. In contrast, an Australian rock climber who had the ghastly experience of putting his hand atop a large funnel-web spider escaped envenomation—no doubt because the spider was taken by complete surprise!

SCORPIONS

Scorpions usually present a nocturnal danger, and, in some parts of the world such as Mexico or the Middle East, may prove rapidly lethal. Some stings are extremely painful, barely relieved by opiates. Severe envenomations should receive antivenin. To avoid scorpion stings, a flashlight should always be used at night in areas where scorpions are found. Scorpion eradication schemes should be considered in infested areas.

TICKS

Humans are accidental hosts to the tick, which needs to feed on warm-blooded animals to survive.

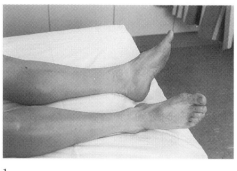

1

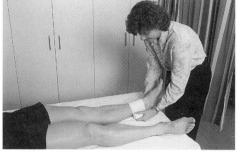

2

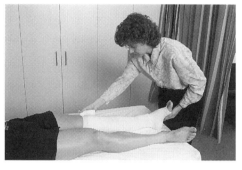

3

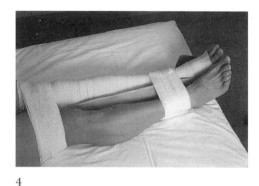

4

1. Snake bite just above ankle

2. Apply a pressure bandage over the bite area
   use a crepe roller bandage over the bite area to apply firm pressure
   tie or tape bandage in place

3. Apply a second bandage upward on the extremity
   bandage the leg upward from the toes to above the knee
   bandage the leg as high as you can
   secure the end of the bandage

4. Apply an improvised splint which extends well above the injured area
   secure this in place with 2 or more ties over padding where there are joints

5. Check the victim's toes to ensure circulation has not been cut off
   look for discoloration of the skin on the foot and toes
   ask the victim if the foot feels cold or numb

5

If the circulation is not restricted
keep the victim at rest and wait for the ambulance

If the victim's circulation is restricted
loosen the bandage slightly, but maintain pressure over the bite site

Monitor the victim until the ambulance arrives

Figure 39-1. The pressure/immobilization method of first aid.

Usually the tiny tick engorges for several days and then falls off. There are many species of ticks, some of which can cause an asymmetrical paralysis. Some carry diseases such as tick typhus and Lyme disease.

Attached ticks should be removed as soon as possible, preferably by mechanical means such as levering it out with curved scissors. When a tick is found, a thorough search for other ticks should be undertaken.

If it is essential to enter tick-infested country, skin exposure should be minimized and insect repellents used to discourage the hungry tick.

LEECHES

Leeches are blood-sucking creatures found in and near damp areas. They can cause two medical problems: allergic reactions to their saliva, and ragged infection-prone wounds when they are improperly removed. The allergy is managed by strict avoidance of further contact.

Leeches are best removed by the application of either a lighted cigarette or salt to the creature. As with ticks, the best protection against leeches is effective clothing: tightly laced boots and leggings or gaiters are essential.

SNAKES

Most snakes are harmless, but the bad publicity accorded the highly venomous species has led to widespread fear of them all. Despite their popular image, most snakes, even the most venomous, are generally shy and retiring creatures that will slither away when they sense the approach of larger animals. Most bites occur when the snake is accidentally trodden upon or deliberately attacked. Under such circumstances, a snake can move with surprising speed and will quite naturally attempt to bite the aggressor.

Snake Bite Prevention

Snakes should be left alone. If one must walk in "snake country," stout shoes and adequate clothing should be worn—sandals or thongs give no protection at all. To avoid disturbing hiding snakes, one should never put hands in hollow logs, burrows, or thick grass without thorough prior inspection. When stepping over logs, one should check the ground on the other side.

Many snakes are active on hot summer nights, so one should always use a flashlight around camps or farmhouses at night. Because rodents are snakes' food source, barns and sheds should be kept free of mice and rats. Around playgrounds, sports arenas, and other gathering areas, the grass should be kept well cut. Allowing children to collect snakes may be dangerous; if a young child claims to have had contact with a snake, it is important to believe the story and investigate.

First Aid for Snake Bite

The first aid and management of a snake bite stress a rational approach: just because there are fang marks or a series of fang marks on the victim does not mean sufficient venom has been injected to cause a serious illness. Indeed, in Australia only 1 in 10 snake bite victims requires antivenin therapy.

Bearing in mind that severe poisoning is uncommon, it is important to reassure the patient and not do any harm. Incision of the bitten area is at best a dubious exercise. Likewise, an arterial tourniquet is only a short term, very painful solution, and it is liable to cause vascular complications. There is no point in washing the bite site; indeed, in some countries this area may be needed later to be swabbed for use in venom detection kits.

Most authorities agree that absolute immobilization of the envenomed limb is highly desirable. The Australian experience has indicated that the pressure/immobilization type of first aid has proven highly beneficial to the snake bite victim (see Fig 39-1). This type of first aid may be used for several hours, if necessary.

- Apply a firm, broad bandage around the limb, moving from below upwards, including the bitten area. The bandage is bound as tight as for a sprained ankle. Gauze bandages are ideal, but any flexible material can be used such as clothing or old towels torn into strips. Pantyhose has proven satisfactory on a number of occasions.

316 III Special Medical Problems in the Athlete

- The limb must be kept as still as possible by using a splint. The splint could be a piece of timber, a spade, or any rigid object.
- Transport should be brought to the patient whenever possible, and the bandages and splint must be left on until medical care is reached.

Experimental and clinical experience has demonstrated that this procedure keeps the venom components trapped at the bite site and allows the patient to reach the hospital protected from the systemic effects of the venom.

Antivenin Administration

Snake venoms contain a complex mixture of toxic proteins, of which the effects can vary from one snake to another. Some venoms cause severe local tissue damage and lesser systemic effects, whereas others are rich in neurotoxins or blood-destroying proteins. Antivenins specifically neutralize these toxins.

If an antivenin is indicated, the sooner it is given, the better. Symptoms and signs of significant envenomation may include headache, vomiting, difficulty in breathing, collapse, or hemorrhaging. When the amount of venom injected by the snake is unknown, it is preferable to use an excess of antivenin.

A patient clearly suffering from significant effects of snake venom should receive adequate antivenin as soon as possible. Reactions to antivenin cannot be predicted by history, or skin or conjunctival testing. The latter tests also delay vital therapy.

The Australian experience is that most reactions to antivenins occur in patients with no prior exposure to equine protein. This has led to the use of premedication by subcutaneous adrenaline dose in most instances. Adrenaline results in an apparent abolition of severe life-threatening reactions to antivenin therapy 3. The incidence of delayed serum sickness and its severity has been markedly reduced by the use of prednisone therapy (50 mg per day for 5 days) commencing after antivenin infusion.

REFERENCES

1 Fisher M. Treating anaphylaxis with sympathomimetic drugs. Br Med J 1992;305:1107–1108.
2 Sutherland SK. Venomous creatures of Australia. Melbourne: Oxford UP, 1994.
3 Sutherland SK. Antivenom use in Australia: premedication, adverse reactions and the use of venom detection kits. Med J Aust 1992;157:734–739.

Chapter 40
Exercise and Pregnancy

M. Patrice Eiff

Exercise and physical fitness are a way of life for an increasing number of women. Most women who exercise regularly plan to continue exercise during pregnancy (1). Once a woman becomes pregnant, many questions arise regarding the benefits, risks, and safety parameters for exercise and competition. The primary care provider needs to be prepared to answer these questions for women who plan to exercise during pregnancy. The pregnant competitive athlete will need guidance on how to minimize disruption in her training regimen. Knowledge of the physiologic responses to exercise in pregnancy and the effect of exercise on pregnancy outcomes is essential in prescribing exercise for pregnant women.

PHYSIOLOGIC RESPONSES TO EXERCISE IN PREGNANCY

Cardiovascular

Pregnancy is characterized by significant changes in the cardiovascular system. Pregnancy causes an increase in blood volume, heart rate, and stroke volume resulting in an increase in cardiac output. The cardiac output rises in early pregnancy, peaks at midpregnancy, and drops significantly in the third trimester (2). For some women there may be an enhanced exercise tolerance during the first half of pregnancy due to the increased cardiovascular reserve. The increase in cardiac output is partially balanced by a decrease in blood pressure due to decreased systemic vascular resistance and venous dilation.

During sustained exercise, vasoconstriction results in a decrease in blood flow through the splanchnic bed while vasodilation increases flow to muscle and skin. The magnitude of decrease in blood flow in the splanchnic circulation is directly related to the intensity and duration of exercise and the level of fitness. A poorly conditioned woman exercising in hot humid weather will have even more flow diverted from the splanchnic vessels to the skin and extremities.

Uterine blood vessels are part of the splanchnic circulation, and research shows that uterine blood flow falls during exercise in pregnancy (3). Concern has been raised that the reduction in flow associated with vigorous activities such as running and cross-country skiing may impair oxygen or nutrient delivery to the fetus or stimulate premature uterine contractions.

Respiratory

As the uterus enlarges during pregnancy, the diaphragm elevates. The chest diameter increases as a compensatory mechanism. The result is a significant decrease in expiratory reserve volume and a decrease in the functional residual capacity. Vital capacity remains normal despite these changes. In the pregnant state, tidal volume increases by 40% and there is a modest increase in oxygen consumption. The increase in tidal volume results in both hyperventilation and a mild maternal alkalosis, which facilitates placental gas exchange and prevents fetal acidosis (4).

Although there is a small increase in $\dot{V}o_2max$ achieved in pregnancy at lower exercise levels than in the nonpregnant state, this can be explained on the basis of progressive weight gain (4). When $\dot{V}o_2max$ is measured as liters per minute per kilogram, the values are similar for pregnant and nonpregnant women performing similar physical tasks. Practically speaking, it would be very difficult to determine a pure effect of pregnancy on $\dot{V}o_2$max because most women, including elite athletes, decrease the frequency and intensity of exercise as pregnancy progresses.

Thermal

Sustained exercise at typical recreational training intensities often raises rectal temperature above the teratogenic threshold (39.2 °C based on animal studies). Thus, there is obvious concern that exercise-induced hyperthermia in the first trimester will result in congenital abnormalities, particularly central nervous system defects. Human data implicating hyperthermia as a teratogen are for the most part based on retrospective case reports (5). The only prospective data, a study of 165 women exposed to first trimester hyperthermia, failed to implicate hyperthermia as a teratogen (6).

Metabolic

Pregnancy is a relative diabetogenic state during which many hormones induce maternal glucose production and reduce peripheral utilization to provide a steady supply of glucose to the fetus. The mobilization and use of carbohydrate and fat increase markedly during moderate exercise and remain increased for a period of time after exercise (7). This is important for the pregnant athlete because glucose is a major fetal fuel that is dependent on maternal levels, and glucose use by exercising muscle may limit fetal glucose availability.

Musculoskeletal

During weightbearing exercise, vertical impact forces usually exceed twice an individual's body weight. Sudden movements often generate significant torque. Increased estrogen and relaxin levels in pregnancy cause ligament and joint relaxation. Other biomechanical changes include weight gain, an accentuated lumbar lordosis, and an anteriorly displaced center of gravity, all of which may alter balance. Despite a suspected increased susceptibility to injury due to these changes, injury rates during exercise are similar in pregnant women compared to nonpregnant women.

EFFECT OF EXERCISE ON PREGNANCY OUTCOMES

Early Pregnancy

Concern has been raised that strenuous exercise early in pregnancy will lead to an increased incidence of spontaneous abortion, but studies have failed to show such an association (1,8). An ongoing prospective study of well-conditioned athletes who exercise at levels above that recommended by current guidelines shows no difference in the incidence of miscarriage, infertility, congenital anomalies, or placental abnormalities compared to carefully matched controls (9).

Labor and Delivery

Exercise causes a release of catecholamines which in turn could stimulate myometrial activity. Because of this, the possibility that exercise might induce premature labor exists. Of particular concern are the effects of exercise on women who are at risk of preterm labor. Studies have not confirmed any increased incidence of preterm labor or rupture of membranes in women who exercise regularly, even in the latter half of pregnancy (8–11). One study found that gestational age at the time of delivery was unaffected by the total number of miles run in women who ran an average of 470 miles during their pregnancy (8). Data from an ongoing prospective study have shown that women who continue to exercise throughout their pregnancy more often deliver before or on their "due date" (72% versus 50% for the controls) (12).

It has been suggested that women who exercise during their pregnancies have shorter labors, especially during the second stage. However, the majority of studies report that exercise has no effect on the length of labor (11,13,14).

Fetal Well-Being and Growth

Changes in fetal heart rate (FHR) during maternal exercise have been used as an indicator of fetal well-being. In general, FHR increases 10 to 30 beats per minute during maternal exercise, and this increase appears to be independent of exercise intensity and gestational age. The return to baseline heart rate levels, however, is related to exercise intensity. Fetal heart rate returns to pre-exercise levels within 15 minutes after mild to moderate exercise. Increases in FHR in response to strenuous exercise may persist for more than 30 minutes.

Of greater concern is fetal bradycardia, which may indicate fetal hypoxia during exercise. Several review articles have summarized the numerous reports of transient fetal bradycardia during and after exercise (12,13,15–18). Despite the fact that episodes of bradycardia occur with regular frequency, no adverse fetal outcome has ever been linked to exercise-induced bradycardia in women with normal pregnancies. Further prospective studies of various exercise intensities are needed to answer questions about the effects of prolonged bradycardia and the long-term effects of repeated transient bradycardia on the fetus.

A number of studies have examined the effect of various exercise regimens on birth weight (1,12–15,19). No changes, increases, or decreases of birth weight have been found in infants born to exercising mothers. The one prospective study that demonstrated a lower birth weight found that this reduction resulted from a slightly shorter gestational length and reduced body fat (12). The incidence of intrauterine growth retardation is not increased in women who exercise throughout their pregnancy. Despite the lack of consistent findings in the research to date, it is prudent to monitor fetal growth closely in pregnant women who exercise. Strenuous physical activity combined with an inadequate diet, a combination not uncommon in some female athletes, may result in low birth weight and other adverse effects on fetal development.

Maternal Well-Being

The lack of controlled prospective longitudinal studies of the maternal benefits of exercise leaves only speculation regarding the positive effects for exercising pregnant women. It is postulated that exercise results in less physical discomfort during pregnancy, faster and easier labors, less gestational diabetes, quicker recovery postpartum, and improved self-esteem (14,16,17,20). Eliminating selection bias by using well-matched controls is essential in future studies. It is possible that women who exercise during their pregnancies may represent a select group who are more prone to positive outcomes for reasons other than the fact that they exercise regularly.

Summary

In 1990, a statistical summary of all the available research to date concerning the effect of exercise on pregnancy outcome was performed (13). The authors cautiously concluded that in the studies reviewed there is little evidence that the quantity of exercise performed is associated with adverse maternal or fetal effects. The overall results of this meta-analysis indicate that a pregnant woman can exercise up to three times per week for approximately 45 minutes at a heart rate of about 140 beats per minute without apparent harm to herself or her fetus.

Because of the differing study designs, protocols, and exercise regimens, it may be difficult to draw conclusions from such a summary analysis, but subsequent research seems to confirm the meta-analysis findings (11,12,21). All authors conclude that well-designed prospective studies with adequate sample sizes are needed before we can make firm guidelines regarding safe limits to exercise in pregnancy. Despite this lack of outcome-based research, primary care providers can still individualize exercise for sedentary women and elite athletes by using available information coupled with a common sense approach to safety, goal-setting, and training.

EXERCISE PRESCRIPTION GUIDELINES

Contraindications to Exercise

Common sense dictates that the presence of certain medical and obstetrical conditions would preclude an exercise program during pregnancy. Sanctioned guidelines in the past were much more restrictive and were not necessarily based on a critical analysis of available data concerning the effect of exercise on pregnancy. The 1994 American College of Obstetricians and Gynecologists (ACOG) Guidelines for Exercise During Pregnancy are less conservative and emphasize an individual and flexible approach to exercise in pregnancy (22). The contraindications to exercise are listed in Table 40-1.

Table 40-1   Contraindications to Exercise
in Pregnancy

Pregnancy-induced hypertension
Preterm rupture of membranes
Preterm labor during the prior or current
pregnancy or both
Incompetent cervix/cerclage
Persistent second or third trimester bleeding
Intrauterine growth retardation
Current uterine bleeding
Hemodynamically significant heart disease
Uncontrolled hypertension
Uncontrolled diabetes
Uncontrolled renal disease

Initiation of Exercise During Pregnancy

Medical authorities in the past have stated that
pregnancy is an inappropriate time to begin a new
aerobic exercise program (23). However, available
scientific data suggest that a previously sedentary
woman can participate safely in a progressive, individualized prescribed aerobic exercise regimen
during her pregnancy (15,16,24). The type of exercise selected should be consistent with the woman's fitness level, and she should be counseled to
stop exercising if she experiences any signs of overexertion, hyperthermia, dehydration, or fetal distress. An active cool-down following exercise is especially important for a pregnant woman because
the venous pooling that may occur with abrupt cessation of activity is accentuated by the growing
uterus.

As the pregnancy progresses, some women experience light headedness while exercising in the
supine position due to occluded venous return
from the gravid uterus. The ACOG Guidelines
state that women should avoid any exercise in the
supine position after the first trimester (22). This
restriction may not be realistic for certain elite athletes, but these women need to be educated about
the possibility of a hypotensive response and counseled to avoid those positions that produce symptoms.

Prescribing Exercise During Pregnancy

Widespread disagreement exists regarding the optimal intensity, duration, and frequency of exercise

for pregnant women (16). As there is no unanim-
ity concerning the best exercise prescription for
pregnant women, a flexible, individual approach
coupled with attention to guiding principles is suggested. The ACOG Recommendations for Exercise in Pregnancy and Postpartum emphasize this
approach (Table 40-2). The primary care provider
should keep in mind the following when prescribing exercise for a pregnant patient:

1 Exercise should be timed relative to food intake
and environmental conditions such that reactive hypoglycemia and heat stress are minimized.

Table 40-2   American College of Obstetricians
and Gynecologists Guidelines for Exercise
During Pregnancy

For women who do not have any additional risk factors for adverse maternal or perinatal outcome, the
following recommendations may be made:
1 Women can continue to exercise and derive health
benefits even from mild to moderate exercise routines. Regular exercise (at least three times per
week) is preferable to intermittent activity.
2 Avoid exercise in supine position after first trimester. Prolonged periods of motionless standing
should also be avoided.
3 Modify the intensity of exercise according to symptoms. Stop exercising when fatigued and do not exercise to exhaustion. Weight-bearing exercises may
under some circumstances be continued at intensities similar to those prior to pregnancy.
4 Avoid exercise in which loss of balance could be
detrimental to maternal or fetal well-being, especially in third trimester. Exercise with the potential
for even mild abdominal trauma should be
avoided.
5 Women who exercise in the first trimester should
augment heat dissipation by ensuring adequate hydration, appropriate clothing, and optimal environmental surroundings during exercise.
6 Prepregnancy exercise routines should be resumed gradually in the postpartum period.

SOURCE: American College of Obstetricians and Gynecologists. Exercise during pregnancy and the postpartum
period (Technical Bulletin 189). Washington, DC, ©
ACOG, February 1994.

2 Serious competition with all-out effort is best avoided until more research is completed.

3 Look for signs of overtraining including fatigue, poor weight gain or weight loss, or increased injuries.

4 Learning a new sport during pregnancy is not recommended.

5 Make sure usual pregnancy milestones, especially weight gain and fundal height growth, are achieved in the same manner as in the sedentary pregnant woman.

6 Vigorous exercise should be undertaken regularly and consistently rather than intermittently in order to prevent injury, exertion beyond safe limits, and wide fluctuations in conditioning,

Realistic Goal-Setting and Monitoring

Development of a sensible, goal-oriented training plan for a pregnant woman who wants to maintain or improve her fitness level requires education and ongoing monitoring. Women athletes should be apprised of the theoretical risks of exercise during pregnancy as well as the available outcome data. Matching the intensity of monitoring with the intensity of training will help the athlete exercise safely throughout her pregnancy. Parameters to be monitored include caloric intake (quantity and mix), hydration (morning weight, urine color), weight gain, musculoskeletal symptoms, and uterine activity during and after exercise. Overtraining should be avoided with the same attention as used in nonpregnant athletes.

Questions arise when considering what physiologic index to use to monitor exercise intensity. Some authors believe heart rate is an accurate reflection of demands on the cardiovascular system (25). Others question the reliability of heart rate as an index of exercise intensity given the significant alterations of cardiovascular dynamics in the pregnant state (18). An alternative indicator of maternal exercise intensity is the use of ratings of perceived exertion (RPE). Though its use is not as familiar to athletes as checking their heart rate during exercise, RPE may be a better monitor because it is not significantly changed during the course of gestation (26). An example of a rating scale of perceived exertion is shown in Table 40-3. Appropriate methods for monitoring exercise dur-

Table 40-3   Rating Scale of Perceived Exertion

0	Nothing at all
1	Very weak
2	Weak
3	Moderate
4	Somewhat strong
5	Strong
6	
7	Very strong
8	
9	
10	Very, very strong

SOURCE: American College of Sports Medicine. Guidelines for exercise testing and prescription. 3rd ed. Philadelphia: Lea & Febiger, 1986:23.

ing pregnancy are still under debate, and further research is necessary to resolve the controversy.

SPECIAL CONSIDERATIONS

Sport-Specific Recommendations

Jogging   There is disagreement as to whether it is safe or advisable for a woman to start jogging during pregnancy. If a running program is initiated, it should be started at low intensity and frequency with close monitoring for any adverse symptoms. Studies of women runners who continue to run while pregnant have failed to show any harmful maternal or fetal effects (8,13). The majority of women runners will progressively decrease the number of miles run per week during each trimester as the pregnancy progresses. Upper limits for mileage should be set based on the level of perceived exertion, adequate weight gain and caloric intake, and musculoskeletal comfort. Progress should be closely monitored and overtraining avoided.

Aerobics   Low-impact aerobics should be well tolerated throughout the entire pregnancy. Concern has been raised that the bouncing or jerking movements associated with higher level aerobics put too much shear-stress force on the pregnant uterus, which may cause premature contractions, membrane rupture, placental separation, or fetal injury. This is a theoretical risk and not based on scientific data. Trained instructors or athletes who wish to continue vigorous aerobics during pregnancy should be advised of warning signs of uterine or musculoskeletal injury. The introduction of new complex maneuvers that require a high degree of coordination and balance probably should be avoided in middle and late pregnancy.

Swimming   Swimming can be safely initiated or maintained during the entire pregnancy. Because swimming is nonweightbearing and places little stress on joints, it is considered a particularly attractive form of exercise for a pregnant woman. The same guidance given to joggers regarding their training mileage applies to competitive swimmers. Swimming in excessively cold or warm water should be avoided.

Cycling   Cycling is a sport that women can continue throughout their entire pregnancy. Musculoskeletal symptoms may be minimized because it is a nonweightbearing activity. A stationary bicycle is probably safer, especially during middle to late pregnancy because of the increased difficulty maintaining balance as the pregnancy progresses. Off-road cycling should be avoided in the second and third trimesters due to the risk of falls resulting in blunt abdominal trauma.

Racket Sports   Tennis, racquetball, and squash are considered fairly safe during pregnancy. The intensity of play should be gradually reduced to maintain a similar perceived level of exertion throughout pregnancy and avoid injuries due to changes in balance and coordination.

Skiing   The risks associated with downhill or nordic skiing are almost entirely related to the risk of falling. This risk is even greater later in pregnancy due to the shift in center of gravity and balance. Experienced skiers probably fall less than novices, but the force of impact may be greater due to the higher speeds achieved. Competitive downhill skiers should ski with great caution during pregnancy and consider discontinuing their sport during the second and third trimester. Switching to a flatter terrain will allow the competitive nordic skier to continue her sport longer.

Contact Sports   Collision and contact sports such as volleyball, basketball, field hockey, gymnastics, and horseback riding are not recommended during pregnancy because of the potential for abdominal trauma.

Weight Training   The effect of weight training on pregnant women has not been adequately studied. The only published study was nonrandomized and did not assess prepregnancy strength levels (14). Strength training may enable the pregnant woman to tolerate her increased body weight and altered center of gravity, and to avoid lower back pain from weak back and abdominal muscles. Despite concerns about the increased laxity of joints and ligaments during pregnancy, there are no specific reports of weight-training–associated injuries during pregnancy.

Some experts dissuade women who have never participated in a weight training program from starting one during pregnancy; others encourage it as part of a balanced exercise program (27). Until further research on injury risk and the long-term effects of weight training during pregnancy is available, a more cautious approach will maximize safety. Women who have never had weight training experience should seek instruction from an exercise specialist at a health club or YMCA. Beginning with light weights (5 to 10 lbs) lifted for 10 to 15 repetitions is suggested with a very gradual increase. Overhead lifting of heavy weights and squatting-type exercises should probably be avoided to minimize the risk of back injury. Strength maintenance during pregnancy should be the goal for competitive athletes and women with previous experience with weight training. These women should work on upper body and abdominal strength, be conservative with lower body exercises, and avoid squat lifts. For all pregnant women, breath holding should be avoided during weight training because of its potential for decreasing uterine blood flow.

Prenatal Nutrition for the Exercising Woman

The recommended dietary intake for pregnant women has been estimated at 300 calories extra per day to meet the increased basal metabolic needs above prepregnancy requirements. In the postpartum period, lactating women will require 400 to 600 calories per day to meet the increased metabolic demands. The nutritional needs of physically active pregnant women are not well defined. An exercising pregnant woman must take in enough calories to provide energy for herself, her pregnancy, and her training program. In terms of calories, this equates to approximately 2000 calories for herself plus 300 calories for her pregnancy plus calories needed to replace the energy expenditure of her exercise (e.g., 300 calories for jogging or walking 3 miles). A competitive athlete will likely need to consume in excess of 3000 calories per day during her pregnancy.

The appropriate amount of weight gain for a woman who exercises during pregnancy should be the same as that for a sedentary woman, approximately 12.5 kg. Many athletes will begin pregnancy underweight. Increased concern over body image and lack of understanding of the energy requirements of pregnancy are additional risks that lead women athletes to consume inadequate low-calorie diets during their pregnancies.

Nutritional counseling is important early in pregnancy to ensure maternal and fetal well being. The physically active pregnant woman should be encouraged to eat a diet rich in complex carbohydrates to replace muscle glycogen lost during exercise. Women have additional needs for protein, iron, calcium, and folate during pregnancy. Exercise may increase the protein and iron requirements further. The active pregnant woman's daily requirement is 75 grams of protein, 40 mg of elemental iron, 1200 mg of calcium, and 1 mg of folic acid. Pregnant women who exercise, especially in hot climates, should be encouraged to drink 2.5 to 3 liters of fluid per day.

Exercise During Lactation

After pregnancy, many women want to increase their activity to prepregnancy levels. This is especially true for competitive athletes. Questions arise regarding the suitability of exercise for lactating mothers. A randomized prospective study of exercise for lactating mothers concluded that activity sufficient to improve cardiovascular fitness did not alter the content and volume of breast milk nor the weight gain of infants (28). The exercise program in this study consisted of up to 45 minutes of aerobic exercise, at 60% to 70% of heart rate maximum, performed an average of 4.5 times per week for a total of 12 weeks. Thus, the conclusions of this study apply to recreational athletes, and the effects of the more vigorous training regimens of competitive athletes on lactation performance are unknown.

Is Pregnancy Ergogenic?

Published reports in the popular press and professional journals have suggested that pregnancy may be performance-enhancing for some women athletes (15,29,30). It is unknown whether the increased performance is the result of physiologic changes of pregnancy or from psychological effects. A prospective cohort study designed to test the training effect of pregnancy concluded that pregnancy is followed by a small but significant increase in $\dot{V}O_2$max in recreational athletes who maintain a moderate to high level of exercise performance during and after pregnancy (31). The reasons why pregnancy might produce a training effect are complex and poorly understood. Athletic performance is influenced by many factors, and these factors need to be investigated in women athletes during and after pregnancy to answer fully whether or not pregnancy is ergogenic.

REFERENCES

1 Clapp JF III, Dickstein S. Endurance exercise and pregnancy outcome. Med Sci Sports Exerc 1984;16:556–562.
2 Wallace JP, Wiswell RA. Maternal cardiovascular response to exercise during pregnancy. In: Artal RM, Wiswell RA, Drinkwater BL, eds. Exercise in pregnancy. Baltimore: Williams & Wilkins, 1991: 197.
3 Clapp JF. The effects of exercise on uterine blood flow. In: Rosenfeld CR, ed. The uterine circulation. Ithaca, NY: Perinatology, 1989:299–310.
4 Liboratore SM, Pistelli R, Patalano F, et al. Respiratory function during pregnancy. Respiration 1984;46:145–150.
5 Shiota K. Neural tube defects and maternal hyperthermia in early pregnancy: epidemiology in a human embryonic population. Am J Med Genet 1982;12:281–288.
6 Clarren SK, Smith DW, Harvey MA, et al. Hyperthermia—a prospective evaluation of a possible teratogenic agent in man. J Pediatr 1979;95:81–83.
7 Clapp JF III, Wesley M, Sleamaker RH. Thermoregulatory and metabolic responses to jogging prior to and during pregnancy. Med Sci Sports Exerc 1987;19:124–130.

8 Jarrett JC II, Spellacy WN. Jogging during pregnancy: an improved outcome? Obstet Gynecol 1983;61:705–709.

9 Clapp JF III. Exercise and fetal health. J Dev Physiol 1991;15:9–14.

10 Clapp JF III. The course of labor after endurance exercise during pregnancy. Am J Obstet Gynecol 1990;163:1799–1805.

11 Sternfeld B, Quesenberry CP Jr, Eskenazi B, Newman LA. Exercise during pregnancy and pregnancy outcome. Med Sci Sports Exerc 1995; 27;634–640.

12 Clapp JF III. A clinical approach to exercise during pregnancy. Clin Sports Med 1994;13:443–458.

13 Lokey EA, Tran ZV, Wells CL, et al. Effects of physical exercise on pregnancy outcomes: a meta-analytic review. Med Sci Sports Exerc 1991; 23:1234–1239.

14 Hall DC, Kaufmann DA. Effects of aerobic and strength conditioning on pregnancy outcomes. Am J Obstet Gynecol 1987;157:1199–203.

15 Sady SP, Carpenter MW. Aerobic exercise during pregnancy. Special considerations. Sports Med 1989;7:357–375.

16 Wolfe LA, Hall P, Webb KA, et al. Prescription of aerobic exercise during pregnancy. Sports Med 1989;8:273–301.

17 Artal R. Exercise and pregnancy. Clin Sports Med 1992;11:363–377.

18 McMurray RG, Mottola MF, Wolfe LA, et al. Recent advances in understanding maternal and fetal responses to exercise. Med Sci Sports Exerc 1993;25:1305–1321.

19 Hatch MC, Shu XO, McLean DE, et al. Maternal exercise during pregnancy, physical fitness, and fetal growth. Am J Epidemiol 1993;137:1105–1114.

20 Wallace AM, Boyer DB, Dan A, Holm K. Aerobic exercise, maternal self-esteem, and physical discomforts during pregnancy. J Nurse Midwifery 1986;31:255–262.

21 Beckmann CR, Beckmann CA. Effect of a structured antepartum exercise program on pregnancy and labor outcome in primiparas. J Reprod Med 1990;35:704–709.

22 Exercise during pregnancy and the postpartum period. ACOG Technical Bulletin Number 189—February 1994. Int J Gynaecol Obstet 1994;45:65–70.

23 American College of Obstetricians and Gynecologists. Exercise during pregnancy and the postnatal period. Washington, DC: American College of Obstetricians and Gynecologists, 1985.

24 Paisley JE, Mellion MB. Exercise during pregnancy. Am Fam Physician 1988;38:143–150.

25 Morton MJ, Paul MS, Campos GR, et al. Exercise dynamics in late gestation: effects of physical training. Am J Obstet Gynecol 1985;152:91–97.

26 Ohtake PJ, Wolfe LA, Hall P, McGrath MJ. Physical conditioning effects on exercise heart rate and perception of exertion in pregnency. Can J Sport Sci 1988;13:71P–73P.

27 Work JA. Is weight training safe during pregnancy? Physician Sports Med 1989;17:256–259.

28 Dewey KG, Lovelady CA, Nommsen-Rivers LA, et al. A randomized study of the effects of aerobic exercise by lactating women on breast-milk volume and composition. N Engl J Med 1994;330:449–453.

29 Boss S. A star runner sets fast pace in motherhood. New York Times, June 4, 1986.

30 Korcok M. Pregnant jogger: what a record! [news] JAMA 1981;246:201.

31 Clapp JF III, Capeless E. The $\dot{V}o_2$max of recreational athletes before and after pregnancy. Med Sci Sports Exerc 1991;23:1128–1133.

Chapter 41
Drugs and Athletes

Chris N. Christakos

Drug abuse is epidemic in modern society, and athletes mirror society as a whole. The deaths and disqualifications of prominent professional and Olympic athletes underscore the importance of this problem. One difference in athletes is that much of their drug use is directed toward improving performance. Anabolic steroids are the best known performance-enhancing drugs that are used. From the first reported use of anabolic steroids by both male and female Soviet athletes in the 1950s to the steroid-positive disqualification of Canadian sprinter Ben Johnson in the 1988 Olympics, anabolic steroids have been seen in sports at all levels and at all ages. Of the illegal drugs abused, cocaine has led to widely publicized deaths and to problems in a number of professional sports.

This chapter deals with three different classes of drugs abused by athletes and discusses how these drugs affect athletic performance. The first class of drugs is the ergogenic drugs, including the androgenic anabolic steroids (AAS), human growth hormone, stimulants, and the beta 2-agonist clenbuterol. The second class comprises those drugs that are commonly used and abused in society: alcohol, caffeine, tobacco, cocaine, amphetamines, and marijuana. The third class encompasses drugs that are used primarily for medicinal purposes but also offer advantages for sports performance, including beta-blockers, beta 2-agonists, and erythropoietin.

ERGOGENIC DRUGS

Ergogenic drugs are drugs that athletes take to enhance performance. Drugs of this type have been used since ancient times to improve endurance, strength, or aggressive behavior.

Androgenic Anabolic Steroids

Androgenic anabolic steroids (AAS) are testosterone-like synthetic drugs with both anabolic and androgenic effects when taken either orally or parenterally. *Anabolism* is defined as "constructive metabolism." Typical androgenic effects include enhanced development of male secondary sexual characteristics such as facial hair growth, male-pattern baldness, deepening voice, and increased muscle mass (1). Their use in sport is banned by the International Olympic Committee (IOC).

AAS were first developed in the 1930s to help restore positive nitrogen balance to starvation victims in World War II. German storm troopers reportedly had used AAS to increase aggressive behavior. In the 1950s both male and female Soviet athletes began using AAS to enhance performance (1). Since that time, many studies have been done to determine the prevalence of AAS use at all levels of competition, but many of these studies have found variable results because they have relied on athlete questionnaires for their data. The range of reports on high school students questioned on AAS use from 1986 to 1991 varied from 0% to 18% in males and 0% to 2.5% in females (2–7).

The oral forms of AAS are alkylated at the 17-alpha position and are absorbed rapidly, with slow hepatic inactivation and a higher risk of hepatotoxicity compared to the parenteral forms. The parenteral forms of AAS are 19-nortestosterone derivatives and testosterone esters, which are administered intramuscularly and absorbed slowly (Table 41-1).

AAS have known medical benefits for patients with anemia of renal disease, breast cancer, bone marrow failure, hypogonadism, and Turner's syn-

Table 41-1 Types of Androgenic Anabolic Steroids (AAS)

Oral Preparations
1 Ethylestrenol (Maxibolin)
2 Fluoxymesterone (Android-F, Halotestin)
3 Mesterolone (Proviron)
4 Methandrostenolone (Dianabol)
5 Norethandrolone (Nileyar)
6 Oxandrolone (Anavar)
7 Oxymetholone (Anadrol)
8 Stanozolol (Winstrol)

Parenteral Preparations
1 Boldenone (Finajet)
2 Hexoxymestrolun (Equipoise)
3 Methandrostenolone (Enoltest-ovis)
4 Methenolone (Primabolin)
5 Nandrolone (Durabolin, Deca-Durabolin)
6 Stanozolol (Winstrol V)
7 Stenobolone (Anatrofin)
8 Testosterone and related compounds (Delatestryl, Ardronaq-LA, Depo-Testosterone, Oretone, and others)
9 Trenbolone (Oreton)

drome, to name but a few. The known effects of AAS include increased protein synthesis, prevention of the catabolic effects of glucocorticoids, and increased aggression. Side effects of AAS are well known, and notably not all are reversible with discontinuation of the drug (Table 41-2) (8).

Athletes use AAS to improve strength, endurance, and muscle mass. There has been no evidence to date that AAS drugs increase aerobic capacity, and some controversy exists whether AAS actually produce the benefits athletes seek. Walder noted that the "consensus is that [AAS] definitely [enhances strength] in some individuals, provided the users of these drugs are experienced weightlifters, performing high-intensity workouts while on high-protein diets" (2).

Athletes augment the effectiveness of AAS by *stacking*, using more than one type of AAS at a time, often in both oral and parenteral forms. *Cycling*, using AAS in 4- to 18-week blocks and then being drug free for 8 to 12 weeks, is also promoted anecdotally as the "safest" way to use AAS. The theory behind cycling is that the athlete should receive the benefit of the AAS while minimizing the risk of unwanted side effects.

AAS drugs are used at all levels of competition, and there are also reports of nonathletes using them to improve appearance. AAS usage continues to increase despite opposition from sports governing bodies. In addition to the health concerns, there is the ethical concern that "the use of AAS by athletes is contrary to the rules and ethical principles of athletic competition" (8).

Table 41-2 Potential Side Effects of Androgenic Anabolic Steroids (AAS)

Hirsutism
Decrease in testicular size and firmness
Oligospermia/azospermia
Decrease in LH, FSH, testosterone
Gynecomastia
Prostate cancer
Deepening voice
Increase in clitoral size
Oligomenorrhea
Amenorrhea
Acne
Male-pattern baldness
Peliosis hepatitis
Hepatic tumors
Increase in liver function tests
Jaundice
Increase in LDL, triglycerides
Decrease in HDL
Increase in blood pressure
Myocardial infarction
Psychosis
Mania
Increase in aggression
Increase/decrease in libido
Depression
Euphoria
Withdrawal symptoms/dependence
Weakened tendons
HIV
CVA
Tumors
Increase in blood urea nitrogen/creatinine
Edema
Wilms' tumor
Increased urinary frequency
Urethritis
Striae
Folliculitis

Human Growth Hormone

Human growth hormone (HGH), called somatotropin, is a polypeptide neurohormone secreted by the anterior lobe of the pituitary gland. HGH increases protein anabolism, enhances tissue repair, and accelerates lipolysis. HGH works by causing a high positive nitrogen balance, which stimulates skeletal and soft tissue growth. This hormone also decreases glucose metabolism through an anti-insulin effect (inhibiting cellular uptake of glucose). HGH helps maintain linear growth from birth until the attainment of adult height. Typically the pituitary stores 5 to 10 mg of HGH, and the hormone is produced at a rate of 0.4 to 1.0 mg per day. HGH release is triggered by sleep, intense exercise, fasting (hypoglycemia), and intravenous amino acids (particularly arginine). HGH may be administered orally or parenterally (1).

In the 1950s, researchers first realized that HGH stimulated somatomedin, the active form of HGH. But it was not until 1985 that synthetic HGH became available commercially as Protropin. Shortly thereafter, in 1987, Humatrope was produced as the second synthetic HGH. These synthetic preparations were developed primarily for the treatment of growth hormone deficient conditions in children.

HGH is banned by the IOC, but the lack of a method for detecting HGH in drug testing makes it an attractive alternative to anabolic steroids. The prevalence of HGH abuse by athletes is unknown. Of 224 male and 208 female high school students in Arkansas, 5% of males and one female admitted to using HGH (2). Although HGH has been shown to increase height, body weight, and mass, its use by athletes comes from an unproven belief that HGH produces improved performance.

One deterrent from widespread abuse is the expense, as HGH use costs in the United States approximately $1000 per week. Another deterrent is the side-effect profile that has been noted in patients using HGH for medicinal purposes and in people with endogenous overproduction (acromegaly) (Table 41-3). The advent of synthetic HGH has potentially eliminated the most serious treatment side effect in past times, the transmission of Creutzfeldt-Jakob disease harbored in cadaveric pituitary glands. Synthetically derived

Table 41-3 Potential Side Effects of Human Growth Hormone (HGH)

Acromegaly
- Coarsening of bones of the face, hands, and feet
- Diabetes mellitus
- Arthritis/arthralgias
- Myopathies

Hypothyroidism (due to antibodies to HGH)
Hyperglycemia
Hyperlipidemia
Heart disease
- Congestive heart failure
- Cardiomyopathy

Impotence
Decreased life span
Creutzfeldt-Jakob disease (from cadaveric HGH)

HGH poses the risk of antibody formation in 30% to 40% of users (8). As currently no reliable tests exist to check for HGH abuse, the team physician must be aware of potential side effects such as acromegalic change and metabolic disorders to help identify the suspected user.

In addition to directly using HGH, certain athletes may choose drugs known to stimulate endogenous release of HGH, including levodopa, clonidine, vasopressin, and propranolol. It is questionable whether oral amino acids (including arginine, lysine, ornithine, and tryptophan) truly stimulate HGH production (9).

Stimulants

The use of stimulants dates to ancient times. Gladiators used them to fight when they were fatigued. Inca tribesmen used stimulants to work longer in the fields (the "divine plant of the Incas"). In more recent times, these medications were first used in the 1930s to treat congestion, narcolepsy, and obesity. Their positive effects on energy levels were soon discovered by athletes who began using them during endurance sports. Drugs with psychomotor and central nervous system effects include amphetamines, caffeine, cocaine, and nicotine.

Amphetamines are one of several classes of drugs used as stimulants. Sympathomimetic amines such as ephedrine, pseudoephedrine, phenylephrine, and phenylpropanolamine are also

Table 41-4   Potential Risks of Stimulant Abuse

Anorexia
Insomnia/sleep disturbances
Psychosis
Rebound depression
Seizure
Hypertension
Decreased arrhythmia threshold
Heat stroke
Dependence
Death
Stroke

stimulants. Their availability in over-the-counter decongestant products make them widely accessible for abuse.

Athletes feel euphoric while using amphetamines and have a heightened sense of alertness, aggressiveness, confidence, and a reduction in fatigue. Although the symptomatic benefits have been well documented, the proof that stimulants aid athletic performance remains limited. Controversy exists as to whether they decrease fatigue or merely mask it (5). Amphetamine effects may be more sport-specific than they are general: one study showed enhanced performance in simple and repetitive skills but no improvement in more complex maneuvers (1).

There have been several reports of stimulant-related deaths. As early as 1886 a cyclist died while using a stimulant (2). Since then, several other deaths among cyclists have been attributed to stimulant use. In spite of known risks, one survey of intercollegiate athletes revealed an 8% usage rate (1). The potential risks of stimulants are listed in Table 41-4, the most serious of which are stroke or death. While amphetamines are usually obtained illicitly, sympathomimetic amines are found in over-the-counter decongestants and other cold preparations. Stimulants are banned by the IOC.

Clenbuterol

Clenbuterol is a beta 2-agonist available by prescription for asthma in some European countries and Mexico. The livestock industry first used clenbuterol in animals to increase lean muscle mass while retarding adipose tissue deposition, which is called a "repartitioning effect." This effect appears to support some of the alleged benefits of clenbuterol that have been reported by athletes using it as a performance enhancer. The physiologic effects include enhanced muscle growth with decreased body fat, and for this reason, clenbuterol is banned by the IOC and other sports governing bodies. Although no data exist about the prevalence of clenbuterol abuse, it is known to have gained popularity among athletes as an ergogenic substitute for AAS.

Clenbuterol is primarily administered by inhaler in the treatment of asthma, but athletes typically use the oral form at twice the recommended dose for performance enhancement. It is completely absorbed when taken orally; with a half-life of approximately 27 hours, it generally clears the system within 5 days. Some individuals develop a tolerance to clenbuterol. The main side effects of clenbuterol are those seen with other beta 2-agonists: tachycardia, palpitations, nervousness, myalgia, muscle tremors, headaches, dizziness, nausea, and fever. Side effects unique to clenbuterol include myocardial hypertrophy, hyperthermia, and malaise. An anecdotal report links clenbuterol to the sudden deaths of two European bodybuilders (10). Athletes using clenbuterol might be identified by one of the side effects listed above. Physicians should caution athletes that the evidence of ergogenic benefits is limited, but the side effects are common.

"RECREATIONAL" DRUGS

Alcohol

In Western societies, ethanol-containing beverages are the most common drugs of abuse—in the United States an estimated 70% of adults drink alcohol, and alcoholism is a major health problem in 10% of men and 3.5% of women (1,8). Generally, athletes mimic nonathletes of the same age group when it comes to the use of recreational drugs, but tobacco and nicotine are usually the exceptions. However, in some sports drinking is a part of the culture, and peer pressure may lead to abuse.

At one time, alcohol was thought to enhance endurance by altering the perception of fatigue, but further research has shown that alcohol is actually a depressant. Alcohol worsens psychomotor skills such as reaction time, hand–eye coordination, accuracy, balance, and complex coordination. It also has diuretic properties. Alcohol does not directly inhibit physical performance, but high doses are toxic to striated muscle. Alcohol also can affect temperature regulation, increasing the risks of exercising in hot or cold climates. Alcohol is subject to certain restrictions under IOC antidoping provisions.

Cocaine

Cocaine, a naturally occurring alkaloid derivative from the leaves of the *Erythroxylon coca* plant, is classified as a central nervous system stimulant. Its primary medical use is as a topical anesthesia. Usage occurs through inhalation ("snorting"), smoking (freebasing or crack cocaine), or intravenous injection. Cocaine's stimulant activity comes from a twofold physiologic action, which causes enhanced release and blocked reuptake of norepinephrine in the nervous system. It is banned by the IOC.

Athletes use cocaine both recreationally and as an ergogenic aid. Anderson and McKeag (1) reported that 17% of U.S. intercollegiate athletes admitted to having used cocaine within the preceding year. Performance enhancement has been attributed to a sense of euphoria and an increase in peripheral reflex speed. However, the numerous deleterious effects include an increase in blood pressure, a decrease in seizure threshold, ventricular arrhythmias, local irritation to the respiratory tract (i.e., nasal septal necrosis, bronchitis, epistaxis, and several other potentially life-threatening conditions) (Table 41-5). Athletes who become acidotic face a greater risk of cocaine-induced seizures.

Caffeine

Caffeine, a central nervous system stimulant, occurs naturally as a plant alkaloid found in the aqueous extracts of *Coffea arabica*, *Thea sinensis*, and *Cola acuminata*. Because of their caffeine content, coffee, tea, soft drinks, and chocolate are widely used by athletes and others to increase work and decrease fatigue. Some research demonstrates that caffeine increases lipolysis, thus releasing free fatty acids into the blood. More rapid breakdown of fat provides calories and spares carbohydrates to

Table 41-5   Potential Adverse Effects of Cocaine Use

Life Threatening
  Ventricular arrhythmias
  Coronary vasospasm with thrombosis
  Myocardial infarction
  Aortic rupture
  Sudden death
  Cerebral vascular accident
Psychiatric Disturbances
  Dependence/rapid addiction
  Agitation
  Psychosis
  Insomnia
  Tremulousness
  Depression
  Paranoia
  Dysphoria
  Mania

potentially improve performance. Caffeine may also affect glycogen metabolism by inhibiting glycogen phosphorylase, thus potentially sparing the utilization of muscle glycogen and enhancing endurance performance. The psychological benefits of caffeine are thought to relate to increased epinephrine levels following usage.

A caffeine level greater than 12 μg/mL (about 5 times average daily consumption) is banned by the IOC, National Collegiate Athletic Association (NCAA), and other sports governing bodies (11). Caffeine is highly addictive and tapering off slowly helps athletes avoid withdrawal headaches.

Tobacco

Tobacco is a legal drug that contains the highly addictive chemical nicotine. Tobacco can be smoked in cigarettes, pipes, or cigars, as well as taken orally as chewing tobacco or dipped as snuff. There have been no proven benefits of tobacco in enhancing athletic performance. Societal usage is common, but generally athletes tend to use tobacco less often. For example, Forman et al. (4) found that 27.9% of adolescent athletes admitted to smoking cigarettes compared with 65.7% of their nonathletic counterparts.

In some sports cultural factors influence usage. Surveys of U.S. professional baseball show that 30% to 40% of major and minor league baseball players dip or chew tobacco (12). Unfortunately, many adolescent athletes emulate their professional idols. For this reason, a major effort to limit tobacco usage in U.S. baseball is underway. The NCAA has banned tobacco use during collegiate baseball tournament play. In 1992, Major League Baseball banned oral tobacco for all minor league players in its Rookie and Class A leagues. Similar bans now exists for Little League, Babe Ruth, American Legion, and U.S. Olympic baseball. While these efforts are underway in the United States, usage rates in Asia, Africa, and parts of Europe are at all-time high levels, and some areas are showing a steady increase.

The adverse effects of tobacco are many, including cancer (lung, oral cavity, bladder), heart disease, and lung disease. Because smoking, dipping, and chewing tobacco are such addictive habits, team physicians must play a role in discouraging use. Most users start in early adolescence when sports participation is also high. Evidence suggests that tobacco hinders rather than helps performance, and thus many teams prohibit use among participants.

Marijuana

Marijuana is a drug derived from the dried leaves of the marijuana plant (*Cannabis sativa*). The active ingredient in marijuana is delta-9-tetrahydrocannabinol or THC. Marijuana, a widely abused drug in society, is usually smoked or sometimes ingested. Forman et al. (4) surveyed adolescent males and found that 18.5% of the athletes admitted to using marijuana compared with 43.7% of their nonathletic counterparts. To date, no evidence suggests that marijuana enhances athletic performance. Marijuana is an illegal drug in the United States and thus is banned by the NCAA. The IOC includes provisions on marijuana use in competition in its antidoping regulations.

DRUGS USED FOR MEDICAL BENEFITS

Beta-Blockers

Beta-blockers are a class of drugs which are synthetic beta-1 selective (cardioselective) adrenoreceptor blocking agents used in the treatment of hypertension and coronary artery disease. Exam-

ples of commonly prescribed beta-blockers include atenolol, propranolol, metoprolol, and nadolol. The side effects of beta-blockers, which some competitors find beneficial, include bradycardia and suppression of tremor. Thus, athletes in sports requiring a steady hand, such as biathlon and archery target shooting, can benefit from beta-blocker use, whereas athletes who rely on quickness and speed are hindered. These drugs are banned by both the NCAA and the IOC for specific sports in which they may confer an advantage (e.g., rifle sports).

Beta 2-Agonists

Beta 2-agonists are a class of drugs used primarily as bronchodilators in individuals with reactive airway disease and as a tocolytic in women in preterm labor. Many athletes with asthma or exercise-induced asthma rely on beta 2-agonists to enable them to compete in their chosen sport. The beta 2-agonist most noted as an ergogenic drug is clenbuterol, as previously discussed in this chapter. Other examples of this class of drug include albuterol, terbutaline, pirbuterol, salmeterol, and similar compounds.

Some athletes use these drugs in hopes of increasing lung function and thus theoretically enhancing athletic performance. Reports of increased power after beta-agonist usage have not been consistently duplicated in physiologic studies. Without stonger evidence that these products enhance performance, these drugs remain permitted by the IOC in aerosol or inhalant form for the treatment of asthma, but written medical confirmation of necessity is expected.

Erythropoietin

Erythropoietin (EPO) is a naturally occurring glycoprotein produced primarily by the kidneys. Once produced, EPO acts on the bone marrow to produce red blood cells. EPO is produced in such small quantities that not enough can be obtained from human sources to be used by others. In 1985, the first synthetic EPO was made available after the gene that codes for EPO was cloned. In 1987, recombinant EPO (rEPO) was produced, and by 1989 the FDA had made it available in the United States. The main medicinal purpose of EPO is in the treatment of patients with EPO-deficient anemia (e.g., acquired immunodeficiency syndrome anemia, malignancies, chronic renal failure, and rheumatoid arthritis).

EPO is usually administered intravenously, but it may also be given subcutaneously. After administration of EPO, red blood cell production is stimulated for 2 weeks. Athletes once relied on blood doping, the process of increasing one's hematocrit by reinfusing autologous blood 1 to 3 months after withdrawing it, as a way to increase $\dot{V}O_2$max, and enhance endurance. Now some athletes are using rEPO as a substitute for blood doping because it is easy to administer and difficult to detect with the drug screenings available today.

Because rEPO increases the hematocrit, it also increases the viscosity of the blood by way of the drug-induced erythrocythemia. When the blood viscosity increases greatly (hematocrit greater than 55%) the risk of vascular accidents such as cerebrovascular occlusion, myocardial infarctions, splenic infarction, or other organ damage rises. These risks may be more than theoretical—certain unexplained deaths in athletes have been associated with higher than expected hematocrit levels (2).

CONCLUSION

Drug use by athletes, particularly for performance enhancement, dates to the earliest sports competitions. The "win at all cost" attitude instilled in many athletes at an early age is one of the reasons athletes resort to drug use. Ergogenic drugs and some of the drugs used for medical benefit do indeed provide an edge to those who use them, and this short-term benefit only serves to reinforce their abuse. Even though tragic and fatal side effects make the news headlines, athletes continue to view the success stories as much more common than the tragedies. This one-sided view, coupled with the general feeling of invincibility that pervades the adolesent psychology, undoubtedly contributes to growing use.

Peer pressure encouraging recreational use, the desire to "escape" stress with the euphoria of drugs, or addictive personality traits are all factors in drug use. The abuse of alcohol, cocaine, marijuana, tobacco, and similar drugs relates more to societal norms than to sport performance, thus athletes tend to mirror patterns seen in non-athletes. The culture that surrounds sports themselves can also encourage excessive use patterns in athletes—as seen with smokeless tobacco use in baseball.

One might hope that athletes and society in general would conclude that the risks of recreational or ergogenic drug use outweigh any potential benefits, but history suggests this has not been the case. Thus, team physicians, coaches, trainers, and others concerned need to play an ongoing role in identifying the athlete engaged in dangerous or unethical drug use. Education in younger athletes and disqualification in older athletes remain the standard methods of controlling this problem.

REFERENCES

1 Puffer JC, Green GA. Drugs and doping in athletes. In: Mellion MB, Walsh WM, Shelton GL, eds. The team physician's handbook. Philadelphia: Hanley & Belfus 1990:111–125.
2 Wadler GI. Drug use update. Med Clin North Am 1994;78:439–455.
3 Tanner SM, Miller DW, Alongi C. Anabolic steroid use by adolescents: Prevalence, motives and knowledge of risks. Clin J Sports Med 1995;5:108–115.
4 Forman ES, Dekker AH, Javors JR, Davison DT. High-risk behaviors in teenage male athletes. Clin J Sports Med 1995;5:36–42.
5 McKeag DB, Hough DO. Primary care sports medicine. Dubuque, IA: Brown & Benchmark, 1993:43–47.
6 Yesalis CE, Wright JE, Lombardo JA. Anabolic—androgenic steroids: a synthesis of existing data and recommendations for future research Clin Sports Med 1989;1:109–134.
7 Yesalis CE, Buckley WE, Anderson WA, et al. Athletes' projections of anabolic steroid use. Clin Sports Med 1990;2:155–171.
8 Epperly T. Drugs and sports. In: Lillegard WA, Rucker KS, eds. Handbook of sports medicine. Boston: Butterworth-Heinemann, 1993:249–257.
9 Fitch KD, Haynes SP. Doping. In: Bloomfield J, Fricker P, Fitch K, eds. Science and medicine in sport. 2nd ed. Melbourne: Blackwell Science, 1996:596.
10 Prather ID, Brown DE, North P, Wilson JR. Clenbuterol: a substitute for anabolic steroids? Med Sci Sports Exerc 1995;27:1118–1121.

11 Benson MT. NCAA banned-drug classes, 1994-95. In: NCAA drug-testing education programs. July 1993:8.

12 Orleans CT, Connolly GN, Workman S. Beat the smokeless habit—game plan for success. National Cancer Instititute 1992;Sept:2.

Chapter 42
International Olympic Committee Provisions Against Doping

Peter A. Fricker

This chapter briefly reviews the provisions of the International Olympic Committee (IOC) that relate to the practice of doping by athletes; and to those coaches, trainers, medical and paramedical practitioners, and officials who work with, or treat, athletes participating in, or preparing for, sports competitions of the Olympic Games; or to those competitions patronized or supported by the IOC. Most sport governing bodies or associations work within these provisions, particularly with respect to drug testing; as such, these provisions are seen as the gold standard where drugs and athletes are concerned. For example, the National Collegiate Athletic Association (NCAA) of the United States uses IOC provisions and relates these to various responsibilities of the NCAA.

The principle underlying drugs in sport is that doping is cheating, and that athletes should be allowed to compete in good health and on "a level playing field"—where honest physical and mental effort are the only two factors used in performance and competition.

PROHIBITED CLASSES OF SUBSTANCES

The IOC states specifically that the rules governing drug use (and the various methods of artificially enhancing performance) do change, and that the IOC publishes its list of prohibited substances and prohibited methods of doping. This list comes into effect as of February 1 of each year, unless otherwise agreed by the IOC executive board (1). The prohibited classes of substances under IOC rules are stimulants, narcotics, anabolic agents, diuretics, peptide and glycoprotein hormones, and their analogues (Table 42-1).

Stimulants

Stimulants include the amphetamines caffeine, cocaine, ephedrine, and pseudoephedrine, the beta 2-agonists including terbutaline and salbutamol, and others. Inadvertent doping most often results from athletes taking ephedrine or pseudoephedrine in over-the-counter medication for the relief of symptoms arising from the common cold, sinusitis, or other upper respiratory conditions. The athlete and coach must be ever-vigilant in taking care with any such medication. It can be devastating if a positive dope test is returned from a simple error in judgment or as a result of well-meaning but ill-informed advice from a coach, relative, or friend.

For caffeine, the definition of a positive result on a dope test depends on finding a concentration of caffeine in the urine of 12 micrograms per milliliter (12 μg/mL) or greater. Caffeine is found in coffee and cola drinks in particular; for example, a positive test can result from drinking six cups of American coffee.

Terbutaline and salbutamol, widely used in the treatment of asthma, are permitted for use as inhaled medication only. In the context of Olympic competition or dope testing where IOC provisions apply, such medication must be declared in writing to the relevant medical or testing authority prior to competition.

Similarly, all imidazole preparations are acceptable for topical use (e.g., oxymetazoline). For ex-

Table 42-1   Prohibited Substances

Stimulants	norphenfluramine	dihydrotestosterone	bunolol
amineptine	parahydroxyamphetamin	drostanolone	metoprolol
amfepramone	pemoline	fluoxymesterone	oxprenolol
amphetamine	phendimetrazine	formebolone	propranolol
caffeine	phentermine	mesterolone	sotalol
cathine	phenylephedrine	methandienone	**Diuretics**
cocaine	phenylpropanolamine	metenolone	acetazolamide
cropropamide	pholedrine	methandriol	bendroflurmethiazide
crotethamide	prolintane	methyltestosterone	bumetanide
ephedrine	propylhexedrine	nandrolone	canrenone
etamivan	pseudoephedrine	norethandrolone	chlortalidone
etilamphetamine	salbutamol	oxandrolone	furosemide
etilefrine	strychnine	oxymesterone	hydrochlorothiazide
fencamfamine	**Narcotics**	oxymetholone	indapamide
fenetylline	dextropropoxyphene	stanozolol	spironolactone
fenfluramine	ethylmorphine	testosterone	triamterene
heptaminol	hydrocodone	trenbolone	**Masking Agents**
mdea	morphine	**Beta Agonists**	epitestosterone
mefenorex	pentazocine	all oral agents	probenecid
mephentermine	pethidine	clenbuterol	**Peptide Hormones**
mesocarb	propoxyphene	**Beta-Blockers**	HCG
methamphetamine	**Anabolic Agents**	acebutolol	hGH
methoxyphanamine	boldenone	alprenolol	erythropoietin (rEPO)
methylephedrine	clostebol	atenolol	ACTH
methylphenidate	danazol	betaxolol	
nikethamide	dehydrochlormethyltest	bisoprolol	

This is not an exhaustive list of prohibited substances. It is provided only to give the reader a more comprehensive list of banned substances. Many drugs that do not appear on this list are considered banned under the term "related substances." SOURCE: IOC Medical Code, 1995: Section 3, Chapter 3.

ample, a vasoconstrictor (such as 1% adrenaline) may be administered together with local anesthetic agents (such as Xylocaine) for suture repair.

Topical preparations of phenylephrine can be used in the treatment of nasal and/or ophthalmologic conditions.

Narcotics

Narcotic drugs include diamorphine (heroin), dextromoramide, morphine, pethidine, methadone, pentazocine, dextropropoxyphene, and related substances. Permitted medications include codeine, dextromethorphan, dihydrocodeine, diphenoxylate, and pholcodine. The banned narcotics all produce degrees of euphoria and analgesia that can enhance performance and thus provide an unfair advantage in competition. The reader

should note that codeine has recently been removed from the banned list by the IOC.

Anabolic Agents

Anabolic agents are a class of prohibited substances that includes the anabolic androgenic steroids (AAS) and the beta 2-agonists. AAS drugs include methandienone, nandrolone, stanozolol, fluoxymesterone, metenolone, oxandrolone, clostebol, testosterone, and related substances. AAS is a subject in its own right, as much of the medical, scientific, sporting, and lay literature discusses this topic on a daily basis. Some sports are particularly prone to AAS abuse because of the capacity of these drugs to increase muscle size, strength, and power when associated with particular training and dietary practices.

The side effects of AAS are well known and include acne, hirsutism, deepening of the voice, clitoral enlargement, gonadal atrophy, decreased sperm count, lipid changes, hypertension, accelerated risk of heart disease, liver disease; an increased risk of hepatic cancer; and psychological disturbances such as rage attacks and altered perceptions of vulnerability.

Most drug testing both outside and during competition includes screening for anabolic steroids. The definition of a positive test for AAS is the presence of a testosterone (T) to epitestosterone (E) ratio of greater than six to one in the urine of a competitor, unless there is evidence that this ratio is due to a physiologic or pathologic condition such as low epitestosterone excretion, a tumor producing androgen(s), or enzyme deficiencies (1).

The beta 2-agonists include clenbuterol, salbutamol, terbutaline, salbutamol, fenoterol, and related substances. Salbutamol and terbutaline are accepted for use by inhaler only, provided written notification of their use is received by the relevant medical authority prior to competition when testing is being carried out.

Diuretics

Athletes have used diuretics in competition to lose weight and facilitate entry into contests governed by weight divisions. They hope that competing under weight will provide a competitive advantage. Diuretics have also been used to expedite clearance of anabolic agents by the kidneys. This group of banned agents includes acetazolamide, chlorthalidone, furosemide, ethacrynic acid, spironolactone, triamterene, and related substances. There is no acceptable use of diuretics in competition.

Peptide and Glycoprotein Hormones and Analogues

The prohibited drugs in the category of peptide and glycoprotein hormones and analogues include (human) chorionic gonadotrophin (HCG), corticotrophin (ACTH), (human) growth hormone (HGH, somatotrophin) and the releasing factors for these substances, together with erythropoietin (EPO).

- HCG promotes fetal growth and is an anabolic agent. It stimulates production of testosterone.
- ACTH stimulates corticoid production from the adrenal cortex; consequently, it is capable of producing an euphoric effect and enhancing performance.
- HGH is an anabolic agent that works by promoting amino acid transport and protein synthesis, thus increasing lean body weight and accelerating cellular growth, linear bone growth, and lipolysis. It can induce diabetes mellitus (because of its anti-insulin properties), and is well known for its acromegalic side effects. Recombinant techniques now produce HGH, eliminating the risk of Creutzfeldt-Jakob disease that accompanied the use of pituitary-extract HGH. Abuse of this agent is common among athletes in strength and power sports.
- EPO is a polypeptide of renal origin, but is now manufactured using recombinant techniques. It stimulates the production of red blood cells and thus is capable of enhancing aerobic performance. Side effects include hypertension, electrolyte abnormalities, seizures, thrombosis, and bone pain (2).

PROHIBITED METHODS

Blood doping and the use of any agent or method to enhance circulating red cell mass and/or volume are banned. Physical, chemical, or pharmaceutical manipulation in relation to prohibited methods describes the use of substances and maneuvers that alter, or attempt to alter, the integrity and validity of urine samples used in doping control (drug tests). Such practices include the substitution of urine for tests, the use of catheters, and the use of agents such as probenecid to block testosterone excretion by the kidney. The IOC emphasizes that the success or failure of such methods is not material with respect to penalties imposed.

CLASSES OF DRUGS SUBJECT TO OTHER RESTRICTIONS

Alcohol

Alcohol may be used as a relaxant to improve performance in contests conducted for target sports.

Testing (by breath analysis) may be requested by any international sports federation, with sanctions imposed accordingly.

Marijuana

In agreement with international sports federations and the responsible authorities, urine tests may be conducted for cannabinoids, and sanctions may be imposed. Many professional sporting bodies not aligned with the IOC conduct such tests during competition seasons.

Local Anesthetics

Injectable local anesthetics are permitted under the following conditions:

- Lignocaine (Xylocaine), bupivacaine, mepivacaine, procaine, but not cocaine, may be used (in conjunction with vasoconstrictor agents such as adrenaline).
- Only local or intra-articular injections may be used.
- Local anesthetics are permitted in competition only when medically justified. Notification in writing must be provided to the relevant medical authority.

Corticosteroids

The use of corticosteroids is banned except for topical use (aural, dermatologic, ophthalmologic, but not rectal), by inhalation (notably for the treatment of asthma), or by intra-articular or local injection. The IOC has introduced mandatory reporting for athletes requiring corticosteroids by inhalation during competitions. Written notification must be provided to the relevant medical authority prior to competition (1).

Beta-Blockers

Beta-blockers suppress physiologic tremor, reduce sweating, and slow the heart rate. They are banned for competition because they enhance performance in sports such as diving, freestyle skiing, and target shooting. They hinder performance in endurance activities because of their capacity to limit heart rate responses to exercise, and because they counter glycogenolysis, gluconeogenesis, and lipolysis (all necessary for substrate metabolism during endurance events). Examples of beta-blockers are acebutolol, alprenolol, atenolol, labetolol, metoprolol, nadolol, oxprenolol, propranolol, and sotalol. In agreement with the rules of particular international sports federations, tests are conducted during competition.

PERMITTED USES OF BANNED DRUGS

Since 1992, the IOC Medical Commission has had a subcommittee that examines applications by athletes who believe they have justifiable grounds for taking banned substances. The principles underlying approval of such use by this subcommittee are that

- significant impairment of health and performance would be experienced should the drug be withheld
- no enhancement of performance would result from taking the drug
- the athlete would not be denied the drug if he or she were not a competitive athlete

A number of countries including Australia, Finland, Norway, and the United States also have mechanisms that permit the medical use of banned drugs in exceptional circumstances (3). Enquiries should be directed to the appropriate national Olympic body.

DRUG TESTING

The IOC has a strict set of guidelines that govern drug tests both in and out of competition times. These guidelines cover the notification of the athlete selected for testing; the chaperoning of the athlete and supervision of the production of a urine sample; the sealing and delivery of the urine sample to the appropriate IOC accredited testing laboratory; the analysis of the sample; and the notification of the results. Procedures then apply with respect to penalties imposed under the auspices of the sports' governing bodies.

At the time of writing, research is being conducted on methods to enable the detection of illicit use of EPO, growth hormone, and autologous blood transfusion.

CONCLUSION

Perhaps the most important aspect of countering the abuse of drugs and the practices that provide an unfair advantage to competitors is education of our athletes. Performance-enhancing drugs and doping methods are cheating, and medical practitioners must carry this message with conviction into every arena of athletic competition.

The abuse of recreational drugs by athletes is outside the scope of this chapter, but the problem is sizeable. The appropriate texts and specialist medical practitioners can assist the treating practitioner in this context.

REFERENCES

1 Medical code and explanatory document. Lausanne: International Olympic Committee, June 1995.
2 Fitch KD, Haynes SP. Doping. In: Bloomfield J, Fricker P, Fitch K, eds. Science and medicine in sport. 2nd ed. Melbourne: Blackwell Science, 1996:596–597.
3 Fitch KD, Haynes SP. Doping. In: Bloomfield J, Fricker P, Fitch K, eds. Science and medicine in sport. 2nd ed. Melbourne: Blackwell Science, 1996:599.

Chapter 43
Implementation of a Drug Testing Program*

James Moriarity
Prentiss Jones

DRUG TESTING

The National Collegiate Athletic Association (NCAA), recognizing the increasing use and dangers of drug use in athletes, began drug testing in 1986. Initially, only championship events were subject to testing, but by 1991, testing was expanded to a year-round format for football and track athletes. The sanctions imposed by the NCAA for discovered AAS use are formidable, with a minimum of a one-year suspension of eligibility. Still, athletes are willing to risk loss of eligibility for performance enhancement as indicated by the cor.tinued presence of positive test results in NCAA statistics.

Deterrence of drug use is one reason given for testing athletes. In their 1991 analysis on the impact of drug testing in 500 college athletes, Coombs and Coombs (2) reported several beneficial outcomes of drug testing. One-fourth of the athletes reported decreased "partying." One-third described drug testing as educational, and said that it had enhanced their awareness of the dangers of drug use. One-half of the respondents credited the program as providing a socially acceptable way to refuse offered drugs. Other authors have suggested that athletes subjected to suspicionless, unannounced, random drug testing are more likely to view testing as a deterrent than are those athletes in programs where testing is done only on "reasonable suspicion" (2).

Finally, drug testing may play a role in preserving the reputations of sport at large and the institutions responsible for its conduct. Reports of drug usage by athletes are hot news for sports publications and television, and this type of negative publicity encourages athletic administrators to implement athletic drug testing (3). Only 54% of schools conducting drug testing programs screen for performance-enhancing agents, so illicit drugs appear to be the greater concern in university settings. A university regent or trustee may view cocaine use as the most serious problem, but Olympic officials are more apt to view anabolic steroid use by an athlete as a serious transgression.

The Case for Not Testing Athletes

Caught in the enthusiasm to do the right thing, many institutions embark on a testing program before fully considering the ramifications. Table 43-1 lists some of the issues that must be addressed before a testing program can begin. One of the most convincing arguments against drug testing of athletes is the assertion that athletes use illicit drugs less frequently than nonathletes. Studies partially funded by the NCAA to investigate drug usage in college athletes and nonathletes support this contention (4). Alcohol is the most commonly abused drug by athletes and nonathletes, but most programs do not test athletes for alcohol use. Table 43-2 compares athlete and nonathlete usage rates of illicit drugs in 11 NCAA schools.

Another argument against testing athletes concerns the hypocrisy of the "level playing field." Athletes using AAS may stop their usage prior to competition testing and resume once testing is over. This is especially true in programs that do not test in and out of season. This practice allows athletes to benefit from the higher level of training afforded by steroid use prior to the competitive season, entering with a strength advantage. Secondly,

*Based on the National Collegiate Athletic Association Standards.

Table 43-1   Factors in Drug Testing Athletes

Cost
Confidentiality
Logistics of collection
Sanctions
Legal defense
False positives
False negatives
Peptide hormones

the class of anabolic agents known as peptide hormones—which includes erythropoietin, growth hormone, human chorionic gonadotropin, and ACTH—are either undetectable in urine samples or not routinely tested for.

Finally, the difficulty of determining the definition of an ergogenic agent sends mixed messages to athletes who must attempt to reconcile this with the "harmless" ergogenic vitamins, potions, and questionable nutritional supplements that flood the marketplace. Should a substance be banned if it is found to be ergogenic but not harmful to the athlete? Is a naturally occurring agent illegal if it is supplied in supra-physiologic amounts? The use of psychoactive compounds in sport has not been extensively discussed, but Hoberman (5) has explored the ethical dilemma of using Prozac for the depression that sometimes ensues from overtraining.

Drug testing of athletes is expensive, and one of the often overlooked issues of creating a testing program is the outcome of positive test results: Can sanctions for a positive test be applied equally to a graduating senior and a first-semester freshman? How does an institution judge an alleged false-positive test for marijuana from secondhand smoke, or a testosterone/epitestosterone ratio of 6? Should athletes discovered to be using AAS be allowed to practice or play? Are coaches entitled to know of positive test results? Should parents be notified of positive test results? What happens to the records of the drug testing program after the student has left school. Are the records part of the permanent medical file of the athlete or are they the property of the institution? These are issues that arise from testing that must be anticipated before testing begins.

Recent Legal Decisions and Drug Testing
The legality of drug testing of athletes varies by nation, and it has been challenged in the courts of the United States. The lessons to be learned from U.S. cases are important to the success of a drug testing program. Institutions must realize that drug testing is an invasion of privacy that is subject to the scrutiny of the legal system. To justify this intrusion, institutions should possess a clearly stated drug policy that emphasizes the goals and objectives of a testing program and is consistent with the overall mission of the institution. Court decisions favoring drug testing in the public school environment will not protect those institutions from legal challenge whose testing programs are punitive in nature, unnecessarily invasive, devoid of reasonable confidentiality, and sloppily administered.

KEY ELEMENTS IN A SUCESSFUL DRUG TESTING PROGRAM

Planning is the first and most important step in the implementation of drug testing, and, as noted in

Table 43-2   Illicit Drug Use by Athletes and Nonathletes During Previous 12 Months

Drugs	Varsity Athletes		Nonathletes	
	% Male (n = 1552)	% Female (n = 730)	% Male (n = 520)	% Female (n = 700)
Alcohol	90	87	93	90
Amphetamines	3	3	7	7
Cocaine/Crack	6	4	19	14
Marijuana/Hashish	29	25	41	34

Table 43-3   Key Elements of a Successful Drug Testing Program

> Formulation of a mission statement
> Identification of drugs subject to testing
> Designation of a drug testing coordinator
> Association with approved laboratories
> Establishment of chain of custody
> Selection of athletes
> Conduct of testing
> Disposition of positive results

Table 43-3, a number of key elements require consideration.

Mission Statment

A formalized, written document that accurately details the policies and procedures of drug testing is an absolute necessity. This document should include a mission statement that outlines in a concise, descriptive, purposeful manner the intended goals of the institution's testing program, that clearly explains the rationale for testing, and that is consistent with the overall mission of the institution. If problems with previous drug usage are identified, there should be documented evidence available to support this assertion. Within reason, a mission statement should reflect the collective opinion of administration, coaching, faculty, athletes, and parents in the spirit of collaborative effort. Above all, institutions should frequently review the drug testing program to see if it serves the mission it was created for.

Personnel

Additional key factors in a successful drug testing program include the choice of a qualified coordinator and the association with a quality laboratory. Someone with a medical background who understands and can evaluate the testing methodology is critical to the role of coordinator. Most physicians need special training and access to the latest information on both the substances tested and the laboratory techniques employed (Table 43-4).

The laboratory itself should have appropriate certification and evidence of ongoing quality control programs. The testing facility should employ the highest standards of tests available for detecting a particular substance, including enzyme immunoassay, fluorescence polarization immunoassay, radioisotope immunoassay, and thin-layer chromatography. Confirmatory testing for positive screens should be possible with gas chromatography or a coupled use of gas chromatography with mass spectrometry (GC/MS) (Table 43-5).

Table 43-4   Forensic Urine Drug Screening: South Bend Medical Foundation

Drug	Positive EMIT Cutoff (Screening)	Positive GC/MS Cutoff (Confirmation)	Duration of Positive
Amphetamines	1000 ng/mL	500 ng/mL	2–4 days
Cocaine	300 ng/mL	150 ng/mL	2–4 days
Marijuana	50 ng/mL	15 ng/mL	Single use, 1–3 days Chronic use, 21–27 days
Opiates	300 ng/mL	300 ng/mL	2–4 days
PCP	25 ng/mL	25 ng/mL	7–14 days
Barbiturates	200 ng/mL	200 ng/mL	
Short Acting			24 hours
Intermediate			48–72 hours
Long Acting			7–14 days
Propoxyphene	300 ng/mL	300 ng/mL	1–3 days
Benzodiazepines	200 ng/mL	200 ng/mL	2–4 days
Ethanol	Alcohol dehydrogenase cutoff 40 mg	Gas chromatography cutoff 40 mg	0.015% to 0.020% per hour = average metabolism

Table 43-5   Screening and Confirmatory
Techniques

Screening Techniques
   Enzyme immunoassay
   Fluorescence polarization immunoassay
   Radioisotope immunoassay
   Thin-layer chromatography
Confirmatory Techniques
   Gas chromatography
   Gas chromatography/Mass spectrometry

Chain of Custody

The *chain of custody* begins with the specimen collection and requires the assurance of the laboratory to athletes that their urine specimens will remain safeguarded and free from possible contamination or alteration at all times. A proper chain of custody must reflect who had possession of the specimen at all times. Failure to document the chain of custody or irregularities in the process pose a potential legal challenge to a positive test. In choosing a laboratory to perform drug analysis, the capability to establish legally defensible chain of custody is essential.

Given the emotional sensitivity and legal volatility associated with drug testing, reports must be handled in a manner that maintains donor confidentiality and provides easily understood results. The tests should use a specimen identification number, and all information should be clearly recorded, including the tests performed, date of specimen receipt, and the cutoff levels for each substance analyzed.

Candidate Selection

The conduct of urine testing encompasses the selection of athletes to be tested, their notification, and registration to initiate chain of custody, and the observation of urination. The selection pool of athletes to be tested can be made by team, by class year, by gender, or from the entire athletic population. In general, the courts favor randomized, suspicionless selection of athletes as opposed to selection based on a screening physical examination, speculation of drug use, or misconduct. To the extent possible, all bias should be removed from the

selection process. It should be assumed that 100% of athletes selected will be tested.

Candidate Notification

Notification of athletes to be tested is a critical issue. Notification is more than just the *revelation* of the names of the athletes selected. Rather, it is the *acknowledgment* on the part of the athlete that she or he is to be tested. Once acknowledgment has taken place, collection should begin as soon as possible to maximize the "window of detection" and to prevent urine manipulation and ingestion of masking agents. Ideally, it is desirable to notify athletes of selection at a time when they may be tested with minimal delay such as during a practice session or after a team meeting.

Registration

When the registration or signing-in process at the site of drug testing begins, so does the chain of custody. The sign-in form should be in triplicate, and only the top copy should have any name identification. This is the copy kept by the drug coordinator. The bottom two copies are retained by the laboratory and contain only identification numbers and recent drug history.

The athletes enter their name and social security number, and list any medications taken over the last 7 days. Identification of all medication taken during the last 2 weeks in an important step in the registration process. Cross reactivity between permissible medications and the screening drug tests may result in a false-positive result. Likewise, an athlete may have appropriately ingested a medication that contains a banned substance. Methylphenidate (Ritalin) is an example of a banned drug with appropriate medical use that should be declared on the registration form at sign-in. Oral contraceptives have been implicated in false-positive tests for anabolic steroids, although the likelihood of a false-positive test is minimal. It is unnecessary for a nonelite high school or college athlete to declare oral contraceptives on the registration forms when the disclosure may be socially uncomfortable.

Specimen Collection

Beaker   The athlete chooses a numbered urine beaker that identically matches the number next to his or her signature. Once the urine is collected and satisfies the pH and specific gravity requirements, the beaker is sealed by the athlete with evidence tape, initialed, and dated, and given to the laboratory personnel for safekeeping.

Observation The observed collection of urine is fundamental to the integrity of a drug testing program. Athletes should not be allowed to provide urine behind closed doors as drug testing officials have noted many "creative efforts" of athletes to substitute fraudulent urine. No extraneous items, books, bags, or containers should be allowed in the collection sites. All specimens should be examined for foreign material or unusual color.

For athletes with a "shy bladder," accommodations can be made. Often removal of the athlete to a quieter location will ease the tension. In rare occasions, an athlete may be allowed to produce a urine specimen behind closed doors after first disrobing to assure no fraudulent urine is being carried on the athlete's person. Obviously, the age and sophistication of the athlete should be considered. A gentle, tolerant manner with a frightened, timid younger athlete will establish a better rapport with and respect for the drug testing process than a brusque, stentorian approach. A word of caution concerning athletes unable to produce a specimen in spite of an urge to urinate: it is not wise to force fluids on these individuals. Invariably, the resulting specimen in athletes who have forced fluids is unacceptably dilute and continues to be so for 1 to 3 hours.

TEST RESULTS

Confidentiality of test results is a debated topic between those who advocate complete public disclosure as part of the deterrent process and the public's "right to know" and those who believe in total patient privacy. College athletes of NCAA member institutions sign the Buckley Amendment consent authorizing the NCAA *limited* disclosure of positive test results. The drug testing policy should specifically state the parties with access to positive test results and the disposition of drug testing results once the athlete has left the institution.

Positive Tests

If the presence of an illegal substance is identified in the urine of an athlete and confirmed by GC/MS, the laboratory director notifies the drug testing coordinator of the positive result. Upon receipt of the identifying identification number from the lab, the drug coordinator searches the original registration forms for the matching number and name of the athlete. If the athlete has indicated recent medications taken, the drug coordinator must determine if the ingested medication is responsible for the positive test, and if the usage was legitimate. If the positive test is validated as illegal use, the athlete and the appropriate institutional authorities are notified according to the protocol of the drug testing policy.

False-Positive Tests

There are three types of false-positive tests that may lend confusion and controversy to the drug testing process.

The first type of false-positive test occurs when a screening test such as the EMIT identifies a banned substance in the urine but the GC/MS analysis fails to confirm. In this situation, another agent is cross reacting with the enzyme/antibody complex initiating a false result. An example of this type of false-positive test occurs in the presence of the nonsteroidal agent oxaprozin (Daypro), which gives a false-positive test for benzodiazepines (6).

The second type of false-positive screening test is a positive GC/MS for an agent the athlete denies knowingly ingesting. In this scenario, the athlete has unwittingly used a compound containing the illegal substance or a metabolite of the substance. As an example, some poppy seeds contain appreciable amounts of morphine and lesser amounts of codeine and may result in a true-positive test result for opiates. Likewise, some herbal teas contain metabolites of Ephedrine, and, if ingested in sufficient amount, can cause a false-positive EMIT result for amphetamines.

The third type of false-positive test concerns the case of testosterone/epitestosterone (T/E) ratios in the urine. Testosterone is the prototypic anabolic steroid. Synthetic anabolic steroids have unique, identifiable, and detectable chemical structures, and their presence in urine is always illegal. In contrast, testosterone is naturally occurring, and an expected finding in urinalysis making exogenous use difficult to determine.

The T/E ratio has been used as the sole criterion for illegal testosterone usage in athletes since 1984 (7). The basis of the test is as follows. The male testes synthesize and secrete into the bloodstream 5 to 10 mg of testosterone per day. Metabolism takes place within the liver, with approximately 1% appearing in the urine. Epitestosterone is the inactive molecular mirror image of testosterone; its secretion is only 3% that of testosterone, but its excretion into the urine is 30% (compared to the 1% for testosterone). The net result is an approximate 1:1 ratio of testosterone to epitestosterone in the urine.

The T/E ratio is not affected by urine specific gravity or volume, thus it can be obtained from a single collected urine specimen. The T/E ratio changes significantly only if exogenous testosterone or epitestosterone is administered. Commercially available testosterone is identical to endogenously produced testosterone and contains no epitestosterone. Accordingly, if an athlete were to inject testosterone, the T/E urine ratio would be elevated during the time the systemic level of testosterone was increased, providing indirect evidence for illegal exogenous use.

Although the "normal" ratio of T to E is roughly 1, there is considerable variation among individuals. In his original investigations, Donike used medical students as a control and found T/E ratios ranging from 0.12 to 4.4 (8). An arbitrary cutoff ratio of 6:1 was adopted as the upper limit of normal, and values above 6:1 were considered to indicate illegal testosterone use.

Though the 6:1 ratio is useful, it is not infallible. There are a small number of athletes who will consistently test near or slightly over the 6:1 level, thus drawing suspicion of testosterone use. In such individuals, additional investigative testing analyzing serum testosterone, urinary testosterone to luteinizing hormone (LH) ratios, and serum LH measurements fail to confirm exogenous use. This small number of individuals with elevated T/E ratios are thought to have reduced levels of epitestosterone glucuronide (EG), which is the fraction most commonly tested for in most analyzing laboratories. Alternatively, these athletes metabolize epitestosterone to a sulfate metabolite (ES) that is not measured in most assays (9–14). The result is a falsely high T/E ratio. If one were to add together the EG and ES fractions in computing the E denominator, the ratio wold more closely approximate 1:1.

Sophisticated athletes may attempt to fool the T/E testing by simultaneously administering both T and E in a mixture calculated to give a 1:1 ratio. Urinary levels of E > 150 ng/mL in athletes with highly concentrated urines with specific gravities >1.030 normalized with repeat testing following rehydration to a specific gravity of 1.020.

It should be emphasized that physiologic high T/E ratios are rare, with a predicted rate of occurrence less than 1% (15). A testing laboratory that is blinded to the identity of an athlete does not have the luxury of assessing likelihood of drug use in an athlete with an elevated T/E ratio, but a drug coordinator does. If suspicion is low that an individual is a steroid user, the drug coordinator may choose to obtain another urine T/E ratio at a later unannounced time. If the T/E ratio is still near 6:1, the athlete is likely to be one of the small percentage of individuals with altered E metabolism. If the T/E ratio on repeat testing is now 1:1 or significantly greater than 6:1, the probability of illegal use is high. Other methods of evaluating elevated T/E ratios or E levels >150 ng/mL include use of oral ketoconazole, which is known to quickly and temporarily suppress endogenous testosterone production (16).

False-Negative Tests

Urine was chosen as the most desirable body fluid for drug testing because of its ready accessibility and its physiologic ability to concentrate drug metabolites. Any process that prevents excretion of offending drugs into the renal tubule, prevents concentration of urine, or interferes with analytical testing may result in false-positive urine tests. Probenecid is an example of a drug that interferes with tubular excretion of anabolic steroids, and for that reason this popular masking agent is banned. Diuretics may interfere with tubular excretion of drugs and increase free water in the urine, resulting in a nonconcentrated, dilute specimen. Thus, diuretics are also banned agents.

A number of common substances can be used by athletes to prevent drug detection because they interfere with enzyme immunoassays (17). A popular masking agent sold to athletes for use before a drug test is Golden Seal tea. The presumed mechanism of inhibition is alteration in pH or direct inhibition of antibody/drug binding. Popular adulterants added to the urine sample itself include vinegar, bleach, Visine, Drano, soap, and salt.

The most effective method for preventing the adulteration of urine specimens is to minimize the time between notification and collection of urine specimens. Observation of urination is also critical. Specimens with nonphysiologic pH, low specific gravity, or a physical appearance suggestive of contamination should be discarded.

REFERENCES

1 Coombs RH, Coombs CJ. The impact of drug testing on the morale and well-being of mandatory participants. Int J Addict 1991;26:981–992.
2 Albrecht RR, Anderson WA, McGrew CA, et al. NCCA institutionally based drug testing: do our athletes know the rules of this game? Med Sci Sports Exerc 1992;24:242–246.
3 Fields L, Lange WR, Kreiter NA, Fudala PJ. A national survey of drug testing policies for college athletes. Med Sci Sports Exerc 1994;26:682–686.
4 Anderson WA, Albrecht RR, McKeag DB, et al. A national survey of alcohol and drug use by college athletes. Physician Sports Med 1991;19:91–104.
5 Hoberman J. Listening to steroids. Sports WQ 1995:Winter.
6 Jones P, Matuch-Hite T, Moriarity J. Interference of Oxaprazin with Benzodiazepines via enzyme immunoassay technique. J Analyt Toxicol 1995; 19:130.
7 Donike M, Barwald K, Klostermann K, et al. Nachweis von exogenem Testosteron. In: Heck H, Hollmann W, Liesen H, Rost R, eds. Sport: Leistung und Geshundeit. Koln: Deutscher Artze-Verlag, 1983:9293–9300.
8 Price CP, Newman DJ. Principles and practice of immunoassay. New York: Stockton, 1991.
9 Brooks RV, Jeremiah G, Webb WA, Wheeler M. Detection of anabolic steroid administration to athletes. J Steroid Biochem 1979;11:913–917.
10 Kicman AT, Brooks RV, Collyer SC, et al. Criteria to indicate testosterone administration. Br J Sports Med 1990;24:253–264.
11 Cowan DA, Kicman AT, Walker CJ, Wheeler MJ. Effect of administration of human chorionic gonadotrophin on criteria used to assess testosterone administration in athletes. J Endocrinol 1991;131:147–154.
12 Dehennin L. Detection of simultaneous self-administration of testosterone and epitestosterone in healthy men. Clin Chem 1994;40:106–109.
13 Dehinnin L. On the origin of physiologically high ratios of urinary testosterone to epitestosterone: consequences for reliable detection of testosterone administration by male athletes. J Endocrinol 1994;142:353–360.
14 Dehennin L, Matsumoto AM. Long-term administration of testosterone enanthate to normal men: alterations of the urinary profile of androgen metabolites potentially useful for detection of testosterone misuse in sport. J Steroid Biochem Mol Biol 1993;44:179–189.
15 Catlin DH, Hatton CK. Use and abuse of anabolic and other drugs for athletic enhancement. Adv Intern Med 1991;36:399–424.
16 Kicman AI, Oftebro H, Walker C, et al. Potential use of ketoconazole in a dynamic endocrine test to differentiate between biological outliers and testosterone use by athletes. Clin Chem 1993; 39:1798–1803.
17 Mikkelsen SL, Ash KO. Adulterants causing false negative in illicit drug testing. Clin Chem 1988; 34:2333–2336.

Chapter 44
Blood Doping and Erythropoietin

Greg Hickey

Over the past 20 years, the use of performance-enhancing drugs has been one of the most controversial areas in sports. Extensive methods toward detection of banned agents have been developed. Blood doping and the use of recombinant human erythropoietin (rEPO) have become stumbling blocks for researchers attempting to develop reliable methods of detecting ergogenic substances.

In ancient times, warriors drank the blood of slain enemies and hunters drank the blood of animal victims, as it was believed that power and strength were enhanced by this practice. In the 20th century some athletes have adopted similar methods as a means of improving their performance. Convincing evidence suggests that both blood doping and the use of rEPO can enhance endurance performance (1,2). Both treatments result in an elevated hematocrit and increased oxygen carrying capacity, and both are banned under International Olympic Committee (IOC) guidelines

Blood doping has doubtless been used on many occasions over the past 20 years in endurance sports. Its use at the 1984 Olympics was admitted by several medal winning cyclists (3), which led to its ban by the IOC in April 1985. rEPO has been implicated in a series of deaths in elite European cyclists in recent years, and was banned in 1990.

BLOOD DOPING

Blood doping (also known as blood boosting, blood packing, or induced erythrocythemia) is the process by which blood is infused to elevate the hemoglobin concentration. Blood can be transfused from a matched donor (homologous transfusion), or reinfused from the same individual after removal and a period of storage (autologous transfusion).

Autologous Infusion In autologous transfusion, the athlete has two units of blood removed, stored, then reinfused several days before competition. The removal of the blood is performed at least 4 to 8 weeks prior to competition, which allows time for the athlete's hemoglobin level to return to normal. By using the athlete's own blood, the risk of transfusion reactions or blood-borne diseases is minimized. The athlete, however, experiences some reduction in performance because of the voluntary blood loss that may persist for several weeks during training.

Homologous Infusion In homologous infusion, the athlete receives blood from a matched donor, thereby avoiding the detraining effect of venesection. However, the risk of transfusion reactions or blood-borne infection increases.

Blood Storage

Blood storage uses *high glycerol freezing*, an unconventional method of blood storage (citrate addition and refrigeration at 4 °C) that has the advantages of providing longer storage time (indefinite) and smaller loss of erythrocytes from cell destruction (only 15%). With conventional refrigeration, progressive loss of red cells occurs (up to 40%), and thus blood stored using this method loses effectiveness after 3 to 4 weeks. The high glycerol freezing method is used routinely for rare blood types. The blood is centrifuged and glycerol is added and then frozen at −80 °C in liquid nitrogen. For reinfusion, the erythrocytes are thawed then resuspended in normal saline, to be reinfused over 1 to 2 hours. This process is complex and requires the use of sophisticated equipment and skilled technicians.

Efficacy

Research into blood doping began in 1947 (4) and continues today with variable results. Positive results demonstrate that endurance exercise capacity and maximal aerobic capacity ($\dot{V}o_2$max) can both be improved after infusing at least 900 mL of blood. In clinical trials, blood doping has been shown to improve 10 km race times (5). These findings reflect that $\dot{V}o_2$max appears to be directly related to total red cell mass rather than blood volume or hemoglobin concentration (6).

Theoretically, blood doping enhances performance in three ways: increased oxygen transport, enhanced lactic acid buffering, and improved thermoregulation (7).

Increased Oxygen Transport   Improved oxygen transport is undoubtedly the main benefit of blood doping. Increasing the number of red blood cells delivers more oxygen to exercising muscle.

Enhanced Lactic Acid Buffering   The accumulation of lactic acid in exercising muscle inhibits enzyme systems and thus limits the contractile performance of the muscle. Hemoglobin has a major role in the maintenance of pH levels in blood. Increasing the amount of hemoglobin improves the body's ability to cope with higher levels of lactic acid. This permits more anaerobic exercise before the pH fall inhibits muscle activity; or, in other words, it allows a greater "oxygen debt."

Improved Thermoregulation   One of the functions of blood during exercise is heat dissipation. To accomplish this, a significant portion of the cardiac output is diverted to the skin. If a smaller proportion of the blood volume is required by exercising muscle, a larger proportion is available for cutaneous circulation and heat dissipation.

Adverse Effects

Homologous transfusions carry two primary risks: transfusion reactions and blood-borne infection (e.g., HIV/AIDS, hepatitis). However, any intravenous infusion carries risks of septicemia, embolism, phlebitis, and venous thrombosis. These risks increase if the transfusion is given in less than ideal surroundings and by inexperienced personnel.

Elevated hematocrit and increased blood viscosity theoretically expose the athlete to risks of events associated with hypercoagulability such as stroke, heart failure, hypertension, venous thrombosis, and pulmonary embolism. This risk may be significantly increased during exercise if the athlete develops dehydration. For example, a blood-doped athlete who starts an endurance event with an elevated hematocrit (e.g., 55%) with dehydration during competition may experience a rise in hematocrit to 65% or more.

Finally, in an ironic twist, it has been reported that one athlete who had used both blood doping and anabolic steroids to enhance performance tested positive for anabolic steroids, despite stopping the steroid well before competition. The steroid had been present in the blood at the time of venesection, and then was reintroduced with the stored blood prior to competition, producing the positive test at competition.

ERYTHROPOIETIN

Erythropoietin is a glycoprotein produced in response to low oxygen tension by the interstitial cells of the kidney. It prompts the production of erythrocytes in the bone marrow by stimulating the growth and development of cells committed to the erythroid pathway while having no effect on other cell lines. Using modern techniques, the erythropoietin gene has been identified and rEPO has been developed. This became commercially available for medical use in 1985; it has been used with great success for the anemia in chronic renal failure and shows potential for use in other chronic anemias. rEPO is indistinguishable from natural human erythropoietin in biological activity and immunologic reactivity.

Dosage

rEPO is generally administered as a subcutaneous or intravenous injection three times a week. A clinically significant rise in hemoglobin is usually not seen for 2 weeks. Oral iron supplementation is taken concurrently with rEPO administration.

Efficacy

Studies have shown that rEPO administration over a 6-week period increases $\dot{V}o_2$max and hemoglobin concentration to a level comparable with that seen following autologous blood transfusion (8). One study showed a significant improvement in a 20-minute race performance following a 6-week period of rEPO administration.

Compared with blood doping, the use of rEPO is less complicated for the athlete: it requires little expertise to use, no support team, and can be administered in private, providing confidentiality. rEPO also eliminates the detraining effect of the venesection in blood doping. Currently, rEPO is very expensive, but may become cheaper in the future.

Adverse Effects

The use of rEPO has been associated with flu-like symptoms, bone pain, and chills in 7.6% of users. Hypertension has been seen in about 30% of chronic renal failure patients who were treated with rEPO. Whether this side effect also occurs in rEPO users who have normal renal function is unclear. Seizures have also occurred in association with rEPO usage in chronic renal failure patients (9).

The greatest danger associated with rEPO usage in athletes appears to be the risk of hyperviscosity syndromes such as thrombosis, cardiac failure, stroke, myocardial infarction, or other catastrophic events. This appears to be the most logical explanation for the recent spate of unexplained deaths noted in elite European cyclists.

A particular concern is that athletes may self-administer rEPO without supervision or monitoring, and may dangerously elevate their hematocrit. In the context of a race situation and consequent dehydration, the hematocrit may become dangerously high, just as in blood doping, and perhaps may trigger a fatal event.

DETECTION OF BLOOD DOPING AND rEPO USE

Currently no reliable methods detect blood doping or rEPO usage. The difficulty is that rEPO is a naturally occurring substance, and the detection of a higher than normal level of hematocrit certainly does not prove any wrongdoing.

The IOC continues to fund research in this area. Berglund et al. (10) showed that hemoglobin, serum iron, and serum bilirubin are high and serum erythropoietin is low after autologous transfusion using refrigerated blood. By using this method, the study was able to detect 50% of blood-doped athletes (10), but the method is less reliable in those athletes who use frozen blood.

Casoni and co-workers (8) found that athletes treated with rEPO differed from a control group: rEPO treatment resulted in higher volumes for hematocrit, mean corpuscular volume (MCV), and hypochromic macrocytes (Macro Hypo). Wide and co-workers (11) reported research on the detection of rEPO using electrophoresis and radioimmunoassay. This research is in its early stage but shows promise as a method of rEPO detection in urine or serum.

Despite the fact that some blood testing was performed at the 1994 Winter Olympic Games at Lillehammer, at present the examination of blood samples from athletes is not allowed due to the many medicolegal issues. If it were allowed, it would increase the ability of the authorities to monitor drug use in athletes. Researchers could also better define normal values for the athlete population and potentially could develop fail-safe methods of detecting blood doping and rEPO abuse.

Recommendations of the placement of a chemical label or marker on rEPO that would enable testers to distinguish natural from manufactured EPO and allow easy detection of its use have not met with enthusiasm by the manufacturers.

SUMMARY

Blood doping and rEPO use improve endurance performance and maximal aerobic capacity by increasing the oxygen carrying capacity of the blood, improving lactic acid buffering, and enhancing thermoregulation. At present, both methods of performance enhancement are banned under IOC guidelines, but are difficult to detect. Blood doping and rEPO have specific medical risks, and contravene our ideals of fair play. The key to lessening their use lies with the researchers who are striving to develop reliable detection methods to combat such doping practices.

REFERENCES

1 Berglund B, Hemmingson P. Effect of reinfusion of autologous blood on exercise performance in cross-country skiers. Int J Sports Med 1987;8:231–233.

2 Ekblom B, Berglund B. Effect of erythropoietin administration on maximal aerobic power. Scand J Sci Sports 1991;1:88–93.

3 Rostaing B, Sullivan R. Triumphs tainted with blood. Sports Illustrated 1985;January 21.

4 Pace N, Lozner EL, Consolazio WV, et al. The increase in hypoxic tolerance of normal men accompanying the polycythemia induced by transfusion of erythrocytes. Am J Physiol 1947;148:152–63.

5 Brian AJ, Simon TL. The effects of red blood cell infusion on 10 km race time. JAMA 1987;257:2761–2765.

6 Kanstrup IL, Ekblom B. Blood volume and haemoglobin concentration as determinants of maximal aerobic power. Med Sci Sports Exerc 1984;16:256–262.

7 Jones M. Blood doping—a literature review. Br J Sports Med 1989;23:84–88.

8 Casoni I, Ricci G, Ballarin E, et al. Hematological indices of erythropoietin administration in athletes. Int J Sports Med 1993;14:307–311.

9 Erslev AJ. Erythropoietin. N Engl J Med 1991;324:1339–1344.

10 Berglund B, Hemmingsson P, Birgegard G. Detection of autologous blood transfusions in cross-country skiers. Int J Sports Med 1987;8:66–70.

11 Wide L, Bengtsson C. Molecular charge heterogeneity of human serum erythropoietin. Br J Haematology 1990:76:121–127.

Chapter 45
Nutritional Strategies for Athletic Performance

Louise M. Burke
John A. Hawley

Over the last 20 years, sports nutrition has developed into a credible science, underpinned by a sophisticated knowledge of exercise biochemistry and physiology. Sports nutrition encompasses issues related to the health of the athlete, as well as nutritional practices aimed at improving training and performance. In the competition setting, special dietary strategies before, during, and after the event have been shown to reduce the detrimental effects of fatigue, thereby enhancing performance. While these factors are important considerations for elite athletes, they apply equally to the much larger number of highly motivated recreational athletes.

It is evident from studies of dietary habits of top athletes, and from the observations of sports nutritionists, that many athletes do not achieve sound dietary practices for optimal health and sports performance. Factors contributing to this include poor nutrition, dietary extremism, and reduced access to food due to a busy lifestyle and frequent travel. This chapter addresses the major dietary issues that impact on the athlete and provides practical scientific guidelines for optimizing health and sporting performance.

GOALS OF EVERYDAY NUTRITION: THE "TRAINING DIET"

The major determinant of an athlete's nutritional needs is his or her training program, as this factor impacts significantly on both energy expenditure and lifestyle. At the elite level, training is a daily commitment, with some athletes expending up to 40% of their total daily energy expenditure in one or more sessions each day. Such a program not only affects the athlete's energy and nutrient requirements, but also affects social and lifestyle factors, including eating habits. Specific nutritional needs vary between sports and individuals, but the goals of everyday eating that are common to all athletes are summarized in Table 45-1.

Although athletes tend to focus on their immediate competition pursuits, it should be remembered that there is life after a sporting career! Therefore, athletes are included in the community nutrition goals proposed for long-term health. Population dietary guidelines recommend a reduced intake of fats and oils, increased intake of nutrient-rich carbohydrate foods, and moderation with salt and alcohol intake. These principles are identical to, or are at least compatible with, the strategies for optimal training nutrition that are discussed in this chapter. Attaining the optimal training nutrition is an incentive for the athlete to follow a healthy training diet, but we should also consider the opportunity for the athlete to provide a role model for the community. High-profile athletes in particular provide a good example of the potential benefits of a well-chosen diet.

Current eating patterns may require some modification, but athletes are encouraged to avoid both extreme dietary changes and the exclusion of all favorite foods. Although moderation and variety are key elements in preserving nutritional adequacy, the pleasures derived from food and eating should not be neglected. Dietary extremism and frustration, rather than flexibility and enjoyment, arise most often in relation to issues of body fat and weight, but they may simply reflect the rigid and perfectionist personalities of many elite athletes.

Table 45-1   The Goals of Sports Nutrition

Training

1 To enjoy food and the pleasure of social eating opportunities.
2 To maintain ideal body mass and body fat levels by balancing energy intake and exercise.
3 To meet all nutrient requirements including any additional needs arising from heavy training.
4 To enhance adaptation and recovery between training sessions by providing all the nutrients associated with these processes.
5 To incorporate healthy eating guidelines that reduce the risk of the chronic diseases of affluent Western countries.
6 To experiment with intended competition nutrition practices so that beneficial strategies can be identified and fine-tuned.

Competition

1 In weight-classed sports, to achieve the weigh-in target without sacrificing fuel stores and body fluid levels.
2 To "fuel up" or maximize body carbohydrate stores prior to the event.
3 To minimize dehydration during the event by practical fluid-intake strategies before, during, and after the event.
4 During prolonged events or other events where body carbohydrate stores become depleted, to supply additional carbohydrates during the event.
5 To achieve gastrointestinal comfort during the event.
6 To promote recovery after competition, particularly in sports played as a series of heats and finals, or as a tournament.

SOURCE: Adapted from Burke LM, Read RSD. Sports nutrition: approaching the nineties. Sports Med 1989;8:80–100.

IDEAL BODY MASS AND BODY FAT

Determining "Ideal" Body Mass and Body Fat for an Athlete

Generally, elite competitors in a given sport exhibit most of the physical characteristics that promote optimal performance in that event/discipline. Characteristics such as muscle mass, body fat level, and bone density are determined by the genetic predisposition that has helped to select athletic potential, and also by the changes achieved through the conditioning effect of high-level training and diet.

Most of the information currently used to identify body fat and body mass goals for various sports is provided by anthropometric studies of groups of elite athletes. The considerable variability in characteristics between elite athletes even in the same sport creates an inherent danger in using this information to establish rigid prescriptions for individuals. Instead, nominating a range of acceptable values for body fat and body mass within a sport, then monitoring the health and performance of the athlete within this range, is the preferable route.

Some athletes easily achieve the body composition that is suited to their sports; others may need to manipulate characteristics such as muscle mass or body fat levels through changes in diet and training. Athletes must be able to identify suitable and realistic body fat goals, take appropriate measures to achieve the desired changes in a suitable time period, and have an appropriate means of measuring the results. Changes in body mass do not distinguish between muscle mass or body fat; however, many athletes judge the suitability of their size or body shape by this simple measure. Athletes might be advised that the only valuable use of a weight scale is to determine short-term changes in hydration levels—weighing oneself before and after a workout allows an estimate of body fluid losses that must be replaced.

Much has been written about the various methods of body composition assessment in athletes (1). The criteria for choosing a technique include the validity, reliability, and sensitivity of the method within the typical range of body composition of the athlete, as well as the expense and the ease of access by the athlete. Regular monitoring of athletes should play an important role in both determining athletes goals and observing their success in achieving them.

Strategies for Losing Body Fat

Although it might sound incongruous that an athlete could be overweight, in fact many athletes seek or desire to lose weight, or more precisely, to lose body fat (2). This is particularly true in sports with specific weight divisions for competition (e.g., weight-lifting, lightweight rowing, and judo), or in sports where low body mass—in particular, low body fat levels—are considered necessary for optimum performance. The main physical advantage of a low body fat level is an increased power-to-weight ratio, which will often result in an improved performance in weightbearing sports such as distance running. However, low body fat levels are also important in sports such as diving, gymnastics, and figure skating where judging involves an athlete's appearance as well as skill. Low levels of body fat are typical in the latter sports, and may sometimes even correlate with performance within a group, but overconcern about body fat by individual athletes may often be misguided and harmful. The optimal body fat level for an athlete can be obtained from each individual history and should be associated with consistent good performances and the promotion of good health. The athlete must be able to achieve these goals while consuming adequate energy and nutrients.

Many studies report that athletes have problems in choosing safe and realistic body fat goals. Many athletes set goals of minimal body fat levels per se, or aim for the low body fat levels seen in another (elite) competitor. However, in many cases individuals will not improve their performances simply by achieving a lower level of body fat, especially when this is not their natural body physique. In fact, such athletes may suffer performance and health disadvantages as a result of the tactics used to lose body fat. Most importantly, the low body fat levels of elite athletes may not be natural or even necessary for serious recreational athletes.

The situation seems worse for female athletes than for males, reflecting the general dissatisfaction of females in the community with their body shape, as well as the biological predisposition for female athletes to have higher absolute and relative levels of body fat than male athletes (despite undertaking the same training program). Many studies report a higher prevalence of eating disorders or disordered eating behaviors and body perceptions among athletes in weight-division sports or in sports in which success is associated with low body fat levels (3).

Even where clinical eating disorders do not exist, many athletes appear to eat considerably less than their expected energy requirements in an attempt to "squeeze" into a smaller and leaner body shape. An adequate intake of energy is a prerequisite for many of the nutritional goals that we discuss in this chapter, and in many cases is the first nutritional strategy that should be recommended by the sports physician or dietitian. Many athletes report intakes of energy, carbohydrates, and nutrients that are inadequate to meet basic daily requirements, let alone the needs of training and competition. While low energy intakes may reflect underreporting errors in dietary survey methodology, there is considerable evidence that many athletes are restrained eaters (4).

There are situations when an athlete is clearly overfat because of hereditary or lifestyle factors or because they have been in a situation of sudden energy imbalance (energy intake exceeds expenditure). Common examples include athletes coming back from an injury or a break from training, or participants in sports that may involve hours of skill and practice without extensive energy expenditure (e.g., golf or archery). Loss of body fat by an athlete, where it is warranted, should be achieved by a gradual program of sustained and moderate energy deficit that results from a decrease in dietary energy intake and perhaps an increase in energy expenditure through aerobic exercise or activity (Table 45-2).

Strategies to Gain Muscle Mass

Gain of muscle mass is desired by many athletes whose performance is linked to size, strength, or power. Increases in muscle mass and strength appear during adolescence, particularly in males, but many athletes pursue additional muscle hypertrophy gains through a program of progressive muscle overload. The main nutritional require-

Table 45-2 Strategies for Eating to Lose Body Fat

1 The athlete should identify individual "ideal" body fat and body mass targets that are consistent with good health and performance and are achievable.

2 If loss of body fat is required, the athlete should plan for a realistic rate loss of about 0.5 kg per week, and set both short-term and long-term goals.

3 The athlete's current exercise and activity plans should be examined: If training is primarily skill or technique-based, or a sedentary lifestyle between training sessions is observed, the athlete may benefit from scheduling in some aerobic exercise activities. This should always be done in conjunction with the coach.

4 By keeping a food diary for a period (e.g., a week), the athlete is allowed an objective look at what they are really eating. Many athletes who feel that they "hardly eat anything" will be amazed at their hidden eating activities.

5 The aim is to reduce typical energy intake by an amount that is appropriate to produce loss of body fat (e.g., 500–1000 kcal/per day) but still ensures adequate food and nutrient intake. An athlete should not reduce his or her energy intake below 1200–1500 kcal/day unless supervised by a sports dietitian. Meals should not be skipped; rather, food should be spread over the day, particularly to allow for efficient refueling after training sessions.

6 Occasions of overeating should be targeted for special attention. Useful techniques include making meals filling by choosing high-fiber forms of foods, fighting the need to finish everything on the plate, and spreading food intake over the day so that there is no need to approach meals feeling extreme hunger.

7 The athlete should also focus on opportunities to reduce intake of fats and oils. Such strategies include choosing low-fat versions of nutritious protein foods; minimizing added fats and oils in cooking and food preparation, and enjoying high-fat snack and sweet foods as occasional treats rather than everyday foods.

8 Moderation with alcohol (and, perhaps, sugar) is advised since these may represent "empty" calories. Since alcohol intake is associated with relaxation, it is often associated with unwise eating.

9 The athlete should focus on nutrient-rich foods so that nutrient needs can be met from fewer kilocalories. A broad-range low-dose vitamin/mineral supplement should be considered if energy intake is to be restricted below 1500 kcal/day for prolonged periods.

10 The athlete should be aware of inappropriate eating behavior. This includes eating when bored or upset, or eating too quickly. Stress or boredom should be handled using alternative activities.

11 The athlete should be wary of supplements that promise weight loss. There are no special pills, potions, or products that produce safe and effective weight loss. If something sounds too good to be true, it probably is.

12 A sports dietitian can assist athletes who are having difficulties with their weight loss goals, or would like a supervised program. Expert advice is needed for those who are struggling with an eating disorder or disordered eating behavior.

SOURCE: Adapted from Burke LM. Practical issues in nutrition for athletes. J Sports Sci 1995;13:S83–S90.

ment for gain of muscle mass while undertaking a strength-training program is additional energy. Additional energy is required for the manufacture of new muscle tissue and other tissues needed to support it, as well as to provide fuel for the training program that supplied the stimulus for this muscle growth. Dietary strategies for muscle gain are summarized in Table 45-3. It should be noted that despite long-standing historical interest, there is little rigorous scientific study of the amount of energy required, the optimal ratio of macronutrients supplying this energy, and the requirements for micronutrients to enhance muscle size. However, there is some evidence that athletes may not automatically achieve a sufficiently positive energy balance to optimize muscle gains during a strength-training program.

Many strength-trained athletes believe that muscle gain is optimized by very high protein intakes (>2–3 grams per kilogram of body mass per

Table 45-3 Strategies for Eating to Increase Muscle Mass

1 Ensure that the athlete is following a well-devised weight-training program that will stimulate muscle development and growth.

2 The athlete should set goals for weight and strength gain that are practical and achievable. Continued increases of 1-2 kg/month are generally considered a good return.

3 The athlete must be organized. Athletes need to apply the same dedication to their eating program as is applied to training, in order to increase their intake of nutrient-dense foods and supply a daily energy surplus of approximately 500–1000 kcal. This additional food should supply carbohydrate to fuel the training sessions and adequate protein and micronutrients for the development and support of new tissue.

4 The athletes should increase the number of times that he or she eats rather than the size of meals. This will enable greater intake of food with less risk of "overfilling" and gastrointestinal discomfort. This will require a supply of nutritious high-carbohydrate snacks to be available between meals, particularly after training sessions.

5 The energy content of high-carbohydrate foods can be increased by adding sugar or low-fat protein. For example, jams and syrups may be added to toast or pancakes, and sandwiches may have 2 or 3 layer fillings. This adds extra kilocalories to a nutritious meal, without adding greatly to the bulkiness of the food.

6 The athlete should avoid excessive intake of fiber, and include the use of "white" cereals with less bulk (e.g., white rice, white bread). It is often impractical to consume a diet that is solely based on whole-grain and high-fiber foods.

7 High-energy fluids such as milkshakes, fruit smoothies, or commercial liquid meal supplements are useful. These drinks provide a compact and low-bulk source of energy and nutrients, and can be consumed with meals or as snacks—including before or after a training session.

8 Many athletes do not eat as much—or more importantly, as often—as they think. It is useful to examine the actual intake of athletes who fail to gain weight yet report "constant eating." Commitments such as training, sleep, medical/physiotherapy appointments, work, or school often interfere with eating opportunities. A food record will identify the hours and occasions of minimal food intake. This information should be used to reorganize the day or to find creative ways to make nutritious foods and drinks part of the activity.

SOURCE: Adapted from Burke LM. Food selection and guidance for physically active people. Asia Pacific J Clin Nutr 1995;4(suppl):39–44.

day), which is in excess of 2–3 times the protein Recommended Dietary Allowances (RDAs) for age-matched sedentary people. The role of protein in enhancing muscle mass remains one of the most controversial issues facing sports nutritionists. Since protein forms the most significant structural component of muscle, it is tempting to conclude that additional protein will stimulate muscle gain. However, if muscle is typically composed of 15% to 20% protein, then the gain of 0.5 kg of muscle per week would mean the addition of approximately 15 grams per day of protein. Protein requirements for athletes are discussed later; however, the value of very high protein intakes in optimizing muscle gains remains unsupported by the scientific literature (5).

MEETING NUTRIENT REQUIREMENTS, INCLUDING ADDITIONAL NEEDS ARISING FROM HEAVY TRAINING

The increased energy intake associated with the energy requirements of training, combined with a variety of nutritious food choices, can generally provide the athlete with macro- and micronutrient intakes well in excess of the population's RDAs. Athletes at the highest risk of inadequate nutrient intake are those with reduced energy intakes, such as restrained eaters on chronic weight loss or maintenance diets. This also applies to those who limit their food variety, such as those with eating disorders, and those following vegetarian or other restrictive diets.

Protein Requirements

The increase in protein requirements during times of muscle gain following strength training has already been discussed. However, exercise also increases daily protein requirements in order to cover the contribution of protein catabolism to the fuel requirements of exercise and the repair and recovery processes following muscle damage or adaptation (5).

The results of nitrogen balance studies generally agree that the protein requirements of heavily training athletes in both strength and endurance are on the order of 1.2 to 1.6 grams per kilogram per day, provided that both carbohydrate and energy requirements are also met (5). Dietary surveys of a variety of athletic groups demonstrate that, with the increased energy intakes that are typically associated with an increased training load and the protein intakes typical of Western diets (i.e., 12% to 15% of total energy intake), there seems little problem in reaching these targets (6). However, athletes who chronically reduce their energy intakes are at risk. Not only is total protein intake restricted by energy intake, but, indirectly, inadequate total energy and/or inadequate carbohydrate intake may increase protein requirements.

Vitamin Requirements

To date, numerous scientific studies have failed to support a beneficial effect of vitamin supplementation on athletic performance, except in the cases of athletes with a preexisting vitamin deficiency (7). Some athletes, particularly females and those undertaking restrictive diets, may benefit from dietary counseling to increase total energy intake and/or dietary variety, thus achieving the full nutrient intake potential from food sources. Nevertheless, problems remain for those athletes who continue to be chronic low-energy consumers. In such cases, a low-dose broad-range vitamin/mineral supplement may be necessary. Athletes who travel extensively may also benefit from a similar supplement as a precaution against uncertain and irregular food supplies.

Iron Requirements

Inadequate iron status may reduce endurance exercise performance because of the role of iron in oxygen transport and in aerobic energy produc-tion. Although it is apparent that some athletes are at risk of low iron status due to increased iron requirements (to cover menstrual losses, growth, and pregnancy), increased iron losses due to exercise (red blood cell trauma, sweat loss of iron, and gastrointestinal blood loss), and poor dietary intake of bioavailable iron, there is currently a lack of consensus about what constitutes optimal iron status. Key questions concern the optimal iron status for an athlete (i.e., whether a reduced but not clinically anemic hemoglobin level, or low ferritin status, reduces performance), and how to distinguish reduced iron status from exercise-mediated changes in iron metabolism (8).

Athletes at high risk for reduced iron status—such as female athletes, endurance athletes in heavy training, adolescent and pregnant athletes, and athletes following low energy or vegetarian diets—should be monitored for early detection of reduced iron status. Serum ferritin levels provide a useful source of information when piecing together the clinical picture of a tired athlete; athletes with ferritin levels below 20 ng/mL who complain of fatigue and poor performance often respond to an increase in iron intake.

Therapy may include iron supplementation, but this should be part of a clinical management decision for individual athletes, rather than a mass-supplementation program. Management plans may also include strategies to reduce excessive iron losses, and most importantly, education to improve dietary iron intake from bioavailable sources. Many athletes find it difficult to integrate several nutritional goals and may be assisted by practical guidelines for iron-rich eating such as those summarized in Table 45-4.

Calcium Requirements

Recent studies reporting low bone density and stress fractures in female athletes have focused attention to the calcium status of sports people. However, the concern should widen to include consideration of menstrual function and estrogen status of these athletes, as evidence of a link between secondary amenorrhea and reduced bone density has strengthened in recent years.

Although the causes of menstrual dysfunction appear to be multifactorial (9), dietary assessment

Table 45-4   Strategies to Meet Iron and Calcium Needs

1 The athlete should include heme iron-rich foods (red meats, shellfish, liver) regularly in his or her meals—at least 3–5 times per week. These can be added to high-carbohydrate meals (e.g., meat sauce on a pasta dish; liver pate in a sandwich).

2 The absorption of non-heme iron (found in wholegrains, cereal foods, eggs, leafy green vegetables, etc.) can be enhanced by including a vitamin C food at the same meal. For example, a glass of orange juice may be consumed with breakfast cereal.

3 Be aware that some foods (excess bran, strongly brewed tea) interfere with iron absorption from non-heme iron foods. Athletes who are at risk of iron deficiency should avoid these items, or eat them separately from meals.

4 Iron supplements should be taken only on the advice of a sports dietitian or physician. They may be useful in the supervised treatment and prevention of iron deficiency, but are not a substitute for dietary improvements.

5 The athlete should eat at least three helpings of dairy foods a day, where one helping is equal to a glass of milk or a carton of yogurt. Low-fat and reduced-fat types are available. Dairy products can be added to a high-carbohydrate meal (e.g., milk on breakfast cereal, cheese in a sandwich).

6 Extra calcium is needed for athletes who are growing, having a baby, or breastfeeding. Dairy intake should be increased to 4–5 helpings a day. Female athletes who have irregular menstrual cycles also require extra calcium and should seek expert advice from a sports physician.

7 Fish eaten with its bones (e.g., tinned salmon, sardines) is also a useful calcium source, and can also accompany a high carbohydrate meal (e.g., salmon casserole with rice).

8 Athletes who are vegetarian, or unable to eat dairy products and red meat in these amounts, should seek the advice of a sports dietitian. With assistance they may find creative ways or the use of other foods to meet iron and calcium needs (such as fortified soy products), or to use mineral supplements correctly.

SOURCE: Adapted from Burke LM. Practical issues in nutrition for athletes. J Sports Sci 1995;13:S83–S90.

and nutritional advice are important for athletes with menstrual dysfunction to optimize their intake of energy, calcium, and other nutrients, and also to correct disordered eating habits. These problems may either contribute to the underlying menstrual problems, or may reduce calcium status and bone integrity. Optimal nutrition plays an important role in the treatment or prevention of bone complications. Table 45-4 summarizes practical guidelines for meeting calcium goals within the athlete's diet.

The Need for Supplements

Reviews of the practices of athletes show that approximately half of the athletic population currently reports the use of supplements (10). These supplements include vitamins and minerals, special carbohydrate and liquid meal drinks, and products containing unusual substances such as free-form amino acids, ferulic acid, creatine, and ginseng. There is a continuous supply of products in healthfood shops, and advertisements in sports magazines claim these supplements can make the

athlete leaner, bigger, stronger, fatter, more enduring, or whatever is required to improve performance.

These products may be divided into two groups: dietary supplements that meet known nutritional or physiologic requirements of athletes, and nutritional ergogenic aids that propose a direct ergogenic effect on exercise performance (10).

- **Dietary Supplements:** Dietary supplements, including products such as sports drinks, liquid meal supplements, and iron supplements, may provide a convenient or practical means for an athlete to achieve nutritional goals, particularly during and after exercise when access to food is difficult or gastrointestinal comfort may be compromised by the consumption of solid food. The case for sports drinks will be discussed later in this chapter.
- **Ergogenic Aids:** There is evidence of beneficial effects on performance resulting from the use of nutritional ergogenic aids such as caffeine, bicarbonate, and creatine in specific individu-

als or situations. However, research supporting the benefits of most other products remains scarce (10).

Carbohydrate Requirements for Performance and Recovery in Training

A major challenge during a heavy training program is to replenish fuel stores depleted during prolonged workouts, particularly when these losses are substantial and where there may be only 8 to 24 hours between sessions. An athlete training strenuously may need to set a special schedule of carbohydrate intake to promote optimal recovery since typical Western eating patterns are unlikely to provide adequate carbohydrate. Failure to consume sufficient carbohydrate to match the demands of training may lead to chronically depleted muscle and liver glycogen stores, which may interfere with optimal training performance and adaptation.

It has been somewhat difficult to show a chronic reduction in training capacity when athletes consume moderate carbohydrate diets (5 grams per kilogram per day) compared with a high carbohydrate intake (10 grams per kilogram per day) (11). However, failure to consume sufficient carbohydrate to match the demands of training may lead to chronically depleted muscle and liver glycogen stores, which may interfere with optimal training performance and adaptation. Therefore nutrition guidelines for the athlete in general training recommend that carbohydrate intakes should be increased above the levels typical of the current Western diet (i.e., from about 45% to above 55% of total energy intake), and that this should be achieved principally by increasing the consumption of nutrient-dense carbohydrate foods (12). These recommendations are similar to the healthy nutrition guidelines aimed at the general community. In the case of the endurance athlete or athlete undertaking prolonged high-intensity training, carbohydrate-intake guidelines have been set to maximize the capacity for daily carbohydrate refueling. These recommendations are best made on the basis of the carbohydrate intake believed to be the threshold for daily glycogen storage (8 to 10 grams per kilogram per day). Such intakes typically require 50% to 70% of total energy intake.

The focus on nutritious carbohydrate-rich foods may assist the athlete to meet requirements for both protein and micronutrients simultaneously. Nevertheless, sugar and refined carbohydrate foods offer the advantages of being compact and pleasant to eat, and can provide a useful but smaller contribution to the athlete's total carbohydrate intake. Carbohydrate-containing drinks (e.g., juices, fruit smoothies, special sports supplements) may also provide a compact and practical way to help achieve the very high carbohydrate requirements of some athletes in heavy training. These attributes may be most appreciated during or immediately after exercise. There is some evidence that the rate of glycogen storage is slightly enhanced during the first 1 to 2 hours after exercise. Certainly, providing carbohydrate to the depleted muscle (1 gram per kilogram of carbohydrate in the first 1 to 2 hours) is a useful strategy in initiating rapid recovery between workouts (12). Practical guidelines for high-carbohydrate eating are presented in Table 45-5; snacks that might be useful in the postexercise situation are summarized in Table 45-6.

GOALS OF THE COMPETITION DIET

Eating for competition is a challenging area of practice for the sports dietitian or doctor. There is considerable pressure on the athlete (and the sports medicine professional) to succeed, and the outcome may be very definite, public, and carry significant financial implications. The nutritional requirements of a sports competition are unique to the specific event, and the practitioner requires a good understanding of the exercise requirements of the event, the environmental conditions, and the practical factors that may influence the development of a nutrition plan. The latter may include the time of the day of the event, access to food and fluid at a competition venue, competition rules governing intake during an event, and the individual response of the athlete to various nutrition strategies. All nutrition strategies should be practiced during training to allow the athlete to identify and fine-tune successful practices, and in some cases, learn to tolerate food and fluid intake before and during exercise.

Table 45-5   Strategies for a High-Carbohydrate Training Diet

1   The athlete should be prepared to eat differently—a Western diet is not a high-carbohydrate diet.
2   Base meals and snacks around nutritious carbohydrate foods, such that these take up at least half of the room on the plate:
   - whole-grain breads and breakfast cereals
   - rice, pasta, noodles, and other grain foods
   - fruits
   - starchy vegetables, such as potatoes, corn
   - legumes (lentils, beans, soy-based products)
   - sweetened dairy products (e.g., fruit-flavored yogurt, fruit smoothies)
3   Many foods commonly believed by athletes to be carbohydrate-rich are actually high-fat foods (e.g., cakes, fast food, chocolates, and pastries). Keep to low-fat eating strategies.
4   Sugar and sugar-rich foods are useful for the athlete, especially when added to a nutritious carbohydrate food meal or when needed during and after exercise.
5   When carbohydrate and energy needs are high, the athlete should increase the number of meals and snacks that he or she eats rather than the size of the meals. This requires organization to have snacks on hand during a busy day.
6   Lower-fiber choices of carbohydrate-rich foods may be useful when energy needs are high or when the athlete needs to eat just before exercise.
7   Carbohydrate drinks (e.g., fruit juices, soft drinks, fruit/milk smoothies) are also a compact source for special situations or high-carbohydrate diets. This category includes many of the supplements made especially for athletes, such as sports drinks or liquid meal supplements.
8   Postexercise recovery of muscle fuel stores is enhanced by eating a high-carbohydrate meal or snack within 15 to 30 minutes of lengthy training sessions. Nutritious carbohydrate-rich foods and drinks can provide protein and other nutrients that may also be useful in recovery.
9   Carbohydrates should be consumed during lengthy training and competition sessions when additional fuel is needed. Sports drinks and other sugary drinks will look after fluid and carbohydrate needs simultaneously; sports drinks are especially designed to rapidly deliver these nutrients.

SOURCE: Adapted from Burke LM. Practical issues in nutrition for athletes. J Sports Sci 1995;13:S83–S90.

Preparation for Competition

Preparing Adequate Fuel Stores   Preparation for competition should aim to maximize body carbohydrate stores of liver and muscle glycogen for the anticipated fuel needs of the event (13). This can be achieved by a high carbohydrate intake, in conjunction with a reduction in exercise volume and intensity for the 24 to 36 hours before an event. Normalized glycogen stores are thought to be sufficient for most sports events, particularly events lasting less than 60 minutes.

An exercise-diet regimen known as glycogen loading (or carbohydrate loading) has been used by endurance athletes to increase glycogen availability prior to endurance exercise events anticipated to last longer than 60 minutes. The original protocol, as described by Scandinavian researchers in the late 1960s, used extremes of diet and exercise to deplete then supercompensate glycogen stores. Recent work has demonstrated that trained athletes need only to taper their training and ensure a high carbohydrate intake (8 to 10 grams per kilogram per day) over the 72 hours prior to an event to achieve similar increases in muscle glycogen. Some studies have reported that athletes do not have sufficient practical nutrition knowledge to achieve such carbohydrate intakes. A menu suitable for carbohydrate loading is provided in Table 45-7 (13).

The Pre-Event Meal   The optimal pre-event meal varies between individual athletes, and is influenced by factors such as the time of day of competition and the degree to which the athlete has prepared or recovered fluid and fuel status since the last exercise session. An athlete who is well-tapered and has been consuming high-carbohydrate

Table 45-6   Eating Before and After Exercise

Suitable Pre-event Meal Choices
Breakfast cereal + low-fat milk + fresh/canned fruit
Muffins or crumpets + jam/honey
Pancakes + syrup
Toast + baked beans (note that this is a high-fiber choice)
Creamed rice (made with low-fat milk)
Rolls or sandwiches with banana filling
Fruit salad + low-fat fruit yogurt
Spaghetti with tomato or low-fat sauce
Baked potatoes with low-fat filling
Fruit smoothie (low-fat milk + fruit + yogurt/ice cream)
Liquid meal supplements (e.g., Sustagen Sport, Exceed Sports Meal, GatorPro)
Suitable Postexercise Recovery Snacks
(Note: these servings provide 50 grams of carbohydrate.)
800–1000 mL sports drink
500 mL fruit juice or soft drink
250 mL high-carbohydrate supplement (e.g., Exceed High Carbohydrate Source, Gatorlode)
250–350 mL fruit smoothie
250–350 mL liquid meal supplement (e.g., Sustagen Sport, Exceed Sports Meal, GatorPro)
50 grams of jelly beans or hard candies
70–80 gram chocolate bar
1 round jam or honey sandwich (thick-sliced bread + lots of jam or honey)
3 muesli bars
3 medium-large pieces of fruit (e.g., apple, orange, banana)
2 cups breakfast cereal + skim milk
Two 200 gram cartons low-fat fruit yogurt
Cup of thick vegetable soup + large breadroll
2 cups fruit salad + ½ carton of low-fat fruit yogurt
1 large bread roll + banana filling

SOURCE: Adapted from Burke LM. Eating for Sydney 2000: nutrition for the athlete. Mod Med Aust 1996;39(2):78–88.

meals over the last 2 to 3 days may only need to top-up liver glycogen stores after an overnight fast. Conversely, pre-event meals eaten 1 to 4 hours prior to exercise may increase carbohydrate availability if this is less than optimal due to inadequate preparation time (13).

A high-carbohydrate low-fat meal is generally advised, with reduced fiber and protein content being an additional recommendation for those who experience gastrointestinal discomfort. Some athletes may be able to comfortably consume a larger meal or snack 3 to 4 hours prior to competition, but those involved in early morning events may prefer to consume a smaller snack 1 to 2 hours prior. In cases where athletes experience difficulty in consuming solid foods prior to exercise, fruit smoothies or commercially available liquid meal supplements may be useful. The athlete is advised to experiment with various pre-event routines during training to define an optimal strategy. Some suitable pre-event meal choices are summarized in Table 45-6.

Fluid and Carbohydrate Needs During Exercise   Evaporation of sweat from the skin provides a major mechanism of heat loss, thus maintaining body temperature. An athlete's sweat rate is determined principally by exercise intensity, the state of heat acclimation, and the prevailing environmental conditions. Sweat rates as high as 2 to 3 liters per hour have been reported in some athletes exercising at high power outputs in hot and humid conditions. However, during more prolonged, moderate-intensity exercise (running, cycling), sweat rates in most athletes are closer to 1.0 to 1.2 liters

Table 45-7   Sample Carbohydrate-Loading Diet

These menu plans provide about 500 grams of carbohydrate per day, providing the recommended carbohydrate intake of 8 to 10 grams per kilogram body mass per day for a 50 to 55 kg athlete. They need to be adapted for athletes outside this weight range. These menus are proposed for carbohydrate-loading days only, because although they meet carbohydrate-intake goals, they do not meet all the nutrient requirements for everyday eating.

Day 1: (498 grams CHO, 2620 kcal CHO = 75% of energy)
- Breakfast:
     1 cup wheat flake cereal + 200 mL skim milk
     1 cup sweetened canned peaches
     250 mL sweetened fruit juice
- Snack:
     2 thick slices toast + scrape margarine and 1 tbsp honey on each
     250 mL sports drink
- Lunch:
     2 breadrolls with light salad
     375 mL can of soft drink
- Snack:
     Large coffee roll (unbuttered)
- Dinner:
     2 cups of boiled rice (as stir fry, with small amount of lean ham, peas, corn, and onion)
     250 mL sweetened fruit juice
- Snack:
     2 crumpets + scrape margarine and 1 tbsp jam on each
- Extra water during day

Day 2: (501 grams CHO, 2750 kcal CHO = 73% of energy)
- Breakfast:
     1 cup oatmeal + 200 mL skim milk
     1 banana
     250 mL sweetened fruit juice
- Snack:
     2 muffins + scrape margarine and 1 tbsp jam on each
- Lunch:
     Stack of 2 large pancakes + 60 mL maple syrup + small scoop frozen yogurt
     250 mL sweetened fruit juice
- Snack:
     50 grams of jelly beans
- Dinner:
     2 cups cooked pasta + 1 cup tomato pasta sauce
     2 slices bread
     250 mL sports drink
- Snack:
     1 cup fresh fruit salad
     200 gram carton low-fat fruit yogurt
- Extra water during day

Day 3:
- The athlete may like to switch to a low-residue diet to reduce gastrointestinal contents and improve comfort during the event.
- Use menus for Day 1 or 2, switching to white bread, white cereals, etc.
- From lunch onward, replace some or all of solid food with 500 mL snacks of commercial carbo-loader or liquid meal supplements.

SOURCE: Adapted from Burke LM, Hargreaves M. Eating for peak performance. In: Zuluaga D et al., eds. Sports physiotherapy. Melbourne: Churchill Livingstone, 1995:707–719.

per hour. Unless this fluid is replaced, the athlete will become dehydrated.

Dehydration of as little as 2% of an athlete's body mass has been shown to reduce high-intensity exercise capacity (14). Furthermore, the effects on exercise response appear to be directly related to the degree of dehydration; contrary to the belief prevalent in some sports, an athlete cannot acquire a tolerance to dehydration. It appears that the effects of dehydration on exercise performance are related to the type of event or sport being undertaken. Aerobic exercise, particularly in the heat, is impaired at such low levels of dehydration, but events requiring strength and power do not seem to be affected by such small fluid losses. However, as minimal dehydration may negatively impact on mental function, it should therefore be avoided in those sports that involve skill and decision-making processes. As dehydration has also been shown to reduce the rate of gastric emptying, which may further compromise exercise performance, the athlete should aim to minimize net fluid losses during all types of exercise.

In terms of optimal fluid balance, the athlete might be advised to consume fluids to keep pace with sweat losses, or at least 80% of sweat loss rate. In general, athletes appear to be able to drink 400 to 800 mL of fluid per hour under most sports conditions. Whether replenishment is done at aid stations, during formal breaks between quarters or halves of a game, or from drink bottles carried by the athlete varies according to the sport. Athletes should be encouraged to establish a drinking routine that takes into account their sweat losses and their opportunities to drink fluid. Some routines may not be optimal when sweat losses greatly exceed the general rate of gastric emptying (about 1 liter per hour), but the athlete should aim to minimize dehydration. Drinking early and frequently should be part of this plan (e.g., 150 to 250 mL every 15 to 20 minutes). In a practical sense, athletes who need to consume fluids during events while literally on the run (as with marathon runners, cyclists, cross-country skiers, or triathletes) may need to balance their intake against the possibility of gastrointestinal discomfort or upset, as well as the time lost while eating or drinking (as when slowing down to approach an aid station or to handle fluids or food). Fluids that are palatable are likely to be consumed in larger quantities; for this reason, cool and sweet-tasting drinks are promoted.

It is difficult to produce guidelines for optimal fluid intake strategies for all sports which take into account fluid needs and opportunities to consume fluid during various sports. General guidelines are summarized in Table 45-8. However, during the organization of endurance events, particularly those conducted in hot environments, special attention must be given to the provision of competition food and fluid intake for athletes. In events where rules allow athletes to provide their own refreshments during formal and informal breaks in play, such practices should be strongly encouraged.

During prolonged intense exercise, fatigue may result from carbohydrate depletion, through muscle glycogen depletion and/or hypoglycemia. Even though competition preparation may have increased body glycogen stores, many endurance and ultra-endurance events challenge the athlete's carbohydrate reserves. Carbohydrate intake during such exercise may benefit performance, both by preventing hypoglycemia in those individuals susceptible to small changes in blood glucose concentration and by supplying additional fuel for muscle glucose oxidation. Numerous studies have reported benefits to endurance capacity and/or performance in prolonged exercise events when carbohydrate is consumed.

Both solid foods and carbohydrate drinks have been used successfully to supply carbohydrates during exercise. Carbohydrate drinks are particularly useful because they decrease the risk of gastrointestinal side effects and simultaneously meet fluid requirements. Although early studies warned against the inhibition of gastric emptying following intake of carbohydrate drinks greater than 2.5% in concentration, there are now many studies that report that carbohydrate drinks of 5% to 7% concentration are emptied rapidly and do not interfere with fluid replacement (15). Today, commercial sports drinks are manufactured using a combination of carbohydrate types (glucose, sucrose, glucose polymers, etc.) to achieve a palatable beverage with a carbohydrate content of 5% to 7% and a moderate sodium level (10–25 mmol/L). These sports drinks provide a practical

Table 45-8   Guidelines for Fluid and Carbohydrate Requirements During Various Sports

Sports	Fluid Needs	CHO Needs	Comments
Weight-division sports (e.g., lightweight rowing, wrestling, boxing)	Variable	Generally not needed	The athlete is encouraged to "make weight" without resorting to severe dehydration and fasting. There may be some opportunity to top-up fluid and fuel levels after the weigh-in. If the athlete is still dehydrated, extra care should be taken with fluid intake needs/opportunities during the event.
Brief events (e.g., sprints, throwing events)	Not applicable	Not applicable	There is generally no need or opportunity to replace fluids and carbohydrates during an event. For multiple events spread over the day, the athlete is encouraged to rehydrate and re-fuel between events with appropriate fluids and foods.
Nonendurance events <60 min (e.g., 5 or 10 km run)	Variable (e.g., minimal at 1 liter per hour)	Generally not needed	Sweat losses will vary with the length and intensity of the event and the environmental conditions. The athlete should make use of opportunities during the event to keep fluid deficits below a liter (approximately). Fluid replacement with water will generally be adequate; however sports drinks are suitable and often preferable. Remaining fluid deficits should be replaced after the event, and rapid fuel recovery can be assisted by immediate intake of carbohydrate-containing foods and fluids.
Team events (e.g., basketball, soccer, football)	Variable (e.g., 500 to 1000 mL per hour, or more)	May be useful (e.g., 30 to 50 grams per hour)	Sweat losses will vary between sports and players, according to the intensity of individual play and the environmental conditions. In tournament conditions, there may be inadequate time for complete recovery of fluid and fuel needs between games. In this situation, aggressive intake of a carbohydrate-containing fluid (e.g., sports drink) during the game will provide an advantage.
Endurance events >90 min (marathon, road cycle, Olympic distance triathlon)	500 to 1000+ mL per hour (more in extreme conditions)	Approximately 50 grams per hour	Opportunities for regular intake of carbohydrate-containing fluids should be encouraged in these sports (via aid stations, breaks in play). Sweat losses may be extreme. Carbohydrate needs will vary according to preexisting glycogen stores and the length and intensity of the event. The athlete is advised to keep pace with sweat losses as well as possible. Rehydrate full and refuel after the event.
Ultra-endurance events >4 hours (e.g., ironman triathlons)	500 to 1000 + mL per hour (more in extreme conditions)	Approximately 50 grams per hour	Same as for endurance events. In addition, the sodium in sports drinks may be useful in reducing the risk of hyponatremia in susceptible athletes. Solid forms of carbohydrate may be eaten to prevent or alleviate hunger as well as continue to supply additional fuel.

SOURCE: Adapted from Burke LM, Hargreaves M. Eating for peak performance. In: Zuluaga D et al., eds. Sports physiotherapy. Melbourne: Churchill Livingstone, 1995:707–719.

way to achieve both carbohydrate and fluid needs during exercise and for rehydration after exercise. The athlete should experiment with carbohydrate intake strategies during training to perfect a competition plan. Guidelines to general carbohydrate intake requirements are summarized in Table 45-8.

Recovery After Exercise

In some sports, competition is conducted as a series of events or stages. Examples include track and field and swimming events where athletes may compete in a number of brief events or heats and finals in the one day. In events such as tennis tournaments and cycle tours, competitors may be required to undertake one or more lengthy bouts each day, with the competition extending for 1 to 3 weeks. The value of rapid recovery between events is clear, and recovery strategies must consider the extent and type of nutritional stresses involved as well as the time interval between competition bouts. Even where athletes compete in a weekly fixture, optimal recovery is desired to allow the athlete to undertake training between matches or races.

The issues underlying rapid restoration of fuel and fluid balance are well documented (16). Immediate intake of carbohydrate food has already been identified as a key strategy in promoting glycogen storage in muscle and liver. Despite the intake of fluid during exercise most athletes will finish the session at least mildly dehydrated. From a practical standpoint, the success of postexercise rehydration is dependent on how much the athlete drinks, and then how much of this is retained and reequilibrated within body fluid compartments. Flavored drinks may encourage greater intake than plain water, in addition to the benefits of carbohydrate content on muscle fuel needs. The inclusion of sodium in the drink or the concurrent consumption of salty foods can help to minimize, although not entirely prevent, the amount of fluid that is lost as urine in postexercise recovery. Caffeine and alcohol also promote diuresis, so consumption of large amounts of alcoholic and caffeine-containing drinks may also impair rapid fluid restoration. The current practices of some athletes, particularly in team sports, to consume

excessive amounts of alcohol after competition requires re-education but appears resistant to change. Disadvantages include impairment of rehydration and thermoregulation, exacerbation of soft tissue damage, and behavior that might be considered a high risk for accidents.

When a single competition or competition season extends beyond a couple of days, the athlete must also consider overall nutrient goals such as requirements for protein, vitamins, and minerals. Eating for optimal competition recovery may simply represent an extension of everyday nutrition patterns, but it is important to remember the practical implications of the competition situation. Athletes are often competing away from their home base, including overseas, so some consideration may need to be given to ensuring access to suitable foods supplies at the competition venue. Also, the postevent phase is often a time of conflicting priorities, with the athlete being bombarded with requests for drug testing, equipment checks, travel, media interviews, and team activities. It is vital that the athlete is aware of the importance of recovery nutrition, and that creative and practical ways of achieving this can be organized. Nutrient-dense supplements in liquid or solid form (e.g., sport-bars) may provide a practical alternative to food in some situations.

PRACTICAL ISSUES OF EATING WELL WHILE TRAVELING

Travel is an integral part of the lifestyle of most elite athletes. Many travel nationally and internationally to compete, or train in special facilities or situations (e.g., for altitude training or heat acclimation). Being away from home provides a number of challenges to sound nutritional practices, including reduced access to suitable food while eating in hotels, restaurants, on planes; reduced supervision by parents or coaches; and disruptions to the usual routine caused by travel. An unusual food supply in a foreign country, and problems with food hygiene and a safe water supply in some countries are additional problems. Athletes may also find it difficult to identify acute changes in nutritional needs caused by a sudden change in training load or environmental conditions.

Table 45-9   Strategies for Eating Well While Traveling

1 The athlete should investigate the food resources at the trip destination before departure. People who have traveled previously to that country, competition, or accommodation facility may be able to provide warnings of likely problems and allow a plan to be prepared in advance.
2 Special menus and meals in restaurants, airplanes, or hotels often can be organized in advance.
3 It is important to find out about food hygiene and water safety in unfamiliar countries. It may be necessary to restrict fluid intake to bottled or boiled drinks and avoid foods that are at high-risk for contamination (e.g., unpeeled fruits and vegetables).
4 The athlete should take some food supplies if important foods are likely to be unavailable or expensive. Foods that are portable and low in perishability include breakfast cereals, milk powder, tinned and dehydrated foods, and special sports supplements.
5 The athlete should be aware of the special nutritional requirements in the new location and should be prepared to meet any increased requirements for fluids, carbohydrates, and other nutrients.

SOURCE: Adapted from Burke LM. Practical issues in nutrition for athletes. J Sports Sci 1995;13:S83–S90.

Failure to meet these challenges may result in unwanted weight loss or gain, chronic dehydration, inadequate carbohydrate recovery, nutrient deficiencies, and gastrointestinal upsets including traveler's diarrhea. An organized nutrition plan may assist athletes to eat well while traveling, thus reducing the risk of these problems and promoting optimal performance at these key times. Table 45-9 summarizes strategies for the traveling athlete.

SUMMARY

Sports nutrition combines science and practice to assist athletes to be healthy, train effectively, and compete at their best. The special nutritional needs of athletes must be met within a busy daily timetable and in conjunction with other nutritional goals. Special fluid and food intake strategies before, during, and after exercise may assist the athlete to perform optimally and recover quickly.

REFERENCES

1 Kerr D. Kinanthropometry. In: Burke LM, Deakin V, eds. Clinical sports nutrition. Sydney: McGraw-Hill, 1994:74–103.
2 Burke LM. Sport and body fatness. In: Hills AP, Wahlqvist ML, eds. Exercise and obesity. London: Smith-Gordon:217–231.
3 Brownell KD, Rodin J, Wilmore JH, eds. Eating, body weight and performance in athletes: disorders of modern society. Philadelphia: Lea and Febiger, 1992.
4 Barr SI. Women, nutrition and exercise: a review of athletes' intakes and a discussion of energy balance in active women. Prog Food Nutr Sci 1987;11:307–361.
5 Lemon PW. Effect of exercise on protein requirements. J Sports Sci 1991;9:53–70.
6 Burke LM, Inge K. Protein requirements for training and bulking up. In: Burke LM, Deakin V, eds. Clinical sports nutrition. Sydney: McGraw-Hill, 1994:124–150.
7 van der Beek EJ. Vitamins and endurance training. Food for running or faddish claims? Sports Med 1985;2:175–197.
8 Deakin V. Iron deficiency in athletes: identification, prevention and dietary treatment. In: Burke LM, Deakin V, eds. Clinical sports nutrition. Sydney: McGraw-Hill, 1994:174–199.
9 Loucks AB, Horvath SM. Athletic amenorrhea: a review. Med Sci Sports Exerc 1985;17:56–72.
10 Burke LM, Heeley P. Dietary supplements and nutritional ergogenic aids in sport. In: Burke LM, Deakin V, eds. Clinical sports nutrition. Sydney: McGraw-Hill, 1994:227–284.
11 Sherman WM, Wimer GS. Insufficient dietary carbohydrate during training: does it impair athletic performance? Int J Sport Nutr 1991;1:28–44.
12 Coyle EF. Timing and method of increased carbohydrate intake to cope with heavy training, competition and recovery. In: Williams C, Devlin JT, eds. Foods, nutrition and sports performance. London: E & FN Spon, 1992:35–63.
13 O'Connor H. Competition nutrition issues: preparation and recovery. In: Burke LM, Deakin V, eds. Clinical sports nutrition. Sydney: McGraw-Hill, 1994:307–332.
14 Sawka MN, Pandolf KB. Effects of water loss on

physiological function and exercise performance. In: Gisolfi CV, Lamb DR, eds. Perspectives in exercise science and sports medicine, vol 3. Carmel, IN: Benchmark Press, 1990:1–38.

15 Hawley JA, Dennis SC, Noakes TD. Carbohydrate, fluid and electrolyte requirements during prolonged exercise. In: Kies CV, Driskell JA, eds. Sports nutrition, minerals and electrolytes. Boca Raton, FL: CRC, 1995:235–265.

16 Burke LM. Nutrition for post-exercise recovery. Aust J Sports Sci Med Sport 1997;29:8–10.

FURTHER READING

Burke LM. The complete guide to food for sports performance. 2nd ed. Sydney: Allen and Unwin, 1995.

Williams C, Devlin JT, eds. Foods, nutrition and sports performance. London: E&FN Spon, 1992.

Wolinsky I, Hickson JF, eds. Nutrition in exercise and sport. 2nd ed. Boca Raton, FL: CRC, 1994.

Chapter 46
Eating Disorders

Peter N. Gilchrist
Kieran E. Fallon

Athletes suffer the same range of ills to which all of us are prey, and among these are disorders that have underlying psychological processes, such as eating disorders. This chapter discusses the classic conditions anorexia nervosa and bulimia nervosa and their strict diagnostic criteria, and also less well-defined abnormal eating behaviors. Pathologic eating behaviors appear to be more common than anorexia nervosa and bulimia nervosa in both athletes and the nonexercising population.

Studies that compare the incidence of eating disorders in athletes and nonathletes (particularly females) do testify to the belief that elite athletes are at increased risk of eating disorders (1), and that some sports such as distance running, gymnastics, ballet, and diving attract athletes who wish to be thin and believe they will be rewarded for being so (2).

ANOREXIA NERVOSA

Anorexia nervosa is characterized by an intense pursuit of thinness, a preoccupation with body image, and a refusal to maintain a normal body weight. It is not a new condition, although its incidence would appear to be increasing. Sufferers are usually female and present in their teenage years. Weight loss is achieved by abstaining from food, although additional methods of weight loss such as vomiting, abuse of laxatives, diuretics, and excessive exercise may be used. Individuals with this disorder have a fear of gaining weight; even after significant weight loss they continue to protest that they are too fat. Body image disturbance may focus on parts of their bodies such as thighs or lower abdomen, usually referred to by patients as their

stomachs, or maybe a general dissatisfaction with the body. As the anorexic condition develops, an individual may spend more time preparing food for others, but go to great lengths to avoid consuming food. They become experts at concealing their behavior.

Anorexic patients may become preoccupied with the calorie content of food, and not infrequently keep extensive records of the calorie content of meals as a means of controlling their food intake. What may begin as an attempt to follow a "healthy diet," quickly becomes inappropriately restrictive in the amount and types of food. Despite dramatic weight loss and change in behavior, the anorexic protests that nothing is wrong, to the frustration of family and friends. Unfortunately, confrontation may lead to more secretive behavior.

Amenorrhea in postmenarcheal females occurs with weight loss; excessive thinness delays menarche in prepubertal girls. The occurrence of menstrual periods induced by the use of the oral contraceptive pill may be used by some to deny the consequences of starvation.

Findings on physical examination and laboratory investigation depend on the degree of weight loss and weight-loss strategies used. There may be cold blue peripheries, hypotension, bradycardia, hypothermia; in some, lanugo (a fine downy hair) appears. Swollen parotid glands and the deterioration of dental hygiene are often associated with vomiting. Laboratory investigations may be unremarkable but commonly reveal a metabolic alkalosis from vomiting, a metabolic acidosis from laxative abuse, hypokalemia, and a leukopenia. With more dramatic weight loss, increasing disturbances of body biochemistry occur, including low luteinizing hormone, low to below normal T_3 (tri-iodo thyronine), and possible increases in serum urea, carotene, cholesterol, and transaminase. Symptoms and signs are consistent with starvation and malnutrition. The ECG may show bradycardia, low voltage QRS complexes, low inverted T waves, and a prolonged QT interval.

BULIMIA NERVOSA

Although only recently described as a clinical entity, bulimia nervosa is not a new condition. Bulimia nervosa has as its essential features a loss of control of appetite, the consumption of large quantities of food (usually readily digestible sweet foods), and the use of a variety of strategies to avoid the feared weight gain. The commonest techniques used to avoid weight gain are induced vomiting or regurgitation. As with anorexia nervosa, patients with bulimia nervosa have a body image disturbance and believe that they are too fat when they are not. The bulimic may be of normal weight, although this may fluctuate significantly—a useful clinical sign if suspicions are aroused. Eating patterns may be concealed and the condition only suspected by complications of behavior, such as a medical complication of purging or chance discovery of the individual during a binge or purge.

Physical examination may be unremarkable, but there may be swollen parotid glands, deterioration in dental hygiene, or calluses on the dorsum of the second and third metacarpophalangeal joints (from abrasions through inducing vomiting by stimulating the gag reflex). Laboratory investigations may demonstrate electrolyte disturbances such as hypokalemia, hyponatremia, and hypochloremia. Metabolic alkalosis may result from vomiting and metabolic acidosis from laxative abuse. Rare complications include hematemesis from vomiting-induced esophageal tears, gastric rupture, and cardiac arrhythmias.

ATHLETES AND EATING DISORDERS

Studies suggest that there is a greater risk of eating disorders (according to rigid diagnostic criteria) in athletes, but more so of abnormal eating behaviors, particularly in female athletes, than in the general population.

Pathogenic weight control behavior such as self-induced vomiting, laxative abuse, frequent use of diet pills and diuretics, and fasting are often used. Approximately one-third of university-level female athletes report use of at least one of these methods (3). High-risk sports are those where rigid body weight standards are enforced, or a low body weight level is seen as important in maximizing performance, or aesthetics and bodily appearance play a part in performance. These sports include distance running, gymnastics, diving, figure skating, ballet, and light-weight rowing. Sports at lower risk are those where leanness can provide an advantage in performance, such as basketball, high jumping, and netball.

Athletes striving to improve performance or to maintain an elite level may focus on diet and appearance and become increasingly obsessed with these issues. Psychological risk factors for eating disorders are common in successful athletes and include perfectionist attitudes, competitiveness, and a willingness to tolerate personal discomfort in order to achieve a set goal. Other potential risk factors include prolonged periods of dieting and weight fluctuation, dieting at an early age, unsupervised dieting, a fear of reaching menarche and developing of secondary sex characteristics too early, and early onset of sport-specific training (4).

A number of trigger factors specific to sport have been identified and these include loss of a coach, illness or injury, and casual negative comments regarding weight by coaches, parents, or others (2).

Presentation of Eating Disorders in Athletes

A sports physician should maintain a high level of suspicion of an eating disorder in high-risk athletes, but must also remember that eating disorders may be present in athletes of either gender, involved in all sports. Physical examination may be unremarkable if there has not been significant weight loss, or weight loss may be justified as part of a program in preparation for competitions. Abnormalities on routine laboratory investigations should alert the physician to the possibility of laxative or diuretic abuse, or vomiting. Often presentations are by referral from concerned peers, coaches, or relatives who may be familiar with eating disorders. Reports of changes in an individual's behavior—such as exercising in excess of the required demands or against coaches' or physicians' advice, changes in dietary intake, or the use of diuretics, laxatives, or appetite suppressants—must be investigated.

Management

The development of an eating disorder is multi-determined and involves biological as well as psychological factors. An eating disorder should be seen as a desperate solution to a number of significant personal problems. Recurring themes in such individuals are issues of self-worth and of establishing a sense of control in their lives. These are the keys to therapy. To hope that eating disorders will just go away is wishful thinking.

Early, accurate assessment is important to good outcome. Once identified, the individual should be confronted and a definite diagnosis made. This usually involves referral to a specialized eating disorder unit or to a professional familiar with these conditions. Treatment relies on a combination of counseling, psychological therapy, and sometimes pharmacology. Whether athletes should be discouraged from competing depends on the individual's age, the severity of the condition, and the risk of physical sequelae, as well as the level of insight that the individual has to his or her condition. Whatever decision is made, the athlete must understand that the eating disorder is *not* simply a weight or dietary problem but an indication of severe psychopathology. Treatment is often difficult, prolonged, and sometimes unsuccessful.

CONCLUSION

Classic cases of eating disorders are easily recognized. The diagnosis is more problematic in the subclinical group. Denial of the problem and the athlete's behavior may be justified as part of his or her preparation for competition. Changes in an athlete's behavior such as unnecessary exercise, the inability to reduce training, an alteration in diet without supervision, or unexplained physical problems should alert the physician to the possibility of such conditions.

REFERENCES

1 Wilmore JH. Eating and weight disorders in female athletes. Int J Sport Nutr 1991;1:104–117.
2 Sundgot-Borgen J. Eating disorders in female athletes. Sports Med 1994;17:176–188.
3 Rosen LW, Hough DO. Pathogenic weight control behaviors of female college gymnasts. Physician Sports Med 1988;16:141–144.
4 Sundgot-Borgen J. Risk and trigger factors for the development of eating disorders in female elite athletes. Med Sci Sport Exerc 1994;26:414–419.

Chapter 47
Physical Activity and Mental Health: Anxiety, Depression, and Burnout in Athletes

M. Anne Duncan
William A. Hensel
Kori A. Graves

The goal of this chapter is to provide physicians with a general understanding of the relationship between physical activity and mental health. Specifically discussed are the areas of stress and anxiety, depression, and the phenomenon of "burnout" within the context of the normal growth and development of athletes. We begin with the definitions of these mental health concerns, then proceed to the discussion of a developmental approach that starts with childhood and ends with older adulthood. We describe the mental health concerns commonly encountered at the various developmental stages, and conclude with general treatment recommendations for the athlete who suffers from anxiety or mood problems.

BACKGROUND CONCEPTS

Stress and Anxiety

Stress is a double-edged sword. The positive aspects of stress include stimulation of growth, change, and improvement (1). This beneficial dimension is apparent in competitive sports when precompetition stress is successfully converted into an energetic athletic performance. Stress has a negative, potentially pathologic side. When the stress exceeds the individual's ability to cope, the physiologic symptoms of anxiety will ensue. Among the most common expressions of anxiety are rapid heartbeat and respiration, sweaty palms, heightened arousal, increased muscle tension, and a feeling of "jitteriness" (2).

Research has often documented the adverse effects of stress (3). Physiologic symptoms relate to catecholamine release and the physical changes accompanied by emotional features such as uneasiness, fear, and rage (4). The constellation of physiologic and psychological effects have been termed the "stress response" (5).

Anxiety has been classified as a "state" or "trait" depending on the onset and severity of symptoms. *Trait anxiety* refers to the anxiety an individual experiences as ongoing and chronic. In contrast, *state anxiety* refers to a transient and situationally induced type of anxiety. "Performance anxiety" is state anxiety that interferes with the ability to perform optimally (2). For instance, a basketball player who suffers from performance anxiety will typically play better in practice than during competition, perhaps shooting 80% of free throws during practice but only 50% during a game.

Certain individuals may be particularly vulnerable to performance anxiety. The athlete with fragile self-confidence may shy away from the intense situations encountered in competitive athletics (6). Athletes with a hereditary predisposition toward anxiety may also be more vulnerable to performance anxiety. Research indicates that there is a significant genetic component in many of the anxiety disorders, and a family history positive for anxiety disorders is a good predictor of this tendency (7).

Even though uncontrolled anxiety has a detrimental effect on athletic performance, successfully modulated anxiety can be useful in certain sports (8). Moderately high levels of prerace anxiety in sprinters may enable an explosive start. Similarly, in sports that emphasize speed and skill, such as tennis and basketball, a moderate level of anxiety can help sharpen the athlete's focus without interfering with hand–eye coordination. If a critical level of stress is exceeded, however, the player will lose control of a shot. In sports that demand precision, such as golf and archery, every effort is made to decrease any anxiety that can interfere with fine motor control.

Depression

The term *depression* has variable meanings to the public but is narrowly defined by physicians and mental health professionals. The physician should distinguish feeling "blue" or "down" from the presentation of a depressive disorder. Virtually everyone experiences periods of sadness and disappointment, most commonly in the face of loss, a difficult transition, or disillusionment. For instance, athletes may describe themselves as "seriously depressed" following a poor performance, yet may rebound a short time later after a good performance. In contrast to the transient nature of such negative emotional states, clinical depression is characterized by the enduring expression of a specific cluster of symptoms, including a pervasive disorder of mood, the loss of joy and optimism, and sleep and appetite disturbance.

As with other patients suffering from depression, the presenting complaints of athletes may be nonspecific, such as a general sense of fatigue or loss of motivation and enthusiasm. When athletes present with such vague symptoms, they should be screened for depression. Another clinical scenario that should prompt the clinician to consider depression would be athletes who have somatic complaints out of proportion to their injury. As with the anxiety disorders, the athlete's family history should be reviewed because depression has a significant genetic component (9). Depression is also more prevalent in females.

Burnout

There is no universal definition of burnout, but general agreement exists that burnout is the result of accumulated stress and is characterized by a predictable set of physical and psychological reactions (10). Burnout typically follows failed attempts to meet the demands of sport participation, leading to a psychological, emotional, and physical withdrawal (11). It is not a specific medical diagnosis, but burnout is a common reason for athletes quitting sports before the natural end of their careers. For our purposes, *burnout* is defined as the negative psychological experience that causes an athlete to prematurely leave a sport. In this context, the athlete who "burns out" has psychological reasons for withdrawing. Burnout has a heterogenous group of causes; therefore, interventions should be based on the reasons an individual athlete has left or is considering leaving a sport.

Because preventing athletes from quitting is easier than getting them to return to their sport, early recognition of the symptoms of burnout is paramount. As with depression, burnout symptoms are often nonspecific, including irritability, anger, feelings of excessive fatigue, somatic complaints, and the loss of enthusiasm for the sport. Identification of these symptoms should prompt the physician to ask more in-depth questions that will lead to a specific diagnosis.

Recreational and Competitive Athletes

The relationship of athletics and mental health varies greatly according to the level of competition. For our purposes, a *recreational athlete* is an individual who competes casually, participates in sport for general health benefits, or participates just for fun. A *competitive athlete* is an individual who participates in sport to achieve excellence, with performance during competition being the measure of that excellence.

It is useful to differentiate between the recreational and competitive athlete when assessing whether the level of stress is excessive. Competitive athletes are under far more pressure to perform than recreational athletes. That pressure may be generated internally, as with the fierce desire to excel, or externally, as with a coach's demand that performance improve or the athlete will be cut from the team. Consequently, competitive athletes are more susceptible than recreational athletes to burnout and performance anxiety.

DEVELOPMENTAL ISSUES IN THE MENTAL HEALTH OF ATHLETES

Athletes, like all people, go through predictable developmental stages. With each stage, athletes face new obstacles. Because many athletes are children or adolescents, parents and coaches often play a large role in their lives. Therefore, an athlete's depression, anxiety, or loss of enthusiasm for the sport may be best explained by understanding his or her stage of development and relationship with significant others, particularly parents, coaches, and teammates. For that reason, this section discusses the problems of anxiety, depression, and burnout within a developmental context and highlights the role of parents and coaches.

Childhood

Play holds an important place in the early development of children. Through involvement in play, games, and sports, children learn about their own physical abilities and about the complexities of social interchange, such as taking turns and following a set of rules. The physical games of childhood are a precursor to organized athletics. As such, attitudes developed during childhood play may have an effect on later sports participation. In general, children who participate in sport for enjoyment and companionship are at low risk for depression, pathologic stress or anxiety, and burnout (12).

Readiness for competitive sports depends on the individual child's level of emotional maturity and his or her level of interest. Competitive sport offers children valuable lessons; but there are many traps to avoid at this early stage of development.

One potential trap involves the family, which is inevitably the emotional center of a child's world. Children are exquisitely sensitive to their parents' attitudes and have a deep need to feel supported by their parents while pursuing their own goals. Parents, however, walk a fine line between encouraging and pushing their child. Parental pressure to perform can be a major source of pathologic stress at a time when children have not yet gained the skills or emotional maturity to cope with this pressure.

Physicians need to be aware of family dynamics when encountering a child athlete who is expressing symptoms of anxiety or depression. It is not unusual to find that the child has become the holder of the unrealized hopes and dreams of their parents. Here, an important principle has been violated: goals are important, but the child athlete, not the parent, must set those goals. Many parents need to be taught to help their children set goals and to refrain from imposing their own expectations.

A second potential trap involves the role of the coach. At the beginning level, most sports programs rely on volunteer coaches who are well-intentioned but may be misdirected in their approach to coaching children. Volunteer coaches may recall high school playing days when their coaches yelled at them (i.e., increased stress as an attempt to motivate the players) and automatically use that tactic with children. Unfortunately, for most children this approach is more stressful than motivational. The primary physician may wish to confer with the parents if the child is being subjected to this unhealthy coaching approach.

Coaches are extremely influential in the lives of impressionable young athletes. Often, they are the major teachers of the values of sport. In children's sports, coaches need to help athletes put competition and winning into a healthy, balanced perspective. Coaches need to reward improvement, attitude, team effort, and fair play, not simply performance. Children prefer to play on a losing team than to sit on the bench for a winning team; thus, fair distribution of playing time is crucial.

Children's athletics present a preventive medicine opportunity. If the child learns to value effort and achievement, if the parents learn to support and encourage but not push their child, and if the coach motivates and instills proper values in the athlete, problems later in life may be minimized. Community youth programs that have guidelines about coaching behavior, sportsmanship, and guaranteed participation will offer children the best introduction to sports. Physicians who are willing to help set up those fair play guidelines can have a positive influence on the community's youth.

Adolescence

Adolescence is a time of physical, social, and emotional transition. Serious psychological problems may go undetected because parents, teachers, and other professionals assume that dramatic mood shifts, sudden changes in peer groups, and wide variations in school performance are expected during adolescence. More often these behaviors are indications of underlying emotional problems.

Many adolescents are involved in competitive athletics and benefit from sports participation. In addition to the obvious health benefits, sports involvement may provide adolescents with a peer group, and help them develop a firmer identity and higher self-esteem. Adolescent athletes demonstrate fewer high-risk characteristics and drug-use tendencies (12). In addition, athletes on average scored 7 percentage points lower (less depressed) than nonathletes on the Children's Depression Inventory (13).

Dedication to a sport also provides adolescents with a greater understanding of the importance of self-discipline and consistent hard work. Team sports help adolescents understand the benefits of cooperation, communication, and allegiance. Sports also provide adolescents with another avenue for testing relationships with authority figures, such as coaches and referees.

Although the advantages of sports participation outweigh the disadvantages, potential problems do exist. One such problem is that the level of stress increases as performance expectations escalate on competitive school teams. Most athletes adapt, but some experience performance anxiety that may negate many of the positive features of participation.

Depression is a serious issue for adolescents. Teens have alarmingly high rates of depressed mood and of attempted suicide (14). One major issue with teenage depression involves their lack of long-term perspective. For instance, when a romance ends, the rejected teen commonly feels that all is lost and the world is coming to an end. The adolescent has little sense that love will exist again and thus may consider suicide. This crisis mentality and poor long-term perspective makes teens very sensitive to disappointment. Adolescent competitive sport must be understood in this context. In the athletic arena where there are winners and losers, vulnerable teens may experience loss as deeply disappointing, and depression may be experienced as the exaggerated response to defeat.

So, even though athletes experience less depression than the general population, adolescent athletes are not immune to depression or, in extreme circumstances, suicide.

Self-esteem in adolescents tends to be fragile and a blow may lead a vulnerable teen into depression. Sports participation is no longer assured, as it was in childhood. Adolescents may feel the pain of rejection when they try out for a team and are cut. Being excluded or sitting constantly on the bench can damage a fragile self-esteem. Many adolescents are able to view defeat within a larger perspective and use setbacks as a motivation to improve. However, those who are unable to cope well may personalize loss, experience a decrease in self-esteem, and respond with depression.

Depression may have a particular presentation in adolescence. In addition to the classic vegetative symptoms, physicians should look for the following symptoms:

1 Abrupt change in friends
2 Withdrawal and isolation
3 Abrupt decline in school performance
4 Truancy, vandalism, drug or alcohol use, or other illegal behavior
5 Changing behavior in sports (i.e., a teen who is suddenly argumentative or hostile to coaches or officials).

Because of the prevalence of attempted suicide in teens, suspected depression must be treated as an urgent matter. The role of the physician is to clarify the diagnosis of depression and to assess suicide potential. Because counseling is usually the primary therapeutic modality, referral to a mental health professional is often necessary.

Burnout, like depression, must be considered within the larger context. Burnout arises from a heterogeneous cluster of problems, so understanding the issues that caused a teen to quit a sport is necessary to identify and treat the real problem. One caveat: when a teen quits a sport, it is not always due to burnout, nor necessarily a bad decision. Part of adolescent development involves learning to make independent life choices. A teen may make a healthy choice to quit a sport in order to pursue other interests. Problems occur when the teen and parents have conflicting ideas about the importance of continuing a sport. In such cases, the physician may chose to convene the family to discuss the issue.

Collegiate and Other Highly Competitive Athletes

Psychological issues play a greater role as the level of competition increases for several reasons. First, athletes are under increased pressure to perform, and the level of stress may exceed the point necessary for optimal performance. This situation may lead to anxiety-related problems. Second, in high-level sport, coaches and athletes look for any edge to improve performance and will often turn to sports psychologists for help, even if there is no particular problem with performance. Many U.S. elite amateur athletes have consulted with sports psychologists in preparation for and during Olympic competition. For instance, at the 1988 Summer Olympic Games, sport psychologist consultations were held with 40 U.S. athletes and coaches (15). Third, a transformation in an athlete's attitude toward his or her sport may occur as expectations change; for instance, the athlete who had participated in a sport for fun now finds that it has become work.

Highly competitive athletes, typically in their late teens or early twenties, usually become less impulsive and more future oriented than they were in early teens. Greater maturity does not mean that stress, anxiety, depression, and burnout are no longer problems—they just assume different forms.

The same nonpharmacologic interventions for stress and anxiety recommended for teens are also appropriate in this age group. However, the differential diagnosis of anxiety symptoms should encompass drug use. For example, stimulants such as amphetamines or excessive caffeine will produce the same symptoms as anxiety. Athletes may use these drugs as a part of social experimentation or in an effort to enhance performance. The physician should discourage such drug use and educate the athlete about the detrimental effects.

Depression   High-level athletes may present with unique aspects of depression. Athletes may experience failure for the first time as they enter more competitive arenas. Perhaps they were "stars" in high school but now find that they are simply mediocre in college. Because of their previous history of success, these athletes may not have developed the skills needed to cope with defeat. These athletes may benefit from cognitive interventions to help them reframe their experience, rediscover the joy and worth of sport, and recapture an intrinsic motivation to excel.

Depression is often triggered by loss, and athletes may experience important losses at this level. They may lose their dream, perhaps realizing that they will never qualify for the Olympics or compete in professional sport. Further, all athletes begin to understand that their competitive careers will soon end. Considering that training occupies an enormous amount of time at this level of competition, and that these athletes have been involved in their sport for much of their lives, the impending end of their competitive days may leave a huge void in the athlete's life. Counseling may help the athlete deal with this transition, remake his or her identity, and move to a new phase of life.

Another form of loss occurs when an athlete is injured. In particular, athletes who base their identity on sport involvement may suffer depression in the wake of an injury. These individuals may experience depression even though no limitation in their daily pursuits has resulted (16). Smith et al. (17) conducted a study comparing the pre- and post-injury mood state of competitive athletes and found significant increases in depression following an injury.

Depressed athletes may need additional encouragement from the physician to enter counseling because seeking help may be interpreted as a sign of weakness that is inconsistent with their self-image of mental toughness. The physician must establish rapport, dispel any myths about depression, and educate the athlete about the condition. Like other patients who have difficulty acknowledging depression, athletes may present to the physician with somatic complaints. The task of the primary care physician is to recognize this presentation as depression and effectively communicate and educate the athlete patient about the diagnosis. Only then can the physician successfully encourage the patient to seek counseling with a mental health professional, preferably one who is knowledgeable about athletes.

Burnout The presenting complaints of athletes suffering from burnout tend to fall into two categories. Vague complaints such as fatigue, difficulty sleeping, or change in appetite represent the first symptom group. The second symptom group consists of somatic complaints that seem to be out of proportion to objective findings. In both categories, burnout is part of a differential diagnosis that should also include depression and overtraining syndrome. Once the diagnosis of burnout is established, the physician or mental health professional must attempt to understand the unique reasons prompting the individual athlete to consider leaving the sport.

Overtraining syndrome deserves additional comment. Intense training regimens push highly competitive athletes to the very limit of their physical endurance. If that threshold is exceeded, the athlete suffers symptoms of overtraining, including fatigue, decreased performance, a depressed mood, weight loss, and decreased enthusiasm for the sport. The diagnosis of overtraining syndrome is based on clinical suspicion, and there are no consistent laboratory abnormalities that will verify the condition. Confirmation of this clinical diagnosis occurs when a lighter training regimen produces a resolution of symptoms.

Adult Recreational Athletes

Depending on the intensity of their competitiveness, adults may be prone to the same stress, anxiety, depression, and burnout that affect younger athletes. Because the number of highly competitive athletes wanes in the adult age group, the focus of this section will be on the recreational athlete.

Stress Recreational sports can be a good way for adults to relieve the general stresses of daily living. Physicians now understand that exercise causes the release of endorphins and has other favorable effects on neurotransmitters, thus improving mood. Exercise may be particularly useful for individuals who have trouble managing stress (18). Although indicated for a wide variety of stress- and anxiety-related disorders, exercise is not sufficient therapy for the most severe causes of anxiety (2). It can be recommended as adjunct therapy in addition to the primary therapy of counseling and/or pharmacotherapy.

Physicians need to be aware that recreational sport can actually add stress to a patient's life. Weekend warriors and Type A patients who cannot tolerate losing often fall into this category. Ironically, many of these people most need a healthy outlet for their stress. The physician may want to direct such patients toward noncompetitive sports or help them find ways to downplay competition within their chosen sport.

Depression Depression may also be improved by exercise when used as an adjunct treatment, with counseling and/or drug therapy as the primary intervention. The National Institute of Mental Health has issued a consensus statement that provides a summary of the effects of exercise on both depression and anxiety-related disorders (19) (Table 47-1).

Table 47-1 Exercise and Mental Health: The National Institute of Mental Health Consensus Statement

1 Physical fitness is positively associated with mental health and well-being.
2 Exercise is associated with the reduction of stress emotions, such as state anxiety.
3 Anxiety and depression are common symptoms of failure to cope with mental stress, and exercise has been associated with a decreased level of mild-to-moderate depression and anxiety.
4 Long-term exercise is usually associated with reductions in traits such as neuroticism and anxiety.
5 Severe depression usually requires professional treatment, which may include medication, electroconvulsive therapy, and/or psychotherapy, with exercise as an adjunct.
6 Appropriate exercise results in reductions in various stress indices, such as neuromuscular tension, resting heart rate, and some stress hormones.
7 Current clinical opinion holds that exercise has beneficial emotional effects across all ages and in both sexes.
8 Physically healthy people who require psychotropic medication may safely exercise when exercise and medications are titrated under close medical supervision.

SOURCE: Morgan WP, Goldston GE, eds. Exercise and mental health. Washington, DC: Hemisphere, 1985:156. Reproduced with permission. All rights reserved.

Burnout   Burnout does not constitute a problem for the adult recreational athlete; however, other psychological issues may need to be addressed. Sporting careers come to an end, and with each passing year the adult athlete is confronted with evidence of the loss of youth. Age and infirmity may require these adult athletes to modify or change their sport in order to continue exercising. It is the physician's role to help athletes recognize the alternatives available to them and ease the transition. For example, progressive arthritis of the knees may end an adult's bicycling endeavors, but should not prevent him or her from pursuing other activities such as aquatic sports. Above all, physicians should consistently encourage adult patients to remain active throughout their lives.

TREATMENT OPTIONS

As is evident from the developmental discussion, anxiety, depression, and burnout must be treated within the greater context. In most cases, nonpharmacologic treatments are indicated. However, patients who present with more severe problems may benefit from a combination of approaches that include pharmacologic interventions. In virtually all cases, exercise may be continued as an adjuvant treatment.

Nonpharmacologic Treatments
Various nonpharmacologic treatments, such as relaxation training, visualization, and basic cognitive interventions, have been used to treat athletes who suffer from mood and anxiety problems. Often the physician will want to use a multidimensional approach to understand and treat mood and anxiety symptoms in athlete populations.

Stress and the Relaxation Response   In contrast to the stress response described earlier, the *relaxation response* is characterized physiologically by a decrease in heart rate, lower blood pressure, and vasodilation (5). Emotional features include comfort and a sense of well being, accompanied by a heightened capacity for social interaction and bonding (4). Behavioral relaxation techniques, which diminish the stress response and enhance the relaxation response, can be useful in treating an athlete's anxiety.

Relaxation Techniques   The cornerstone of relaxation training is *diaphragmatic breathing*. This simple but powerful technique involves taking regular deep breaths, inhaling through the nose and exhaling through the mouth. Slower breathing has a calming effect. The physician can teach the athlete patient to use diaphragmatic breathing as the first step in a more extensive relaxation training or as a useful technique on its own. For instance, a few deep slow breaths may help the anxious basketball player to achieve calm before taking free throws.

After breathing has slowed, the next step in relaxation training is typically a guided journey through the major muscle groups of the body. *Progressive muscle relaxation* involves purposefully tensing and releasing each area. This exercise is particularly helpful for patients who are chronically tense and need to learn the sensation of "letting go." Another approach to relaxation involves mentally scanning each area of the body and calling upon the power of the mind to focus in and release tension. The coupling of diaphragmatic breathing and muscle relaxation may help athletes feel generally more relaxed and it can also be used at specific times of elevated stress. For example, slow breathing and muscle relaxation may help a tense athlete unwind and get to sleep the night before the big game.

Many athletes use *visualization* to focus attention and enhance performance. The physician may help the athlete apply visualization techniques to alleviate stress that exceeds the optimal amount needed for peak performance. The patient should be encouraged to identify times when visualization might be useful and to create a repertoire of imagery cues that inspire relaxation.

Visualization has a wide variety of applications. A brief, situation-specific image may help an athlete become calm and focused immediately before an act. An example of this would be a tennis player "seeing" the shot land precisely where it will be aimed as a mental preparation before serving. Athletes may use more elaborate visual rehearsals as part of their competition day preparation. For instance, swimmers may visualize their best effort, focusing in to "preview" every moment of a race.

Calming visualization may be used by any patient who needs to allay the symptom of generalized anxiety, and may help the athlete who tends to be anxious much of the time. This type of visualization tends to be highly individual, and it is important for the patient to generate the specific imagery. All the senses should be fully engaged with vivid images, sounds, smells, tastes, and sensations. For instance, the patient might envision a clear, azure pool of water in the mountains, feeling the warm mid-day sun and a slight cool breeze, smelling pine in the air, and hearing birds off in the distance.

Cognitive Interventions The physician may use some *cognitive interventions* with athletes who have problems with stress and anxiety. These approaches include the identification of negative, undermining thoughts and the creation of more positive and self-enhancing ways of thinking.

The concept of *reframing* situations may be useful for an athlete who becomes anxious and "chokes" in the face of intense competition. For instance, the basketball player who has responded to anxiety by passing the ball during the last seconds of a game can learn to actually "want the shot" in such pressure-packed situations. This new perspective highlights self-actualization and the intrinsic desire to excel while removing focus from the external pressures to perform.

Cognitive interventions that are used to uncover, question, and challenge maladaptive beliefs about the self and the world have also been successful in treating depression (20). The physician may use this approach with athletes who are having problems with a transient mood disturbance (i.e., reaction to an injury) or in patients with mild depression. Physicians should refer athletes who suffer from severe depression to an experienced mental health professional for more intensive therapy and possibly treatment with an antidepressant medication. Suicide potential should always be assessed in patients with depression.

The Multidimensional Approach

Specific approaches such as relaxation training, visualization, and cognitive interventions serve an important purpose in treating the patient athlete. However, stress, anxiety, depression, and burnout are complex issues, and it is important for the physician to be mindful of the diverse nature of such problems. The experience of stress is highly subjective, being influenced by a myriad of factors including stage of development, personality, and sociocultural variables (21,22), as well as genetic factors and coping style (23). Therefore, we advocate a multidimensional approach to understanding the athlete patient who suffers from mood or anxiety problems.

Example of Multidimensional Intervention Tammy is an 18-year-old, African-American track athlete with fatigue that interferes with her training schedule. Her family physician finds that she also suffers from a disturbance in sleep and loss of appetite. Typically optimistic, Tammy now expresses feelings of hopelessness and voices lessened self-confidence. These problems have been ongoing for several months and indicate a diagnosis of depression. Rather than ending the interview at this point with a prescription for an antidepressant medication, Tammy's physician inquires further to understand the context of the depression. What emerges is that Tammy is at a developmental crossroads. She has been accepted to a prestigious university on a track scholarship that will enable her to move out of her inner-city neighborhood. However, it will also take her far away from her friends, boyfriend, and family—particularly her mother with whom she shares a close relationship. This significant developmental transition is characterized by the loss of a familiar neighborhood, home, and ongoing relationships, and also involves negotiating a new environment that will challenge Tammy mentally, emotionally, socially, and physically. Having treated the family over time, the physician is aware that several other family members have had significant problems with depression, including Tammy's mother who has recently been symptomatic. Ultimately, the physician prescribes an antidepressant and schedules a follow-up appointment. The physician also arranges a meeting with Tammy and her family to discuss this transition and the family history of depression. In addition, the physician encourages Tammy to meet regularly with the physician at the university and contact the counseling center for individual and/or group counseling.

Pharmacologic Treatments

Beta-Blockers Beta-blockers are drugs that diminish the manifestations of anxiety, as they decrease heart rate and tremor. Because these medications lower maximal cardiac output, they can decrease performance capacity for endurance athletes. Unfortunately, some athletes involved in shooting events have abused beta-blockers, using them to steady their trigger finger, and the drugs have been banned by the National Collegiate Athletic Association (NCAA) for riflery and by the International Olympic Committee (IOC) for a number of precision sports.

Tranquilizers Benzodiazepams are minor tranquilizers, commonly used to treat a variety of anxiety-related disorders. These drugs are generally safe but should not be prescribed indiscriminately because of abuse potential. Like beta-blockers, they have been banned from shooting events and are subject to IOC regulation.

Antidepressants Antidepressants fall under three broad categories: tricyclics, selective serotonin reuptake inhibitors (SSRIs), and others. Tricyclics are an older class of drugs that tend to create more side effects than SSRIs. Because many tricyclics have anticholinergic properties, which decrease a patient's ability to sweat, they should be prescribed with caution for athletes who participate in events that subject them to heat stress. Tricyclic antidepressants have been banned by the IOC from shooting events.

Because of their milder side-effect profile, SSRIs have become first-line therapy for mild to moderate depression. Patients who take these drugs and exercise do not have to follow any specific precautions. Currently, there is a debate about whether or not SSRIs enhance performance. Depending on the outcome of this debate, SSRIs may face wider bans. Currently, they are regulated by the IOC and are also banned from shooting events.

The category of other antidepressants is broad. In general, these drugs are not first-line treatments for depression. Before prescribing one of these drugs, the physician needs to determine if it is a banned substance and if the medication has any particular side effects that might jeopardize athletic performance.

Precautions A final caution about prescribing medication for athletes: the physician must be aware that certain medications may lead to changes in thinking, emotions, and behaviors. Anabolic steroids are a prime example of an ergogenic drug that may give rise to rage reactions and other behavioral changes. Similarly, amphetamines can cause anxiety and, with continuous use, psychosis.

Also, individuals may take prescription or nonprescription drugs inappropriately. Alcohol is the most commonly abused drug, and patients who have problems with mood or anxiety may drink in an attempt to soothe their symptoms. Use of any of these substances may negate the benefits of other therapy, and patients should be questioned carefully about this. In the short run, this self-prescribed "therapy" may seem effective, but in the long run it may have disastrous results—actually increasing depression and creating secondary psychological and medical problems. Team physicians need to actively discourage inappropriate drug use and be aware of associated mental health problems.

CONCLUSIONS

The psychological benefits of participation in sports far outweigh the risks. Patients of all ages and abilities should be encouraged by their physicians to participate in athletics. Sport does affect mood and behavior, and the physician needs to understand the positive effects of sports as well as the associated mental health problems. Developmental concerns and interactions with significant figures such as parents, coaches, and teammates need to be considered, as well as the level at which the athlete is competing.

Mental health interventions are primarily nonpharmocologic for athletes, although a clinical approach that includes medication may be useful for patients with more marked difficulties. To serve these athletes, team physicians should develop basic counseling skills, and establish a close working relationship with a psychologist who is knowledgeable about the specific problems athletes face.

REFERENCES

1 Silva, JM. An analysis of the training stress syndrome in competitive athletics. Appl Sport Psychol 1990;2:5–20.

2 Benight CC, Taylor CB. Exercise, emotions, and type A behavior. In: Goldberg L, Elliot DL, eds. Exercise for prevention and treatment of illness. Philadelphia: FA Davis, 1994:319–332.

3 Cohen LS, Biederman J. Further evidence for an association between affective disorders and anxiety disorders: review and case reports. J Clin Psychiatry 1988;49:313–316.

4 Rossi E. The psychobiology of mind-body healing. New York: Irvington, 1993.

5 Benson H. The relaxation response. New York: Times Books, 1976.

6 Roberts GC, Kleiber DA, Duda JL. An analysis of motivation in children's sport: the role of perceived competence in participation. J Sport Psychol 1981;3:206–216.

7 Torgersen S. Genetic factors in anxiety disorders. Arch Psychiatry 1983;40:1085–1089.

8 Krane V, Williams JM. Cognitive anxiety, somatic anxiety, and confidence in track and field athletes: the impact of gender, competitive level and task characteristics. Int J Sport Psychol 1994; 25:203–217.

9 Torgersen S. Comorbidity of major depression and anxiety disorders in twin pairs. Am J Psychiatry 1990;147:1199–1202.

10 Dale J, Weinberg R. Burnout in sport: a review and critique. Appl Sport Psychol 1990;2:67–83.

11 Smith RE. Toward a cognitive-affective model of athletic burnout. J Sport Psychol 1986;8:36–50.

12 Oler MJ, Mainous AG, Martin CA, et al. Depression, suicidal ideation, and substance use among adolescents. Are athletes at less risk? Arch Fam Med 1994;3:781–785.

13 Daino A. Personality traits of adolescent tennis players. Int J Sports Psychol 1985;16:120–125.

14 Gans JE, Blythe DA, Elster AB, Gaveras LL. America's adolescents: how healthy are they? AMA Profiles of Adolescent Health 1990:1.

15 Murphy SM, Ferrante AP. Provisions of sport psychology services to the U.S. team at the 1988 Summer Olympic Games. Sport Psychol 1989;3:374–385.

16 Brewer BW. Self-identity and specific vulnerability to depressed mood. J Pers 1993;61:343–364.

17 Smith AM, Stuart MJ, Wiese-Bjornstal DM, et al. Competitive athletes: preinjury and postinjury mood state and self-esteem. Mayo Clin Proc 1993;68:939–947.

18 Ellickson KA. Psychological aspects of exercise and sport. In: Strauss RH, ed. Sports medicine. Philadelphia: WB Saunders, 1991:299–306.

19 Morgan WP, Goldston GE, eds. Exercise and mental health. Washington, DC: Hemisphere, 1985.

20 Beck AT, Rush AJ, Shaw BF, Emery G. Cognitive therapy of depression. New York: Guilford Press, 1979.

21 Syme SL. Sociocultural factors and disease etiology. In: Gentry WD, ed. Handbook of behavior medicine. New York: Guilford Press, 1984.

22 Temoshok L, Dreher H. The type C connection. New York: Random House, 1992.

23 Temoshok L. On new-old myth and new-old models concerning the role of emotion in health and illness. Advances 1996;12:38–41.

Chapter 48
Exercise and Cancer

Daniel Larson

*In many ways, cancer is a blessing. You see life as a gift
and every day becomes precious—and that's a lesson
you never forget.*
—George Sheehan (1)

Cancer generates understandable feelings of fear
and apprehension, and many people believe the
diagnosis is a veritable death sentence. In developed countries such as the United States, Australia, and Canada, almost one-quarter of the population die from some form of cancer.

Cancer is not a single disease, but rather a collection of different disorders that have certain similarities. The causes of cancer (carcinogens) are
well known in some cases, such as ultraviolet light
and skin cancer or tobacco smoke and lung cancer.
In other cases, there are logical postulates such as
hormonal influences on female reproductive cancers. In many cases the cause is obscure. On a molecular basis, one of the most popular theories of
causality is the generation of free radicals by factors such as chemical carcinogens, viruses, or ultraviolet light.

This chapter addresses the relationship between exercise and cancer. It also reviews some of
the more important scientific studies and presents
reasonable explanations that can be of practical
use to primary care physicians and allied health
professionals.

CANCER AND EPIDEMIOLOGY: SPECIAL CONSIDERATIONS IN ATHLETES

Exercise to prevent malignancy is a topic that generates debate among physicians and patients. A
careful review of the evidence reveals that good
data exist to support the benefits of exercise for
some specific malignancies. Most evidence is encouraging for the active person but discouraging
for the sedentary individual. Some of the more
common and important malignancies are discussed below.

Colon and Colorectal Cancer
An increasing body of evidence suggests a protective benefit of exercise in preventing colon cancer.
Numerous studies consistently indicate a protective effect, strengthened by biological plausibility
and a dose/response relationship.

Initial studies reviewed occupational exertion.
For example, one study examined colon cancer in
textile workers and found that the incidence was
higher in managers, administrators, and execu-
tives than in the more physically active workers (2).
Similar analyses of activity levels of various occupations were performed in the 1980s. One of the best
combined a compelling three-tiered analysis of activity level versus colon cancer risk across numerous occupations. In this data set, sedentary individuals had an age-adjusted relative risk of colon
cancer of 1.8 compared to active individuals. This
relationship persisted across socioeconomic classes (3).

Other studies have related the benefits of exercise to specific characteristics of certain individuals. For example, the ongoing Harvard alumni
study found that the protective effect of exercise
was limited to those alumni with Quetelet's index
greater than or equal to 26 units (weight in kilo-
grams per height in square meters). The association was strong, with a relative risk of 0.19 for the
most active individuals in the heavier subpopula-
tion; the protective effect nearly disappeared for

thinner alumni (4). A study of twins showed that a sedentary twin has a relative risk of 2.78 for colon cancer as opposed to an active twin (5). The nearly identical genetic makeup of twins supports the conclusion that exercise is the operative variable leading to this benefit.

The most probable cause for the protective effect of exercise in colon cancer is that people who exercise have rapid gastrointestinal transit times; thus, the colon is exposed to potential carcinogens for a shorter period of time. This mechanism seems self-evident to anyone who has experienced runner's diarrhea or relief of constipation with exercise. However, this conclusion does not fit well with the Harvard alumni study, which showed that heavier people received a greater benefit from exercise. The fact that the protective effect weakens among thin people may be due to confounding variables, such as the association of thinness with more regular exercise.

Breast Cancer and Female Reproductive Cancers

The risk of breast cancer is related to numerous factors, although general agreement exists that long-term exposure to estrogens and progestins (endogenous or exogenous) is a major factor in the development of breast cancer. Early menarche, nulliparity, and lack of prolonged lactation are all relative risk factors for breast cancer. Genetic risk factors are clearly quite important but cannot be altered for any given individual.

Vigorous exercise often results in anovulation and lower levels of endogenous ovarian hormones. This offers a plausible reason for why regular exercise might be protective against breast cancer. A case-control study of premenopausal breast cancer supported this association: the odds ratio for the most active parous women was 0.28, and the odds ratio was 0.73 for the most active nulliparous women (6). This protective effect persisted even after controlling for confounding variables. Previous studies had found a relative risk of 1.85 for sedentary women, once again controlled for confounding variables such as smoking, alcohol consumption, and body weight (7). Not all studies, however, find a protective effect of exercise, and in certain subsets of the Framingham study a small trend to-ward a sedentary lifestyle being protective against breast cancer was denoted (8).

Hormonal stimulation plays a role in other female reproductive cancers. Female athletes had lower relative risks (0.40) for cancers of the uterus, cervix, vagina, and ovary combined with the strongest association found for cancers of the uterus and cervix (7). In a study of endometrial carcinoma, sedentary lifestyles (9) were associated with a relative risk of 1.9, or, when adjusted for body mass index, 1.5. Similar ratios were found by Levi et al. (10).

Testicular Cancer and Male Reproductive Cancer

Testicular cancer is less common than breast and female reproductive cancers, and it frequently strikes a younger population. Testicular cancer has been found to be significantly more common in sedentary individuals and in those who went through puberty at an early age (11). The common factor is thought to be exposure to higher levels of endogenous hormones. Vigorous exercise is believed to decrease these hormone levels.

Prostate cancer is the most common malignancy in men over 50 years of age in our society, so anything that can be done to lower its incidence has widespread benefit. Public awareness regarding prostate cancer has increased because of laboratory screening for prostate cancer with prostate-specific antigen. The relationship of prostate cancer to exercise is one of the most controversial areas in the exercise oncology literature. The death of prominent runner, author, and physician George Sheehan (1) contributed to the awareness of prostate cancer among exercise enthusiasts.

Studies thus far have reached no consensus regarding prostate cancer and exercise. One large study found no significant relationship between prostate cancer and physical activity (12), another study found conflicting evidence (13), and yet a third study found an insignificant trend toward higher relative risk (1.05) in active men (14).

Other Cancers

Skin Cancer   Skin cancer is linked to ultraviolet light exposure as is common in outdoor sports. Athletes participating in sports in which large areas of skin are exposed are at higher risk. Some cases of skin cancer must relate to solar exposure during exercise, but the limited data to date do not show large increases in active individuals (15).

Certain practices that athletes follow to gain an advantage pose potential risks for cancer. Hepatomas have been reported with increased frequency in athletes who use androgenic steroids. Definitive proof is limited, but the causal relationship of hepatomas to androgenic steroid use is generally accepted (16).

Lung Cancer   Lung cancer is lower among nonsmokers, which include most active endurance exercisers. If one controls for tobacco use, the influence of exercise lessens but it generally indicates a protective effect. A contrasting result was found in a study of active longshoremen (waterside workers) that showed nonsignificant increases in lung cancer compared to sedentary co-workers (17). Exercise, however, may not have been the primary factor leading to the increased cancer rates, as longshoremen may have increased exposure to dockside carcinogens, especially in polluted environments.

MALIGNANCIES OVERALL

Cancer is heterogeneous, occurs at different sites, and leads to varied illnesses; however, exercise may offer protection for most malignancies. One approach to studying the question has been to use resting heart rate as an estimate of overall fitness: the lower the heart rate, the more active the individual. Using this analysis, the relative risk of all cancer in sedentary men was found to be 1.68 in a study of 7735 men. This risk remained consistent after controlling for pulmonary function, underlying ill health, or death within the first 5 years (18). Other large studies show similar protective benefits (7,15).

Exercise indirectly promotes good health habits, such as nonsmoking and avoidance of excessive body weight. It is entirely plausible that the indirect benefits of exercise may be far more important in lessening cancer risks than the direct benefits. Most large epidemiologic studies have attempted to control for confounding variables, but controlling for all lifestyle changes associated with exercise

is not possible. For example, many of the excellent colon cancer studies do not control for aspirin use. This may confuse results, as recent evidence suggests that low-dose aspirin intake may be protective against colon cancer in both men and women.

Recommendations for Prevention

Active, health-conscious patients often request health maintenance advice from medical practitioners. Unfortunately, many of those who most need advice rarely seek it. Nevertheless, health care providers should continue to promote good health habits among the entire population, despite the sometimes frustrating experience of failing to persuade individuals to give up bad health habits.

What credible advice can physicians offer regarding exercise? There is evidence that overall cancer rates are moderately increased among sedentary people. Specifically, colon cancer is more common among sedentary individuals and less common among regular exercisers. Furthermore, female reproductive cancers, including breast cancer, appear more common among sedentary women, although some conflicting data regarding breast cancer exist. There are no definitive findings about prostate cancer. Lung cancer has decreased incidence among exercisers, but most of this effect is probably due to nonsmoking status. In general, strong evidence suggests that a sedentary lifestyle is a mild to moderate risk factor for several malignancies.

Regular, vigorous sport does not imply immunity to cancer, as exercise offers only modest levels of protection. Individuals must still follow the usual medical precautions and undergo accepted cancer screening and diagnostic procedures.

EXERCISE AFTER MALIGNANCY

Athletes typically challenge their body to perform to the limit. Exercising after malignancy presents new challenges to the patient and physician. Communication between the cancer patient and physician is critical if the patient wishes to pursue vigorous or recreational exercise. Treatment regimens, while specific, generally allow room for professional judgment and patient preference. For example, potentially cardiotoxic or pneumotoxic regimens may be a less favorable choice in the endurance athlete with early stage Hodgkin's disease or node negative breast cancer. However, the physician should not offer less efficacious treatment because of the patient's exercise zeal: there should be a balance between quality of care and quantity of life. The patient can make the appropriate decision only when presented with all the information by a compassionate physician who understands each patient's particular lifestyle issues.

Exercise During Treatment

A full discussion of the specific toxicities of antineoplastic agents is beyond the scope of this book, but the basic principles are worth presenting. The primary care physician or sports-related allied health professional must be willing and able to communicate with the oncologist or radiation oncologist regarding the specific treatment advantages and toxicities.

Cardiotoxicity Cardiotoxicity is a potential complication of several chemotherapeutic agents including doxorubicin, daunorubicin, and cyclophosphamide. Much of the cardiotoxicity is dose related. The decision to use these agents and risk their potential side effects must clearly be discussed with the patient who is an athlete. Radiation therapy may also accelerate atherosclerosis.

Pneumotoxicity Long-term pulmonary toxicity of chemotherapeutic agents and radiation therapy must also be considered, especially with the prolonged survival of certain patients. Hodgkin's disease, in particular, presents a number of treatment choices, and studies of the various options (19,20) have shown a number of fairly consistent findings. Mantle irradiation is generally extremely well tolerated by the sedentary individual, and long-term pulmonary function changes are quite small. Mantle irradiation exposes a relatively large volume of lung to radiation when compared with other treatment regimens (21). In the vast majority of cases, the sedentary or casual recreational athlete notes no impairment whatsoever, but subtle changes may be significant to athletes testing the limits of their aerobic capacity. Radiation pneumonitis can occur acutely, and progressive pulmonary changes develop over several years. Both forced expiratory volume in 1 second,

(FEV1) and forced vital capacity (FVC) are decreased approximately 10% to 15% compared with predicted values at 8 years after radiation, with the FEV1 dropping slightly more than FVC. This results in a FEV1/FVC ratio with an approximate 8% deficit at 10 years after radiation. Diffusion capacity (DLCO) also declines 10% 8 years after treatment.

The pulmonary sequelae may be enough for competitive athletes to feel that they have "lost their edge." Unfortunately, standard cytotoxic chemotherapy regimens such as MOPP, when compared to radiation therapy, do not improve long-term physiologic function (22). The type of sport, the precise radiation fields, and the specific chemotherapy courses are all important to the long-term outcome, and choices must be individualized. Following successful treatment of Hodgkin's disease, several athletes have returned to compete at the international level in sports as diverse as wrestling and marathon running.

Potential Physical Limitations Radiation fields are extremely important to the treatment of breast cancer (23). A discussion of lumpectomy plus radiation versus mastectomy for appropriate localized tumors encompasses many issues, including the effects of radiation as well as the physical and psychological impacts of mastectomy. In sport, specific issues arise with regards to lymph node dissection and radiation and their effect on activities that involve the use of the arm and shoulder.

Psychological Benefits The most important benefits of exercise for the cancer patient are probably psychological. Individuals may experience an increased sense of well being, higher self-esteem, and decreased depression. These psychological benefits are specific to exercise and have been found in people without cancer as well as in patients who have a malignancy, are undergoing therapy, or are in remission (24). These effects may positively influence longevity, but the more important results are the enhancement of quality of life, maintenance of independence, and improvement of function.

Precautions Clearly, patients undergoing cancer therapy must take certain precautions. Leukopenia increases the risk of infection and anemia may cause excessive fatigue and susceptibility to cardiovascular disease, as may chemotherapy and radiation therapy. Bony metastases may make a patient more prone to stress fractures.

SUMMARY

Epidemiologic studies associate exercise with a lower risk of malignancy. Some of these effects appear to be directly mediated by exercise, and others occur because of a healthier lifestyle in athletic individuals. Exercise after malignancy may be limited by the illness or treatment but can help in the physical recovery. For certain individuals, high performance sports participation is possible after malignancy. Regardless of physical changes, the psychological benefits of continuing to be physically fit and independent may be among the most important gains for many cancer patients.

REFERENCES

1 Sheehan G. Personal best. Emmaus, PA: Rodale Press, 1989:232.
2 Hoar SK, Blair A. Death certificate case-control study of cancers of the prostate and colon and employment in the textile industry. Arch Environ Health 1984;39:280–283.
3 Garabrant DH, Peters JM, Mack TM, Bernstein L. Job activity and colon cancer risk. Am J Epidemiol 1984;119:1005–1014.
4 Lee IM, Paffenbarger RS Jr, Hsieh C. Physical activity and risk of developing colorectal cancer among college alumni. J Natl Cancer Inst 1991; 83:1324–1329.
5 Gerhardsson M, Floderus B, Norell SE. Physical activity and colon cancer risk. Int J Epidemiol 1988;17:743–746.
6 Bernstein L, Henderson BE, Hanisch R, et al. Physical exercise and reduced risk of breast cancer in young women. J Natl Cancer Inst 1994;86:1403–1408.
7 Frisch RE, Wyshak G, Albright NL, et al. Lower prevalence of breast cancer and cancers of the reproductive system among former college athletes compared to non-athletes. Br J Cancer 1985; 52:885–891.
8 Dorgan JF, Brown C, Barrett M, et al. Physical activity and risk of breast cancer in the Framingham Heart Study. Am J Epidemiol 1994;139:662–669.
9 Sturgeon SR, Brinton LA, Berman ML, et al. Past and present physical activity and endometrial cancer risk. Br J Cancer 1993;68:584–589.
10 Levi F, LaVecchia C, Negri E, Franceschi S. Selected physical activities and the risk of endometrial cancer. Br J Cancer 1993;67:846–861.
11 United Kingdom Testicular Cancer Study Group. Aetiology of testicular cancer: association with congenital abnormalities, age at puberty, infertility, and exercise. Br Med J 1994;308:1393–1399.
12 Lee IM, Paffenbarger RS Jr. Physical activity and its relation to cancer risk: a prospective study of college alumni. Med Sci Sports Exerc 1994; 26:831–837.
13 Sternfeld B. Cancer and the protective effect of physical activity: The epidemiological evidence. Med Sci Sports Exerc 1992;24:1195–1209.
14 Severson RK, Nomura AM, Grove JS, Stemmermann GN. A prospective analysis of physical activity and cancer. Am J Epidemiol 1989;130:522–529.
15 Frisch RE, Wyshak G, Albright NL, et al. Lower prevalence of non-reproductive system cancers among female former college athletes. Med Sci Sports Exerc 1989;21:250–253.
16 Creagh TM, Rubin A, Evans DJ. Hepatic tumours induced by anabolic steroids in an athlete. J Clin Pathol 1988;41:441–443.
17 Paffenbarger RS Jr, Hyde RT, Wing AL. Physical activity and incidence of cancer in diverse populations: A preliminary report. Am J Clin Nutr 1987;45(suppl):312–317.
18 Blair SN, Kohl HW III, Paffenbarger RS Jr, et al. Physical fitness and all-cause mortality: a prospective study of healthy men and women. JAMA 1989;262:2395–2401.
19 Shapiro SJ, Shapiro SD, Mill WB, Campbell EJ. Prospective study of long-term pulmonary manifestations of mantle irradiation. Int J Radiat Oncol Biol Phys 1990;19:707–714.
20 Curran WJ Jr, Moldofsy PHJ, Solin LJ. Analysis of the influence of elective nodal irradiation on postirradiation pulmonary function. Cancer 1990;65:2488–2493.
21 Smith LM, Mendenhall NP, Cicale MJ, et al. Results of a prospective study evaluating the effects of mantle irradiation on pulmonary function. Int J Radiat Oncol Biol Phys 1989;16:79–84.
22 Jensen BV, Carlsen NL, Groth S, Nissen NI. Late effects on pulmonary function of mantle-field irradiation, chemotherapy or combined modality therapy for Hodgkin's disease. Eur J Haematol 1990;44:165–171.
23 Kimsey FC, Mendenhall NP, Ewald LM, et al. Is radiation treatment volume a predictor for acute or late effect on pulmonary function? A prospective study of patients treated with breast-conserving surgery and postoperative irradiation. Cancer 1994;73:2549–2555.
24 Shephard RJ. Physical activity and the healthy mind. Can Med Assoc J 1983;128:525–530.

Index